HANDBOOK OF
DIAGNOSTIC TESTS

HANDBOOK OF
DIAGNOSTIC TESTS

Springhouse Corporation
Springhouse, Pennsylvania

STAFF

Senior Publisher: Matthew Cahill

Clinical Manager: Cindy Tryniszewski, RN, MSN

Art Director: John Hubbard

Senior Editor: Michael Shaw

Clinical Editors: Maryann Foley, RN, BSN; Judith Schilling McCann, RN, BSN; Kate McGovern, RN; Beverly Ann Tscheschlog, RN

Editors: Marcia Andrews, Kathleen M. Angone, Jane V. Cray, Judd L. Howard, Richard J. Koreto, Pat Wittig

Designers: Stephanie Peters (associate art director), Matie Patterson (assistant art director), Lesley Weissman-Cook, Mary Ludwicki

Copy Editors: Cynthia C. Breuninger (manager), Lewis Adams, Priscilla DeWitt, Lynette High, Doris Weinstock

Manufacturing: Deborah Meiris (director), Pat Dorshaw (manager), Anna Brindisi, T.A. Landis

Typography: Diane Paluba (manager), Elizabeth Bergman, Joyce Rossi Biletz, Phyllis Marron, Robin Mayer, Valerie L. Rosenberger

Production Coordination: Patricia McCloskey

Editorial Assistants: Beverly Lane, Mary Madden

Indexer: Barbara Hodgson

The cover photograph depicts cholesterol molecules as seen through a scanning electron microscope.

CONTENTS

PART ONE

PART TWO

CHAPTER 1: HEMATOLOGY AND COAGULATION TESTS

CHAPTER 2: BLOOD CHEMISTRY TESTS

CHAPTER 3: HORMONE TESTS

CHAPTER 4: VITAMIN AND TRACE ELEMENT TESTS

CONTRIBUTORS AND CONSULTANTS

Charol Abrams, MS, MT(ASCP) CLS(NCA), CLSp(H), CLS consultant, Philadelphia

Ellen Digan, MA, MT(ASCP), Professor of Biology; Coordinator, MLT Program, Manchester Community-Technical College, Manchester, Conn.

Stanley J. Dudrick, MD, Clinical Professor of Surgery, The University of Texas, Health Science Center at Houston

Pamela W. Gitschier, MT, MS, Chemistry Supervisor, St. Luke's Hospital, Bethlehem, Pa.

Debra R. Hanna, RN, MSN, CNRN, Neuroscience Clinical Nurse Specialist, Mayo Foundation Hospitals, Rochester, Minn.

Carol McLimans, MA, MT(ASCP), SM, Program Director, Medical Laboratory Technician Program, Mayo Foundation, Rochester, Minn.

Karen E. Michael, RN, MSN, Case Manager, Greater Atlantic Health Service, Philadelphia

Linda T. Raichle, PhD, MT(ASCP), Laboratory Training Advisor, National Laboratory Training Network, Exton, Pa.

Daniele Shollenberger, RN, MSN, Educational Nurse Specialist, Lehigh Valley Hospital, Allentown, Pa.

Deborah Porter Thornton, MEd, MT(ASCP)SC, Assistant Professor, Medical Laboratory Science Program, Department of Molecular and Microbiology, University of Central Florida, Orlando

Patricia Zander, RTR, BS, Clinical Chief Technologist, University of Iowa Hospital and Clinics, Iowa City

FOREWORD

Advances in diagnostic testing are bringing remarkable improvements to the efficiency, accuracy, and timeliness of health care. Imaging techniques, such as magnetic resonance imaging, reveal anatomic details with unprecedented clarity. High-tech laboratory techniques provide test results in minutes, enabling you to respond faster and more effectively. The future will undoubtedly bring more exciting breakthroughs.

If patients are to reap the full benefit of today's sophisticated diagnostic tests, you need to have up-to-date information. No matter what your expertise, you may be called upon to answer questions about tests, to guide patients through them, and to interpret results. For any test, you must know:
• its indications
• how to prepare the patient
• normal findings, as well as the significance of abnormal results
• associated risks and complications.

The *Handbook of Diagnostic Tests* provides all of this and more. This quick reference covers virtually all major diagnostic procedures and laboratory tests. No other manual, text, or reference book offers so much relevant information in such a convenient format. What's more, the book's pocket size makes it ideal for use on the job.

Handbook of Diagnostic Tests presents information from two distinct but vital approaches. Part One provides key diagnostic findings in more than 500 disorders, which are alphabetically organized. Simply look up any major disorder in this section and you'll find all relevant test findings clearly and succinctly summarized.

Part Two, in contrast, provides full details about each test. Organized into 16 chapters, Part Two covers blood and urine tests, endoscopies, X-rays, computed tomography scans, magnetic resonance imaging, and much more. Each of these tests is covered in a consistent format:
• description of the test
• its purpose
• patient preparation
• procedure and posttest care
• reference values or normal findings
• abnormal findings and their significance.

When appropriate, a list of the necessary equipment appears as well. In addition, the handbook emphasizes patient-teaching responsibilities.

With all of these features, the *Handbook of Diagnostic Tests* gets straight to the point. It will prove to be an invaluable asset to any health care professional, especially doctors, nurses, medical technologists, radiographers, respiratory therapists, and other allied health workers. I recommend this handbook enthusiastically. After all, no other diagnostic test book makes it easier and quicker for you to gain the necessary knowledge, skill, and confidence in this critically important area.

STANLEY J. DUDRICK, MD
Clinical Professor of Surgery
The University of Texas
Health Science Center at Houston

PART ONE

KEY DIAGNOSTIC FINDINGS IN MAJOR DISORDERS

Abdominal aortic aneurysm

• Computed tomography scan or ultrasonography reveals the size, shape, and location of the aneurysm.

• Anteroposterior and lateral X-rays of the abdomen may detect aortic calcification, which outlines the mass.

• Aortography shows the condition of vessels proximal and distal to the aneurysm and the extent of the aneurysm but may underestimate aneurysm diameter, because it visualizes only the blood flow channel and not the surrounding clot.

Abnormal premenopausal bleeding

• Serum hormone levels reflect adrenal, pituitary, or thyroid dysfunction.

• Urine 17-ketosteroids reveal adrenal hyperplasia, hypopituitarism, or polycystic ovarian disease.

• Endometrial biopsy rules out malignancy and should be performed in all patients who experience premenopausal bleeding.

• Pelvic examination and Papanicolaou smear rule out local or a malignant cause.

Abruptio placentae

• Mild to moderate vaginal bleeding (usually during second half of pregnancy)

• Amniocentesis reveals "port wine" fluid.

• Coagulation tests reveal a rise in fibrin split product levels.

• Complete blood count reveals decreased hemoglobin level and platelet counts.

• Pelvic ultrasound reveals abnormal echo patterns.

Acceleration-deceleration cervical injuries

• Full cervical spine X-rays indicate absence of cervical fracture.

• If the X-rays are negative for obvious cervical fracture, examination emphasizes motor ability and sensation below the cervical spine to detect signs of nerve root compression.

Acquired immunodeficiency syndrome

• Enzyme-linked immunosorbent assay (ELISA) identifies the HIV-1 antibody.

• Western blot test may also reveal the HIV-1 antibody and should be performed after a positive ELISA to confirm the diagnosis (antibody may not be detected in late stages due to inability to mount an antibody response).

• CD4+ T-lymphocyte assay will reveal a lymphocyte count below 200 cells/μl.

Actinomycosis

• Culture of tissue or exudate reveals *A. israelii*.

• Gram staining of excised tissue or exudates reveals branching gram-positive rods.

• Chest X-ray reveals lesions in unusual locations such as the shaft of a rib.

Acute leukemia

• Bone marrow aspiration indicates a proliferation of immature white blood cells.

• Bone marrow biopsy reveals cancerous cells.

• Complete blood count indicates thrombocytes less than 150,000/μl.

Acute poststreptococcal glomerulonephritis

• History of recent streptococcus infection

• Serum electrolyte studies reveal elevated calcium, chloride, phosphate, potassium, and sodium levels.

• Elevated blood urea nitrogen level

• Elevated serum creatinine levels

- Urinalysis reveals red blood cells, white blood cells, mixed cell casts, and protein.
- Antistreptolysin-O test reveals elevated streptozyme titers of 500 to 5,000 Todd units, indicating a recent streptococcal infection (in 80% of patients).
- Elevated anti-Dnase B titers, indicating a recent streptococcal infection
- Serum complement assay levels are low, indicating recent streptococcal infection.
- Throat culture may show group A beta-hemolytic streptococcus.
- Kidney-ureter-bladder X-rays show bilateral kidney enlargement.
- Renal biopsy reveals histologic changes indicating glomerulonephritis.

Acute pyelonephritis

- Urinalysis reveals sediment containing leukocytes singly, in clumps, and in casts and, possibly, a few red blood cells, as well as low specific gravity and osmolality and a slight alkaline urine pH.
- Urine culture reveals more than 100,000 organisms/mm³ of urine.
- Kidney-ureter-bladder X-rays may reveal calculi, tumors, or cysts in the kidneys and the urinary tract.
- Excretory urography may show asymmetrical kidneys.

Acute renal failure

- History of renal disease
- Blood urea nitrogen level greater than 20 mg/dl and rising
- Serum creatinine level greater than 1.2 mg/dl and rising
- Serum potassium level greater than 5.5 mEq/liter
- Urine sodium level below 20 mEq/liter if oliguria results from decreased perfusion; above 40 mEq/liter if it results from an intrinsic problem
- Arterial blood gas analysis indicates a blood pH less than 7.35 and an HCO_3^- level less than 22 mEq/liter.

Acute respiratory failure in chronic obstructive pulmonary disease

- Arterial blood gas measurements show progressive deterioration when compared with normal values for patient; increased HCO_3^- level may indicate metabolic alkalosis or metabolic compensation for chronic respiratory acidosis.
- Chest X-ray reveals pulmonary pathology such as emphysema, atelectasis, lesions, pneumothorax, infiltrates, or effusions.
- Decreased hemoglobin and hematocrit levels
- Serum electrolyte studies reveal hypokalemia.
- Elevated white blood cell count, if bacterial infection is present
- Electrocardiography indicates arrhythmias that suggest cor pulmonale and myocardial hypoxia.

Acute tubular necrosis

- Urinalysis reveals urinary sediment containing red blood cells and casts, specific gravity of 1.010 or less, and osmolality less than 400 mOsm/kg.
- Urine sodium level between 40 to 60 mEq/liter
- Elevated blood urea nitrogen level
- Elevated serum creatinine level
- Hyperkalemia
- Arterial blood gas analysis indicates blood pH less than 7.25 and HCO_3^- level less than 22 mEq/liter.

Adenoid hyperplasia

- Nasopharyngoscopy or rhinoscopy reveals abnormal tissue mass.
- Lateral pharyngeal X-rays show obliteration of the nasopharyngeal air column.

Adrenal hypofunction

• Decreased plasma cortisol levels (less than 10 mcg/dl in the morning with lower levels in the evening)
• Decreased serum sodium level (in Addison's disease)
• Decreased fasting blood glucose level (in Addison's disease)
• Increased serum potassium level
• Increased blood urea nitrogen level
• Complete blood count reveals increased hematocrit and elevated lymphocyte and eosinophil counts.
• X-rays will reveal a small heart.
• Corticotropin level increased above 60 pg/ml
• Rapid corticotropin test reveals low cortisol levels.
• Sweat test reveals elevated sodium level (30 to 80 mEq/liter) and chloride level (35 to 80 mEq/liter).
• Decreased urine 17-hydroxycorticosteroid levels
• Decreased urine 17-ketosteroid levels

Adrenogenital syndrome

• Physical examination reveals pseudohermaphroditism in females or precocious puberty in patients of either sex.
• Elevated urine 17-ketosteroid (17-KS) levels, which can be suppressed by administering dexamethasone by mouth
• Elevated levels of urine hormone metabolites (particularly pregnanetriol)
• Elevated plasma 17-hydroxyprogesterone levels
• Normal or decreased urine 17-hydroxycorticosteroid levels
• Symptoms of adrenal hypofunction or adrenal crisis in the first week of life strongly suggest congenital adrenal hyperplasia; elevated serum calcium, chloride, and sodium levels (in the presence of excessive levels of urine 17-KS and pregnanetriol) and decreased urine aldosterone levels confirm it.

Age-related macular degeneration

• Indirect ophthalmoscopy reveals gross macular changes.
• I.V. fluorescein angiography reveals leaking vessels.
• Amsler's grid reveals visual field loss.

Albinism

• Family history suggests inheritance pattern.
• Pale skin (in whites) and white-to-yellow hair
• Microscopic examination of the skin and of hair follicles reveals the amount of pigment present.
• Pigmentation testing of plucked hair roots by incubating them in tyrosine distinguish tyrosinase-positive albinism from tyrosinase-negative albinism; tyrosinase-positive hair roots will develop color.

Alcoholism

• History of chronic and excessive ingestion of alcohol
• Liver function studies reveal increased levels of serum cholesterol, lactate dehydrogenase, alanine aminotransferase, aspartate aminotransferase, and creatine phosphokinase in patients with liver damage.
• Elevated serum amylase and lipase levels (in pancreatitis)

Allergic rhinitis

• Personal or family history of allergies
• Sputum and nasal smears reveal a large numbers of eosinophils.
• Positive skin test for specific allergen, supported by tested response to environmental stimuli

Alport's syndrome

• Family history of recurrent hematuria, deafness, and renal failure (especially in men)

- Urinalysis indicates presence of red blood cells.
- Renal biopsy reveals histologic changes characteristic of Alport's syndrome.
- Blood tests reveal immunoglobulins and complement components.
- Eye examination may reveal cataracts and, less commonly, keratoconus, microspherophakia, myopia, nystagmus, and retinitis pigmentosa.

Alzheimer's disease

- History of progressive personality, mental status, and neurologic changes
- Positron emission tomography scan reveals alteration in the metabolic activity of the cerebral cortex.
- EEG and a computed tomography scan may help diagnose later stages of illness.
- Autopsy reveals neurofibrillary tangles, neuritic plaques, and granulovascular degeneration.

Amebiasis

- Culture of feces, sputum, or aspirates from abscesses, ulcers, or tissue reveal *Entamoeba histolytica* (cysts and trophozoites).

Amputation, traumatic

- History and examination reveal trauma to an extremity.
- Complete blood cell count reveals decreased hemoglobin and hematocrit, indicating hemorrhage.

Amyloidosis

- Histologic examination of tissue specimen (rectal mucosa, gingiva, skin, or nerve biopsy) or abdominal fat pad aspiration using a polarizing or electron microscope and appropriate tissue staining reveals amyloid deposits.
- Liver function studies are generally normal, except for slightly elevated serum alkaline phosphatase.

- Electrocardiography shows low voltage and conduction or rhythm abnormalities resembling those characteristic of myocardial infarction (with cardiac amyloidosis).
- Echocardiography (M-mode and two-dimensional) may detect myocardial infiltration.

Amyotrophic lateral sclerosis

- Upper and lower motor neuron degeneration occurs without sensory impairment.
- Electromyography may show abnormalities of electrical activity of involved muscles.
- Muscle biopsy may disclose atrophic fibers interspersed among normal fiber.
- Nerve conduction studies are usually normal.
- Cerebrospinal fluid analysis reveals increased protein content in one-third of patients.
- Computed tomography scan and EEG may help rule out other disorders.

Anal fissure

- Digital examination elicits pain and bleeding.
- Gentle traction on perianal skin allows for visualization of fistula.
- Anoscopy reveals longitudinal tear and confirms the diagnosis.

Anaphylaxis

- Patient's history and signs and symptoms establish the diagnosis: They may include a rapid onset of severe respiratory or cardiovascular symptoms after ingestion or injection of a drug, vaccine, diagnostic agent, food, or food additive or after an insect sting.

Ankylosing spondylitis

- Family history
- X-rays reveal blurring of the bony margins of joints (in early stage), bilateral sacroiliac involvement, patchy sclerosis with superficial bony ero-

sions, squaring of vertebral bodies, and "bamboo spine" (with complete ankylosis).

• Serum HLA-B27 is present in about 95% of patients with primary disease and 80% of patients with secondary disease.

• Blood count reveals slightly elevated erythrocyte sedimentation rate and alkaline phosphatase and creatine phosphatase levels in active disease.

• Serum immunoglobulin A levels may be elevated.

Anorectal abscess and fistula

Examination of rectum helps to distinguish type of abscess:

• Perianal abscess produces a red, tender, localized, oval swelling close to the anus, which may drain pus. Sitting or coughing increases pain.

• Ischiorectal abscess involves the entire perianal region on the affected side of the anus. Digital examination reveals a tender induration bulging into the anal canal, which may not produce drainage.

• Submucous or high intramuscular abscess may produce a dull, aching pain in the rectum, tenderness, and occasionally, induration. Digital examination reveals a smooth swelling of the upper part of the anal canal or lower rectum.

• Pelvirectal abscess produces fever, malaise, and myalgia but no local anal or external rectal signs or pain. Digital examination reveals a tender mass high in the pelvis, perhaps extending into one of the ischiorectal fossae.

• Sigmoidoscopy, barium enema, and colonoscopy may be performed to rule out other conditions.

Anorectal stricture, stenosis, or contracture

• Visual inspection reveals narrowing of the anal canal.

• Digital examination reveals tenderness and tightness.

Anorexia nervosa

• Weight loss of 25% or greater with no organic basis

• History of compulsive dieting and bulimic episodes, or gorging and purging

• Emaciated appearance accompanied by maintenance of physical vigor

• Laxative or diuretic abuse

• Complete blood count reveals low hemoglobin levels, platelet levels, white blood cells, and erythrocyte sedimentation rate.

• Prolonged bleeding time (due to thrombocytopenia)

• Decreased serum creatine, blood urea nitrogen, uric acid, cholesterol, total protein, albumin, sodium, potassium, chloride, and calcium levels

• Decreased fasting blood glucose level

• Electrocardiography will reveal nonspecific ST interval, T-wave changes, prolonged PR interval, and ventricular arrhythmias.

• Additional diagnostic testing may be performed to rule out other disorders that may cause wasting.

Anthrax

• History of exposure to wool, hides, or other animal products

• A large, pruritic, painless skin lesion

• Tissue culture with Gram stain reveals large gram-positive rods.

• Drainage cultures reveal *Bacillus anthracis*.

• Indirect hemagglutination reveals a fourfold rise in titer.

Aortic insufficiency

• Cardiac catheterization shows reduced arterial diastolic pressure, aortic insufficiency, and valvular abnormalities.

• Echocardiography reveals left ventricular enlargement and changes in left ventricular function; it may show a dilated aortic root, a flail leaflet, thickening of the cusps, or valve prolapse.

• Doppler echocardiography readily detects mild degrees of aortic insufficiency that may be inaudible. It also shows a rapid, high-frequency, diastolic fluttering of the anterior mitral leaflet that results from aortic insufficiency.
• Electrocardiography may show left ventricular hypertrophy, ST-segment depression, and T-wave inversion.
• Radionuclide angiography helps to determine the degree of regurgitant blood flow and assess left ventricular function.

Aortic stenosis

• Cardiac catheterization reveals the pressure gradient across the aortic valve (indicating the severity of obstruction), increased left ventricular end-diastolic pressures (indicating left ventricular dysfunction), and the number of cusps.
• Chest X-ray shows valvular calcification, left ventricular enlargement, dilation of the ascending aorta, pulmonary venous congestion and, in later stages, left atrial, pulmonary artery, right atrial, and right ventricular enlargement.
• Echocardiography demonstrates a thickened aortic valve and left ventricular wall and possible coexistent mitral valve stenosis.
• Doppler echocardiography allows calculation of the aortic pressure gradient.
• Electrocardiography reveals left ventricular hypertrophy and ST-segment and T-wave abnormalities. As hypertrophy progresses in severe aortic stenosis, left atrial enlargement is noted. Up to 10% of patients have atrioventricular and intraventricular conduction defects.

Aplastic or hypoplastic anemias

• Complete blood count reveals normochromic and normocytic red blood cells with a total count of 1 million or less as well as decreased platelet, neutrophil, and white blood cell counts.

• Elevated serum iron (Hemosiderin is present and tissue iron storage is visible microscopically.)
• Prolonged bleeding time
• Bone marrow biopsy yields a "dry tap" or shows severely hypocellular or aplastic marrow, with a varying amount of fat, fibrous tissue, or gelatinous replacement; absence of tagged iron and megakarocytes; and depression of erythroid elements.

Appendicitis

• History of right upper quadrant abdominal pain that eventually localizes in lower right quadrant
• Elevated temperature (99° to 102° F [37.2° to 38.8° C])
• White blood cell count of 12,000 to 15,000/µl, with increased immature cells

Arm and leg fractures

• History of trauma to extremity
• Physical examination reveals pain and difficulty moving parts distal to the injury.
• Anteroposterior and lateral X-ray of extremity reveals fracture.

Arterial occlusive disease

• Arteriography demonstrates the type (thrombus or embolus), location, and degree of obstruction, and the collateral circulation.
• Doppler ultrasonography and plethysmography show decreased blood flow distal to the occlusion.
• Ophthalmodynamometry helps determine degree of obstruction in the internal carotid artery by comparing ophthalmic artery pressure to brachial artery pressure on the affected side. More than a 20% difference between pressures suggests insufficiency.

Asbestosis

• History of occupational, family, or neighborhood exposure to asbestos fibers
• Chest X-ray reveals fine, irregular, and linear diffuse infiltrates; extensive fibrosis results in "honeycomb" or "ground glass" appearance. X-rays also show pleural thickening and calcification, with bilateral obliteration of costophrenic angles.
• Pulmonary function studies reveal decreased vital capacity, forced vital capacity (FVC), and total lung capacity; decreased or normal forced expiratory volume in one second (FEV_1); a normal ratio of FEV_1 to FVC; and reduced diffusing capacity for carbon dioxide.
• Arterial blood gas analysis may reveal decreased PaO_2 and $PaCO_2$.

Ascariasis

• Feces contains ova or roundworm.
• Vomitus contains roundworm.
• Chest X-ray reveals infiltrates, patchy areas of pneumonitis, and widening of hilar shadows.

Aspergillosis

• Chest X-ray reveals crescent-shaped radiolucency surrounding a circular mass.
• History of ocular trauma or surgery
• Exudate culture reveals *Aspergillus.*

Asphyxia

• History of change in mental status and alteration of respiratory pattern.
• Arterial blood gas analysis reveals:
— PaO_2 less than 60 mm Hg
— $PaCO_2$ greater than 50 mm Hg.
• Chest X-ray may reveal presence of foreign body, pulmonary edema, or atelectasis.
• Toxicology screening may reveal abnormal hemoglobins or ingestion of drugs or chemicals.
• Pulmonary function tests may indicate respiratory muscle weakness.

Asthma

• Pulmonary function studies may reveal the following:
— forced expiratory flow of less than 75%
— forced expiratory volume (after 1 second) of 83% or below
— tidal volumes of less than 5 to 7 ml/kg of body weight
— residual volume greater than 35% of total lung capacity.
• Arterial blood gas analysis may reveal:
— PaO_2 less than 75 mm Hg
— $PaCO_2$ greater than 45 mm Hg (indicating severe bronchial obstruction).
• Complete blood count reveals eosinophil count greater than 7%.
• Chest X-ray shows hyperinflation.

Asystole

Electrocardiography reveals a waveform that is almost a flat line. Characteristic findings include the following:
• Usually, atrial rhythm is indiscernible. No ventricular rhythm is present.
• Usually, atrial rate is indiscernible. No ventricular rate is present.
• P wave may or may not be present.
• PR interval is not measurable.
• QRS complex is absent or occasional escape beats are present.
• T wave is absent.
• QT interval is not measurable.

Ataxia-telangiectasia

• Presence of ataxia, telangiectasia, and recurrent sinopulmonary infection
• Serum analysis shows absent or deficient levels of immunoglobulin A (IgA) or IgE.
• Examination of thymic tissue reveals absence of Hassall's corpuscles.

Atelectasis

• Chest auscultation reveals decreased or absent breath sounds.
• Chest X-ray reveals characteristic horizontal lines in the lower lung zones

(in widespread atelectasis), dense shadows (with segmental or lobar collapse) with hyperinflation of neighboring lung.

Atopic dermatitis

• History of clinical manifestations of allergy symptoms such as asthma, hay fever, or urticaria

• Complete blood count reveals eosinophil count greater than 7%.

• Serum analysis shows elevated IgE levels.

• Tissue culture may be performed to rule out bacterial, viral, or fungal superinfections.

Atrial fibrillation

Electrocardiography reveals the following:

• Both atrial and ventricular rhythms are grossly irregular.

• The atrial rate, almost indiscernible, usually exceeds 400 beats/minute. The ventricular rate usually varies from 100 to 150 beats/minute, but can be less than 100 beats/minute.

• P wave is absent. Erratic baseline f (fibrillatory) waves appear instead. These chaotic f waves represent atrial tetanization from rapid atrial depolarizations. When f waves are pronounced, the arrhythmia is called coarse atrial fibrillation. When they are not pronounced, the arrhythmia is called fine atrial fibrillation.

• PR interval is indiscernible.

• Duration and configuration of QRS complex are usually normal. If ventricular conduction is aberrant, the QRS complex may be wide and abnormally shaped.

• T wave is indiscernible.

• QT interval is not measurable.

• Atrial fib-flutter, a rhythm that frequently varies between a fibrillatory line and flutter waves, may appear.

Atrial flutter

Electrocardiography reveals the following:

• Atrial rhythm is regular. Ventricular rhythm depends on the atrioventricular (AV) conduction pattern; it's often regular, although cycles may alternate. An irregular pattern may herald atrial fibrillation or indicate a block.

• Atrial rate is 250 to 400 beats/minute. Ventricular rate depends on the degree of AV block; usually, it's 60 to 100 beats/minute, but it may accelerate to 125 to 150 beats/minute.

• P wave is saw-toothed, referred to as flutter or F waves.

• PR interval is not measurable.

• Usually, duration of QRS complex is within normal limits; however, the complex may be widened if flutter waves are buried within.

• T wave is not identifiable.

• QT interval is not measurable because T wave can't be identified.

• The patient may develop an atrial rhythm that frequently varies between a fibrillatory line and flutter waves. This is called atrial fib-flutter; the ventricular response is irregular.

Atrial septal defect

• Echocardiography measures right ventricular enlargement, may locate the defect, and shows volume overload in the right heart.

• Cardiac catheterization reveals a left-to-right shunt, determines the extent of shunting and pulmonary vascular disease, detects the size and location of pulmonary venous drainage, and the atrioventricular valves' competence.

Atrial tachycardia

Electrocardiography reveals the following:

• Both atrial and ventricular rhythms are regular.

• Atrial rate is characterized by three or more consecutive ectopic atrial beats occurring at a rate between 160 and 250 beats/minute; the rate rarely exceeds 250 beats/minute. The ventricular rate depends on the atrioventricular conduction ratio.

• Usually positive, the P wave may be aberrant, invisible, or hidden in the previous T wave. If visible, it precedes each QRS complex.

• PR interval may be unmeasurable if the P wave can't be distinguished from the preceding T wave.

• Duration and configuration of QRS complex are usually normal.

• T wave usually can't be distinguished.

• QT interval is usually within normal limits, but may be shorter because of the rapid rate.

Atrioventricular block, third-degree

Electrocardiography reveals the following:

• Both atrial and ventricular rhythms are regular.

• Atrial rate, which is usually within normal limits, exceeds the ventricular rate. The slow ventricular rate ranges from 25 to 40 beats/minute, but this rate is determined by the block's location and the origin of the subsidiary impulse.

• P wave has normal size and configuration.

• PR interval is not measurable because the atria and ventricles beat independently (AV dissociation).

• Configuration of the QRS complex depends on where the ventricular beat originates. A high AV junctional pacemaker produces a narrow QRS complex; a pacemaker in the bundle of His produces a wide QRS complex; a ventricular pacemaker produces a wide, bizarre QRS complex.

• T wave has normal size and configuration.

• QT interval may or may not be within normal limits.

B cell deficiency

• History of recurrent infections

• Family history of infection as cause of death

• Decreased levels of immunoglobulin M (IgM), IgA, and IgG (after age 6 months)

• Tissue biopsy may show B cells but no plasma cells (B cells mature to form plasma cells as part of a normal immune response) in acquired hypogammaglobulinemia.

Basal cell carcinoma

• Skin lesions

• Tissue biopsy reveals basal cell carcinoma.

Bell's palsy

• Distorted facial appearance

• Inability to raise the eyebrow, close the eyelid, smile, show the teeth, or puff the cheek

• EEG distinguishes temporary conduction defect from pathologic interruption of nerve fibers (after 10 days).

Benign prostatic hyperplasia

• History of problems with urination

• Rectal examination reveals enlarged prostate gland.

• Prostate biopsy reveals histologic changes characteristic of benign prostatic hyperplasia.

• Excretory urography may indicate urinary tract obstruction, hydronephrosis, calculi, or tumors, and filling and emptying defects in the bladder.

• Elevated blood urea nitrogen and creatinine levels suggest impaired renal function.

• Urinalysis and urine culture show hematuria, pyuria, and, when bacterial count exceeds 100,000/mm³, infection.

• Cystourethroscopy indicates prostate enlargement (usually performed immediately before surgery to help determine the best operative procedure).

Berylliosis

• History of occupational, family, or neighborhood exposure to beryllium dust, fumes, or mists
• In acute berylliosis, chest X-ray reveals acute miliary process or patchy acinous filling, and diffuse infiltrates with prominent peribronchial markings.
• In chronic berylliosis, chest X-ray reveals reticulonodular infiltrates, hilar adenopathy, and large coalescent infiltrates in both lungs.
• Pulmonary function tests reveal decreased lung capacity.

Bladder cancer

• Cystoscopy with biopsy reveals the presence of malignant cells and may reveal that the bladder is fixed to the pelvic wall or prostate.
• Arylsulfatase A levels greater than 19.3 U/liter in males, 11 U/liter in females, or 1 U/liter in children
• Retrograde cystography evaluates bladder structure and integrity and confirms the diagnosis.
• Excretory urography reveals an early-stage or infiltrating tumor, ureteral obstruction, or a rigid deformity of the bladder wall. This test may also delineate functional problems in the upper urinary tract and help assess the degree of hydronephrosis.
• Urinalysis indicates presence of blood and malignant cytology.
• Ultrasonography may detect metastases in tissue beyond the bladder and can distinguish a bladder cyst from a bladder tumor.
• Pelvic arteriography reveals tumor invasion of the bladder wall.
• Computed tomography scan reveals the thickness of the involved bladder wall and detects enlarged retroperitoneal lymph nodes.

Blastomycosis

• Culture of skin lesions, pus, sputum, or pulmonary secretions reveals *Blastomyces dermatitidis.*

Blepharitis

• History of irritated eyes and rubbing of the eyes
• Tissue culture of ulcerated lid margin reveals *Staphylococcus aureus* (with ulcerative blepharitis).
• Presence of nits (with pediculosis)

Blood transfusion reaction

• Crossmatching reveals conflicting blood types.
• Urinalysis reveals hemoglobinuria.
• Antibody screening reveals anti-A or anti-B antibodies in the blood.
• Indirect bilirubin above 1.1 mg/dl
• Serum haptoglobin level 40% below pretransfusion level after 24 hours
• Blood cultures may indicate bacterial contamination.

Blunt and penetrating abdominal injuries

• History of trauma to abdomen or chest area
• Chest X-ray or abdominal X-ray indicate presence of free air.
• Peritoneal lavage reveals blood, urine, bile, stool, or pus.
• Serum amylase level above 220 U/L (pancreatic injury)
• Hemoglobin and hematocrit levels show a serial decrease.
• Excretory urography and retrograde cystography indicate renal and urinary tract damage.
• Computed tomography scan indicates abdominal organ rupture.
• Exploratory laparotomy reveals specific injuries when other clinical evidence is incomplete.

Blunt chest injuries
- History of trauma to chest area
- With hemothorax, percussion reveals dullness.
- With tension pneumothorax, percussion reveals tympany.
- Chest X-ray may indicate rib and sternal injuries, pneumothorax, flail chest, pulmonary contusion, lacerated or ruptured aorta, diaphragmatic rupture, lung compression, or hemothorax.
- Computed tomography scan reveals aortic laceration or rupture, or diaphragmatic rupture.
- Serial aspartate aminotransferase level greater than 20 U/L
- Serial alanine aminotransferase level greater than 37 U/L in men or greater than 27 U/L in women
- Serial lactate dehydrogenase level greater than 115 IU/L
- Serial creatine kinase (CK) level greater than 130 U/L in men or 150 U/L in women
- CK-MB level shows mild elevation.

Bone tumor, primary malignant
- Palpable mass over bony area
- Biopsy reveals malignant cells.
- Bone X-ray and radioisotope bone scan reveal tumor location and size.
- Computed tomography scan reveals tumor location and size
- Magnetic resonance imaging reveals tumor.
- Elevated serum alkaline phosphatase level (in patients with sarcomas)

Botulism
- Identification of an offending toxin in the patient's serum, stool, gastric content, or the suspected food
- Electromyography shows diminished muscle action potential after a single supramaximal nerve stimulus.

Brain abscess
- History of congenital heart disease or infection, especially of the middle ear, mastoid, nasal sinuses, heart, or lungs
- Computed tomography scan or magnetic resonance imaging reveals site of abscess.
- Arteriography highlights the abscess with a halo.
- Culture of drainage reveals causative organism, such as *Staphylococcus aureus, Streptococcus viridans,* or *Streptococcus hemolyticus.*

Breast cancer
- Abnormal breast examination
- Mammography, ultrasonography, or thermography indicates presence of mass.
- Surgical biopsy reveals malignant cells.
- Carcinoembryonic antigen levels greater than 5 ng/ml
- Presence of human chorionic gonadotropin in serum or urine of woman who is not pregnant

Bronchiectasis
- History of recurrent bronchial infections, pneumonia, and hemoptysis
- Chest X-ray reveals pleural thickening, areas of atelectasis, and scattered cystic changes.

Bronchitis, chronic
- Chest X-rays may show hyperinflation and increased bronchovascular markings.
- Pulmonary function studies demonstrate increased residual volume, decreased vital capacity and forced expiratory flow, and normal static compliance and diffusing capacity.
- Arterial blood gas analysis reveals decreased PaO_2 and normal or increased $PaCO_2$.
- Sputum culture reveals the presence of microorganisms and neutrophils.

- Electrocardiography may detect atrial arrhythmias; peaked P waves in leads II, III, and aV_F and, occasionally, right ventricular hypertrophy.
- Bronchography reveals location and extent of disease.

Brucellosis

- History of contact with animals
- Agglutinin titers of 1:160 or more within 3 weeks of illness
- Multiple blood cultures, bone marrow culture, and biopsy of infected tissue indicate presence of *Brucella* bacteria.

Buerger's disease

- History of intermittent claudication of the instep
- Doppler ultrasonography reveals diminished circulation in the peripheral vessels.
- Plethysmography reveals decreased circulation in the peripheral vessels.

Burns

- History of exposure to heat, electricity, or chemicals
- Examination reveals depth of skin and tissue damage and area affected.
- Urinalysis may reveal myoglobinuria and hemoglobinuria.
- Arterial blood gas analysis reveals reduced respiratory function.
- Fiber-optic bronchoscopy may reveal epithelial damage to the trachea and bronchi.
- Serum protein studies show increased albumin levels.
- Increased blood urea nitrogen level due to increased protein catabolism
- Increased fibrin split products
- Serum magnesium levels are suppressed.
- High osmotic fragility (increased tendency to hemolysis)
- Changes in serum electrolyte levels, including elevated potassium and decreased sodium levels

- White blood cell count reveals leukocytosis.

Calcium imbalance

- Hypocalcemia:
— Serum calcium level less than 4.5 mEq/liter.
- Hypercalcemia:
— Serum calcium level greater than 5.5 mEq/liter.
— Urinalysis reveals increased calcium precipitation.
   Note: Because approximately one-half of serum calcium is bound to albumin, changes in serum protein must be considered when interpreting serum calcium levels.

Cancer of the vulva

- Papanicolaou test reveals abnormal cells.
- Tissue biopsy reveals malignant cells.
- Vulva staining (with toluidine blue dye) indicates diseased tissues.

Candidiasis

- Culture of skin, vaginal scrapings, pus, sputum, blood, or tissue reveals *Candida albicans.*

Cardiac tamponade

- Chest X-ray reveals slightly widened mediastinum and cardiomegaly.
- Echocardiography reveals pericardial effusion with signs of right ventricular and atrial compression.
- Pulmonary artery monitoring reveals increased right atrial pressure, right ventricular diastolic pressure, and central venous pressure.

Cardiogenic shock

- Auscultation detects gallop rhythm, faint heart sounds, and a holosystolic murmur (with ruptured ventricular septum or papillary muscles).
- Pulmonary artery pressure monitoring reveals the following:
— increased pulmonary artery pressure

— increased pulmonary capillary wedge pressure
— increased systemic vascular resistance
— increased peripheral vascular resistance
— decreased cardiac output.
• Invasive arterial pressure monitoring reveals hypotension.
• Increased creatine kinase levels
• Arterial blood gas analysis may show metabolic acidosis and hypoxia.
• Electrocardiography shows acute myocardial infarction, ischemia, or ventricular aneurysm.

Carpal tunnel syndrome
• Decreased sensation to light touch or pinpricks in the affected fingers
• Positive Tinel's sign
• Wrist-flexion test reveals positive Phalen's sign.
• Compression test provokes pain and paresthesia along the distribution of the median nerve.
• Electromyography detects a median nerve motor conduction delay of more than 5 milliseconds.

Cataract
• Eye examination reveals the white area behind the pupil (unnoticeable until the cataract is advanced).
• Ophthalmoscopy or slit-lamp examination reveals a dark area in the normally homogeneous red reflex.

Celiac disease
• Tissue biopsy of the small bowel reveals a mosaic pattern of alternating flat and bumpy areas on the bowel surface (due to an almost total absence of villi) and an irregular, blunt, and disorganized network of blood vessels (usually prominent in the jejunum).
• Stool samples (after 72-hour collection) reveal excess fat.
• Human leukocyte antigen test reveals presence of HLA-B8 antigen.

• D-xylose absorption test reveals depressed blood and urine D-xylose levels.
• Upper GI series followed by a small bowel series demonstrates protracted barium passage: Barium shows up in a segmented, coarse, scattered, and clumped pattern; the jejunum shows generalized dilation.
• Glucose tolerance test indicates poor glucose absorption.
• Low serum carotene levels, indicating malabsorption
• Complete blood count indicates decreased hemoglobin and hematocrit levels as well as white blood cell and platelet counts.
• Decreased serum albumin, sodium, potassium, cholesterol, and phospholipid levels
• Prothrombin time may be decreased.

Cerebral aneurysm
• History of headache and change in mental status (usually with rupture or leakage)
• Angiography reveals location and size of unruptured aneurysm.
• Computed tomography scan reveals location of clot, hydrocephalus, areas of infarction, and extent of blood spillage within the cisterns around the brain.

Cerebral contusion
• History of head trauma
• Computed tomography scan reveals ischemic tissue and hematoma.
• Skull X-ray indicates fracture is absent.

Cerebral palsy
Infant displays the following characteristics:
• difficulty sucking or keeping food in his mouth
• infrequent voluntary movement
• arm or leg tremors with movement

• crossing legs when lifted from behind rather than pulling them up or "bicycling"
• legs difficult to separate to change diapers
• persistent use of one hand, or ability to use hands well but not legs.

Cerebrovascular accident
• Motor or sensory impairment
• Computed tomography scan detects structural abnormalities, edema, and lesions, such as nonhemorrhagic infarction and aneurysms.
• Cerebral angiography reveals disruption or displacement of the cerebral circulation by occlusion or hemorrhage.
• Digital abstraction angiography evaluates the patency of the cerebral vessels and identifies their position in the head and neck. It also detects and evaluates lesions and vascular abnormalities.
• Positron emission tomography provides data on cerebral metabolism and cerebral blood flow changes, especially in ischemic stroke.
• Single-photon emission tomography identifies cerebral blood flow and helps diagnose cerebral infarction.
• EEG may detect reduced electrical activity in an area of cortical infarction.
• Transcranial Doppler studies examine the size of intracranial vessels and the direction of blood flow.
• Magnetic resonance imaging allows evaluation of the lesion's location and size.

Cervical cancer
• Abnormal Papanicolaou (Pap) test
• Cone biopsy of cervical tissue reveals malignant cells.
• Colposcopy determines the source of the abnormal cells seen on the Pap test.

Cesarean birth
The following test findings indicate the need for cesarean birth:

• X-ray pelvimetry may reveal cephalopelvic disproportion and malpresentation.
• Ultrasonography may reveal pelvic masses that interfere with vaginal delivery and fetal position.
• Amniocentesis may reveal Rh isoimmunization, fetal distress, or fetal genetic abnormalities.
• Auscultation of fetal heart rate (fetoscope, Doppler unit, or electronic fetal monitor) may reveal acute fetal distress.

Chalazion
• Visual examination and palpation of the eyelid reveal a small bump or nodule.
• Tissue biopsy rules out meibomian gland cancer.

Chancroid
• History of sexual contact with a partner with chancroid
• Tissue culture of ulcer exudate, bubo aspirate, or blood reveals *Haemophilus ducreyi.*

Chlamydial infections
• History of sexual contact with partner with chlamydial infection
• Culture of site indicates *Chlamydia trachomatis* (findings may reveal urethritis, cervicitis, salpingitis, endometritis, or proctitis).
• Culture of blood, pus, or cerebrospinal fluid reveals *C. trachomatis* (findings may reveal epididymitis, prostatitis, or lymphogranuloma venereum).

Chloride imbalance
• In hypochloremia, serum chloride level less than 98 mEq/liter.
• In hyperchloremia, serum chloride level greater than 108 mEq/liter.

Cholelithiasis and related disorders

• Ultrasound of the gallbladder indicates presence of stones.
• Percutaneous transhepatic cholangiography reveals gallbladder disease.
• Endoscopic retrograde cholangiopancreatography visualizes the biliary tree.
• Hida scan of the gallbladder reveals obstruction of the cystic duct.
• Oral cholecystography shows stones in the gallbladder and biliary duct obstruction.
• Technetium-labeled iminodiacetic acid scan of the gallbladder indicates cystic duct obstruction and acute or chronic cholecystitis if the gallbladder can't be seen.
• Blood studies may reveal elevated serum alkaline phosphatase levels, lactate dehydrogenase levels, aspartate aminotransferase levels, icteric index, and total bilirubin levels.
• White blood cell count is slightly elevated during a cholecystitis attack.

Cholera

• Stool or vomitus culture reveals presence of *Vibrio cholerae*.
• Agglutination and other clear reactions to group- and type-specific antisera provide definitive diagnosis.
• Dark-field microscopic examination of fresh feces shows rapidly moving bacilli.
• Immunofluorescence allows for rapid diagnosis.

Choriocarcinoma

• Radioimmunoassay of human chorionic gonadotropin (hCG) levels, performed frequently, provides early and accurate diagnosis; levels that are extremely elevated for early pregnancy indicate gestational trophoblastic disease.
• Histologic examination of possible hydatid vessels confirms the diagnosis.

• Ultrasonography performed after the third month shows grapelike clusters rather than a fetus.
• Amniography reveals the absence of a fetus (performed only when the diagnosis is in question).
• Doppler ultrasonography demonstrates the absence of fetal heart tones.
• Abnormal hemoglobin, hematocrit, and red blood cell count
• Abnormal fibrinogen levels
• Abnormal prothrombin and partial thromboplastin time
• Increased white blood cell count and erythrocyte sedimentation rate
• Chest X-rays, computed tomography scan, and magnetic resonance imaging may identify choriocarcinoma metastasis.
• Lumbar puncture may detect early cerebral metastasis if hCG is on the cerebrospinal fluid.

Chronic fatigue and immune dysfunction syndrome

• History reveals persistent or relapsing debilitating fatigue or tendency to tire easily.
• Average level of activity is less than 50% of normal for 6 months or more.
• Fatigue doesn't resolve with bed rest
• Diagnostic tests rule out other illnesses, such as Epstein-Barr virus, leukemia, and lymphoma.

Chronic glomerulonephritis

• Urinalysis reveals proteinuria, hematuria, cylindruria, and red blood cell casts.
• Blood urea nitrogen level greater than 20 mg/dl and rising
• Serum creatinine level greater than 1.2 mg/dl and rising
• Kidney X-rays or ultrasound reveals small kidneys.
• Renal biopsy indicates presence of underlying disease.

Chronic granulomatous disease

• History of osteomyelitis, pneumonia, liver abscess, or chronic lymphadenopathy in a young child
• Nitroblue tetrazolium (NBT) test reveals impaired NBT reduction, indicating abnormal neutrophil metabolism.
• Neutrophil function test measures the rate of intracellular killing by neutrophils; in chronic granulomatous disease, killing is delayed or absent.

Chronic lymphocytic leukemia

• Complete blood count reveals numerous abnormal lymphocytes.
• White blood cell count mildly but persistently elevated (early stages)
• Granulocytopenia
• Bone marrow aspiration and biopsy reveal lymphocytic invasion.

Chronic mucocutaneous candidiasis

• Large, circular lesions
• Culture of affected area indicates presence of *Candida*.

Chronic renal failure

• History of chronic progressive debilitation
• Blood urea nitrogen level greater than 20 mg/dl
• Serum creatinine level greater than 1.2 mg/dl
• Serum potassium level greater than 5.5 mEq/liter
• Arterial blood gas analysis reveals a blood pH less than 7.35 and an HCO_3^- level less than 22 mEq/liter.
• Urine specific gravity fixed at 1.010
• Urinalysis may show proteinuria, glycosuria, erythrocytes, leukocytes, and casts.
• Kidney biopsy identifies underlying pathology.

Cirrhosis and fibrosis

• Liver biopsy reveals destruction and fibrosis of hepatic tissue.

• Abdominal X-rays show liver size and cysts or gas within the biliary tract or liver, liver calcification, and massive ascites.
• Computed tomography and liver scans determine the liver size, identify liver masses, and reveal hepatic blood flow and obstruction.
• Esophagogastroduodenoscopy reveals bleeding esophageal varices, stomach irritation or ulceration, or duodenal bleeding and irritation.
• Elevated alanine aminotransferase, aspartate aminotransferase, total serum bilirubin, and indirect bilirubin levels
• Decreased serum albumin and protein levels
• Prolonged prothrombin time
• Decreased hematocrit, hemoglobin, and serum electrolyte levels

Coal worker's pneumoconiosis

• History of exposure to coal dust
• In simple coal worker's pneumoconiosis (CWP), chest X-ray reveals small opacities (less than 10 mm in diameter) prominent in the upper lung fields.
• In complicated CWP, chest X-ray reveals one or more large opacities (1 to 5 cm in diameter, possibly exhibiting cavitation.
• Pulmonary function tests reveal decreased lung capacity.

Coarctation of the aorta

• Resting systolic hypertension, absent or diminished femoral pulses, and wide pulse pressure
• Chest X-ray reveals notching of the undersurfaces of the ribs due to collateral circulation.
• Echocardiography reveals left ventricular muscle thickening, coexisting aortic valve abnormalities, and the coarctation site.
• Aortography locates the site and extent of coarctation.

Coccidioidomycosis

- Skin test indicates a positive reaction for coccidioidin.
- Immunodiffusion of sputum and pus from lesions and tissue biopsy reveal presence of *Coccidioides immitis* spores.
- Complement fixation reveals presence of immunoglobulin G antibodies.
- Serum immunoglobulin levels help establish diagnosis.

Colorado tick fever

- History of recent exposure to ticks
- Serum studies indicate presence of Colorado tick fever virus.

Colorectal cancer

- Hemoccult test (guaiac) reveals blood in stools.
- Proctoscopy or sigmoidoscopy reveals presence of mass.
- Colonoscopy reveals lesion.
- Tissue biopsy reveals malignant cells.
- Barium X-ray reveals lesion.
- Carcinoembryonic antigen level greater than 5 ng/ml

Common variable immunodeficiency

- Normal circulating B-cell count
- Decreased serum immunoglobulin M (IgM), IgA, and IgG levels, suggesting diminished synthesis or secretion
- Antigenic stimulation reveals an inability to produce specific antibodies.
- X-rays may reveal signs of chronic lung disease or sinusitis.

Complement deficiencies

- Low total serum complement level
- Specific assays may confirm deficiency of specific complement components.

Concussion

- History of head trauma, with or without loss of consciousness
- Amnesia with regard to traumatic event
- Headache
- Neurologic examination results normal for patient
- Skull X-ray and computed tomography scan may be negative.

Congenital hip dysplasia

- Positive Ortolani's or Trendelenburg's sign
- Extra thigh fold on affected side; higher buttock fold on the affected side; restricted abduction of the affected hip
- X-ray reveals the location of the femur head and a shallow acetabulum.

Congestive heart failure

- Dyspnea or crackles on auscultation
- Chest X-ray reveals increased pulmonary vascular markings, interstitial edema, or pleural effusion and cardiomegaly.
- Pulmonary artery monitoring reveals elevated pulmonary artery and capillary wedge pressures, left ventricular end-diastolic pressure in left-sided heart failure, and elevated right atrial pressure or central venous pressure in right-sided heart failure.

Conjunctivitis

- Inflammation of the conjunctiva
- Stained smear of conjunctival scrapings reveal monocytes (viral conjunctivitis), polymorphonuclear cells (bacterial conjunctivitis) or eosinophils (allergic conjunctivitis).
- Conjunctival culture reveals causative organism.

Cor pulmonale

- Pulmonary artery pressure measurements reveal:
— increased right ventricular and pulmonary artery pressures
— right ventricular systolic and pulmonary artery systolic pressures greater than 30 mm Hg

— pulmonary artery diastolic pressures greater than 15 mm Hg.

• Chest X-ray reveals large central pulmonary arteries and rightward enlargement of cardiac silhouette.

• Echocardiography reveals right ventricular enlargement.

Corneal abrasion

• History of eye trauma or prolonged wearing of contact lenses

• Fluorescein stain of the cornea turns the injured area green during flashlight examination.

• Slit-lamp examination discloses the depth of the abrasion.

Corneal ulcers

• History of trauma or use of contact lenses

• Flashlight examination reveals irregular corneal surface.

• Fluorescein dye, instilled in the conjunctival sac, stains the outline of the ulcer.

Coronary artery disease

• History of angina and risk factors for coronary artery disease

• Electrocardiography (ECG) reveals ischemia and, possibly, arrhythmias during an anginal attack. ECG returns to normal when pain ceases.

• Coronary angiography reveals coronary artery stenosis or obstruction, collateral circulation, and the arteries' condition beyond the narrowing.

• Myocardial perfusion imaging with thallium-201 during treadmill exercise detects ischemic areas.

Corrosive esophagitis and stricture

• History of chemical ingestion

• Oropharyngeal burns (indicated by white membranes and edema of the soft palate and uvula)

• Endoscopy (in the first 24 hours after ingestion) delineates the extent and location of the esophageal injury and assesses depth of the burn; 1 week after ingestion, this test helps assess stricture development.

• Barium swallow, performed 1 week after ingestion and every 3 weeks thereafter, as ordered, identifies segmental spasm or fistula.

Cri du chat syndrome

• Cat cry, facial disproportions, microencephaly, small birth size, and poor physical and mental development

• Karyotype reveals deleted short arms of chromosome 5.

Crohn's disease

• History of frequent stools and abdominal cramping

• Barium enema reveals the string sign (segments of stricture separated by normal bowel).

• Sigmoidoscopy and colonoscopy reveal patchy areas of inflammation.

• Biopsy of bowel tissue reveals histologic changes indicative of Crohn's disease.

Cryptococcosis

• Sputum, urine, prostatic secretion cultures; bone marrow aspirate or biopsy; or pleural biopsy reveals *Cryptococcus neoformans*.

• Blood culture reveals *C. neoformans* (with severe infection).

• Chest X-ray reveals pulmonary lesion.

Cushing's syndrome

• Consistently elevated serum cortisol levels

• 24-hour urine sample demonstrates elevated free cortisol levels.

• Dexamethasone suppression test reveals a cortisol level of 5 g/dl or greater (failure to suppress).

• Elevated urine 17-hydroxycorticosteroid levels

• Elevated urine 17-ketosteroid levels

- Ultrasonography, computed tomography (CT) scan, or angiography localize adrenal tumors.
- CT scan of the head identifies pituitary tumors.

Cutaneous larva migrans
- Characteristic migratory lesions
- History of contact with warm, moist soil within the past several months

Cystic fibrosis
- Pulmonary disease or pancreatic insufficiency (absence of trypsin)
- Family history of the disorder
- Sweat test reveals:
— sodium level above 60 mEq/liter
— chloride level above 60 mEq/liter.
- Deoxyribonucleic acid testing may locate the Delta 508 deletion and help to confirm the diagnosis.
- Pulmonary function tests evaluate lung function.
- Sputum culture allows the detection of concurrent infectious disease.
- Arterial blood gas analysis helps determine pulmonary status.
- Chest X-ray helps diagnose respiratory obstruction and monitor its progress.

Cystinuria
- Family history of renal disease or kidney stones
- Chemical analysis of calculi shows cystine crystals, with a variable amount of calcium.
- Elevated clearance of cystine, lysine, arginine, and ornithine
- Urinalysis with amino acid chromatography indicates aminoaciduria, as evidenced by the presence of cystine, lysine, arginine, and ornithine.
- Urine pH is usually less than 5.
- Microscopic examination of urine shows hexagonal, flat cystine crystals.
- Positive cyanide-nitroprusside test
- Excretory urography or kidney-ureter-bladder X-rays reveal size and location of calculi.

Cytomegalovirus infection
- Culture of urine, saliva, throat, or blood or biopsy specimens reveal virus.
- Indirect immunofluorescent test reveals immunoglobulin M antibody.

Dacryocystitis
- History of constant tearing
- Culture of discharge from tear sac reveals *Staphylococcus aureus* and, occasionally, *beta-hemolytic streptococci* in acute dacryocystitis; culture reveals *S. pneumoniae* or *Candida albicans* in the chronic form.
- Dacryocystography locates the atresia.

Decompression sickness
- History of rapid decompression
- Physical examination reveals incapacitating joint and muscle pain, and neurologic and respiratory disturbance.

Dermatitis
- Family history of allergy and chronic inflammation
- Characteristic distribution of skin lesions
- Elevated serum immunoglobulin E levels

Dermatophytosis
- Skin lesions
- Microscopic examination or culture of lesion scrapings reveals infective organism.
- Wood's light examination may reveal types of tinea capitis.

Diabetes insipidus
- Urinalysis reveals almost colorless urine of low osmolality (between 50 and 200 mOsm/kg, less than that of plasma) and low specific gravity (less than 1.005). Urine volume will decrease hourly and specific gravity will increase after subcutaneous injection of 5 units of aqueous vasopressin.

Diabetes mellitus

- In nonpregnant adults:
— symptoms of uncontrolled diabetes and a random blood glucose level greater than or equal to 200 mg/dl
— fasting plasma glucose level above 140 mg/dl on at least two occasions
— in a patient with normal fasting glucose, a blood glucose level above 200 mg/dl during the first 2 hours and on at least one other occasion during the glucose tolerance test.
- Ophthalmologic examination may show diabetic retinopathy.
- Urinalysis reveals presence of acetone.

DiGeorge's syndrome

- History of facial anomalies in infant
- T-lymphocyte assay shows decreased or absent T cells.
- B-lymphocyte assay shows elevated B cells.
- Absent thymus
- Serum calcium levels below 8 mg/dl

Dilated cardiomyopathy

- Chest X-ray reveals cardiomegaly, usually affecting all heart chambers.
- Chest X-ray may show pulmonary congestion, pleural or pericardial effusion, or pulmonary venous hypertension.
- Echocardiography reveals left ventricular thrombi, global hypokinesia, and degree of left ventricular dilation.

Diphtheria

- Characteristic thick, patchy grayish green membrane over the mucous membranes of the pharynx, larynx, tonsils, soft palate, and nose
- Throat culture or culture of other suspect lesions reveals *Corynebacterium diphtheriae*.

Dislocated or fractured jaw

- History of trauma to jaw or face

- Abnormal maxillary or mandibular mobility
- X-ray of the jaw shows fracture.

Dislocations and subluxations

- Joint deformity
- X-ray negative for fracture
- Arthroscopy reveals dislocation or subluxation.

Disseminated intravascular coagulation

- Abnormal bleeding in the absence of a known hematologic disorder
- Platelets less than $100,000/mm^3$
- Fibrinogen less than 150 mg/dl
- Prothrombin time greater than 15 seconds
- Partial prothrombin time greater than 60 seconds
- Fibrin split products will reveal fibrin degradation products greater than 100 mcg/ml.
- Positive D-dimer test (a specific fibrinogen test for disseminated intravascular coagulation)

Diverticular disease

- Upper GI series reveals barium-filled pouches in the esophagus and upper bowel.
- Barium enema reveals barium-filled pouches in the lower bowel; barium outlines diverticula filled with feces.

Down's syndrome

- Hypotonia at birth
- Karyotype reveals chromosome abnormality.
- Prenatal ultrasonography may suggest Down's syndrome if a duodenal obstruction or an atrioventricular canal defect is present.
- Reduced maternal serum alpha-fetoprotein levels
- Amniocentesis reveals the translocated chromosome.

Dysfunctional uterine bleeding
- History of excessive vaginal bleeding
- Organic, systemic, psychogenic, and endocrine causes of bleeding are ruled out.
- Dilation and curettage and biopsy reveal endometrial hyperplasia.

Dysmenorrhea
- History of abdominal pain related to menstruation
- In primary dysmenorrhea, secondary cause of pain is ruled out; in secondary dysmenorrhea, pain during menstruation is due to underlying disorder.
- Pelvic examination may reveal the physical cause.
- Laparoscopy may reveal an underlying cause such as endometriosis or uterine leiomyoma.
- Dilatation and curettage may reveal an underlying cause such as cervical stenosis or pelvic inflammatory disease.

Dyspareunia
- History of discomfort during sexual intercourse
- Pelvic examination may reveal a physical disorder as underlying cause of discomfort.

Ectopic pregnancy
- Serum pregnancy test shows presence of human chorionic gonadotropin.
- Real-time ultrasonography (performed if serum pregnancy test is positive) reveals intrauterine pregnancy or ovarian cyst.
- Culdocentesis reveals free blood in the peritoneum (performed if ultrasonography detects the absence of a gestational sac in the uterus).
- Laparoscopy (performed if culdocentesis is positive) reveals pregnancy outside the uterus.

Electric shock
- History reveals electrical contact, voltage, and length of contact.
- Physical examination reveals electrical burn.
- Electrocardiography reveals ventricular fibrillation or other arrhythmias that progress to fibrillation or myocardial infarction.
- Positive urine myoglobin test

Emphysema
- Examination reveals barrel chest, pursed-lip breathing, and use of accessory muscles; palpation may reveal decreased tactile fremitus and decreased chest expansion; percussion may reveal hyperresonance; auscultation may reveal decreased breath sounds, crackles and wheezing on inspiration, prolonged expiratory phase with grunting respirations, and distant heart sounds.
- In advanced disease, chest X-rays may show a flattened diaphragm, reduced vascular markings at the lung periphery, overaeration of the lungs, a vertical heart, enlarged anteroposterior chest diameter, and large retrosternal air space.
- Pulmonary function tests indicate increased residual volume and total lung capacity, reduced diffusing capacity, and increased inspiratory flow.
- Arterial blood gas analysis usually shows reduced PaO_2 and normal $PaCO_2$ until late in the disease.
- Electrocardiography may reveal tall, symmetrical P waves in leads II, III, and aV_F; a vertical QRS axis; and signs of right ventricular hypertrophy late in the disease.
- Red blood cell count usually demonstrates an increased hemoglobin level late in the disease, when the patient has persistent severe hypoxia.

Encephalitis
• Lumbar puncture reveals elevated cerebrospinal fluid (CSF) pressure and clear CSF, with slightly elevated white blood cell and protein levels.
• CSF or blood culture reveals virus.
• Serologic studies (in herpes encephalitis) may show rising titers of complement-fixing antibodies.
• EEG reveals abnormalities such as generalized slowing of waveforms.

Endocarditis
• Auscultation reveals a loud, regurgitant murmur.
• Blood cultures (three or more during a 24- to 48-hour period) reveal infecting organism.
• White blood cell count greater than 10,000/μl
• Elevated erythrocyte sedimentation rate
• Elevated serum creatinine level
• Echocardiography or transesophageal echocardiography reveals valvular damage and endocardial vegetation.

Endometriosis
• Pelvic examination reveals multiple tender nodules on uterosacral ligaments or in the rectovaginal septum, which enlarge and become more tender during menses.
• Palpation may uncover ovarian enlargement in patients with endometrial cysts on the ovaries or thickened, nodular adnexa (as in pelvic inflammatory disease).
• Laparoscopy shows small, blue, powder burns on the peritoneum or the serosa of any pelvic or abdominal structure.
• Barium enema rules out malignant or inflammatory bowel disease.

Enterobiasis
• Collecting a sample from the perianal area with a cellophane tape swab leads to identification of the *Enterobius* ova.

• History reveals pruritus ani as well as recent contact with infected person or infected articles.
• Stool culture for ova and parasites is ova- and worm-free.

Enterocolitis
• Stool Gram stain reveals numerous gram-positive cocci and polymorphonuclear leukocytes with few gram-negative rods.
• Stool culture reveals *Staphylococcus aureus* as the causative organism.
• Blood studies reveal leukocytosis, moderately increased blood urea nitrogen level, and decreased serum albumin level.

Epicondylitis
• History of traumatic injury or strain associated with athletic activity
• Examination reveals pain with wrist extension and supination with lateral involvement, or with flexion and pronation with epicondyle involvement.
• X-rays are normal at first, but later bony fragments, osteophyte sclerosis, or calcium deposits appear.
• Arthrography is normal with some minor irregularities on the tendon undersurface.
• Arthrocentesis identifies causative organism if joint infection is suspected.

Epidermolysis bullosa
• Skin biopsy of a freshly induced blister reveals type of epidermolysis bullosa.
• Fetoscopy and biopsy provide prenatal diagnosis of the severe scarring forms (at 20 weeks' gestation).

Epididymitis
• History reveals unilateral, dull aching pain radiating to the spermatic cord, lower abdomen, and flank.
• Physical examination shows characteristic waddle, as an attempt to protect the groin and scrotum when walking.

• Urinalysis reveals increased white blood cell count.
• Urine culture and sensitivity tests reveal causative organism.
• White blood cell count greater than 10,000/µl indicates infection.

Epiglottitis

• Throat examination reveals a large, edematous, bright red epiglottis.
• Direct laryngoscopy reveals swollen, beefy-red epiglottis (not done if significant obstruction is suspected or immediate intubation is not possible).
• Lateral neck X-rays show an enlarged epiglottis and distended hypopharynx.

Epilepsy

• Computed tomography scan provides brain density readings indicating abnormalities in internal structures.
• EEG may show paroxysmal abnormalities and helps classify the disorder.
• Magnetic resonance imaging helps identify the cause of the seizure by providing clear images of the brain in regions where bone normally hampers visualization.

Epistaxis

• History of trauma to the nose, chemical irritation, sinus infection, or coagulopathy
• Inspection with a bright light and nasal speculum locates the site of bleeding.

Erectile dysfunction

• Detailed sexual history reveals persistent or recurrent partial or complete failure to attain or maintain erection until completion of sexual activity or a persistent or recurrent lack of a subjective sense of sexual excitement and pleasure during sexual activity.
• Urologic screening rules out urogenital problems.
• Neurologic evaluation rules out neurologic dysfunction.

• Drug history rules out medication use as a causative factor.

Erysipeloid

• History reveals occupational exposure to *Erysipelothrix insidiosa* and skin injury.
• Isolation of *E. insidiosa* from a full-thickness skin biopsy taken from the edge of the lesion

Erythroblastosis fetalis

• Maternal history reveals risk factors for incompatibility of fetal and maternal blood such as erythroblastotic stillbirths, abortions, previously affected children, previous anti-Rh titers, and blood transfusions.
• Maternal blood typing indicates mother is Rh-negative (titers determine changes in the degree of maternal immunization).
• Amniocentesis reveals an increase in bilirubin levels (indicating possible hemolysis) and elevations in anti-Rh titers.
• Radiologic studies may show edema and, in hydrops fetalis, the halo sign (edematous, elevated, subcutaneous fat layers) and the Buddha position (fetus's legs are crossed).
• Direct Coombs' test of umbilical cord blood to measure red blood cells (Rh-positive) antibodies in the newborn (Results are positive only when the mother is Rh-negative and the fetus is Rh-positive.)
• An umbilical cord hemoglobin count of less than 10 g signals severe disease.
• Stained red blood cell examination reveals many nucleated peripheral red blood cells.

Esophageal cancer

• X-rays of the esophagus, with barium swallow and motility studies, reveal structural and filling defects and reduced peristalsis.

• Chest X-rays or esophagography reveal pneumonitis.
• Esophagoscopy, punch-and-brush biopsies, and exfoliative cytologic tests confirm esophageal tumors.
• Bronchoscopy may reveal tumor growth in the tracheobronchial tree.
• Endoscopic ultrasonography (combined with endoscopy and ultrasonography) identifies depth of penetration of tumor.
• Mediastinoscopy reveals lesion and extent of disease.
• Esophageal biopsy reveals malignant cells.

Esophageal diverticula
• Barium swallow reveals characteristic out-pouching in esophagus.
• Esophagoscopy rules out other lesions as cause.

Exophthalmos
• Physical examination reveals forward displacement of the eyeballs.
• Exophthalmometer readings reveal the degree of anterior projection and asymmetry between the eyes to be greater than 12 mm.
• X-rays show orbital fracture or bony erosion by an orbital tumor.
• Computed tomography scan identifies lesions in optic nerve, orbit, or ocular muscle within the orbit.

Extraocular motor nerve palsies
• Neuro-ophthalmologic examination reveals third nerve palsy (ptosis, exotropia, pupil dilation, and unresponsiveness to light, inability to move and accommodate) fourth nerve palsy (diplopia and inability to rotate eye downward and upward), or sixth nerve palsy (one eye turning, with the other eye unable to abduct beyond midline).
• Skull X-rays rule out intracranial tumor.

• Computed tomography scan and magnetic resonance imaging rule out tumor.
• Cerebral angiography rules out vascular abnormalities.
• Blood studies rule out diabetes.
• Culture and sensitivity tests reveal infective organism (for sixth nerve palsy resulting from infection).

Extrapulmonary tuberculosis
• Acid-fast smear reveals *Mycobacterium tuberculosis.*
• Positive Tuberculin skin test
• Chest X-ray reveals primary pulmonary nodular infiltrates and cavitations (often, however, chest X-ray is negative in extrapulmonary tuberculosis).
• Fluid specimen culture (urine, synovial fluid) reveals *M. tuberculosis.*

Fallopian tube cancer
• History reveals unexplained postmenopausal bleeding.
• Papanicolaou test reveals abnormal cells.
• Ultrasound defines tumor mass.
• Chest X-ray rules out metastasis.
• Barium enema rules out intestinal obstruction.
• Laparotomy and biopsy reveal malignant cells.

Fanconi's syndrome
• 24-hour urine testing reveals excessive excretion of glucose, phosphate, amino acids, HCO_3^-, and potassium.
• Elevated phosphorus and nitrogen levels (with increased renal dysfunction)
• Elevated serum alkaline phosphatase levels (with rickets)
• Serum potassium level less than 3.8 mEq/liter
• Serum HCO_3^- level less than 22 mEq/liter

Fatty liver

• Examination reveals large, tender liver.
• Liver function studies reveal low albumin, elevated globulin, elevated total bilirubin, low aminotransferase, and, commonly, elevated cholesterol levels.
• Prothrombin time is prolonged.
• Liver biopsy reveals excessive fat.

Femoral and popliteal aneurysms

• Palpation reveals a pulsating mass above or below the inguinal ligament (in femoral aneurysm) or in popliteal space (in popliteal aneurysm).
• Arteriography or ultrasonography reveals location and size of aneurysm.

Folic acid deficiency anemia

• Serum folate level less than 4 mg/ml
• Decreased reticulocyte count
• Positive Schilling test
• Serum blood studies show macrocytosis, increased mean corpuscular volume, and abnormal platelets.

Folliculitis, furunculosis, and carbunculosis

• Examination reveals pustule, painful nodule, or abscess on areas with hair growth.
• Wound culture reveals *Staphylococcus aureus*.
• Complete blood count may reveal leukocytosis.
• In carbunculosis, patient history reveals preexistent furunculosis.

Galactorrhea

• History reveals milk secretion more than 21 days after weaning.
• Breast palpation results in expression of secretions.
• Microscopic examination reveals fat droplets in fluid.
• Prolactin levels are 100 to 300 ng/ml.
• Computed tomography scan and mammography rule out tumor.

Galactosemia

• Deficiency of the enzyme galactose-1-phosphate uridyl transferase in red blood cells (RBCs), indicating classic galactosemia; decreased RBC levels of galactokinase (galactokinase deficiency)
• Increased serum and urine galactose levels
• Ophthalmoscopy reveals punctate lesions in the fetal lens nucleus.
• Liver biopsy reveals acinar formation.
• Elevated liver enzyme levels (aspartate aminotransferase and alanine aminotransferase)
• Urinalysis reveals presence of albumin.
• Amniocentesis provides prenatal diagnosis (recommended for heterozygous and homozygous parents).

Gallbladder and bile duct carcinoma

• Liver function test may show elevated urobilirubin levels and may show elevated levels of bile and bilirubin.
• Elevated serum bilirubin levels (5 to 390 mg/dl)
• Prolonged prothrombin time
• Consistently elevated serum alkaline phosphatase levels
• Liver-spleen scan identifies abnormality.
• Cholecystography shows stones or calcifications.
• Magnetic resonance imaging may show areas of tumor growth.
• Cholangiography outlines common bile duct obstruction.
• Ultrasonography of the gallbladder shows a mass.
• Endoscopic retrograde cholangiopancreatography identifies tumor site.
• Biopsy reveals malignant cells.

Gas gangrene

• History reveals recent surgery or a deep puncture wound with rapid onset of pain and crepitation around the wound.

• Anaerobic cultures of wound drainage reveal *Clostridium perfringens*.

• Gram stain of wound drainage reveals large, gram-positive, rod-shaped bacteria.

• X-rays reveals gas in tissues.

• Blood studies reveal leukocytosis and, later, hemolysis.

Gastric carcinoma

• Barium X-rays with fluoroscopy reveal tumor or filling defect in the outline of the stomach, loss of flexibility and distensibility, and abnormal gastric mucosa with or without ulceration.

• Gastroscopy with fiber-optic endoscope visualizes mucosal lesions and allows gastroscopic biopsy (biopsy reveals malignant cells).

• Photography with fiber-optic endoscope provides a permanent record of gastric lesions that may help determine disease progression and effect of treatment.

• Computed tomography scans, chest X-rays, liver and bone scans, and liver biopsy may rule out specific organ metastasis.

Gastritis

• History reveals gastric discomfort or bleeding.

• Gastroscopy demonstrates inflammation of mucosa and confirms diagnosis.

• Stools or vomitus may contain occult blood.

• Hemoglobin and hematocrit levels are decreased if bleeding has occurred.

Gastroenteritis

• History reveals acute onset of diarrhea accompanied by abdominal pain and discomfort.

• Stool or blood culture reveals causative bacteria, parasites, or amoebae.

• Barium enema reveals inflammation.

Gastroesophageal reflux

• Barium swallow with fluoroscopy may be normal except in patients with advanced disease; in children, barium esophagography under fluoroscope reveals reflux.

• Esophageal acidity test reveals pH of 1.5 to 2.0.

• Acid perfusion test elicits pain or burning.

• Gastroesophageal reflux scanning detects radioactivity in the esophagus.

• Endoscopy and biopsy identify pathologic mucosal changes.

Gaucher's disease

• Bone marrow aspiration reveals Gaucher's cells.

• Direct assay of glucocerebrosidase activity, which can be performed on venous blood, shows absent or deficient activity.

• Liver biopsy reveals increased glucosylceramide accumulation.

• Increased serum acid phosphatase levels

• Decreased platelet count and serum iron level

Genital herpes

• History reveals oral, vaginal, or anal sexual contact with an infected person or other direct contact with lesions.

• Examination reveals vesicles on the genitalia, mouth, or anus.

• Tissue culture and histologic biopsy of vesicular fluid reveals herpes simplex II virus.

Genital warts

• Dark-field examination of scrapings from wart cells shows marked vascularization of epidermal cells, which helps to differentiate genital warts from condylomata lata.

• Applying 5% acetic acid (white vinegar) to the warts turns them white, indicating papillomas.

Giardiasis

• History reveals risk factors such as recent travel to an endemic area, participation in sexual activity involving oral-anal contact, ingestion of suspect water, or institutionalization.
• Stool specimen shows cysts.
• Duodenal aspirate or biopsy shows trophozoites.
• Small bowel biopsy shows parasitic infection.

Glaucoma

• Gradual loss of peripheral vision
• Tonometry (using an applanation, Schiøtz, or pneumatic tonometer) reveals intraocular pressure greater than 21 mm Hg.
• Gonioscopy determines the angle of the anterior chamber of the eye, differentiating between chronic open-angle glaucoma and acute closed-angle glaucoma.
• Ophthalmoscopy reveals cupping and atrophy of the optic disk.
• Slit-lamp examination visualizes anterior structures of the eye, demonstrating effects of glaucoma.
• Perimetry or visual field tests evaluate the extent of visual field loss of open-angle deterioration.
• Fundus photography reveals changes in the optic disk.

Glycogen storage diseases

• Type Ia:
— Liver biopsy reveals normal glycogen synthetase and phosphorylase enzyme activities but reduced or absent glucose-6-phosphatase activity.
— Liver biopsy reveals glycogen structure is normal, but amounts are elevated.
— Serum glucose levels are low.
— Plasma studies reveal high levels of free fatty acids, triglycerides, cholesterol, and uric acid.
— Injection of glucagon or epinephrine increases pyruvic and lactic acid levels but does not increase blood glucose levels.
— Glucose tolerance test curve reveals depletional hypoglycemia and reduced insulin output.
• Type II (Pompe's):
— Muscle biopsy reveals increased concentration of glycogen with normal structure and decreased alpha-1,4-glucosidase level.
— Electrocardiography (in infants) shows large QRS complexes in all leads, inverted T waves, and a shortened PR interval.
— Electromyography (in adults) demonstrates muscle fiber irritability and myotonic discharges.
— Amniocentesis reveals a deficiency in alpha-1,4-glucosidase level.
— Placenta or umbilical cord examination shows an alpha-1,4-glucosidase deficiency.
— Liver biopsy shows deficient debranching activity and increased glycogen concentration.
• Type III (Cori's):
— Laboratory tests (in children only) may reveal elevated aspartate aminotransferase or alanine aminotransferase levels and an increase in erythrocyte glycogen.
• Type IV (Andersen's):
— Liver biopsy demonstrates deficient branching enzyme activity and that the glycogen molecule has longer outer branches.
• Type V (McArdle's):
— Serum studies indicate no increase in venous levels of lactate in sample drawn from extremity after ischemic exercise.
— Muscle biopsy reveals a lack of phosphorylase activity and an increased glycogen content.
• Type VI (Hers'):
— Liver biopsy shows decreased phosphorylase beta activity and increased glycogen concentration.

• Type VII:
— Serum studies indicate no increase in venous levels of lactate in sample drawn from extremity after ischemic exercise.
— Muscle biopsy shows deficient phosphofructokinase and a marked rise in glycogen concentration.
— Blood studies reveal low erythrocyte phosphofructokinase activity and reduced half-life of red blood cells.
— Muscle biopsy shows deficient phosphofructokinase with a marked rise in glycogen concentration with normal structure.
• Type VIII:
— Liver biopsy shows deficient phosphorylase beta activity and increased liver glycogen.
— Blood studies show deficient phosphorylase beta kinase in leukocytes.

Goiter, simple

• History reveals residence in an area known for nutritionally related risk factors (such as iodine-depleted soil or malnutrition) or ingestion of goitrogenic medications or foods.
• High or normal serum thyroid-stimulating hormone or triiodothyronine concentration
• Low to normal or normal serum thyroxine concentrations
• Normal or increased ^{131}I uptake
• Low to normal or normal protein-bound iodine
• Low urinary excretion of iodine

Gonorrhea

• History reveals sexual contact with a partner with gonorrhea.
• Culture from site of infection (urethra, cervix, rectum, pharynx) reveals *Neisseria gonorrhoea.*
• Culture of joint fluid and skin lesions reveals gram-negative diplococci (gonococcal arthritis).
• Culture of conjunctival scrapings confirms gonococcal conjunctivitis.

• Complement fixation and immunofluorescent assays of serum reveal antibody titers four times the normal rate.

Goodpasture's syndrome

• Immunofluorescence of alveolar basement membrane shows linear deposition of immunoglobulin as well as C3 and fibrinogen.
• Immunofluorescence of glomerular basement membrane (GBM) shows linear deposition of immunoglobulin combined with detection of circulating anti-GBM antibody.
• Lung biopsy shows interstitial and intra-alveolar hemorrhage with hemosiderin-laden macrophages.
• Chest X-ray reveals pulmonary infiltrates in a diffuse, nodular pattern.
• Renal biopsy reveals focal necrotic lesions and cellular crescents.
• Serum creatinine and blood urea nitrogen levels typically increase two to three times normal.
• Urinalysis may reveal red blood cells and cellular casts, granular casts, and proteinuria.

Gout

• Microscopic analysis of synovial fluid obtained by needle aspiration reveals needlelike intracellular crystals of sodium urate; presence of monosodium urate monohydrate crystals confirms diagnosis.
• Serum uric acid levels are normal, but may be increased; the higher the level, especially when it rises above 10 mg/dl, the more likely a gout attack.
• Urine uric acid levels are increased (in approximately 20% of patients).
• X-rays reveal damage of the articular cartilage and subchondral bone (in chronic gout).

Granulocytopenia
• Markedly reduced neutrophil count (less than 500/µl leads to severe bacterial infections)
• White blood cell count less than 2,000/µl
• Complete blood count reveals few observable granulocytes.
• Bone marrow aspiration reveals a scarcity of granulocytic precursor cells beyond the most immature forms.

Guillain-Barré syndrome
• History reveals minor febrile illness 1 to 4 weeks before current symptoms.
• Examination reveals progressive muscle weakness.
• Cerebrospinal fluid analysis reveals normal white blood cell count, rising protein levels (peaks in 4 to 6 weeks), and increasing pressure.
• Electromyography reveals repeated firing of the same motor unit instead of widespread sectional stimulation.
• Electrophysiologic studies may reveal marked slowing of nerve conduction velocities.

Haemophilus influenza infection
• Blood culture reveals *H. influenza* infection.
• Complete blood count reveals polymorphonuclear leukocytosis (15,000 to 30,000/µl) and, in young children with severe infection, leukopenia (2,000 to 3,000 /µl).

Hearing loss
• Audiometry identifies and quantifies hearing loss.
• The Weber, the Rinne, and the Schwabach tests differentiate between conductive and sensorineural hearing loss.
• Auditory brain stem response and behavioral tests may help to identify neonatal or infant hearing loss.
• Computed tomography scan evaluates vestibular and auditory pathways.

• Magnetic resonance imaging detects acoustic tumors and lesions.

Hemochromatosis
• Serum or plasma iron concentration is greater than 180 mcg/100 ml.
• Transferrin levels are increased to 70% to 100% saturation.
• 24-hour urine collection shows iron excretion 10 mg or more after administration of deferoxamine, an iron-chelating agent.

Hemophilia
• History suggests disorder runs in family.
• History of prolonged bleeding after surgery or trauma or of episodes of spontaneous bleeding into muscles or joints
• Hemophilia A:
— Factor VIII assay 0% to 30% of normal
— prolonged activated partial thromboplastin time
— normal platelet count and function, bleeding time, and prothrombin time.
• Hemophilia B:
— Factor IX assay deficient
— prolonged activated partial thromboplastin time.
• Hemophilia C:
— Assay testing reveals deficient Factor XI.
— Assay testing reveals normal Factors VIII and IX levels (rules out hemophilias A and B).
— prolonged partial thromboplastin time.
• Degree of severity:
— Mild hemophilia shows factor levels 5% to 40% of normal.
— Moderate hemophilia shows factor levels 1% to 5% of normal.
— Severe hemophilia shows factor levels less than 1% of normal.

• Computed tomography scan rules out intracranial bleeding.
• Arthroscopy rules out joint bleeding.
• Endoscopy rules out GI bleeding.

Hemorrhoids

• History reveals intermittent rectal bleeding after defecation.
• Examination reveals hemorrhoids protruding from rectum.
• Proctoscopy reveals internal hemorrhoids.
• Anoscopy and flexible sigmoidoscopy identify internal hemorrhoids and rule out polyps or fistulae.

Hemothorax

• History reveals recent trauma to chest area.
• Chest percussion reveals dullness.
• Chest auscultation reveals decreased to absent breath sounds on the affected side.
• Thoracentesis reveals blood or serosanguineous fluid.
• Chest X-ray reveals pleural fluid with or without mediastinal shift.
• Arterial blood gas studies show respiratory failure.
• Hemoglobin levels may be decreased depending on the degree of blood loss.

Hepatic encephalopathy

• History reveals liver disease, with symptoms beginning with slight personality changes progressing to mental confusion and coma.
• Serum ammonia levels greater than 50 µg/dl
• EEG shows slowing waves as the disease progresses.

Hepatitis, viral

• A hepatitis profile identifies serum antigens and antibodies (serum markers) specific to the causative virus, establishing the type of hepatitis (Types A, B, C, D, and E).

• Prolonged prothrombin time (more than 3 seconds longer than normal indicates liver damage)
• Elevated aspartate aminotransferase and alanine aminotransferase levels
• Elevated serum alkaline phosphatase levels
• Elevated serum and urine bilirubin levels (with jaundice)
• Decreased serum albumin and increased serum globulin
• Patchy necrosis on liver biopsy and liver scan

Hereditary hemorrhagic telangiectasia

• History reveals an established family pattern of bleeding disorders.
• Examination reveals localized aggregations of dilated capillaries on the skin of the face, ears, scalp, hands, arms, and feet, and under the nails; characteristic telangiectases are raised or flat, non-pulsatile, violet in color, and blanche under pressure and bleed easily.
• Bone marrow aspiration shows depleted iron stores (confirms secondary iron deficiency anemia).
• Platelet count may be abnormal.

Herniated disk

• History reveals unilateral low back pain radiating to the buttocks, legs, and feet; often associated with a previous traumatic injury or back strain.
• X-rays show degenerative changes and rule out other abnormalities.
• The LeSegue's test causes resistance and pain, as well as loss of ankle or knee-jerk reflex.
• Myelography pinpoints the level of herniation and reveals spinal canal compression by herniated disk material.
• Computed tomography scan identifies soft tissue and bone abnormalities.
• Electromyelography confirms nerve involvement.

• Neuromuscular tests identify motor and sensory loss and leg muscle weakness.

Herpangina
• Examination reveals vesicular lesions on the mucous membranes of the soft palate, tonsillar pillars, and throat.
• Cultures of mouth washings or feces reveal the coxsackieviruses.
• Elevated antibody titers

Herpes simplex
• Examination reveals edema with small vesicles on an erythematous base that rupture leaving a painful ulcer followed by yellow crusting.
• Isolation of virus from local lesions and biopsy reveal *Herpesvirus hominis*.

Herpes zoster
• Examination reveals small red, nodular skin lesions that spread unilaterally around the thorax or vertically over the arms or legs and vesicles filled with clear fluid or pus.
• Examination of vesicular fluid and infected tissue reveals eosinophilic intranuclear inclusions and varicella virus.
• Lumbar puncture shows increased cerebrospinal fluid (CSF) pressure; CSF analysis shows increased protein levels and possibly, pleocytosis (with central nervous system involvement).

Hiatal hernia
• Chest X-ray reveals air shadow behind the heart (with large hernia).
• Barium swallow with fluoroscopy reveals outpouching at lower end of the esophagus and identifies diaphragmatic abnormalities.
• Serum hemoglobin and hematocrit levels may be decreased (with paraesophageal hernia).
• Endoscopy and biopsy rule out varices and other small gastroesophageal lesions.

• Esophageal motility studies reveal esophageal motor or lower esophageal pressure abnormalities.
• pH studies reveal reflux of gastric contents.
• Acid perfusion test reveals heartburn resulting from esophageal reflux.

Hirschsprung's disease
• Rectal biopsy reveals absence of ganglion cells.
• Barium enema studies reveal a narrowed segment of distal colon with a sawtooth appearance and a funnel-shaped segment above it; barium is retained longer than the usual 12 to 24 hours.
• Rectal manometry detects failure of the internal anal sphincter to relax and contract.
• Upright films of the abdomen show marked colonic distention.

Histoplasmosis
• History reveals an immunocompromised condition or exposure to contaminated soil in an endemic area.
• Tissue biopsy and sputum culture reveal *Histoplasma capsulatum* (in acute primary and chronic pulmonary histoplasmosis).
• Histoplasmosis skin test is positive.
• Complement fixation test results are increased, and agglutination titers are greater than 1:32.

Hodgkin's disease
• Lymph node biopsy reveals Reed-Sternberg's abnormal histiocyte proliferation and nodular fibrosis and necrosis.
• Computed tomography scan shows lymph node abnormality.
• Lymphangiography shows lymph node abnormality.
• Bone marrow, liver, mediastinal, and spleen biopsies, abdominal computed tomography scan, and lung and bone scans identify organ involvement.

• Blood studies show normochromic anemia (in 50% of patients) and elevated, normal, or reduced white blood cell count and differential showing any combination of neutrophilia, lymphocytopenia, monocytosis, and eosinophilia.

• Increased serum alkaline phosphatase levels

Hookworm disease

• Stool specimen reveals hookworm ova.

• Blood studies show hemoglobin of 5 to 9 g/dl (in severe cases), white blood cell count as high as 47,000/ μl, and eosinophil count of 500 to 700/μl.

Huntington's disease

• History reveals family inheritance pattern along with progressive chorea and dementia, with usual onset between ages 35 and 40.

• Positron emission tomography identifies disease.

• Deoxyribonucleic acid analysis identifies marker for gene linked to the disease.

• Evoked potential studies reveal bilateral abnormal P100 latencies.

• Pneumoencephalography reveals the characteristic butterfly dilation of the brain's lateral ventricles.

• Computed tomography scan reveals brain atrophy.

Hydatidiform mole

• History reveals vaginal bleeding, ranging from brownish red spotting to bright red hemorrhage.

• Examination reveals an abnormally enlarged uterus; pelvic examination reveals grapelike vesicles.

• Histologic identification of hydatid vesicles after passage helps confirm diagnosis.

• Ultrasonography shows grapelike structures rather than a fetus; use of a Doppler ultrasonic flowmeter demonstrates the absence of fetal heart tones.

• Amniography reveals the absence of a fetus.

• Increased white blood cell count and erythrocyte sedimentation rate

• Hemoglobin, hematocrit levels, red blood cell count, prothrombin time, partial thromboplastin time, fibrinogen levels, and hepatic and renal function studies are abnormal.

• Serum human chorionic gonadotropin levels are elevated 100 or more days after the last menstrual period.

• Serum human placental lactogen levels are subnormal.

Hydrocephalus

• Examination reveals an abnormally large head size for age.

• Skull X-rays reveal thinning of the skull with separation of sutures and widening of the fontanelles.

• Ventriculography reveals enlargement of the brain's ventricles.

• Angiography, computed tomography scan, or magnetic resonance imaging of brain reveal areas of altered density and rule out intracranial lesions.

Hydronephrosis

• Kidney-ureter-bladder X-rays reveal bilateral kidney enlargement.

• Renal ultrasound reveals large, echo-free, central mass that compromises the renal cortex.

• Excretory urography reveals abnormal kidneys.

• Urine studies reveal the inability to concentrate urine, a decreased glomerular filtration rate, and possibly, pyuria (if infection is present).

Hyperaldosteronism

- Persistently low serum potassium levels (in the absence of edema, diuretic use, gastrointestinal loss, or abnormal sodium intake).
- Elevated serum aldosterone levels
- Low plasma renin level after volume depletion by diuretic administration and upright posture and a high plasma aldosterone level after volume expansion by salt loading (confirms primary hyperaldosteronism in a hypertensive patient without edema)
- Elevated serum HCO_3^- level with ensuing alkalosis resulting from the loss of hydrogen and potassium in the distal tubules
- Increased serum and urine aldosterone levels
- Adrenal angiography or computed tomography scan reveals adrenal tumor.
- Plasma volume levels increased to 30% to 50% above normal
- Suppression testing reveals decreased plasma aldosterone and urine metabolites (secondary hyperaldosteronism) or normal plasma aldosterone and urine metabolites (primary hyperaldosteronism).
- Electrocardiography reveals ST-segment depression and the presence of U waves indicating hypokalemia.
- Chest X-ray shows left ventricular hypertrophy from chronic hypertension.
- Computed tomography scan, ultrasonography, or magnetic resonance imaging identifies tumor location.

Hyperbilirubinemia

- Examination reveals jaundice.
- Serum bilirubin levels greater than 12.0 mg/dl

Hyperemesis gravidarum

- History reveals uncontrolled nausea and vomiting that persists beyond the first trimester of pregnancy.

- Examination reveals substantial weight loss.
- Decreased serum sodium, chloride, potassium, and protein levels
- Blood urea nitrogen level greater than 20 mg/dl
- Urinalysis reveals ketonuria and proteinuria.

Hyperlipoproteinemia

- Type I (Fredrickson's hyperlipoproteinemia, fat-induced hyperlipemia, idiopathic familial):
— chylomicrons (very-low-density lipoproteins [VLDL], low-density lipoproteins [LDL], high-density lipoproteins [HDL]) in plasma 14 hours or more after last meal
— high elevated serum chylomicron and triglyceride levels; slightly elevated serum cholesterol levels
— decreased serum lipoprotein lipase levels
— leukocytosis.
- Type II (familial hyperbetalipoproteinemia, essential familial hypercholesterolemia):
— increased plasma concentrations of LDL
— elevated serum LDL and cholesterol levels
— increased LDL levels detected by amniocentesis.
- Type III (familial broad-beta disease, xanthoma tuberosum):
— abnormal serum beta-lipoprotein levels
— elevated cholesterol and triglyceride levels
— slightly elevated glucose levels.
- Type IV (endogenous hypertriglyceridemia, hyperbetalipoproteinemia):
— elevated plasma VLDL levels
— moderately increased plasma triglyceride levels
— normal or slightly elevated serum cholesterol levels
— mildly abnormal glucose tolerance
— early coronary artery disease.

• Type V (mixed hypertriglyceridemia, mixed hyperlipidemia):
— chylomicrons in plasma
— elevated plasma VLDL levels
— elevated serum cholesterol and triglyceride levels.

Hyperparathyroidism
• Increased serum parathyroid hormone levels
• Increased serum calcium levels
• Urine cyclic adenosine monophosphate test reveals failure to respond to parathyroid hormone
• X-rays show diffuse demineralization of bones, bone cysts, outer cortical bone absorption, and subperiosteal erosion of the radial aspect of the middle fingers.
• X-ray spectrophotometry demonstrates increased bone turnover.
• Radioimmunoassay shows increased concentration of parathyroid hormone with accompanying hypercalcemia.
• Increased serum phosphorus levels
• Increased serum and urine chloride, uric acid, creatinine, and alkaline phosphatase levels; basal acid secretion
• Increased serum immunoreactive gastrin levels

Hyperpituitarism
• Growth hormone (GH) immunoassay shows increased plasma GH levels.
• Glucose suppression test shows failure to suppress GH level to below accepted norm of 5 mg.
• Skull X-rays, computed tomography scan, arteriography, and pneumoencephalography reveal the presence and extent of a pituitary lesion.
• Bone X-rays reveal a thickening of the cranium (especially of frontal, occipital, and parietal bones) and of the long bones, as well as osteoarthritis in the spine.

Hypersplenism
• I.V. infusion of chromium-labeled red blood cells or platelets reveals high spleen-liver ratio of radioactivity, indicating splenic destruction or sequestration.
• Complete blood count shows decreased hemoglobin levels (as low as 4 g/dl), white blood cell count less than 4,000/µl, platelet count less than 125,000/mm^3, and an elevated reticulocyte count.
• Examination reveals splenomegaly.

Hypertension
• Serial blood pressure measurements on a sphygmomanometer of more than 140/90 in a patient under age 50 or 150/95 in patient over age 50
• Urinalysis reveals presence of protein, red blood cells, white blood cells, or glucose.
• Excretory urography may reveal renal atrophy.
• Serum potassium levels less than 3.5 mEq/liter indicating adrenal dysfunction
• Blood urea nitrogen levels are normal or elevated to more than 20 mg/dl and serum creatinine levels are normal or elevated to more than 1.5 mg/dl; elevated levels suggest renal disease.

Hyperthyroidism
• Radioimmunoassay shows increased serum thyroxine and triiodothyronine levels.
• Thyroid scan reveals increased uptake of ^{131}I.
• Thyroid-releasing hormone (TRH) stimulation test reveals failure of the thyroid-stimulating hormone level to rise within 30 minutes after administration of TRH.
• Autoantibody tests reveal presence of thyroid-stimulating immunoglobulin.

Hypervitaminoses A and D
• History reveals accidental or misguided use of supplemental vitamin preparations.
• Serum vitamin A level greater than 90 mcg/dl (hypervitaminosis A)
• Serum vitamin D level greater than 100 ng/ml (hypervitaminosis D)
• X-rays showing calcification of tendons, ligaments, and subperiosteal tissues (hypervitaminosis D).
• Serum carotene level greater than 250 mcg/dl (hypercarotenemia)

Hypoglycemia
• Blood glucose studies (children and adults) reveal abnormally low levels: less than 40 mg/dl before a meal and less than 50 mg/dl after a meal.
• C-peptide assay identifies fasting hypoglycemia.

Hypogonadism
• Serum and urine gonadotropin levels:
— increased in primary, or hypergonadotropic, hypogonadism
— decreased in secondary, or hypogonadotropic, hypogonadism.
• Chromosomal analysis identifies cause.
• Testicular biopsy and semen analysis reveal impaired spermatogenesis and low testosterone levels.
• X-rays and bone scans show delayed closure of epiphyses and immature bone age.

Hypoparathyroidism
• Radioimmunoassay shows decreased serum parathyroid hormone levels.
• Decreased urine and serum calcium levels
• Serum phosphorus levels are increased to more than 5.4 mg/dl.
• Decreased urine creatinine levels
• X-rays show increased bone density and malformation.

• Cyclic adenosine monophosphate test demonstrates a ten- to twentyfold increase (3.6 to 4.0 micromoles).
• Electrocardiography shows increased QT and ST intervals due to hypercalcemia.

Hypopituitarism
• Radioimmunoassay shows decreased plasma levels of some or all pituitary hormones.
• Decreased serum thyroxine (T_4) levels (with thyroid dysfunction)
• Arginine test reveals failure of human growth hormone (hGH) levels to rise after arginine infusion (with pituitary dysfunction).
• Insulin tolerance test reveals failure of stimulation or a blunted response of hGH levels (with hypothalamic-pituitary-adrenal axis dysfunction).
• Decreased urine 17-ketosteroid levels (with hypoadrenalism)
• Decreased levels of serum pituitary hormones (follicle-stimulating hormone, luteinizing hormone, and thyroid-stimulating hormone)
• Computed tomography scan, pneumoencephalography, or cerebral angiography confirms the presence of tumors inside or outside the sella turcica.

Hypothermic injuries
• History reveals severe and prolonged exposure to cold.
• Core body temperature below 95° F (35° C)
• Physical examination shows burning, tingling, numbness, swelling, pain, and mottled blue-gray skin in exposed areas.

Hypothyroidism in adults
• Radioimmunoassay shows low serum levels of thyroid hormones.
• Decreased serum triiodothyronine and thyroxine levels
• Serum thyroid-stimulating hormone level may be increased (due to thyroid

insufficiency) or decreased (due to hypothalamic or pituitary insufficiency).
- Radioactive iodine uptake test reveals below normal percentages of iodine uptake.
- Radionuclide thyroid imaging reveals "cold spots."
- Thyroid ultrasonography identifies cysts or tumors.
- Elevated serum antithyroid antibodies (in autoimmune thyroiditis)

Hypothyroidism in children
- Elevated serum thyroid-stimulating hormone level, associated with low triiodothyronine and thyroxine levels
- Thyroid scan (^{131}I uptake test) shows decreased uptake levels and confirms the absence of thyroid tissue in athyroid children.
- Gonadotropin levels are increased and compatible with sexual precocity in older children.
- Hip, knee, and thigh X-rays reveal absence of the femoral or tibial epiphyseal line and delayed skeletal development that is markedly inappropriate for the child's chronologic age.

Hypovolemic shock
- History reveals recent loss of blood volume.
- Blood pressure auscultation reveals mean arterial pressure under 60 mm Hg in adults and a narrowing pulse pressure.
- Blood studies show low hemoglobin and hematocrit levels, low red blood cell count, and low platelet levels.
- Serum potassium, sodium, lactate dehydrogenase, creatinine, and blood urea nitrogen levels are elevated.
- Urine specific gravity greater than 1.020
- Elevated urine osmolality
- Decreased urine creatinine levels
- Arterial blood gas measurements show decreased pH, decreased PaO_2, and increased $PaCO_2$ levels.

Idiopathic hypertrophic subaortic stenosis
- Echocardiography shows increased thickness of the intraventricular septum and abnormal motion of the anterior mitral leaflet during systole, occluding left ventricular outflow in obstructive disease.
- Cardiac catheterization reveals elevated left ventricular end-diastolic pressure and, possibly, mitral insufficiency.
- Electrocardiography usually demonstrates left ventricular hypertrophy, T-wave inversion, left anterior hemiblock, Q waves in precordial and inferior leads, ventricular arrhythmias, and, possibly, atrial fibrillation.
- Phonocardiography confirms an early systolic murmur.

Idiopathic thrombocytopenic purpura
- Platelet count less than 20,000/mm^3
- Prolonged bleeding time
- Bone marrow studies show an abundance of megakaryocytes (platelet precursors) and a shortened circulating platelet survival time.

IgA deficiency
- Serum immunoglobulin A (IgA) levels below 5 mg/dl
- IgA usually absent from secretions
- Low-molecular-weight IgM (7S) detected in serum (normally absent)

Impetigo
- Characteristic lesions
- Microscopic visualization, Gram stain or culture of exudate reveals *Staphylococcus aureus* infection.
- White blood cell count may be elevated.

Inactive colon

- History reveals dry, hard, infrequent stools.
- Digital rectal examination reveals stools in the lower portion of the rectum and a palpable colon.
- Proctoscopy reveals unusually small colon lumen, prominent veins, and an abnormal amount of mucous.
- Upper GI series and barium enema rule out tumor.
- Fecal occult blood test is negative.

Inclusion conjunctivitis

- Examination reveals swollen, reddened lower eyelids, excessive tearing, and a moderately purulent discharge.
- History reveals sexual contact with a partner infected with *Chlamydia trachomatis*.
- Conjunctival scraping reveals cytoplasmic inclusion bodies in conjunctival epithelial cells and many polymorphonuclear leukocytes; culture for bacteria is negative.

Infantile autism

- Denver Developmental Screening Test shows delayed development, especially of social and language skills.
- IQ testing shows retardation in 70% of patients (low IQ scores may reflect inability to cooperate with testing).
- History reveals symptom development before age 30 months.
- Evaluation reveals impairment in social interaction skills, verbal and nonverbal communication, and imaginative activity and a markedly restricted range of activities and interests.

Infectious mononucleosis

- Leukocyte count 10,000 to 20,000/µl during second and third week of illness, with lymphocytes and monocytes 50% to 70% of white blood cells (10% of lymphocytes are abnormal)
- Heterophil agglutination tests indicate the presence of heterophil antibodies; testing at 3- to 4-week intervals reveals a rise to four times normal levels.
- Indirect immunofluorescence shows antibodies to Epstein-Barr virus and cellular antigens.
- Liver function studies are abnormal.

Infectious myringitis

- Otoscopic examination shows small, reddened inflamed blebs in the ear canal, on the tympanic membrane, and in the middle ear (with bacterial invasion).
- Exudate culture reveals infective organism.

Infertility, female

- History reveals inability to achieve pregnancy after having regular intercourse, without contraception, for at least 1 year.
- Endometrial biopsy provides histologic evidence that ovulation has occurred.
- Progesterone blood levels reveal a luteal phase deficiency.
- Decreased follicle-stimulating hormone levels
- Hysterosalpingography reveals tubal obstruction and uterine abnormalities.
- Endoscopy shows tubal obstruction or uterine abnormalities.
- Laparoscopy visualizes abdominal and pelvic areas and may reveal peritubular adhesions or ureterotubal obstruction.
- Postcoital test (Sims-Huhner test) shows inadequate motile sperm cells in cervical fluid following intercourse.
- Immunologic or antibody testing detects spermicidal antibodies in the sera of the female.

Infertility, male

- History reveals abnormal sexual development, delayed puberty, or infertility in previous relationships
- Medical history reveals prolonged fever, mumps, impaired nutritional status, previous surgery, or trauma to genitalia.

- Semen analysis reveals subnormal sperm counts, decreased sperm motility, abnormal morphology, or absence of viable spermatozoa.
- Decreased urine 17-ketosteroid levels
- Decreased serum testosterone levels

Influenza
- Nose and throat culture reveals the causative virus
- Elevated cold agglutinin titers
- Increased serum antibody titers
- White blood cell count is decreased and lymphocytes are increased (uncomplicated cases).

Inguinal hernia
- History reveals sharp or "catching" pain when lifting or straining, with excessive coughing, or following a recent pregnancy.
- Examination reveals a swelling or lump in the inguinal area.
- Palpation of the inguinal area, while the patient is performing Valsalva's maneuver, reveals pressure against the fingertip (indirect hernia) or pressure against the side of the finger (direct hernia).
- Abdominal X-ray rules out obstruction.
- White blood cell count may be elevated.

Insect bites and stings
- Tick:
— History reveals exposure in woods and fields and complaints of itching.
— After several days, tick paralysis (acute flaccid paralysis, starting as paresthesia and pain in legs and resulting in respiratory failure from bulbar paralysis).
- Bee, wasp, or yellow jacket:
— History reveals painful sting.
— Examination reveals protruding stinger (bees), edema, urticaria, or pruritus.
— Systemic reaction (anaphylaxis), indicating hypersensitivity, usually appears within 20 minutes and may include weakness, chest tightness, dizziness, nausea, vomiting, abdominal cramps, and throat constriction.
- Brown recluse (violin) spider:
— History reveals exposure to dark areas (outdoor privy, barn, woodshed) in south-central United States with reaction within 2 to 8 hours of the bite.
— Examination reveals localized vasoconstriction with ischemic necrosis at bite site with small, reddened puncture wound forming a bleb and becoming ischemic, proceeding to a dark, hard center in 3 to 4 days and an ulcer within 2 to 3 weeks.
— Pain is minimal initially, but increases over time
— Commonly, fever, chills, malaise, weakness, nausea, vomiting, edema, seizures, joint pains, petechiae, cyanosis, and phlebitis develop.
— Rarely, thrombocytopenia and hemolytic anemia develop and lead to death within 24 to 48 hours (usually in a child or patient with previous history of cardiac disease).
- Scorpion:
— In nonlethal types, history reveals symptoms lasting from 24 to 78 hours and including local swelling and tenderness, sharp burning sensation, skin discoloration, paresthesia, lymphangitis with regional gland swelling, and anaphylaxis (rare).
— In lethal types, history reveals symptoms including immediate sharp pain, hyperesthesia, drowsiness, itching (nose, throat, mouth), impaired speech, and generalized muscle spasms (including jaw muscle spasms, laryngospasm, incontinence, seizures, nausea, and vomiting).
- Black widow spider:
— History reveals exposure to dark areas (outdoor privy, barn, woodshed) in southern United States between April

and November and report of pinprick sensation, followed by dull, numbing pain.

— Examination reveals edema and tiny, red bite marks, rigidity of stomach muscles, and severe abdominal pain (10 to 40 minutes after bite).

— Muscle spasms develop in extremities.

— Ascending paralysis occurs, causing difficulty in swallowing and labored, grunting respirations.

— Other symptoms include extreme restlessness, vertigo, sweating, chills, pallor, seizures (especially in children), hyperactive reflexes, hypertension, tachycardia, thready pulse, circulatory collapse, nausea, vomiting, headache, ptosis, eyelid edema, urticaria, pruritus, and fever.

Intestinal obstruction

• History reveals progressive, colicky, abdominal pain and distention.

• Abdominal X-ray reveals the presence and location of intestinal gas or fluid.

• In X-ray, small bowel obstruction appears as a typical "stepladder" pattern of alternating gas and fluid levels.

• In X-ray, large bowel obstruction reveals a distended, air-filled colon or a closed loop of sigmoid with extreme distention.

• Serum sodium, chloride, and potassium levels may decrease because of vomiting.

• White blood cell count may be normal or slightly elevated if necrosis, peritonitis, or strangulation occurs.

• Serum amylase level may increase.

• Sigmoidoscopy, colonoscopy, or barium enema may help identify the cause of obstruction.

Intussusception

• Barium enema reveals characteristic coiled spring sign and delineates the extent of intussusception.

• Upright abdominal X-rays may show a soft-tissue mass and signs of complete or partial obstruction, with dilated loops of bowel.

• White blood cell count up to 15,000/µl indicates obstruction; greater than 15,000/µl, strangulation; more than 20,000/µl, bowel infarction.

Iodine deficiency

• Serum thyroxine levels are low, with high ^{131}I uptake.

• 24-hour urine collection reveals low iodine levels.

• High levels of serum thyroid-stimulating hormone

• Radioiodine uptake test traces ^{131}I in the thyroid 24 hours after administration.

Iron deficiency anemia

• Bone marrow studies reveal depleted or absent iron stores and normoblastic hyperplasia.

• Hemoglobin levels less than 12 g/dl in men or less than 10 g/dl in women

• Hematocrit levels less than 47 mg/dl in men and less than 42 mg/dl in women

• Serum iron levels low, with high binding capacity

• Serum ferritin levels low

• Red blood cell count low, with microcytic and hypochromic cells

• GI studies rule out or confirm the bleeding.

Irritable bowel syndrome

• History reveals diarrhea alternating with constipation.

• Bowel upset related to diet or psychological stress

• Sigmoidoscopy may reveal spastic contraction.

• Barium enema may reveal colonic spasm and tubular appearance of descending colon.

- Colonoscopy, rectal examination, or rectal biopsy may rule out other disorders.
- Fecal tests for occult blood, parasites, and pathogenic bacteria are negative.

Junctional tachycardia

Electrocardiography findings include the following:
- Atrial and ventricular rhythms are usually regular. The atrial rhythm may be difficult to determine if the P wave is absent or hidden in the QRS complex or preceding T wave.
- Atrial and ventricular rates exceed 100 beats/minute (usually between 100 and 200 beats/minute). The atrial rate may be difficult to determine if the P wave is absent or hidden in the QRS complex, or precedes the T wave.
- P wave is usually inverted. It may occur before or after the QRS complex, be hidden in the QRS complex, or be absent.
- If the P wave precedes the QRS complex, the PR interval is shortened (less than 0.12 second). Otherwise, the PR interval can't be measured.
- Duration of QRS complex is within normal limits. The configuration is usually normal.
- T-wave configuration is usually normal, but may be abnormal if the P wave is hidden in the T wave. Fast rate may make the T wave indiscernible.
- QT interval is usually within normal limits.

Juvenile angiofibroma

- Nasopharyngeal mirror or nasal speculum reveals a blue mass in the nose or nasopharynx.
- Nasal X-rays reveal a bowing of the posterior wall of the maxillary sinus.
- Angiography reveals the size and location of the tumor and also shows the source of vascularization.

Keratitis

- Slit-lamp examination reveals one or more small branchlike (dendritic) lesions (caused by herpes simplex virus).
- Touching the cornea with cotton reveals reduced corneal sensation.
- History reveals a recent infection of the upper respiratory tract accompanied by cold sores.

Kidney cancer

- Renal ultrasonography and computed tomography scan identify renal tumor.
- Excretory urography, nephrotomography, and kidney-ureter-bladder X-ray identify renal tumor.
- Liver function studies show increased alkaline phosphatase, bilirubin, and transaminase levels.
- Prolonged prothrombin time
- Blood studies show anemia, polycythemia, hypercalcemia, and increased erythrocyte sedimentation rate.
- Urinalysis reveals hematuria.
- Antegrade urography and cytologic studies reveal malignancy.
- Renal biopsy reveals malignant cells.
- Radionuclide renal imaging reveals malignant tumor.

Klinefelter syndrome

- Karyotype obtained by culturing lymphocytes from the patient's peripheral blood shows chromosome abnormality.
- Testosterone level is depressed after puberty.
- Decreased urine 17-ketosteroid levels
- Increased follicle-stimulating hormone levels

Kyphosis
• History reveals severe pain.
• Examination reveals curvature of the thoracic spine and bone destruction.
• X-rays reveal vertebral wedging, Schmorl's nodes, irregular plates, and possibly mild scoliosis of 10 to 20 degrees.

Labyrinthitis
• History reveals nausea and vomiting, hearing loss, and severe vertigo from any movement of the head.
• Examination reveals spontaneous nystagmus with jerking movements of the eyes toward the unaffected ear.
• Drainage culture reveals infective organism.
• Audiometry reveals sensorineural hearing loss.
• Computed tomography scan rules out brain lesion.

Laryngeal cancer
• History reveals hoarseness that lasts longer than 2 weeks.
• Laryngoscopy reveals lesion.
• Laryngeal tomography, computed tomography scan, or laryngography defines the borders of a lesion.
• Laryngeal biopsy reveals malignant cells.
• Chest X-ray identifies metastasis.

Laryngitis
• History reveals hoarseness, ranging from mild to complete loss of voice.
• Indirect laryngoscopy reveals red, inflamed and, occasionally, hemorrhagic vocal cords, with rounded rather than sharp edges, and exudate; bilateral swelling may be present, which restricts movement but doesn't cause paralysis.

Lassa fever
• Throat washings, pleural fluid, or blood cultures reveal Lassa virus.
• History reveals recent travel to an endemic area.
• Antibody titer reveals Lassa immunoglobulins.

Legg-Calvé-Perthes disease
• Examination reveals restricted abduction and rotation of the hip.
• Hip X-rays (taken every 3 to 4 months) reveal flattening of the femoral head or deformity, new bone formation, and eventually regeneration of the joint.
• Bone scan reveals involvement of anterolateral portion of the femoral head.
• Aspiration and culture of synovial fluid rule out joint sepsis.

Legionnaires' disease
• Respiratory tract secretions and tissue culture reveal *Legionella pneumophila*.
• Direct immunofluorescence testing reveals *L. pneumophila*.
• Indirect fluorescent serum antibody testing shows convalescent serum with a fourfold or greater rise in antibody titer for *L. pneumophila*.
• Chest X-ray reveals patchy, localized infiltration, which progresses to multilobar consolidation, pleural effusions, and, in fulminant disease, opacification of the entire lung.
• Blood studies show leukocytosis, increased erythrocyte sedimentation rate, and increases in alkaline phosphatase, alanine aminotransferase, and aspartate aminotransferase levels.
• Arterial blood gas measurements show decreased PaO_2 and, initially, decreased $PaCO_2$.
• Bronchial washings, blood and pleural fluid cultures, and transtracheal aspirate studies rule out pulmonary infections.

Leishmaniasis
• Scrapings from edges of lesion reveal species of *Leishmania*.
• Positive *Leishmania* skin test

Leprosy
• Examination reveals skin lesions and muscular and neurologic deficits.
• Biopsy of skin lesions, peripheral nerves, or smear of skin or ulcerated mucous membranes allows identification of *Mycobacterium leprae*.

Lichen planus
• Examination reveals generalized eruptions of flat, glistening purple papules marked with white lines or spots appearing linearly or coalescing into plaques.
• Skin biopsy reveals lichen planus.

Listeriosis
• Cultures of blood, cerebrospinal fluid, cervical or vaginal lesion drainage, or lochia from a mother with an infected fetus reveal *Listeria monocytogenes*.
• Complete blood count reveals monocytosis.

Liver abscess
   Liver scan reveals filling defects at the area of the abscess longer than ¾" (1.9 cm).
• Hepatic ultrasonography reveals defects caused by abscess.
• Computed tomography scan reveals low-density, homogenous area with well-defined borders.
• Chest X-ray reveals the diaphragm on the affected side to be raised and fixed.
• Blood tests show elevated levels of aspartate aminotransferase, alanine aminotransferase, alkaline phosphatase, and bilirubin.
• Decreased serum albumin
• Elevated white blood cell count
• Blood cultures and percutaneous liver aspiration identify causative organism.
• Stool cultures and serologic and hemagglutination tests isolate *Entamoeba histolytica* (in amoebic abscesses).

Liver cancer
• Needle biopsy or open biopsy reveals malignant cells.
• Alpha-fetoprotein levels rise above 500 mcg/ml
• Liver scan shows filling defects.
• Liver function tests are abnormal.
• Chest X-rays rule out metastasis to lungs.
• Arteriography may define large tumors.
• Serum electrolyte measurements show increased levels of sodium.
• Decreased serum glucose levels
• Decreased cholesterol levels

Lower urinary tract infection
• Microscopic urinalysis reveals red blood cell and white blood cell counts greater than 10/high-power field.
• Clean-catch urinalysis reveals bacterial count of more than 100,000/ml.
• Voiding cystoureterography or excretory urography shows congenital anomalies predisposing the patient to urinary tract infections.

Lung abscess
• Auscultation of the chest may reveal crackles and decreased breath sounds.
• Chest X-ray shows a localized infiltrate with one or more clear spaces, usually containing air-fluid levels.
• Percutaneous aspiration of an abscess or bronchoscopy may be used to obtain cultures to identify the causative organism.
• Blood and sputum cultures and Gram stain identify causative organism.
• White blood cell count above 10,000/µl

Lung cancer
• Chest X-ray reveals lesion or mass.
• Sputum cytology reveals malignant cells.
• Bronchoscopy reveals site of mass.
• Biopsy reveals malignant cells.

• Tissue biopsy reveals evidence of metastasis.

Lupus erythematosus
• Examination reveals classic butterfly rash occurring over the nose and cheeks.
• Positive antinuclear antibody, anti–deoxyribonucleic acid, and lupus erythematosus cell tests.
• Urine studies may show red blood cells and white blood cells, urine casts and sediment, and protein loss greater than 3.5 g/24 hours.
• Chest X-ray reveals pleurisy or lupus pneumonitis.
• Blood studies may show decreased serum complement (C3 and C4) levels indicating active disease; erythrocyte sedimentation rate is usually elevated; leukopenia, mild thrombocytopenia, and anemia also may be evident.
• Electrocardiography may show a conduction defect (with cardiac involvement or pericarditis).
• Renal biopsy identifies progression of and extent of renal involvement.

Lyme disease
• History reveals travel to endemic areas or exposure to ticks.
• Examination reveals the classic skin lesion called erythema chronicum migrans, beginning as a red macule or papule at the tick bite site growing in size to as large as 2″ (5 cm), described as hot and pruritic, with bright red outer rims and white centers.
• Mild anemia and elevated erythrocyte sedimentation rate, leukocyte count, serum immunoglobulin M level, and aspartate aminotransferase level support the diagnosis.
• Antibody titers, enzyme-linked immunosorbent assay, or blood culture may reveal *Borrelia burgdorferi*; lumbar puncture with cerebrospinal fluid allows for identification of antibodies

to *B. burgdorferi* (if Lyme disease involves the central nervous system).

Lymphocytopenia
• Lymphocyte count less than 1500/µl in adults (less than 3000/µl in children)
• Bone marrow aspiration and lymph node biopsies identify the cause.

Magnesium imbalance
• Hypomagnesemia:
— serum magnesium levels less than 1.5 mEq/liter
— decreased serum potassium and calcium levels
— Electrocardiogram showing tachyarrhythmias, slightly prolonged PR interval, prolonged QT interval, slightly prolonged QRS complex, ST-segment depression, prominent U waves, and broad flattened T waves.
• Hypermagnesemia:
— serum magnesium levels greater than 2.5 mEq/liter
— elevated serum potassium and calcium levels
— Electrocardiogram showing prolonged PR interval, prolonged QRS complex, and elevated T wave.

Malaria
• History reveals travel to an endemic area, recent blood transfusion, or I.V. drug use.
• Blood smears reveal parasites in red blood cells.
• Indirect immunofluorescent serum antibody tests reveal malaria (2 weeks after onset).
• Complete blood count shows decreased hemoglobin level and a normal or decreased white blood cell count as low as 3,000/µl.
• Urinalysis reveals protein and white blood cells in urine sediment.
• Serum blood studies show a reduced platelet count of 20,000 to 50,000/mm³, prolonged prothrombin time of 18 to 20 seconds, prolonged partial thrombo-

plastin time of 60 to 100 seconds, and decreased plasma fibrinogen levels (in falciparum malaria).

Malignant brain tumor
• Skull X-ray, brain scan, computed tomography scan, or magnetic resonance imaging reveals lesion.
• Biopsy of lesion reveals malignant cells.
• Lumbar puncture shows the following:
— increased protein levels and decreased glucose levels in cerebrospinal fluid
— increased cerebrospinal fluid pressure indicating increased intracranial pressure
— occasionally, tumor cells in cerebrospinal fluid.

Malignant lymphomas
• Examination reveals enlarged lymph nodes.
• Biopsy of lymph nodes, tonsils, bone marrow, liver, bowel, or skin reveals malignant cells.
• Chest X-ray; lymphangiography; liver, bone, and spleen scans; computed tomography scan of the abdomen; and excretory urography show disease progression.
• Serum uric acid level may be normal or elevated.
• Serum calcium level may be elevated, indicating bone lesions.

Malignant melanoma
• Examination reveals skin lesion or nevus with recent changes in appearance.
• Excisional biopsy and full-depth punch biopsy reveal malignant cells.
• Urine test reveals melanin.

Mallory-Weiss syndrome
• History reveals recent bout of forceful vomiting followed by vomiting

blood or passing blood rectally (after a few hours to several days).
• Endoscopy identifies esophageal tear.
• Angiography reveals bleeding site.
• Decreased serum hematocrit level (Measurements help to quantify blood loss.)

Marfan syndrome
• History reveals disease in close relatives.
• Examination reveals skeletal deformities and ectopia lentis.
• X-rays reveal skeletal abnormalities.
• Echocardiography detects aortic root dilation.

Mastitis and breast engorgement
• History reveals breast discomfort or other symptoms of inflammation (lactating woman).
• Examination reveals redness, swelling, warmth, hardness, tenderness, cracks or fissures of the nipple, and enlarged lymph nodes.
• Cultures of expressed milk reveal infective organism (generalized mastitis).
• Cultures of breast skin reveal infective organism (localized mastitis).

Mastoiditis
• X-rays of the mastoid area reveal hazy mastoid air cells, and the bony walls between the cells appear decalcified.
• Otoscopy reveals a dull, thickened, and edematous tympanic membrane, if the membrane isn't concealed by obstruction.
• Culture and sensitivity tests reveal causative organism.
• Audiometry shows a conductive hearing loss.

Medullary cystic disease
• Family history reveals relatives with medullary cystic disease.
• Arteriography and excretory urography demonstrate small kidneys.

• Kidney biopsy shows structural abnormalities.
• Blood studies show profound anemia.
• Elevated serum alkaline phosphatase level (in young patients)

Medullary sponge kidney

• Excretory urography reveals a characteristic flowerlike appearance of the pyramidal cavities when they fill with contrast material.
• Urinalysis is normal, but may show increased white blood cell count and casts (with infection) or an increased red blood cell count (with hematuria).

Melasma

• Inspection shows large, brown, irregular patches symmetrically distributed on forehead, cheeks, and sides of nose.

Ménière's disease

• History reveals vertigo, tinnitus, and hearing loss or distortion.
• Audiometric studies indicate a sensorineural hearing loss and loss of discrimination and recruitment.
• Magnetic resonance imaging rules out brain lesions or tumors.
• Auditory brain stem response test rules out cochlear or retrocochlear lesion as the cause of hearing loss.

Meningitis

• Lumbar puncture reveals cloudy cerebrospinal fluid (CSF), elevated CSF pressure, high protein level, and depressed glucose concentration.
• CSF culture and sensitivity tests reveal gram-positive or gram-negative organisms.
• Chest X-rays show pneumonitis or lung abscess, tubercular lesions, or granulomas (secondary to fungal infection).
• Sinus and skull X-rays may help identify cranial osteomyelitis, paranasal sinusitis, or skull fracture.

• White blood cell count shows leukocytosis.
• Computed tomography scan rules out cerebral hematoma, hemorrhage, or tumor.
• Positive Brudzinski's sign and Kernig's sign

Meningococcal infection

• Blood, cerebrospinal fluid, or lesion culture reveals *Neisseria meningitidis.*
• Decreased platelet and clotting levels (with skin or adrenal hemorrhages)

Menopause

• History reveals menstrual cycle irregularities.
• Papanicolaou test results show changes indicating the influence of estrogen deficiency on vaginal mucosa.
• Radioimmunoassay blood studies show estrogen level of 0 to 14 ng/dl, plasma estradiol level of 15 to 40 pg/ml, and estrone level of 25 to 50 pg/ml.
• Radioimmunoassay urine studies show estrogen level of 6 to 18 mcg/24 hours, and pregnanediol level of 0.3 to 0.9 mg/24 hours.
• Pelvic examination, endometrial biopsy, and dilatation and curettage rule out suspected organic disease.
• Serum follicle-stimulating hormone level is 50 to 100 mIU/ml.
• Plasma luteinizing hormone level is greater than 50 mIU/ml.

Mental retardation

• Standardized IQ testing reveals:
— IQ of 51 to 69, mild retardation
— IQ of 36 to 50, moderate retardation
— IQ of 20 to 35, severe retardation
— IQ of less than 20, profound retardation (ranges may vary slightly depending on test used).
• Developmental screening tests reveal functional level in comparison to normal level for that chronological age.
• Adaptive Behavior Scale reveals self-help skills, physical and social develop-

ment, language, socialization, and time and number concepts.

Metabolic acidosis
• Arterial blood gas levels:
— pH below 7.35 (in severe acidosis, pH may fall to 7.10)
— $PaCO_2$ may be normal or less than 34 mm Hg
— HCO_3^- level may be less than 22 mEq/liter.
• Anion gap greater than 14 mEq/liter
• Urine pH is 4.5 (in the absence of renal disease).
• Serum potassium levels are usually elevated.
• Blood glucose levels and serum ketone body levels increase (in diabetes mellitus).
• Plasma lactic acid levels are elevated (in lactic acidosis).

Metabolic alkalosis
• Arterial blood gas levels:
— pH greater than 7.45
— HCO_3^- level greater than 29 mEq/liter
— $PaCO_2$ may be greater than 45 mm Hg (indicating respiratory compensation).
• Serum electrolyte levels usually show decreased potassium, calcium, and chloride levels.
• Electrocardiography shows a low T wave merging with a P wave and atrial or sinus tachycardia.

Mitral insufficiency
• Cardiac catheterization may indicate signs of mitral insufficiency, including increased left ventricular end-diastolic volume and pressure, increased atrial and pulmonary artery wedge pressures, and decreased cardiac output.
• Chest X-rays may demonstrate left atrial and ventricular enlargement, pulmonary venous congestion, and calcification of the mitral leaflets.

• Echocardiography may reveal abnormal motion of the valve leaflets, left atrial enlargement, and a hyperdynamic left ventricle.
• Electrocardiography may show left atrial and ventricular hypertrophy, sinus tachycardia, or atrial fibrillation.

Mitral stenosis
• Cardiac catheterization shows a diastolic pressure gradient across the mitral valve and elevated left atrial and pulmonary artery pressures. It also shows an elevated pulmonary artery wedge pressure that exceeds 15 mm Hg. Catheterization may also reveal elevated right ventricular pressure, decreased cardiac output, and abnormal contraction of the left ventricle. Note that this test may not be indicated in patients who have isolated mitral stenosis with mild symptoms.
• Chest X-ray shows left atrial and left ventricle enlargement (in severe mitral stenosis), straightening of the left border of the cardiac silhouette, enlarged pulmonary arteries, dilation of the pulmonary veins of the upper lobes of the lungs, and mitral valve calcification.
• Echocardiography may disclose thickened mitral valve leaflets and left atrial enlargement.
• Electrocardiography can reveal atrial fibrillation, right ventricular hypertrophy, left atrial enlargement (in sinus rhythm), and right axis deviation.

Motion sickness
• History reveals nausea, vomiting, dizziness, headache, fatigue, diaphoresis, or difficulty breathing related to a sensation of motion.

Multiple endocrine neoplasia

• Family history reveals inheritance pattern.
• Evaluation of signs and symptoms suggests multiple endocrine neoplasia.
• Diagnostic tests reveal hyperplasia, adenoma, or carcinoma in two or more endocrine glands.

Multiple myeloma

• Complete blood count shows moderate to severe anemia; differential may show 40% to 50% lymphocytes but seldom more than 3% plasma cells.
• Rouleaux formation is seen on differential smear results.
• Analysis of urine proteins reveals Bence Jones protein, proteinuria, and hypercalciuria.
• Serum calcium levels are greater than 10.1 mg/dl.
• Serum electrophoresis shows an elevated globulin spike, which is electrophoretically and immunologically abnormal.
• Excretion tests show phenolsulfonphthalein level greater than 25% in 15 minutes, greater than 80% in 2 hours.
• Bone marrow aspiration detects myelomatous cells.
• Kidney-ureter-bladder radiography reveals bilateral renal enlargement.
• X-rays reveal multiple, sharply circumscribed osteolytic lesions, especially on the skull, pelvis, and spine.

Multiple sclerosis

• History reveals multiple neurologic attacks with characteristic remissions and exacerbations.
• EEG results are abnormal.
• Cerebrospinal fluid analysis reveals elevated gamma globulin fraction of immunoglobulin G (with normal serum gamma globulin levels).
• Magnetic resonance imaging reveals multifocal white matter lesions resulting from demyelination.

• Evoked potential studies show slowed conduction of nerve impulses (in 80% of patients).
• Computed tomography scan may show lesions within the brain's white matter.

Mumps

• History reveals inadequate immunization and exposure to person infected with mumps.
• Examination reveals swelling and tenderness of the parotid glands and one or more of the other salivary glands.
• Antibody titer increases fourfold 3 weeks after acute phase of illness.
• Serum amylase level may be elevated.

Muscular dystrophy

• History reveals progressive muscle weakness and evidence of genetic transmission.
• Muscle biopsy reveals fat and connective tissue deposits, degeneration and necrosis of muscle fibers, and in Duchenne's and Becker's dystrophies, a deficiency of muscle protein dystrophin.
• Electromyography shows short, weak bursts of electrical activity in affected muscles.
• Genetic testing identifies the gene defect (in some patients).
• Elevated urine creatinine, serum creatine kinase, lactate dehydrogenase, asparate aminotransferase, and alanine aminotransferase levels

Myasthenia gravis

• History reveals progressive muscle weakness and muscle fatigability that improves with rest.
• Tensilon test is positive, showing improved muscle function after an I.V. injection of edrophonium or neostigmine.
• Serum acetylcholine receptor antibodies test is positive in symptomatic adults.

• Electromyography reveals motor unit potentials that are initially normal but progressively diminish in amplitude with continuing contractions.
• Chest X-ray or computed tomography scan may show a thymoma.

Mycosis fungoides

• History reveals multiple, varied, and progressively severe skin lesions.
• Biopsy of lesions reveals lymphoma cells.
• Fingerstick smear reveals Sézary cells (abnormal circulating lymphocytes), found in the erythrodermic variants of mycosis fungoides (Sézary syndrome).

Myelitis and acute transverse myelitis

• White blood cell count may be normal or slightly elevated.
• Cerebrospinal fluid analysis may show normal or increased lymphocyte and protein levels and allow for isolation of the causative agent.
• Throat washings may reveal the causative virus (in poliomyelitis).
• Computed tomography scan or magnetic resonance imaging rules out spinal tumor.

Myocardial infarction

• History reveals substernal chest pain, with radiation.
• Serial 12-lead electrocardiogram may be normal or inconclusive during the first hours after a myocardial infarction (MI); may reveal serial ST-segment depression (in subendocardial MI) and ST-segment elevation and Q waves (in transmural MI).
• Cardiac enzyme tests reveal creatine kinase (CK) greater than 130 U/L in men or 150 U/L in women, with CK-MB isoenzyme greater than 5% of total CK (or more than 10 U/L) over a 72-hour period.
• Echocardiography shows ventricular wall dyskinesia (with a transmural MI).

• Radioisotope scans using I.V. technetium 99m pertechnetate show "hot spots" indicating damaged muscle.
• Myocardial perfusion imaging with thallium-210 reveals a "cold spot" (in most patients during the first few hours after a transmural MI).

Myocarditis

• History reveals recent febrile upper respiratory tract infection, viral pharyngitis, or tonsillitis.
• Cardiac examination reveals supraventricular and ventricular arrhythmias, S_3 and S_4 gallops, a faint S_1, possibly a murmur of mitral insufficiency, and a pericardial friction rub (in patients with pericarditis).
• Endomyocardial biopsy reveals histologic changes consistent with myocarditis.
• Elevated cardiac enzyme levels, including creatine kinase (CK), CK-MB, serum aspartate aminotransferase, and lactate dehydrogenase
• Elevated white blood cell count and erythrocyte sedimentation rate
• Antibody titers, such as antistreptolysin-O, are elevated.
• Electrocardiography shows diffuse ST-segment and T-wave abnormalities, conduction defects, and other ventricular and supraventricular arrhythmias.
• Cultures of stools, throat, pharyngeal washings, or other body fluids identify the causative bacteria or virus.

Nasal papillomas

• Examination reveals inverted papillomas as large, bulky, highly vascular, and edematous; color varies from dark red to gray; consistency, from firm to friable.
• Examination may also reveal exophytic papillomas that are raised, firm, and rubbery; color varies from pink to gray; papillomas are securely attached by a broad or pedunculated base to the mucous membrane.

• Biopsy reveals histologic findings characteristic of papillomas.

Nasal polyps

• X-rays of sinuses and nasal passages reveal soft tissue shadows over the affected areas.
• Examination with a nasal speculum reveals nasal obstruction and a dry, red surface with clear or gray growths; large growths may resemble tumors.

Near-drowning

• Recent water submersion
• Auscultation of the lungs reveals rhonchi and crackles.
• Arterial blood gas analysis reveals:
— pH less than 7.35
— PaO$_2$ less than 75 mm Hg
— HCO$_3^-$ level less than 22 mEq/liter.
• Electrocardiography may show supraventricular tachycardia, premature ventricular contractions, and nonspecific ST-segment and T-wave abnormalities.

Necrotizing enterocolitis

• Anteroposterior and lateral abdominal X-rays reveal nonspecific intestinal dilation and, in later stages, gas or air in the intestinal wall.
• Platelet count may fall below 50,000/mm^3.
• Serum sodium levels below 135 mEq/L
• Serum bilirubin levels (indirect, direct, and total) may be elevated.
• Blood and stool cultures positive for *Escherichia coli, Clostridia, Salmonella, Pseudomonas,* or *Klebsiella.*
• Hemoglobin level less than 10 g/dl
• Prothrombin time is prolonged (greater than 15 seconds).
• Partial thromboplastin time is prolonged (greater than 60 seconds).
• Fibrin degradation products are increased (greater than 100 mcg/ml).
• Guaiac test detects occult blood in stool.

Nephrotic syndrome

• Consistent proteinuria in excess of 3.5 g/24 hours
• Urinalysis reveals increased number of hyaline, granular, and waxy, fatty casts and oval fat bodies.
• Renal biopsy provides histologic identification of the lesion.
• Triiodothyronine resin uptake percentage is high with a low or normal free thyroxine level.
• Serum protein electrophoresis reveals decreased albumin and gamma globulin levels and markedly increased alpha$_2$ and beta globulin levels.
• Serum triglyceride, phospholipid, and cholesterol levels are elevated.

Neurofibromatosis

• Examination reveals café-au-lait spots and multiple pedunculated nodules (neurofibromas) of varying sizes on the nerve trunks of the extremities and on the nerves of the head, neck, and body.
• X-rays and computed tomography scanning reveal widening internal auditory meatus and intervertebral foramen.
• Myelography reveals spinal cord tumors.
• Lumbar puncture with cerebrospinal fluid analysis reveals elevated protein concentration.

Neurogenic arthropathy

• History of painless joint deformity
• X-rays reveal soft-tissue swelling or effusion (early stage), articular fracture, subluxation, erosion of articular cartilage, periosteal new bone formation, and excessive growth of marginal new bodies or resorption.
• Vertebral examination reveals narrowing of vertebral disk spaces, deterioration of vertebrae, and osteophyte formation.
• Synovial biopsy reveals bony fragments and bits of calcified cartilage.

Neurogenic bladder

• History reveals neurologic disease or spinal cord injury.

• Spinal fluid analysis shows increased protein level indicating cord tumor; increased gamma globulin may indicate multiple sclerosis.

• X-rays of the skull and vertebral column show fracture, dislocation, congenital anomalies, or metastasis.

• Myelography shows spinal cord compression.

• Electromyelography confirms presence of peripheral neuropathy.

• Cystometry reveals abnormal micturition and vesical function.

• External sphincter electromyography reveals detrusor-external sphincter dyssynergia.

• Voiding cystourethrography reveals neurogenic bladder.

• Whitaker test reveals bladder abnormality.

Nezelof syndrome

• History of failure to thrive, poor eating habits, weight loss, and recurrent infections in children.

• T-lymphocyte assay reveals defective T cells that are moderately to markedly decreased in number.

• Familial history may reveal genetic transmission.

Nocardiosis

• Sputum or discharge culture reveals *Nocardia*.

• Biopsy of lung or other tissue reveals Nocardia.

• Chest X-ray shows fluffy or interstitial infiltrates, nodules, or abscesses.

• History reveals progressive pneumonia despite antibiotic therapy.

Nonspecific genitourinary infections

• Cultures of prostatic, cervical, or urethral secretions reveal excess polymorphonuclear leukocytes but few, if any, specific organisms.

• History of sexual contact with partner with a nonspecific genitourinary infection

Nonviral hepatitis

• History reveals exposure to hepatotoxic chemicals or drugs.

• Serum alanine aminotransferase levels greater than 32 U/L

• Serum aspartate aminotransferase levels greater than 20 U/L

• Elevated serum total and direct bilirubin levels (with cholestasis)

• Elevated serum alkaline phosphatase levels

• Differential white blood cell count reveals elevated eosinophils.

Nystagmus

• Involuntary eye movement

• Positional testing causes nystagmus to occur.

• Electronystagmography reveals nystagmus.

Obesity

• Observation and comparison of height and weight to a standardized table reveals weight exceeding ideal body weight by 20% or more. In morbid obesity, body weight greater than 200% of standard range.

• Measurement of the thickness of subcutaneous fat folds with calipers reveals excess body fat.

Optic atrophy

• Slit-lamp examination reveals a pupil that reacts sluggishly to direct light stimulation.

• Ophthalmoscopy shows pallor of the nerve head from loss of microvascular circulation in the disk and deposit of fibrous or glial tissue.

• Visual field testing reveals a scotoma and, possibly, major visual field impairment.

Orbital cellulitis
• Examination reveals eyelid edema and purulent discharge.
• Culture of eye discharge reveals *Streptococcus, Staphylococcus,* or *Pneumococcus* as the causative organism.

Ornithosis
• History reveals recent exposure to birds.
• Recovery of *Chlamydia psittaci* from mice, eggs, or tissue culture inoculated with the patient's blood or sputum.
• Comparison of acute and convalescent serum shows a fourfold rise in antibody titers during convalescent phase.
• Chest X-ray reveals patchy lobar infiltrate.

Osgood-Schlatter disease
• Examination reveals pain during internal rotation of the tibia while extending the knee from 90 degrees flexion, which subsides immediately with external rotation of the tibia.
• X-rays may reveal epiphyseal separation and soft tissue swelling (up to 6 months after onset) and eventual bone fragmentation.

Osteoarthritis
• History reveals deep, aching joint pain, particularly after exercise or weight bearing, usually relieved by rest.
• Examination reveals nodes in the distal and proximal joints that become red, swollen, and tender.
• X-rays reveal narrowing of the joint space or margin, cystlike bony deposits in joint space and margins, sclerosis of the subchondral space, joint deformity due to degeneration or articular damage, bony growths at weight-bearing areas, and fusion of joints.

Osteogenesis imperfecta
• Examination reveals blue sclera and deafness.

• X-rays reveal multiple old fractures and skeletal deformities.
• Skull X-ray shows wide sutures with small, irregularly shaped islands of bone (wormian bones).

Osteomyelitis
• History reveals sudden pain in the affected bone accompanied by tenderness, heat, swelling, and restricted movement.
• Blood cultures reveal *Staphylococcus aureus, Streptococcus pyogenes, Pneumococcus, Pseudomonas aeruginosa, Escherichia coli,* or *Proteus vulgaris* as the causative organism.
• Bone scan shows infection site in early stages of illness.
• X-ray reveals abnormal areas of calcification (may not be evident until 2 to 3 weeks).
• Elevated erythrocyte sedimentation rate (greater than 20 mm/hour)
• White blood cell count reveals leukocytosis.

Osteoporosis
• X-rays reveal typical degeneration in the lower thoracic and lumbar vertebrae; vertebral bodies may appear flattened and more dense than normal.
• Photon absorptiometry reveals deterioration of bone mass.
• Bone biopsy reveals thin, porous, but otherwise normal-looking bone.

Otitis externa
• Examination reveals pain on palpation of the tragus or auricle.
• Otoscopy reveals a swollen external ear canal (sometimes to the point of complete closure), periauricular lymphadenopathy (tender nodes in front of the tragus, behind the ear, or in the upper neck), and, occasionally, regional cellulitis.
• In fungal otitis externa, examination reveals thick, red epithelium after removal of growth.
• Microscopic examination or culture and sensitivity tests identify *Aspergillus*

niger or *Candida albicans* as the causative organism for fungal otitis externa; *Pseudomonas, Proteus vulgaris, Streptococcus,* or *Staphylococcus aureus* as the causative organism for bacterial otitis externa.
• In chronic otitis externa, examination of the ear canal reveals a thick red epithelium.

Otitis media
• In acute suppurative otitis media:
— Otoscopy reveals obscured or distorted bony landmarks of the tympanic membrane.
— Pneumatoscopy may show decreased tympanic membrane mobility.
— Examination shows that pulling on the auricle does not exacerbate the pain.
• In acute secretory otitis media:
— Otoscopy demonstrates tympanic membrane retraction, causing the bony landmarks to appear more prominent, with clear or amber fluid detected behind the tympanic membrane, possibly with a meniscus and bubbles.
— If hemorrhage into the middle ear has occurred, the tympanic membrane appears blue-black.
• In chronic otitis media:
— History discloses recurrent or unresolved otitis media; otoscopy shows thickening and sometimes scarring, and decreased mobility of the tympanic membrane.
— Pneumatoscopy reveals decreased or absent tympanic membrane movement.
• History of recent air travel or scuba diving suggests barotitis media.

Otosclerosis
• Rinne test reveals bone conduction lasting longer than air conduction (normally, the reverse is true); as otosclerosis progresses, bone conduction deteriorates.
• Audiometric testing reveals hearing loss ranging from 60 dB, in early stages, to total loss, as the disease advances.
• Weber's test reveals sound lateralizing to the more affected ear.

Ovarian cancer
• Examination reveals abdominal mass.
• Computed tomography scan shows the abdominal tumor.
• Pelvic ultrasonography reveals mass.
• Exploratory laparotomy with biopsy reveals malignant cells.
• Transvaginal ultrasound shows ovarian enlargement and growth.
• Transvaginal Doppler color flow imaging reveals ovarian growth.
• Carcinoembryonic antigen levels greater than 5 ng/ml
• Serum human chorionic gonadotropin levels greater than 3 mIU/ml in nonpregnant women.
• Barium enema reveals obstruction and size of tumor.

Ovarian cysts
• Pelvic ultrasonography reveals ovarian mass.
• Laparoscopy reveals a bubble on the surface of the ovary, which may be clear, serous, or mucous-filled.
• Highly elevated human chorionic gonadotropin titers (with theca-lutein cysts)
• Elevated progesterone levels

Paget's disease
• X-rays reveal increased bone expansion and density (before overt symptoms appear).
• Bone scan reveals radioisotope concentrates in areas of active lesions (early pagetic lesions).
• Bone biopsy reveals characteristic mosaic pattern.
• Markedly elevated serum alkaline phosphatase level
• Increased urine hydroxyproline levels (greater than 45 mg/24 hours)

Pancreatic cancer

- Ultrasound, computed tomography scan, or magnetic resonance imaging reveals mass size and locations.
- Laparotomy and biopsy reveal malignant cells.
- Barium swallow shows neoplasm or changes in the duodenum or stomach indicating carcinoma of the head of the pancreas.
- Endoscopic retrograde cholangiopancreatography shows mass and abnormalities of the pancreatic ducts.
- Cholangiography shows obstructed bile ducts caused by carcinoma of the pancreas.
- Secretin test reveals an abnormal volume of secretions, HCO_3^-, or enzymes.
- Markedly elevated serum alkaline phosphatase and serum bilirubin levels (with biliary obstruction)
- Plasma insulin immunoassay reveals measurable serum insulin (with islet cell tumors).
- Stool guaiac shows occult blood suggesting ulceration in GI tract or ampulla of Vater.

Parainfluenza

- History reveals symptoms of respiratory illness.
- Serum antibody titers differentiate parainfluenza from other respiratory illnesses.
- Blood culture reveals virus (rarely done).

Parkinson's disease

- History and examination reveal muscle rigidity, akinesia, and pill-roll tremors increasing during stress or anxiety.
- Urinalysis reveals decreased dopamine levels.
- Evoked potential studies reveal bilateral abnormal P100 latencies.

Pediculosis

- In pediculosis capitis, examination reveals oval, grayish nits that can't be shaken loose.
- In pediculosis corporis, examination reveals characteristic skin lesions and nits found on clothing.
- In pediculosis pubis, examination reveals nits attached to pubic hairs, which feel coarse and grainy to the touch.

Pelvic inflammatory disease

- History reveals recent sexual intercourse, intrauterine device insertion, childbirth, or abortion.
- Cultures and Gram stain of secretions from the endocervix or cul-de-sac reveal *Neisseria gonorrhoeae* or *Chlamydia trachomatis* as the infective organism.
- Ultrasonography reveals an adnexal or uterine mass.
- Laparoscopy reveals infection or abscess.

Penetrating chest wounds

- Examination reveals chest wound and a sucking sound during breathing.
- Hemoglobin and hematocrit levels are markedly decreased, indicating severe blood loss.
- Chest X-ray reveals pneumothorax and possible lung laceration.

Penile cancer

- Tissue biopsy reveals malignant cells.
- Examination reveals small circumscribed lesion, pimple, or sore on the penis, which may be accompanied by pain, hemorrhage, dysuria, purulent discharge, and urinary meatal obstruction (in late stages).

Peptic ulcers

- History reveals heartburn, midepigastric pain, or gastric bleeding.
- Endoscopy reveals ulcer.
- Upper GI X-rays show abnormalities in the mucosa.

- Gastric secretory studies show hyperchlorhydria.
- Biopsy rules out malignancy.
- Guaiac stools may be positive for occult blood.

Perforated eardrum

- History reveals trauma to the ear accompanied by severe earache and bleeding from the ear.
- Direct visual inspection of the tympanic membrane with an otoscope confirms perforation; flaccid, thin areas indicate previous perforation.
- Audiometric testing reveals hearing loss.

Pericarditis

- Chest auscultation reveals pericardial friction rub.
- Pericardial fluid culture reveals infecting organism (in bacterial or fungal pericarditis).
- Electrocardiography (ECG) reveals elevation of ST segment in the standard limb leads and most precordial leads without the significant changes in QRS morphology that occur with myocardial infarction.
- ECG may also reveal atrial ectopic rhythms and diminished QRS voltage (with pericardial effusion).
- Echocardiography reveals an echo-free space between the ventricular wall and the pericardium (with pericardial effusion).

Peritonitis

- Examination reveals severe abdominal pain with direct or rebound tenderness.
- Abdominal X-rays reveal edematous and gaseous distention of the small and large bowel, or air in the abdominal cavity (with perforation of a visceral organ).
- Paracentesis reveals bacteria in fluid, exudate, pus, blood, or urine.

- Chest X-ray may show elevation of the diaphragm.
- White blood cell count indicates leukocytosis (greater than 20,000/µl).

Pernicious anemia

- Hemoglobin level is decreased (4 to 5 g/dl).
- Red blood cell levels are decreased.
- Mean corpuscular volume is increased (greater than 120 mm^3).
- Serum vitamin B_{12} assay reveals levels less than 0.1 mcg/ml.
- Schilling test reveals less than 3% excretion of radioactive B_{12} in urine in 24 hours.
- Bone marrow aspiration reveals erythroid hyperplasia with increased numbers of megaloblasts but few normally developing red blood cells.
- Gastric analysis reveals absence of free hydrochloric acid after histamine or pentagastrin injection.

Pharyngitis

- Examination reveals generalized redness and inflammation of the posterior wall of the pharynx, and red, edematous mucous membranes studded with white or yellow follicles.
- Exudate is usually confined to the lymphoid areas of the throat, sparing the tonsillar pillars.
- Throat culture reveals infective organism, most often *Streptococcus*.

Phenylketonuria

- Family history reveals presence of autosomal recessive gene.
- Guthrie screening test reveals elevated serum phenylalanine levels.
- Drops of 10% ferric chloride solution added to a wet diaper turns a deep, bluish-green color, indicating phenylpyruvic acid in the urine.
- Serum tyrosine level less than 0.6 mg/dl
- Urine testing reveals presence of phenylpyruvic acid.

Pheochromocytoma
• History of acute episodes of hypertension, headache, sweating, and tachycardia — particularly in a patient with hyperglycemia, glycosuria, and hypermetabolism
• 24-hour urine test reveals increased excretion of total free catecholamine and its metabolites, vanillylmandelic acid, and metanephrine.
• Total plasma catecholamines may show levels 10 to 50 times higher than normal.
• Angiography reveals an adrenal medullary tumor.
• Excretory urography with nephrotomography, adrenal venography, or computed tomography scan helps localize a tumor.

Phosphorus imbalance
• In hypophosphatemia, serum phosphorus level is less than 1.7 mEq/liter or 2.5 mg/dl; urine phosphorus level is greater than 1.3 g/24 hours.
• In hyperphosphatemia, serum phosphorus level is more than 2.6 mEq/liter or 4.5 mg/dl; serum calcium level is less than 9 mg/dl; urine phosphorus level is less than 0.9 g/24 hours.

Photosensitivity reactions
• History reveals recent exposure to light or certain chemicals.
• Examination reveals erythema, edema, desquamation, and hyperpigmentation (characteristic skin eruptions).
• Photopatch test for ultraviolet A and B may identify the causative light wavelength.

Pilonidal disease
• Examination reveals a series of openings along the midline (of the intergluteal fold) with thin, brown, foul-smelling drainage or a protruding tuft of hair; pressure on the sinus tract produces purulent drainage.

• Culture of discharge from the infected sinus reveals staphylococci or skin bacteria (not usually bowel bacteria).

Pituitary tumors
• Skull X-rays with tomography reveal enlargement of the sella turcica or erosion of its floor and enlargement of the paranasal sinuses and mandible, thickened cranial bones, and separated teeth (if growth hormone predominates).
• Carotid angiogram reveals displacement of the anterior cerebral and internal carotid arteries (with enlarging tumor mass).
• Intracranial computed tomography scan may confirm the existence of the adenoma and accurately depict its size.
• Orbital radiography shows superior orbital fissure enlargement.
• Magnetic resonance imaging of the brain differentiates healthy, benign, and malignant tissues and blood vessels.
• Tangent screen examination reveals bitemporal hemianopia.
• Urine free cortisol levels greater than 108 mcg/24 hours
• Human growth hormone levels greater than 5 ng/ml in men, greater than 10 ng/ml in women, or greater than 16 ng/ml in children
• Urine 17-OHCS levels greater than 12 mg/24 hours in adults or greater than 4.5 mg/24 hours in children

Pityriasis rosea
• Examination reveals slightly raised oval lesion, approximately 2 to 6 cm in diameter, changing to yellow-tan or erythematous patches with scaly edges approximately 0.5 to 1 cm in diameter on the trunk and extremities.

Placenta previa
• History reveals painless bleeding during third trimester.
• Pelvic ultrasound reveals abnormal echo patterns.

- Pelvic examination (performed only immediately before delivery) reveals only cervix and minimal descent of fetal presenting part.

Plague

- History reveals exposure to rodents (bubonic plague).
- Culture of skin lesion reveals *Y. pestis.*
- White blood cell count and differential reveals white blood cells greater than 20,000/µl with increased polymorphonuclear leukocytes.
- Chest X-ray reveals fulminating pneumonia (with pneumonic plague).

Platelet function disorders

- History reveals excessive bleeding or bruising.
- Bleeding time is prolonged.
- Prothrombin time and partial thromboplastin time is normal.
- Platelet count is normal.
- Platelet function tests measure platelet release reaction and aggregation to identify defective mechanism.

Pleural effusion and empyema

- Chest X-ray reveals radiopaque fluid in dependent regions.
- Lung auscultation reveals decreased breath sounds.
- Percussion detects dullness over the effused area, which doesn't change with respiration.
- Pleural fluid analysis reveals:
— transudative effusions with specific gravity less than 1.015 and protein less than 3 g/dl
— exudative effusions with ratio of protein in pleural fluid to serum greater than or equal to 0.5, pleural fluid lactate dehydrogenase (LD) levels greater than or equal to 200 IU, and ratio of LD in pleural fluid to LD in serum greater than or equal to 0.6
— empyema with acute inflammatory white blood cells and microorganisms

— empyema or rheumatoid arthritis with extremely decreased pleural fluid glucose levels.

Pleurisy

- Auscultation of the chest reveals characteristic pleural friction rub — a coarse, creaky sound heard during late inspiration and early expiration, directly over the area of pleural inflammation.
- Palpation may reveal coarse vibration.

Pneumocystis carinii pneumonia

- History reveals immunocompromised condition, such as human immunodeficiency virus infection, leukemia, lymphoma, or procedure such as organ transplantation.
- Histologic studies of sputum specimen confirms presence of *P. carinii.*
- Chest X-ray shows slowly progressing, fluffy infiltrates and occasional nodular lesions or a spontaneous pneumothorax.
- Gallium scan of the chest shows increased uptake over the lungs even if the chest X-ray appears relatively normal.

Pneumonia

- Percussion reveals dullness; auscultation discloses crackles, wheezing, or rhonchi over the affected lung area as well as decreased breath sounds and decreased vocal fremitus.
- Chest X-rays disclose infiltrates, confirming the diagnosis.
- Gram stain and culture of sputum show acute inflammatory cells.
- White blood cell count indicates leukocytosis in bacterial pneumonia and a normal or low count in viral or mycoplasmal pneumonia.
- Blood cultures reflect bacteremia and help determine the causative organism.

Pneumothorax

• History reveals sudden, sharp pain and shortness of breath.

• Chest X-ray reveals air in the pleural space and, possibly, mediastinal shift.

• Examination reveals overexpansion and rigidity of the affected chest side; in tension pneumothorax, examination may reveal neck vein distention.

• Palpation of chest reveals crackling beneath the skin and decreased vocal fremitus.

• Chest auscultation reveals decreased or absent breath sounds on the affected side.

• Arterial blood gas measurements reveal pH less than 7.35, a PaO_2 less than 80 mm Hg, and a $PaCO_2$ greater than 45 mm Hg.

Poisoning

• History reveals ingestion, inhalation, injection of, or skin contact with, a poisonous substance.

• Toxicologic studies (including drug screens) reveal poison in the mouth, vomitus, urine, feces, or blood or on the victim's hands or clothing.

• Chest X-ray (with inhalation poisoning) reveals pulmonary infiltrates or edema, or aspiration pneumonia (with petroleum distillate inhalation).

Poliomyelitis

• Throat washings or stool examination reveals poliovirus.

• Convalescent serum antibody titers rise fourfold from acute titers.

• Cerebrospinal fluid pressure and protein levels may be slightly increased.

• White blood cell count may be elevated initially, mostly due to polymorphonuclear leukocytes, which constitute 50% to 90% of the total count; thereafter, the number of cells is diminished with mononuclear leukocytes accounting for most of them.

Polycystic kidney disease

• Family history of polycystic kidney disease

• Physical examination reveals large bilateral, irregular masses in the flanks.

• Excretory or retrograde urography reveals enlarged kidneys, with elongation of pelvis, flattening of the calyces, and indentations caused by cysts.

• Excretory urography of the newborn shows poor excretion of contrast medium.

• Ultrasonography, computed tomography scan, and radioisotope scans of the kidney show kidney enlargement and presence of cysts. Computed tomography scan also demonstrates multiple areas of cystic damage.

Polycythemia, secondary

• Red blood cell mass is increased.

• Increased hemoglobin, hematocrit, mean corpuscular volume, and mean corpuscular hemoglobin levels

• Elevated urine erythropoietin and blood histamine levels

• Arterial oxygen saturation may be decreased.

• Bone marrow biopsies reveal hyperplasia confined to the erythroid series.

Polycythemia, spurious

• Elevated hemoglobin and hematocrit levels and red blood cell (RBC) count

• Normal RBC mass

• Normal white blood cell count

Polycythemia vera

• Laboratory studies confirm polycythemia vera by showing increased red blood cell mass and normal arterial oxygen saturation in association with splenomegaly or two of the following:

— platelet count above 400,000/mm³ (thrombocytosis)

— white blood cell count above 10,000/mm³ in adults (leukocytosis)

— elevated leukocyte alkaline phosphatase level

— elevated serum B_{12} elevation or unbound B_{12}-binding capacity.

• Bone marrow biopsy reveals panmyelosis.

• Increased serum and urine uric acid levels

Polymyositis and dermatomyositis

• Muscle biopsy reveals necrosis, degeneration, regeneration, and interstitial chronic lymphocytic infiltration.

• Muscle enzymes (creatine kinase, aldolase, aspartate aminotransferase) elevated and not attributable to hemolysis of red blood cells or hepatic or other diseases

• Urine creatine level greater than 150 mg/24 hours

• Electromyography reveals polyphasic short-duration potentials, fibrillation, and bizarre high-frequency repetitive changes.

• Antinuclear antibodies are positive.

• Rheumatoid factor titer 1:20 to 1:80

Porphyrias

• Screening tests reveal porphyrins or their precursors (such as aminolevulinic acid and porphobilinogen) in urine, stool, blood, or skin biopsy.

• Urinary lead level of 0.2 mg/liter (toxic-acquired porphyria)

Potassium imbalance

• Hypokalemia shows serum potassium levels less than 3.5 mEq/liter.

• Hypokalemia electrocardiogram shows flattened T waves, elevated U waves, and depressed ST segment.

• Hyperkalemia shows serum potassium levels greater than 5 mEq/liter.

• Hyperkalemia electrocardiogram shows tall, tented T waves, widened QRS complex, prolonged PR interval, flattened or absent P waves, and depressed ST segment.

Precocious puberty in females

• X-rays of hands, wrists, knees, and hips reveal advanced bone age and possible premature epiphyseal closure.

• Androstenedione level greater than 3 ng/ml

• Radioimmunoassay for estrogen levels and follicle-stimulating hormone levels are abnormally high for age.

• Vaginal smear for estrogen secretion reveals abnormally high levels.

• Urinary test for gonadotropic activity and excretion of 17-ketosteroids show abnormally high levels.

Precocious puberty in males

• Detailed patient history reveals recent growth pattern, behavior changes, family history of precocious puberty, or any hormonal ingestion.

• In true precocious puberty:

— Serum levels of luteinizing and follicle-stimulating hormones and corticotropin are elevated.

— Plasma tests for testosterone demonstrate elevated levels (equal to those of an adult male).

— Evaluation of ejaculate indicates true precocity by revealing presence of live spermatozoa.

— Skull and hand X-rays reveal advanced bone age.

• In pseudoprecocious puberty:

— Chromosome analysis may demonstrate an abnormal pattern of autosomes and sex chromosomes.

— Steroid excretion levels such as testosterone levels and 24-hour 17-ketosteroid levels are elevated.

Pregnancy

• Elevated serum human chorionic gonadotropin (hCG) level

• Elevated urine hCG level

• Pelvic examination reveals changes to uterus consistent with pregnancy.

Pregnancy-induced hypertension
• Mild preeclampsia:
— systolic blood pressure level of 140 mm Hg or a rise of 30 mm Hg or more above the patient's normal systolic pressure (measured on two occasions, 6 hours apart)
— diastolic blood pressure level of 90 mm Hg or a rise of 15 mm Hg or more above the patient's normal diastolic pressure (measured on two occasions, 6 hours apart)
— proteinuria (urine protein level greater than 500 mg/24 hours).
• Severe preeclampsia:
— blood pressure measurements of 160/110 mm Hg or higher (measured on two occasions, 6 hours apart) at bed rest
— increased proteinuria (urine protein level of 5 g/24 hours or more)
— oliguria (urine output less than or equal to 400 ml/24 hours)
— hyperactive deep tendon reflexes.
• Eclampsia:
— History and examination reveal signs of severe preeclampsia and seizure activity.
— Ophthalmoscopic examination may reveal vascular spasm, papilledema, retinal edema or detachment, and arteriovenous nicking or hemorrhage.

Premature labor
• Physical examination reveals rhythmic uterine contractions, cervical dilation and effacement, possible rupture of membranes, expulsion of cervical mucous plug, and bloody discharge occurring prior to expected date of delivery.
• Vaginal examination reveals progressive cervical effacement and dilation.
• Pelvic ultrasound identifies fetus position in the mother's pelvis.

Premature rupture of the membranes
• Passage of amniotic fluid prior to the expected date of delivery

• Examination reveals amniotic fluid in the vagina.
• Nitrazine paper test of fluid from posterior fornix turns deep blue.
• Fluid smeared on slide and allowed to dry takes on a fernlike pattern.

Premenstrual syndrome
• History of menstruation-related symptoms including mild to severe personality changes, nervousness, irritability, fatigue, lethargy, depression, breast tenderness or bloating, joint pain, headache, diarrhea, exacerbations of skin, and respiratory or neurologic problems recorded for 2 to 3 months
• Normal serum estrogen and progesterone levels (normal ruling out hormonal imbalance)

Pressure ulcers
• History of immobility, malnutrition, or skin irritation
• Skin breakdown
• Wound culture and sensitivity reveal the infecting organisms.

Proctitis
• In acute proctitis, sigmoidoscopy reveals edematous, bright-red or pink rectal mucosa that's thick, shiny, friable, and possibly ulcerated.
• In chronic proctitis, sigmoidoscopy reveals thickened mucosa, loss of vascular pattern, and stricture of the rectal lumen.
• Biopsy reveals absence of malignant cells.

Progressive systemic sclerosis
• History reveals Raynaud's phenomenon.
• Antinuclear antibody test is positive, revealing low titer and speckled pattern.
• Hand X-rays reveal terminal phalangeal tuft resorption, subcutaneous calcification, and joint space narrowing and erosion.

• Chest X-ray reveals bilateral basilar pulmonary fibrosis.
• Rheumatoid factor is positive in approximately one-third of patients.
• Elevated erythrocyte sedimentation rate
• Urinalysis reveals proteinuria, microscopic hematuria, and casts (with renal involvement).

Prostatic cancer

• Digital rectal examination reveals small, hard nodule in prostate area.
• Elevated serum prostate-specific antigen levels
• Serum acid phosphatase greater than 1.9 U/L (in two-thirds of men with metastasized prostatic cancer)
• Biopsy reveals malignant cells.
• Serum alkaline phosphatase level is elevated.

Prostatitis

• Examination reveals tender, indurated, swollen, and warm prostate.
• Urine samples, taken at start of voiding, midstream, after doctor massages the prostate, and final specimen, reveal a significant increase in colony count of the prostatic specimens.

Protein-calorie malnutrition

• Examination reveals a small, gaunt, and emaciated appearance with no adipose tissue; dry and "baggy" skin; general weakness; sparse hair and dull brown or reddish yellow eyes; and slow pulse rate and respirations.
• History reveals a poor diet lacking in protein.
• Anthropometry reveals height and weight less than 80% of standard for the patient's age and sex, and below standard arm circumference and triceps skinfolds.
• Serum albumin level is less than 2.8 g/dl.

Pruritus ani

• History of perianal itching, irritation, or superficial burning
• Rectal examination identifies no fissures or fistulas.
• Biopsy rules out carcinoma.

Pseudomembranous enterocolitis

• History reveals sudden onset of copious, watery or bloody diarrhea, abdominal pain, and fever.
• Rectal biopsy reveals histologic changes indicative of pseudomembranous enterocolitis.
• Stool cultures reveals *Clostridium difficile*.

Pseudomonas infections

• Blood, spinal fluid, urine, exudate, or sputum culture reveals the pseudomonas organism.
• Gram stain reveals gram-negative bacillus.

Psoriasis

• Examination reveals dry, cracked, encrusted lesions (erythematous plaques) accompanied by itching on the scalp, chest, elbows, knees, back, or buttocks.
• Skin biopsy reveals psoriasis.
• Serum uric acid level above 8.0 mg/dl in men or 6.0 mg/dl in women, without indications of gout

Psoriatic arthritis

• Examination reveals psoriatic lesions.
• X-rays reveal:
— erosion of terminal phalangeal tufts
— "whittling" of the distal end of the terminal phalanges
— "pencil-in-cup" deformity of the distal interphalangeal joints
— sacroiliitis
— atypical spondylitis with syndesmophyte formation, resulting in hyperostosis and vertebral ossification.
• Nonreactive rheumatoid screening test

• Elevated erythrocyte sedimentation rate
• Increased serum uric acid levels

Ptosis

• Examination reveals drooping of the upper eyelid.
• Measurement of palpebral fissure widths, range of lid movement, and relation of lid margin to upper border of the cornea reveal the severity of illness.

Puerperal infection

• History reveals fever within 48 hours after delivery or abortion.
• A culture of lochia, blood, incisional exudate (from cesarean incision or episiotomy), uterine tissue, or material collected from the vaginal cuff reveals *Streptococcus,* coagulase-negative staphylococci, *Clostridium perfringens, Bacteroides fragilis,* or *Escherichia coli* as the causative organism.
• White blood cell count shows leukocytosis (15,000 to 30,000/μl) and an increased sedimentation rate.
• Pelvic examination reveals induration without purulent discharge (parametritis).
• Culdoscopy shows adnexal induration and thickening.

Pulmonary edema

• Examination reveals respiratory distress.
• Chest auscultation reveals crackles in the lung fields.
• Arterial blood gas analysis usually shows decreased PaO_2 (hypoxia); $PaCO_2$ is variable; profound respiratory alkalosis and acidosis may occur; metabolic acidosis occurs when cardiac output is low.
• Chest X-ray shows diffuse haziness of the lung fields and, often, cardiomegaly and pleural effusions.
• Pulmonary artery catheterization reveals elevated pulmonary wedge pressures.

Pulmonary embolism and infarction

• Lung scan reveals perfusion defects in areas beyond occluded vessels.
• Pulmonary angiography reveals emboli.
• Chest X-ray shows areas of atelectasis, elevated diaphragm and pleural effusion, prominent pulmonary artery, and occasionally, a wedge-shaped infiltrate suggesting pulmonary infarction.
• Electrocardiography may show right axis deviation, right bundle-branch block, tall peaked P waves, depression of ST segment and T-wave inversion, and supraventricular tachycardia.
• Auscultation reveals right ventricular gallop, increased intensity of the pulmonic component of S_2, crackles, and pleural rub at the site of the embolism.
• Arterial blood gas analysis may show decreased PaO_2 and $PaCO_2$ levels.

Pulmonary hypertension

• Pulmonary artery catheterization reveals pulmonary systolic pressure greater than 30 mm Hg; pulmonary artery wedge pressure may be elevated.
• Pulmonary angiography reveals filling defects in pulmonary vasculature.
• Pulmonary function tests may show decreased flow rates and increased residual volume (with underlying obstructive disease); total lung capacity may be decreased (with underlying restrictive disease).
• Arterial blood gas analysis reveals decreased PaO_2.
• Electrocardiography shows right axis deviation and tall or peaked P waves in inferior leads (with right ventricular hypertrophy).

Pulmonic insufficiency

• Cardiac catheterization shows pulmonic insufficiency, increased right ventricular pressure, and associated cardiac defects.

• Chest X-ray shows enlargement of the right ventricle and pulmonary artery.

• Echocardiography shows right ventricular or right atrial enlargement.

• Electrocardiography may be normal in mild cases or show right ventricular or right atrial hypertrophy.

Pulmonic stenosis

• Cardiac catheterization reveals increased right ventricular pressure, decreased pulmonary artery pressure, and an abnormal valve orifice.

• Chest X-ray usually reveals a normal heart size and normal lung vascularity, although the pulmonary arteries may be evident. With severe obstruction and right-sided heart failure, chest X-ray may reveal right atrial and ventricular enlargement.

• Echocardiography reveals the abnormality in the pulmonic valve.

• Electrocardiography results may be normal in mild cases, or they may indicate right axis deviation and right ventricular hypertrophy. High amplitude P waves in leads II, III, aV_F, and V_1 indicate right atrial enlargement.

Rabies

• History reveals animal bite.

• Throat and saliva culture reveals virus.

• Positive serum fluorescent rabies antibody test

• Elevated white blood cell count, with increased polymorphonuclear and large mononuclear cells

• Elevated urine glucose, acetone, and protein levels

Radiation exposure

• History reveals exposure to radiation and nausea and vomiting.

• Complete blood count reveals:

— decreased hemoglobin and hematocrit levels

— decreased white blood cells

— decreased platelet count

— decreased lymphocyte count.

• Bone marrow studies reveal blood dyscrasias.

• X-rays may show bone necrosis.

• Geiger counter measurement reveals the amount of radiation in an open wound.

Rape trauma syndrome

• History reveals rape or attempted rape, accompanied by feelings of anxiety, grief, anger, fear, or revenge.

• Examination shows signs of physical trauma.

• X-rays reveal fractures.

• Vaginal specimen is positive for semen.

• Fingernail and pubic hair scrapings may help to identify alleged rapist.

• Semen analysis may help to identify alleged rapist.

Raynaud's disease

• History and examination reveal changes in skin color induced by cold or stress, bilateral involvement, minimal cutaneous gangrene or absence of gangrene, and clinical symptoms of 2 years duration or more.

• Cold stimulation test demonstrates Raynaud's syndrome.

• Arteriography reveals no underlying secondary disease.

Rectal polyps

• Proctosigmoidoscopy or colonoscopy reveals type, size, and location of polyps.

• Biopsy reveals histologic changes consistent with polyps.

• Barium enema reveals polyps high in the colon.

• Stool guaiac testing reveals presence of occult blood.

Rectal prolapse
• In complete prolapse, visual examination reveals the full thickness of the bowel wall and, possibly, the sphincter muscle protruding and mucosa falling into bulky, concentric folds.
• In partial prolapse, visual examination reveals only partially protruding mucosa and a smaller mass of radial mucosal folds.

Reiter's syndrome
• History reveals venereal or enteric infection.
• Human leukocyte antigen testing reveals presence of the HLA-B27 antigen.
• Analysis of urethral discharge and synovial fluid reveals numerous white blood cells (WBCs), mostly polymorphonuclear leukocytes.
• Synovial fluid analysis reveals increased complement and protein; fluid is grossly purulent.
• Elevated WBC count and erythrocyte sedimentation rate

Relapsing fever
• History reveals recurrent fever for 5 to 15 days.
• Blood smear shows spirochetes.
• White blood cell count greater than 25,000/mm³, with increase in lymphocytes (although it may be within normal limits)
• Increased erythrocyte sedimentation rate

Renal calculi
• Kidney-ureter-bladder X-rays reveal renal calculi.
• Excretory urography reveals size and location of calculi.
• Kidney ultrasonography reveals obstructive changes.
• Urine culture may reveal urinary tract infection.
• Urinalysis may be normal or may show increased specific gravity, acid or

alkaline pH (depending on the type of stone), hematuria, crystals, casts, and pyuria (with or without white blood cells).
• 24-hour urine collection reveals calcium oxalate, phosphorus, or uric acid.

Renal infarction
• Urinalysis reveals proteinuria and microscopic hematuria.
• Elevated urine enzyme levels, especially lactate dehydrogenase (LD) and alkaline phosphatase
• Elevated serum aspartate aminotransferase, LD, and alkaline phosphatase levels
• Excretory urography shows diminished or absent excretion of contrast dye (with vascular occlusion or urethral obstruction).
• Isotopic renal scan demonstrates absent or reduced blood flow to the kidneys.
• Renal arteriography reveals infarction.

Renal tubular acidosis
• Urine studies reveal pH greater than 6, low titratable acids and ammonia content, increased HCO_3^- and potassium levels, and low specific gravity (less than 1.005).
• Blood pH less than 7.35
• Serum HCO_3^- level less than 22 mEq/liter
• Decreased serum potassium and phosphorus levels

Renal vein thrombosis
• Excretory urography reveals enlarged kidneys and diminished excretory function (in acute thrombosis); urography contrast medium seems to "smudge" necrotic renal tissue.
• In chronic thrombosis, excretory urography may show ureteral indentations that result from collateral venous channels.

- Renal venography reveals filling defects.
- Renal biopsy reveals characteristic histologic changes.
- Urinalysis reveals gross or microscopic hematuria, proteinuria (more than 2 g/day in chronic disease), casts, and oliguria.
- Blood studies show leukocytosis, hypoalbuminemia, hyperlipemia, and thrombocytopenia.

Renovascular hypertension
- Isotopic renal blood flow scan and rapid-sequence excretory urography reveal abnormal renal blood flow and discrepancies in kidney size and shape.
- Renal arteriography reveals the arterial stenosis or obstruction.
- Samples from both the right and left renal veins allow for comparison of plasma renin levels with those in the inferior vena cava; renin level is increased in the affected kidney.

Respiratory acidosis
- Arterial blood gas measurements reveal:
— pH less than 7.35
— $PaCO_2$ greater than 45 mm Hg
— HCO_3^- level of 22 to 26 mEq/liter (acute stage); greater than 26 mEq/liter (chronic stage).

Respiratory alkalosis
- Arterial blood gas measurements reveal:
— pH greater than 7.45
— $PaCO_2$ less than 35 mm Hg (in acute stage)
— HCO_3^- level normal (in acute stage) and less than 22 mEq/liter (in chronic stage).

Respiratory distress syndrome, adult
- Initial arterial blood gas (ABG) measurements:
— pH more than 7.45

— PaO_2 less than 60 mm Hg
— $PaCO_2$ less than 35 mm Hg.
- ABG measurements following progression of illness:
— pH less than 7.35
— Decreased PaO_2 (despite oxygen therapy)
— $PaCO_2$ level greater than 45 mm Hg
— HCO_3^- level less than 22 mEq/liter.
- Serial chest X-rays initially show bilateral infiltrates; later X-rays reveal ground glass appearance and eventually "whiteouts" of both lungs.

Respiratory distress syndrome, child
- Chest X-ray reveals fine reticulonodular pattern (may be normal for first 6 to 12 hours after birth).
- Arterial blood gas measurements reveal:
— pH less than 7.35
— PaO_2 less than 75 mm Hg.
- Chest auscultation reveals normal or diminished air entry and crackles (rare in early stages).
- Amniocentesis reveals lecithin-sphingomyelin ratio of less than 2 (used to assess risk of respiratory distress syndrome).

Respiratory syncytial virus infection
- Nasal and pharyngeal secretion cultures reveal respiratory syncytial virus infection (not always reliable).
- Serum antibody titers elevated (maternal antibodies may impair results before 6 months of age)
- Chest X-ray may reveal pneumonia.
- Positive indirect immunofluorescence and enzyme-linked immunosorbent assay tests

Restrictive cardiomyopathy
- Chest X-ray reveals massive cardiomegaly, affecting all four chambers of the heart, pericardial effusion, and pulmonary congestion (advanced stage).

• Echocardiography detects increased left ventricular muscle mass and differences in end-diastolic pressures between the ventricles.
• Carotid palpation reveals blunt carotid upstroke with small volume.
• Cardiac catheterization demonstrates increased left ventricular end-diastolic pressure.
• Electrocardiography may show low-voltage complexes, hypertrophy, atrioventricular conduction defects, or arrhythmias.

Retinal detachment
• Ophthalmoscopy reveals the usually transparent retina to be gray and opaque.
• In severe detachment, ophthalmoscopy reveals folds in the retina and a ballooning out of the area.
• Indirect ophthalmoscopy reveals retinal tears.
• Ocular ultrasound shows a dense sheetlike echo on a B-scan.

Retinitis pigmentosa
• Family history indicates a possible predisposition to retinitis pigmentosa.
• Electroretinography shows a retinal response time slower than normal, or absent.
• Visual field testing (using a tangent screen) detects ring scotoma.
• Fluorescein angiography shows white dots (areas of dyspigmentation) in the epithelium.
• Ophthalmoscopy may initially show normal fundi but later reveals characteristic black pigmentary disturbance.

Reye's syndrome
• History of recent viral disorder with varying degrees of encephalopathy and cerebral edema
• Alanine aminotransferase level is greater than 64 U/L in men or greater than 48 U/L in women.

• Aspartate aminotransferase level is greater than 40 U/L.
• Liver biopsy reveals fatty droplets uniformly distributed throughout cells.
• Prolonged prothrombin time and partial thromboplastin time
• Cerebrospinal fluid (CSF) analysis reveals white blood cells less than $10/mm^3$; in coma, CSF pressure is increased.
• Elevated serum ammonia levels
• Increased serum fatty acid and lactate levels
• Normal or low serum glucose levels

Rheumatic fever and rheumatic heart disease
• History reveals streptococcal infection.
• Examination reveals joint pain and swelling and one or more of the following symptoms: carditis, polyarthritis, chorea, erythema marginatum, or subcutaneous nodules.
• Positive C-reactive protein
• Elevated antistreptolysin-O titer (within 2 months of onset)
• Echocardiography and cardiac catheterization reveal valvular damage.
• Cardiac enzymes may be elevated (in severe carditis).

Rheumatoid arthritis
• Rheumatoid factor titer above 1:80
• X-rays reveal the following:
— bone demineralization and soft-tissue swelling (in early stages)
— loss of cartilage and narrowing of joint spaces
— cartilage and bone destruction, erosion, subluxations, and deformities.
• Synovial fluid analysis reveals increased volume and turbidity but decreased viscosity and complement (C3 and C4) levels, and white blood cell count greater than $10,000/mm^3$.
• Increased erythrocyte sedimentation rate

• Complete blood count shows moderate decrease in red blood cell count, hemoglobin, and hematocrit and slight leukocytosis.

Rheumatoid arthritis, juvenile

• History reveals persistent joint stiffness and pain in the morning or after periods of inactivity.
• Antinuclear antibodies test may be positive in patients who have pauciarticular juvenile rheumatoid arthritis (JRA) with chronic iridocyclitis.
• Rheumatoid factor is present in 15% of patients with JRA, as compared with 85% of patients with rheumatoid arthritis.
• Early X-ray changes include soft-tissue swelling, effusion, and periostitis in affected joints.
• In later X-ray changes, osteoporosis and accelerated bone growth may appear, followed by subchondral erosions, joint space narrowing, bone destruction, and fusion.
• Complete blood count usually shows decreased hemoglobin levels, increased neutrophil count, increased platelet levels, and elevated erythrocyte sedimentation rate.
• Blood studies reveal elevated C-reactive protein, serum haptoglobin, immunoglobulin, and C3 complement levels.
• Human leukocyte antigen (HLA-B27) is present, forecasting later development of ankylosing spondylitis.

Rocky Mountain spotted fever

• History reveals tick bite or travel to a tick-infested area.
• Complement fixation test shows a fourfold rise in convalescent antibodies compared to acute titers.
• Blood culture reveals *Rickettsia rickettsii*.
• Decreased platelet count (12,000 to 150,000/mm^3) indicating thrombocytopenia during second week of illness

• Elevated white blood cell count (11,000 to 33,000/µl) during second week of illness

Rosacea

• Examination reveals vascular and acneiform lesions without the comedones characteristically associated with acne vulgaris; in severe cases, rhinophyma is seen.

Roseola infantum

• History reveals high fever (103° to 105° F [39.4° to 40.4° C]) followed by rash 48 hours after fever subsides.
• Examination reveals maculopapular, nonpruritic rash that blanches on pressure.

Rubella

• History reveals exposure to infected person.
• Examination reveals maculopapular rash, beginning on the face and spreading to the trunk and extremities.
• Examination also reveals lymphadenopathy.
• Cell cultures of throat, blood, urine, and cerebrospinal fluid reveal rubella virus.
• Convalescent serum antibody titers rise fourfold from acute titers.

Rubeola

• History reveals exposure to person infected with the measles virus (patient may be unaware of contact).
• Examination reveals the pathognomonic Koplik's spots.
• Blood, nasopharyngeal, and urine cultures reveal measles virus (during the febrile period).
• Serum antibody titers appear within 3 days after the onset of the rash and reach peak titers 2 to 4 weeks later.

Salmonellosis

• Blood, stool, urine, bone marrow, pus or vomitus culture reveals gram-negative bacilli of the genus *Salmonella*.
• Widal's test reveals a fourfold rise in titer.

Sarcoidosis

• Kveim-Siltzbach skin test confirms discrete epithelioid cell granuloma.
• Chest X-ray reveals bilateral hilar and right paratracheal adenopathy with or without diffuse interstitial infiltrates; occasionally, large nodular lesions appear in lung parenchyma.
• Lymph node, skin, or lung biopsy reveals noncaseating granulomas with negative cultures for mycobacteria and fungi.
• Pulmonary function test shows decreased total lung capacity and compliance and decreased diffusing capacity.
• Tuberculin skin test, fungal serologies, and sputum cultures for mycobacteria and fungi and biopsy cultures are negative.

Scabies

• Visual examination of the contents of the scabietic burrow may reveal itch mite.
• Mineral oil placed over the burrow, followed by superficial scraping and examination of expressed material, reveals ova or mite feces.
• Pediculicide administration to affected area clears skin.

Scarlet fever

• History reveals recent streptococcal pharyngitis.
• Examination reveals strawberry tongue and fine erythematous rash that blanches on pressure.
• Pharyngeal culture reveals group A beta-hemolytic streptococci.
• Complete blood count reveals granulocytosis and, possibly, a reduced red blood cell count.

Schistosomiasis

• History reveals travel to endemic areas.
• Urine, stool, or lesion biopsy reveals ova.
• White blood cell count reveals eosinophilia.

Scoliosis

• Examination reveals unequal shoulder height, elbow levels, and heights of iliac crests and asymmetry of the paraspinal muscles.
• Scoliosometer (an apparatus for measuring curvature of the spinal column) reveals angle of trunk rotation to be abnormal.
• Anterior, posterior, and lateral spinal X-rays reveal degree of curvature and flexibility of the spine.

Septal perforation and deviation

• History and examination reveal whistle on inspiration, rhinitis, epistaxis, nasal crusting, and watery discharge.
• Inspection of the nasal mucosa with bright light and a nasal speculum reveals perforation or deviation.

Septic arthritis

• Synovial fluid Gram stain and culture or biopsy of synovial membrane reveals gram-positive cocci *(Staphylococcus aureus, Streptococcus pyogenes, Streptococcus pneumoniae,* or *Streptococcus viridans)*, gram-negative cocci *(Neisseria gonorrhoeae* and *Haemophilus influenzae)*, or gram-negative bacilli *(Escherichia coli, Salmonella,* or *Pseudomonas)* as the causative organism.
• Joint fluid analysis reveals gross pus or watery, cloudy fluid of decreased viscosity, usually with 50,000/mm^3 or more white blood cells (WBCs), containing primarily neutrophils.
• Skin exudate, sputum, urethral discharge, stools, urine, blood, or naso-

pharyngeal culture is positive for causative organism.

• Skeletal X-rays show distention of joint capsules, followed by narrowing of joint space (indicating cartilage damage), and erosions of bone (joint destruction).

• WBC count may be elevated with many polymorphonuclear cells; erythrocyte sedimentation rate is increased.

Septic shock

• History reveals infection accompanied by fever, confusion, nausea, vomiting, and hyperventilation.

• Blood cultures reveal gram-negative bacteria (*Escherichia coli, Klebsiella, Enterobacter, Proteus, Pseudomonas,* or *Bacteroides)* or gram-positive bacteria *(Streptococcus pneumoniae, Streptococcus pyogenes,* or *Actinomyces)* as the causative organism.

• White blood cell count is greater than $15,000/mm^3$.

• Pulmonary artery catheterization reveals decreased central venous pressure, pulmonary artery pressures, wedge pressure, and cardiac output (may be initially elevated), and systemic vascular resistance.

• Arterial blood gas measurements reveal decreased $PaCO_2$, low or normal HCO_3^- level, and pH above 7.45 (in early stages); as shock progresses, decreasing $PaCO_2$, PaO_2, HCO_3^- level, and pH indicate the development of metabolic acidosis with hypoxemia.

• Serum blood urea nitrogen and creatinine levels increase; creatinine clearance decreases.

• Urine osmolality falls below 400 milliosmoles; ratio of urine osmolality to plasma osmolality is below 1.5.

• Electrocardiography reveals ST-segment depression, inverted T waves, and arrhythmias.

Severe combined immunodeficiency disease

• History reveals overwhelming infections during the first year of life.

• T-cell count and function is severely diminished.

• Lymph node biopsy reveals absence of lymphocytes.

Shigellosis

• Microscopic examination of a fresh stool may reveal mucus, red blood cells, and polymorphonuclear leukocytes.

• Stool culture reveals *Shigella.*

• Hemagglutinating antibodies may be present, indicating severe infection.

Sickle cell anemia

• Family history reveals homozygous inheritance.

• Stained blood smear reveals sickle cells.

• Hemoglobin electrophoresis reveals hemoglobin S.

• Complete blood count reveals decreased red blood cells, elevated white blood cells, and elevated platelet count.

• Decreased erythrocyte sedimentation rate

• Increased serum iron levels

Sideroblastic anemias

• Bone marrow aspirate reveals ringed sideroblasts.

• Microscopic examination reveals red blood cells that are hypochromic or normochromic and slightly macrocytic; red cell precursors may be megaloblastic, with anisocytosis and poikilocytosis.

• Decreased hemoglobin levels

• Increased serum iron and transferrin levels

Silicosis

• History reveals occupational exposure to silica dust.

• Examination reveals decreased chest expansion, diminished intensity of breath sounds, areas of hypo- and hyperresonance, fine to medium crackles, and tachypnea (with chronic silicosis).

• Chest X-ray reveals the following:

— small, discrete, nodular lesions distributed throughout both lung fields but typically concentrated in the upper lung zones

— enlarged hilar lung nodes that exhibit "eggshell" calcification (in simple silicosis)

— one or more conglomerate masses of dense tissue (in complicated silicosis).

• Pulmonary function tests reveal:

— reduced forced vital capacity (in complicated silicosis)

— reduced forced expiratory volume (in obstructed disease)

— reduced maximal voluntary ventilation (in restrictive and obstructive disease)

— reduced diffusing capacity for carbon monoxide when fibrosis destroys alveolar walls and obliterates pulmonary capillaries, or when fibrosis thickens alveolar capillary membrane.

• Arterial blood gas measurements reveal:

— significantly decreased PaO_2 (in the late stages of chronic or complicated disease)

— decreased or normal $PaCO_2$ in early stages, but may increase as restrictive pattern develops.

Sinus bradycardia

• Electrocardiography reveals:

— regular atrial and ventricular rhythm

— atrial and ventricular rates less than 60 beats/minute

— P wave with normal size and configuration; P wave precedes each QRS complex

— PR interval within normal limits and constant

— QRS complex of normal duration and configuration

— T wave of normal size and configuration

— QT interval within normal limits, but possibly prolonged.

Sinus tachycardia

• Electrocardiography reveals:

— regular atrial and ventricular rhythms

— atrial and ventricular rates greater than 100 beats/minute (usually between 100 and 160 beats/minute)

— P wave of normal size and configuration and precedes each QRS complex

— PR interval within normal limits and constant

— QRS complex of normal duration and configuration

— T wave of normal size and configuration

— QT interval within normal limits, but commonly shortened.

Sinusitis

• Nasal examination reveals inflammation and pus.

• Sinus X-rays reveal cloudiness in the affected sinus, air-fluid levels, or thickened mucosal lining.

• Transillumination allows inspection of the sinus cavities by passing a light through them; in sinusitis, purulent drainage prevents passage of light.

Sjögren's syndrome

• Elevated erythrocyte sedimentation rate

• Hypergammaglobulinemia

• Positive rheumatoid factor test (75% to 90% of patients)

• Positive antinuclear antibodies test (50% to 80% of patients)

• Schirmer's tearing test positive for tearing deficiency

• Lower lip biopsy shows salivary gland infiltration by lymphocytes.
• History and examination reveal two of the following three conditions:
— xerophthalmia
— xerostomia (with salivary gland biopsy showing lymphocytic infiltration)
— associated autoimmune or lymphoproliferative disorder.

Skull fractures
• History reveals head trauma.
• Skull X-ray reveals fracture (minor vault fractures may not be visible).
• Neurologic examination reveals cerebral function.
• Cerebral angiography reveals vascular disruption from internal pressure and injury.
• Computed tomography scan, echoencephalography, air encephalography, magnetic resonance imaging, and radioactive scanning reveal cranial nerve injury or intracranial hemorrhage from ruptured blood vessels. These tests also help to localize subdural or intracerebral hematomas.

Snakebites, poisonous
• Examination reveals fang marks.
• Prolonged bleeding time and partial thromboplastin time
• Decreased hemoglobin and hematocrit levels
• Sharply decreased platelet count (less than 200,000/mm³)
• Urinalysis may reveal hematuria.
• Chest X-ray may show pulmonary edema or emboli.
• Electrocardiography may reveal tachycardia and ectopic beats.

Sodium imbalance
• Hyponatremia:
— serum sodium level below 135 mEq/liter
— urine sodium level above 100 mEq/24 hours
— low serum osmolality.

• Hypernatremia:
— serum sodium level above 145 mEq/liter
— urine sodium level below 40 mEq/24 hours
— high serum osmolality.

Spinal cord defects
• Examination reveals a protruding sac on the spine.
• Transillumination of sac reveals meningocele.
• Spinal X-ray reveals bone defect (in spina bifida occulta).
• Computed tomography scan reveals hydrocephalus (in 90% of patients).

Spinal injuries without cord damage
• Patient history reveals trauma, metastatic disease, infection, or endocrine disorder.
• Physical examination reveals the location and level of injury.
• Spinal X-rays reveal fracture.
• Myelography reveals spinal mass.
• Lumbar puncture reveals increased cerebrospinal fluid pressure, indicating spinal trauma or lesion.

Spinal neoplasms
• Lumbar puncture reveals clear yellow cerebrospinal fluid with increased protein levels.
• X-rays show distortions of intervertebral foramina, changes in vertebrae or collapsed areas in the vertebral body, and localized enlargement of the spinal canal indicating an adjacent block.
• Myelography identifies the level of the lesion.
• Computed tomography scan and magnetic resonance imaging show cord compression and tumor location.
• Radioisotope bone scan reveals evidence of metastatic invasion of the vertebrae by showing increased osteoblastic activity.
• Biopsy reveals malignant cells.

Sporotrichosis

- Examination reveals small, painless, movable subcutaneous nodules with discoloration and ulceration.
- Sputum, pus, or bone drainage cultures reveal *Strongyloides schenckii.*

Sprains and strains

- History reveals recent injury or chronic overuse of extremity.
- Examination reveals pain (local with a sprain, sharp and transient with a strain), swelling, and ecchymoses (rapid onset with a sprain; may take several days with a strain).
- X-ray of the extremity does not indicate fracture.

Squamous cell carcinoma

- Examination reveals ulcerated nodule with indurated base.
- Biopsy reveals squamous cell carcinoma.

Staphylococcal scalded skin syndrome

- Examination reveals three-stage progression of erythema, exfoliation, and desquamation.
- Skin lesions are positive for Group 2 *Staphylococcus aureus.*

Stomatitis and other oral infections

- Examination reveals inflammation of the oral mucosa or surrounding area.
- Smear of ulcer exudate reveals fusiform bacillus or spirochete as the causative organism (in Vincent's angina).

Strabismus

- Visual acuity test reveals the degree of visual defect.
- Hirschberg's method detects malalignment.
- Retinoscopy identifies refractive error.
- Maddox rods test identifies specific muscle involvement.

- Convergence test shows distance at which convergence is sustained.
- Duction test reveals limitation of eye movement.
- Cover-uncover test demonstrates eye deviation and the rate of recovery to original alignment.
- Alternate-cover test shows intermittent or latent deviation.

Strongyloidiasis

- Stool specimen reveals *Strongyloides stercoralis* larvae.
- Sputum specimen contains eosinophils and larvae.
- History reveals travel to endemic area.
- Hemoglobin level is decreased to between 6 and 10 g.
- White blood cell count with differential shows eosinophils at 450 to 700/μl.

Stye

- Visual examination reveals abscess of the lid glands.
- Abscess culture reveals a staphylococcal organism.

Sudden infant death syndrome

- Autopsy reveals:
— small or normal adrenal glands
— petechiae over the visceral surface of the pleura, within the thymus, and in the epicardium
— well-preserved lymphoid structures
— pathologic changes suggesting chronic hypoxemia
— edematous, congestive lungs fully expanded in the pleural cavities
— liquid blood in the heart (not clotted)
— curd from the stomach inside the trachea.

Syndrome of inappropriate antidiuretic hormone secretion

- History reveals recent weight gain despite anorexia, nausea, and vomiting.
- Serum osmolality below 280 mOsm/kg of water

- Serum sodium level below 123 mEq/liter
- High urine sodium level (more than 20 mEq/liter) without diuretics

Syphilis

- History reveals sexual contact with partner with syphilis.
- Lesion culture reveals *Treponema pallidum.*
- The fluorescent treponemal antibody absorption test identifies antigens of *T. pallidum* in tissue, ocular fluid, cerebrospinal fluid (CSF), tracheobronchial secretions, and exudates from lesions.
- Venereal Disease Research Laboratory (VDRL) slide test and rapid plasma reagin test are positive, detecting nonspecific antibodies.
- In neurosyphilis:
— CSF reveals total protein level is above 40 mg/dl.
— VDRL slide test is reactive.
— Cell count exceeds five mononuclear cells/mm^3.

Taeniasis

- Laboratory observation reveals tapeworm ova or body segments in feces.
- History reveals travel to endemic areas.
- History reveals exposure to eating undercooked, infected beef, pork, or fish; in dwarf tapeworm, exposure to an infected person.
- In beef tapeworm:
— crawling sensation in perianal area
— intestinal obstruction and appendicitis.
- In pork tapeworm:
— seizures, headaches, personality changes (often overlooked in adults).
- In fish tapeworm:
— anemia (hemoglobin as low as 6 to 8 g).
- In dwarf tapeworm:
— no symptoms (mild infestation)

— anorexia, diarrhea, restlessness, dizziness, and apathy (severe infestation).

Tay-Sachs disease

- Family history reveals Ashkenazic Jewish ancestry or history of the disease; diagnostic screening may detect carriers of autosomal recessive gene.
- Serum analysis shows deficiency of hexosaminidase A.
- Ophthalmic examination reveals optic nerve atrophy and a distinctive cherry-red spot on the retina.

Tendinitis and bursitis

- Examination reveals localized pain and inflammation at joint.
- History reveals unusual strain or injury 2 to 3 days prior to onset of pain or heat-aggravated joint pain
- X-rays (in late stages) reveal bony fragments, osteophyte sclerosis, or calcium deposits.
- Arthrography is usually normal, with occasional small irregularities on the undersurface of the tendon.

Testicular cancer

- Physical examination reveals testicular mass.
- Transillumination confirms tumor.
- Biopsy reveals malignant cells.
- Excretory urography reveals ureteral deviation (indicates node involvement).
- Testosterone levels are greater than 1,200 ng/dl or less than 300 ng/dl.
- Urine testing indicates presence of human chorionic gonadotropin.
- Increased serum alpha-fetoprotein and beta human chorionic gonadotropin levels

Testicular torsion

- Physical examination reveals tense, tender swelling in the scrotum or inguinal canal and hyperemia of the overlying skin.
- Doppler ultrasonography reveals testicular torsion.

Tetanus

• History reveals trauma and absence of tetanus immunization.
• Meningitis, rabies, phenothiazine or strychnine toxicity, or other conditions that mimic tetanus are ruled out.

Tetralogy of Fallot

• Echocardiography reveals septal overriding of the aorta, the ventricular septal defect (VSD), and pulmonary stenosis, and detects hypertrophy of walls of the right ventricle.
• Cardiac catheterization shows pulmonary stenosis, the VSD, and the overriding aorta and rules out other cyanotic heart defects.
• Auscultation reveals a loud systolic heart murmur, which may diminish or obscure the pulmonic component of S_2.
• Palpation may reveal a cardiac thrill at the left sternal border and an obvious right ventricular impulse.
• Electrocardiography shows right ventricular hypertrophy, right axis deviation and, possibly right atrial hypertrophy.
• Chest X-ray reveals decreased pulmonary vascular marking (depending on the severity of pulmonary obstruction) and a boot-shaped cardiac silhouette.

Thalassemia

• Thalassemia major:
— lowered red blood cell and hemoglobin levels
— elevated reticulocyte level
— elevated bilirubin and urinary and fecal urobilinogen levels
— low serum folate level
— X-rays of the skull and long bones show a thinning and widening of the marrow space.
— Hemoglobin electrophoresis reveals a significant rise in Hb F and a slight increase in Hb A_2.
— Peripheral blood smear reveals extremely thin and fragile red blood cells, pale nucleated red blood cells, and marked anisocytosis.
• Thalassemia intermedia:
— hypochromia and microcytic red blood cells.
• Thalassemia minor:
— hypochromia and microcytic red blood cells
— Hemoglobin electrophoresis reveals a significant increase in Hb A2 and a moderate rise in Hb F.

Thoracic aortic aneurysm

• Chest X-ray reveals widening of the aorta.
• Computed tomography scan or magnetic resonance imaging reveals location and size of aneurysm
• Aortography reveals the lumen of the aneurysm, its size and location and, in dissecting aneurysm, the false lumen.

Throat abscesses

• History reveals staphylococcal or streptococcal infection.
• Retropharyngeal abscess, as indicated by:
— history of nasopharyngitis or pharyngitis
— a soft, red bulging of the posterior pharyngeal wall
— X-rays that reveal the larynx pushed forward and a widened space between the posterior pharyngeal wall and vertebrae
— pharyngeal culture that reveals infective organism.
• Examination reveals swelling of the soft palate on the abscessed side of the throat, with displacement of the uvula to the opposite side; red, edematous mucous membranes; and tonsil displacement toward the midline.
• Throat culture reveals streptococcal or staphylococcal infection.

Thrombocytopenia

• Platelet count less than 100,000/mm^3
• Prolonged bleeding time

- Normal prothrombin time and partial thromboplastin time
- Bone marrow studies reveal an increased number of megakaryocytes (platelet precursors) and shortened platelet survival.

Thrombophlebitis
- Positive Homans' sign
- Doppler ultrasonography reveals reduced blood flow to a specific area and obstruction to venous flow.
- Plethysmography reveals decreased circulation distal to affected area.
- Phlebography reveals filling defects and diverted blood flow.

Thyroid cancer
- Examination reveals an enlarged, palpable node in the thyroid gland, neck, lymph nodes of the neck, or vocal cords.
- History reveals exposure to radiation therapy or a family history of thyroid cancer.
- Thyroid scan reveals a "cold," nonfunctioning nodule
- Thyroid biopsy reveals a well-encapsulated, solitary nodule of uniform but abnormal structure.
- Serum calcitonin assay reveals an elevated fasting calcitonin and an abnormal response to calcium stimulation (with medullary cancer).

Thyroiditis
- Autoimmune thyroiditis:
— positive precipitin test
— high titers of thyroglobulin
— microsomal antibodies present in serum.
- Subacute granulomatous:
— elevated erythrocyte sedimentation rate
— increased thyroid hormone levels
— decreased thyroidal radioiodine uptake.

Tic disorders
- Examination reveals recurrent, involuntary movements involving the facial muscles, coughing, sniffling, or jerking head movements.
- History identifies stressors that may be related to symptoms.

Tinea versicolor
- Wood's light examination reveals lesions.
- Microscopic examination of skin scrapings show hyphae and clusters of yeast.

Tonsillitis
- Examination reveals generalized inflammation of the pharyngeal wall and swollen tonsils that project from between the pillars of the fauces and exude white or yellow follicles, with inflamed uvula.
- Purulent drainage appears when pressure is applied to the tonsillar pillars.
- Throat culture reveals infective organism, commonly beta-hemolytic streptococci.

Torticollis
- History reveals painless neck deformity.
- Examination reveals enlargement of the sternocleidomastoid muscle.
- Cervical spine X-rays are negative for bone or joint disease but may reveal an associated disorder such as tuberculosis, scar tissue formation, or arthritis (in acquired torticollis).

Toxic epidermal necrolysis
- Examination reveals scalded skin with no history of burn.
- Nikolsky's sign (skin sloughs off with slight friction) appears in erythematous areas.
- Culture and Gram stain reveal infective organism.
- White blood cell count reveals leukocytosis.

Toxic shock syndrome
• Vaginal discharge or lesions reveal *Staphylococcus aureus.*
• Creatine kinase level greater than 750 U/L
• Blood urea nitrogen level greater than 40 mg/dl
• Serum creatinine level greater than 1.8 mg/dl
• Aspartase aminotransferase and alanine aminotransferase levels greater than 20 U/L
• Platelet count less than 100,000/mm³

Toxocariasis
• History reveals pica, eosinophilia, or recent exposure to a dog.
• Massive leukocytosis (white blood cell count above 100,000/mm³)
• Hypereosinophilia (eosinophil count above 3,000/mm³)
• Antibodies to *Toxocara canis* present in serum
• Liver biopsy reveals *T. canis* larvae.

Toxoplasmosis
• History reveals exposure to a cat or ingestion of uncooked meat.
• Blood, body fluid, or tissue tests positive for *Toxoplasma gondii* antibodies.
• Identification of *T. gondii* in mice after their inoculation with specimens of patient's body fluids, blood, and tissue

Tracheoesophageal fistula and esophageal atresia
• Examination reveals respiratory distress and drooling in a newborn.
• Catheter (#10 or #12 French) meets obstruction when passed through the nose at 4″ to 5″ (10 to 13 cm) distal from the nostrils.
• Chest X-ray demonstrates the position of the catheter and can show a dilated, air-filled upper esophageal pouch, pneumonia in the right upper lobe, or bilateral pneumonitis.
• Abdominal X-ray reveals gas in the bowel in a distal fistula (but none in a proximal fistula or atresia without fistula).
• Cinefluorography defines the upper pouch by allowing visualization on a fluoroscopic screen and differentiates between overflow aspiration from a blind end (atresia) and aspiration due to passage of liquids through a tracheoesophageal fistula.

Trachoma
• Examination reveals follicular conjunctivitis with corneal infiltration and upper lid or conjunctival scarring, with symptoms persisting for 3 weeks.
• Microscopic examination of a Giemsa-stained conjunctival scraping reveals cytoplasmic inclusion bodies, some polymorphonuclear reaction, plasma cells, Leber's cells (large macrophages containing phagocytosed debris), and follicle cells.

Transposition of the great arteries
• Echocardiography reveals the reversed position of the aorta and the pulmonary artery and records echoes from both semilunar valves simultaneously, due to the aortic valve displacement.
• Cardiac catheterization reveals:
— decreased oxygen saturation in left ventricular blood and aortic blood
— increased right atrial, right ventricular, and pulmonary artery oxygen saturation
— right ventricular systolic pressure equal to systemic pressure.
• Dye injection during catheterization reveals the transposed vessels and the presence of any other cardiac defects.
• Chest X-rays show right atrial and ventricular enlargement causing the heart to appear oblong (within days to weeks) and increased vascular markings, except when pulmonary stenosis exists.

• Electrocardiography reveals right axis deviation and right ventricular hypertrophy (may be normal in a neonate).
• Arterial blood gas measurements reveal hypoxia and secondary metabolic acidosis.

Trichinosis
• History reveals ingesting raw or improperly cooked pork or pork products.
• Stools contain mature worms and larvae during the invasion stage.
• Skeletal muscle biopsy reveals encysted larvae 10 days after ingestion.
• Elevated antibody titers during acute and convalescent stage
• During acute stages, elevated serum liver enzymes (aspartase aminotransferase, lactate hydrogenase, and creatine kinase)
• Elevated eosinophil count (up to 15,000 /μl)

Trichomoniasis
• History reveals sexual contact with someone with trichomoniasis.
• Microscopic examination of vaginal or seminal discharge reveals *Trichomonas vaginalis.*
• Examination of clear urine specimens may also reveal *T. vaginalis.*
• Examination reveals vaginal erythema; edema; frank excoriation; a frothy, malodorous, greenish-yellow vaginal discharge; and, rarely, a thin, gray pseudomembrane over the vagina.
• Cervical examination shows punctate cervical hemorrhages, giving the cervix a strawberry appearance.

Trichuriasis
• Stool specimen contains whipworm ova.
• History reveals ingestion of food contaminated with nematoid ova.

Tricuspid insufficiency
• Cardiac catheterization shows markedly decreased cardiac output; mean right atrial and right ventricular end-diastolic pressures may be elevated.
• Chest X-ray reveals right atrial and ventricular enlargement.
• Echocardiography shows right ventricular dilation and paradoxical septal motion. It may show prolapsing or flailing of the tricuspid valve leaflets. Doppler echocardiography provides estimates of pulmonary artery and right ventricular systolic pressure.
• Electrocardiography (ECG) reveals right atrial hypertrophy and right or left ventricular hypertrophy. ECG also may reveal atrial fibrillation or incomplete right bundle-branch block.

Tricuspid stenosis
• Cardiac catheterization shows increased right atrial pressure and decreased cardiac output; it may also show an increased pressure gradient across the tricuspid valve.
• Chest X-ray reveals right atrial and superior vena cava enlargement.
• Echocardiography reveals a thick tricuspid valve with reduced mobility and right atrial enlargement.
• Electrocardiography shows right atrial hypertrophy and right ventricular hypertrophy. Atrial fibrillation may be present. Tall, peaked P waves are seen in lead II and prominent, upright P waves are seen in lead V_1, indicating right atrial enlargement.

Trigeminal neuralgia
• History reveals pain in the superior mandibular or maxillary area, without sensory or motor impairment.
• Examination reveals splinting on the affected side of the face while talking.
• Skull X-rays, tomography, and computed tomography scans rule out sinus or tooth infections and tumors.

Tuberculosis

• Stains and cultures of sputum, cerebrospinal fluid, urine, and abscess drainage reveal heat-sensitive, nonmotile, aerobic, acid-fast bacilla.
• Chest X-ray reveals nodular lesions, patchy infiltrates, cavity formation, scar tissue, and calcium deposits.
• Auscultation reveals crepitant crackles, bronchial breath sounds, wheezes, and whispered pectoriloquy.
• Chest percussion reveals a dullness over the affected area.
• Tuberculin skin test reveals that the patient has been infected with tuberculosis.

Tularemia

• History reveals exposure to animals or ticks.
• Lymph nodes, sputum, or gastric washings reveal *Francisella tularensis*.
• Agglutination test reveals a rise in antibody titers from 1:80 during the second week of illness to a possible high of 1:1,280 in 4 to 6 weeks.
• Skin test (with a diluted specimen of *F. tularensis*) reveals a positive reaction (90% of patients).

Typhus, epidemic

• Weil-Felix reaction reveals a fourfold rise in agglutination titer 8 to 12 days following infection.
• Complement fixation for group-specific typhus antigens is positive 8 to 12 days following infection.

Ulcerative colitis

• History reveals recurrent bloody diarrhea and GI disturbances.
• Sigmoidoscopy reveals increased mucosal friability, decreased mucosal detail, and thick inflammatory exudate.
• Biopsy reveals histologic changes characteristic of ulcerative colitis.
• Colonoscopy identifies the extent of the disease.

• Barium enema identifies the extent of the disease and detects complications.
• Erythrocyte sedimentation rate increases, correlating with severity of attack.
• Decreased serum potassium and magnesium levels
• Complete blood count shows decreased hemoglobin level and leukocytosis.
• Decreased serum albumin level
• Prolonged prothrombin time

Undescended testes

• Examination of scrotum reveals unpalpable testes, either unilateral or bilateral.
• Buccal smear identifies genetic sex by showing a male sex chromatin pattern.
• Serum gonadotropin levels confirm the presence of testes.

Urticaria and angioedema

• History reveals exposure to medications, food, and environmental influences.
• Skin testing reveals specific allergens.
• Decreased level of serum C4 and C1 esterase inhibitors (confirms hereditary angioedema)
• Complete blood count, urinalysis, erythrocyte sedimentation rate, and chest X-ray rule out inflammatory infections.

Uterine cancer

• Endometrial, cervical, and endocervical biopsies reveal malignant cells.
• Schiller's test shows cancerous tissues resisting stain.
• Cervical biopsies and endocervical curettage identifies degree of cervical involvement.
• Barium enema reveals bladder or rectal involvement.

Uterine leiomyomas

- History reveals abnormal endometrial bleeding.
- Pelvic palpation reveals round or irregular mass.
- Ultrasound reveals dense mass.
- Hysterosalpingography reveals asymmetrical uterus.
- Laparoscopy reveals lumps on the uterus.
- Complete blood count reveals decreased red blood cell count and hemoglobin and hematocrit levels.

Uveitis

- Slit-lamp examination reveals a "flare and cell" pattern, which looks like light passing through smoke, and an increased number of cells over the inflamed area.
- Examination with a special lens, slit-lamp, and ophthalmoscope identifies active inflammatory fundus lesions involving the retina and choroid.
- Serologic tests indicate toxoplasmosis (in posterior uveitis).

Vaginal cancer

- Papanicolaou test reveals abnormal cells.
- Vaginal examination, aided by Lugol's solution, reveals lesion.
- Lesion biopsy reveals malignant cells.
- Gallium scan reveals abnormal gallium activity.

Vaginismus

- Pelvic examination reveals involuntary constriction of the musculature surrounding the outer portion of the vagina.
- History and examination rule out physical disorders causing muscle constriction.
- Detailed sexual history reveals involuntary spastic contraction of the lower vaginal muscles, possibly coexisting with dyspareunia, preventing intercourse.

Varicella

- History reveals exposure to person infected with chicken pox (patient may be unaware of contact).
- Examination reveals crops of small, erythematous macules on the trunk or scalp progressing to papules and then clear vesicles on a erythematous base; vesicles become cloudy and break, and then form a scab.
- Vesicular fluid tests positive for herpesvirus varicella-zoster.

Variola

- History reveals exposure to infected person.
- Aspirate from vesicles and pustules reveals variola virus.
- Complement fixation detects antibodies to variola virus.
- Microscopic examination of smears from lesions show variola virus.

Vascular retinopathies

- Central retinal artery occlusion:
— Ophthalmoscopy (direct or indirect) shows emptying of retinal arterioles.
— Slit-lamp examination reveals, within 2 hours of occlusion, clumps or segmentation in the artery. Later examination shows a milky white retina around the optic disk (resulting from swelling and necrosis of ganglion cells caused by reduced blood supply). Other findings include a cherry-red spot in the macula. (This spot subsides after several weeks.)
— Ophthalmodynamometry measures approximate relative pressures in the central retinal arteries and indirectly assess internal carotid artery blockage.
— Ultrasonography reveals blood vessel conditions in the neck.
— Digital subtraction angiography identifies carotid occlusion.

— Magnetic resonance imaging helps identify the reason for obstruction by revealing carotid or other obstruction.

— Contrast-enhanced computed tomography scan discloses the diseased carotid artery.

• Central retinal vein occlusion:

— Ophthalmoscopy (direct or indirect) reveals retinal hemorrhage, retinal vein engorgement, white patches among hemorrhages, and edema around the optic disk.

— Ultrasonography confirms or rules out occluded blood vessels.

• Diabetic retinopathy:

— Slit-lamp examination shows thickening of retinal capillary walls.

— Indirect ophthalmoscopy demonstrates retinal changes, such as microaneurysms (earliest change), retinal hemorrhages and edema, venous dilation and beading, exudates, vitreous hemorrhage, proliferation of fibrin into vitreous from retinal holes, growth of new blood vessels, and microinfarctions of nerve fiber layer.

— Fluorescein angiography shows leakage of fluorescein from dilated vessels and differentiates between microaneurysms and true hemorrhages.

• Hypertensive retinopathy:

— Ophthalmoscopy (direct or indirect) performed in early disease discloses hard and shiny deposits, tiny hemorrhages, narrowed arterioles, nicking of the veins where arteries cross them (referred to as arteriovenous nicking), and elevated arterial blood pressure. The same test in later disease shows cotton wool patches, exudates, retinal edema, papilledema caused by ischemia and capillary insufficiency, hemorrhages, and microaneurysms.

— History reveals hypertension and decreased vision.

Vasculitis

• Polyarteritis nodosa:

— History reveals hypertension, abdominal pain, myalgia, headache, joint pain, and weakness.

— elevated erythrocyte sedimentation rate (ESR)

— leukocytosis

— anemia

— thrombocytosis

— depressed C3 complement

— rheumatoid factor greater than 1:60

— circulating immune complexes

— Tissue biopsy shows necrotizing vasculitis.

• Allergic angiitis and granulomatosis:

— History reveals asthma.

— eosinophilia

— A tissue biopsy may show granulomatous inflammation with eosinophilic infiltration.

• Polyangiitis overlap syndrome:

— History reveals allergy.

— eosinophilia

— Tissue biopsy may show granulomatous inflammation with eosinophilic infiltration.

• Wegener's granulomatosis:

— Tissue biopsy reveals necrotizing vasculitis with granulomatous inflammation.

— leukocytosis

— elevated ESR and immunoglobulin A (IgA) and IgG levels

— low titer rheumatoid factor

— circulating immune complexes.

• Temporal arteritis:

— decreased hemoglobin level

— elevated ESR

— Tissue biopsy shows panarteritis with infiltration of mononuclear cells, giant cells within vessel wall, fragmentation of internal elastic lamina, and proliferation of intima.

• Takayasu's arteritis:

— decreased hemoglobin level

— leukocytosis

— positive lupus erythematosus cell preparation and elevated ESR

— Arteriography shows calcification and obstruction of affected vessels.

— Tissue biopsy shows inflammation of adventitia and intima of vessels and thickening of vessel walls.

• Hypersensitivity vasculitis:
— history of exposure to an antigen such as a microorganism or a drug
— Tissue biopsy may show leukocyto-clastic angiitis usually in postcapillary venules, with infiltration of polymor-phonuclear leukocytes, fibrinoid necro-sis, and extravasation of erythrocytes.

• Mucocutaneous lymph node syndrome:
— History and examination reveal fe-ver; nonsuppurative cervical adenitis; edema; congested conjunctivae; erythe-ma of oral cavity, lips, and palms; and desquamation of finger tips.
— Tissue biopsy may show intimal proliferation and infiltration of vessel walls with mononuclear cells.

Velopharyngeal insufficiency

• Examination reveals unintelligible speech.

• Fiber-optic nasopharyngoscopy per-mits monitoring of velopharyngeal pa-tency during speech and may identify the insufficiency.

• Ultrasonography shows air-tissue overlap reflecting the degree of velo-pharyngeal sphincter incompetence; an opening of greater than 20 mm^2 results in unintelligible speech.

Ventricular aneurysm

• History of persistent arrhythmias, on-set of heart failure, or systemic emboli-zation in a patient with left ventricular failure and a history of myocardial in-farction

• Chest X-ray reveals an abnormal bulge distorting the heart's contour (with large aneurysm).

• Left ventriculography reveals left ventricular enlargement, with an area of akinesia or dyskinesia and diminished cardiac function.

• Echocardiography reveals abnormal motion in the left ventricular wall.

Ventricular fibrillation

• Electrocardiography reveals the fol-lowing:
— Atrial rhythm is not measurable. Ventricular rhythm has no pattern or regularity.
— Atrial and ventricular rates are not measurable.
— P wave is not measurable.
— PR interval is not measurable
— Duration of the QRS complex is not measurable; configuration is wide and irregular.
— T wave is not measurable.

Ventricular septal defect

• Echocardiography or magnetic reso-nance imaging reveals large defect and its location in the septum, estimates the size of a left-to-right shunt, suggests pulmonary hypertension, and identifies associated lesions and complications.

• Cardiac catheterization determines the size and exact location of the defect, calculates the degree of shunting, deter-mines the extent of pulmonary hyper-tension, and detects associated defects.

• Chest X-ray is normal with small de-fects; in large defects, it shows cardio-megaly, left atrial and ventricular en-largement, and prominent pulmonary vascular markings.

• Electrocardiography is normal with small defects; in large defects, it shows left and right ventricular hypertrophy.

Ventricular tachycardia

• Electrocardiography reveals the fol-lowing:
— Atrial rhythm is not measurable. Ventricular rhythm is usually regular, but may be slightly irregular.
— Atrial rate can't be measured. Ven-tricular rate is usually rapid (140 to 220 beats/minute).
— P wave is usually absent. It may be obscured by and is dissociated from the QRS complex. Retrograde and upright P waves may be present.

— PR interval is not measurable.
— QRS complex has a duration greater than 0.12 second, has a bizarre appearance, and usually has increased amplitude.
— T wave occurs in the opposite direction of the QRS complex.
— QT interval is not measurable.

Vesicoureteral reflux

• History reveals symptoms of urinary tract infection.
• Examination reveals hematuria or strong-smelling urine (in infants).
• Palpation may reveal a hard, thickened bladder (if posterior urethral valves are causing an obstruction in male infants).
• Cystoscopy reveals reflux.
• Urinalysis reveals bacterial count greater than 100,000/mm^3, specific gravity less than 1.010, and increased pH.
• Excretory urography may show dilated lower ureter, ureter visible for its entire length, hydronephrosis, calyceal distortion, and renal scarring.
• Voiding cystourethrography identifies and determines the degree of reflux, shows when reflux occurs, and may also pinpoint the cause.
• Bladder catheterization identifies the amount of residual urine.

Vitamin A deficiency

• Dietary history reveals inadequate dietary intake of foods high in vitamin A.
• Ocular examination reveals xerophthalmia, Bitot's spots, perforation, and scarring.
• Serum levels of vitamin A are below 20 mcg/dl.
• Carotene levels are less than 40 mcg/dl.

Vitamin B deficiencies

• Dietary history reveals inadequate dietary intake of foods high in vitamin B.
• 24-hour urine test reveals:
— thiamine deficiency
— riboflavin deficiency
— niacin deficiency, with levels under 0.05 mg/g

— pyridoxine deficiency (if xanthurenic acid is less than 50 mg/day).
• Serum cobalamin levels less than 150 pg/ml
• Serum vitamin B_2 activity index less than 0.9

Vitamin C deficiency

• Dietary history reveals an inadequate intake of ascorbic acid.
• Serum ascorbic acid levels less than 0.2 mg/dl and white blood cell ascorbic acid levels less than 30 mg/dl

Vitamin D deficiency

• Dietary history reveals inadequate dietary intake of preformed vitamin D.
• Low or undetectable serum vitamin D_3 levels
• Plasma calcium serum levels less than 7.5 mg/dl
• Inorganic phosphorus serum levels less than 3 mg/dl
• Serum citrate levels less than 2.5 mg/dl
• Alkaline phosphatase levels less than 4 Bodansky units/dl
• X-rays reveal characteristic bone deformities and abnormalities, such as Looser's zones.

Vitamin E deficiency

• Dietary history reveals diet high in polyunsaturated fatty acids fortified with iron but not vitamin E.
• Serum alpha-tocopherol levels below 0.5 mg/dl in adults and below 0.2 mg/dl in infants
• Increased serum creatinine kinase levels
• Increased platelet levels

Vitamin K deficiency

• Prothrombin time 25% longer than the normal range of 10 to 20 seconds (in the absence of anticoagulant therapy or hepatic disease)
• Positive capillary fragility test

Vitiligo

• Examination reveals stark white skin patches.
• Wood's light examination in a darkened room detects vitiliginous patches; depigmented skin reflects the light, while pigmented skin absorbs it.

Vocal cord nodules and polyps

• History reveals persistent hoarseness.
• Indirect laryngoscopy initially shows small red nodes; later, white solid nodes appear on one or both cords.
• Indirect laryngoscopy shows unilateral or, occasionally, bilateral, sessile or pedunculated polyps of varying size anywhere on the vocal cords.

Vocal cord paralysis

• History and examination reveal hoarseness or airway obstruction.
• Indirect laryngoscopy reveals one or both cords fixed in an adducted or partially abducted position.

Volvulus

• History reveals sudden onset of severe abdominal pain.
• Examination reveals palpable abdominal mass.
• Abdominal X-rays reveal obstruction and abnormal air-fluid levels in the sigmoid and cecum (in midgut volvulus, abdominal X-rays may be normal).
• Barium enema reveals the following:
— In cecal volvulus, barium fills the colon distal to the section of cecum.
— In sigmoid volvulus in children, barium may twist to a point; in adults, barium may take on an "ace of spades" configuration.
• In midgut volvulus, upper GI series reveals obstruction and possibly a twisted contour in a narrow area near the duodenojejunal junction where barium will not pass.
• White blood cell count may be greater than 15,000/µl (in strangulation) or

greater than 20,000/µl (in bowel infarction).

Von Willebrand's disease

• History reveals family inheritance pattern.
• Prolonged bleeding time (greater than 6 minutes)
• Prolonged partial thromboplastin time (more than 45 seconds)
• Factor VIII-related antigens are decreased and Factor VIII activity level is low.
• Normal clot retraction and platelet aggregation

Vulvovaginitis

• Examination reveals vaginal discharge and inflammation of the vulva.
• Vaginal exudate culture reveals presence of *Trichomonas vaginalis, Candida albicans, Gardnerella vaginitis, Neisseria gonorrhoeae,* or *Phthirus pubis.*

Warts

• Visual examination reveals evidence of irregular growth on skin.
• Sigmoidoscopy may rule out internal involvement in recurrent anal warts.

Whooping cough

• Examination reveals forceful coughing that ends in a characteristic whoop.
• Nasopharyngeal swabs and sputum cultures reveal *Bordetella pertussis* (in the early stages of illness).
• White blood cell count greater than 10,000/µl and possibly up to 200,000/µl, with 60% to 90% lymphocytes

Wilms' tumor

• Examination reveals palpable abdominal mass in early childhood.
• Gallium scan reveals abnormal activity.
• Percutaneous renal biopsy reveals malignant cells.
• Excretory urography does not indicate neoplasm or extrarenal mass.

Wilson's disease

• Slit-lamp ophthalmic examination reveals Kayser-Fleischer rings (in advanced disease).
• Liver biopsy reveals excessive copper deposits (250 mcg/g dry weight) and tissue changes indicative of chronic active hepatitis, fatty liver, or cirrhosis.
• Serum ceruloplasmin less than 20 mg/dl
• Serum copper less than 80 mcg/dl
• Urine copper greater than 100 mcg/24 hours (may be as high as 1,000 mcg)

Wiskott-Aldrich syndrome

• History reveals thrombocytopenia, bleeding disorders at birth, and recurrent infections.
• Platelet count below 100,000/mm^3
• Normal or elevated immunoglobulin E (IgE) levels
• Normal IgG and IgA levels
• Decreased IgM levels
• Low or absent isohemagglutinin levels
• Sputum and throat cultures commonly identify *Streptococcus pneumoniae,* meningococci, and *Haemophilus influenzae* as the causative organisms.

Wounds, open trauma

• History reveals injury.
• Examination reveals open wound.
• X-rays reveal bone damage, extent of injury to the area and surrounding tissue, and retention of injuring object.
• Electromyography reveals isolated, irregular motor unit potentials with increased amplitude and duration indicating peripheral nerve injury.
• Nerve conduction studies reveal abnormal nerve conduction time indicating peripheral nerve injury.
• Complete blood count reveals decreased hemoglobin and hematocrit levels and increased white blood cell count (above 10,000 /μl).

X-linked infantile hypogammaglobulinemia

• Serum immunoglobulin M (IgM), IgA, and IgG decreased or absent (in patient at least 9 months old)
• Antigenic stimulation testing confirms an inability to produce specific antibodies, although cellular immunity remains intact.

Yellow fever

• Blood culture reveals presence of arbovirus.
• Increased urine albumin levels (in 90% of patients)
• Elevated antibody titer

Zinc deficiency

• History reveals excessive intake of foods containing iron, calcium, vitamin D, and the fiber and phytates in cereals.
• Serum zinc levels below 121 μg/dl

PART TWO

DIAGNOSTIC TESTS

CHAPTER 1

Hematology and Coagulation Tests

RED BLOOD CELLS

RED BLOOD CELL COUNT

This test, also called an erythrocyte count, is part of a complete blood count. It is used to detect the number of red blood cells (RBCs) in a microliter (cubic millimeter) of whole blood.

Purpose
• To provide data for calculating mean corpuscular volume and mean corpuscular hemoglobin, which reveal RBC size and hemoglobin content
• To support other hematologic tests for diagnosing anemia or polycythemia

Patient preparation
• Explain to the patient that this test is used to evaluate the number of RBCs and to detect possible blood disorders.
• Tell him that a blood sample will be taken and explain who will perform the venipuncture and when.
• Reassure him that drawing a blood sample will take less than 3 minutes.
• Explain that there may be slight discomfort from the tourniquet pressure and the needle puncture.
• If the patient is a child, explain to him (if he is old enough) and his parents that a small amount of blood will be taken from the finger or earlobe.
• Inform the patient that food or fluids need not be restricted before the test.

Procedure and posttest care
• For adults and older children, draw venous blood into a 7-ml *lavender-top* tube.
• For younger children, collect capillary blood in a microcollection device.

• If a hematoma develops at the venipuncture site, apply warm soaks to ease discomfort.

Precautions
• Completely fill the collection tube.
• Invert the tube gently several times to mix the sample and the anticoagulant.
• Handle the sample gently to prevent hemolysis.

Reference values
Normal RBC values vary, depending on the type of sample and on the patient's age and sex, as follows:
• Adult males: 4.2 to 5.4 million RBCs/µl of venous blood
• Adult females: 3.6 to 5.0 million RBCs/µl of venous blood
• Children: 4.6 to 4.8 million RBCs/µl of venous blood
• Full-term infants: 4.4 to 5.8 million RBCs/µl of capillary blood at birth, decreasing to 3 to 3.8 million RBCs/µl at age 2 months, and increasing slowly thereafter.
  Normal values may exceed these levels in patients living at high altitudes.

Abnormal findings
An elevated RBC count may indicate absolute or relative polycythemia. A depressed count may indicate anemia, fluid overload, or hemorrhage beyond 24 hours. Further tests, such as stained cell examination, hematocrit, hemoglobin, red cell indices, and white cell studies are needed to confirm diagnosis.

HEMATOCRIT

A hematocrit (HCT) test may be done separately or as part of a complete blood count. It measures percentage by volume of packed red blood cells (RBCs) in a whole blood sample — for example, 40% HCT indicates 40 ml of packed RBCs in a 100-ml sample. Packing is achieved by centrifuging anticoagulated whole blood in a capillary tube, so that red cells are tightly packed without hemolysis.

Purpose
• To aid diagnosis of polycythemia, anemia, or abnormal states of hydration
• To aid calculation of two red cell indices: mean corpuscular volume and mean corpuscular hemoglobin concentration

Patient preparation
• Explain to the patient that HCT is tested to detect anemia and other abnormal blood conditions.
• Tell him that a capillary blood sample will be taken and explain who will perform the test and when.
• If the patient is a child, explain to him and his parents that a small amount of blood will be taken from the finger or earlobe.
• Inform the patient that food or fluids need not be restricted before the test.

Procedure and posttest care
• Perform a fingerstick, using a heparinized capillary tube with a red band on the anticoagulant end.
• Fill the capillary tube from the red-banded end to about two-thirds capacity, and seal this end with clay.
• If a hematoma develops at the venipuncture site, apply warm soaks to ease discomfort.

Precautions
• Send the sample to the laboratory immediately.
• If you perform the test, place the tube in the centrifuge with the red end pointing outward.

Reference values
HCT is usually measured electronically. The results are 3% lower than manual measurements, which trap plasma in the column of packed RBCs.

Reference values vary, depending on the type of sample, the laboratory performing the test, and the patient's sex and age, as follows:
• Newborns: 55% to 68% HCT
• 1 week old: 47% to 65% HCT
• 1 month old: 37% to 49% HCT
• 3 months old: 30% to 36% HCT
• 1 year old: 29% to 41% HCT
• 10 years old: 36% to 40% HCT
• Men: 42% to 54% HCT
• Women: 38% to 46% HCT.

Abnormal findings
Low HCT suggests anemia, hemodilution, or massive blood loss. High HCT indicates polycythemia or hemoconcentration due to blood loss and dehydration.

RED CELL INDICES

Using the results of the red blood cell (RBC) count, hematocrit, and total hemoglobin tests, the red cell indices (erythrocyte indices) provide important information about the size, hemoglobin concentration, and hemoglobin weight of an average red cell.

Purpose
• To aid diagnosis and classification of anemias

Patient preparation
• Explain to the patient that this test helps determine if he has anemia.
• Tell him the test requires a blood sample. Explain who will perform the venipuncture and when.

COMPARATIVE RED CELL INDICES IN ANEMIAS

	NORMAL VALUES (Normocytic, normochromic)	IRON DEFICIENCY ANEMIA (Microcytic, hypochromic)	PERNICIOUS ANEMIA (Macrocytic, normochromic)
MCV	84 to 99 μ^3	60 to 80 μ^3	95 to 150 μ^3
MCH	26 to 32 pg	5 to 25 pg	33 to 53 pg
MCHC	30% to 36%	20% to 30%	33% to 38%

• Tell him he may experience slight discomfort from the needle puncture and tourniquet pressure but that collecting the sample takes less than 3 minutes.

Procedure and posttest care
• Perform a venipuncture, and collect the sample in a 7-ml *lavender-top* tube.
• If a hematoma develops at the venipuncture site, apply warm soaks.

Precautions
• Completely fill the collection tube, and invert it gently several times to adequately mix the sample and anticoagulant.
• Handle the sample gently to prevent hemolysis.

Reference values
The indices tested include mean corpuscular volume (MCV), mean corpuscular hemoglobin (MCH), and mean corpuscular hemoglobin concentration (MCHC).

MCV, the ratio of hematocrit (packed cell volume) to the RBC count, expresses the average size of the erythrocytes and indicates whether they are undersized (microcytic), oversized (macrocytic), or normal (normocytic). MCH, the hemoglobin-RBC ratio, gives the weight of hemoglobin in an average red cell. MCHC, the ratio of hemoglobin weight to hematocrit, defines the concentration of hemoglobin

in 100 ml of packed red cells. It helps distinguish normally colored (normochromic) red cells from paler (hypochromic) red cells.

The range of normal red cell indices is as follows:
• MCV: 84 to 99 μ^3
• MCH: 26 to 32 pg
• MCHC: 30% to 36%.

Abnormal findings
Low MCV and MCHC indicate microcytic, hypochromic anemias caused by iron deficiency anemia, pyridoxine-responsive anemia, or thalassemia. A high MCV suggests macrocytic anemias caused by megaloblastic anemias, due to folic acid or vitamin B_{12} deficiency, inherited disorders of deoxyribonucleic acid synthesis, or reticulocytosis. Because MCV reflects the average volume of many cells, a value within normal range can encompass RBCs of varying size, from microcytic to macrocytic. (See *Comparative red cell indices in anemias*.)

ERYTHROCYTE SEDIMENTATION RATE

The erythrocyte sedimentation rate (ESR) measures the degree of erythrocyte settling in a blood sample during a specified time period. The ESR is a sensitive but nonspecific test that is frequently the earliest indicator of disease when other chemical or physical signs are normal. The ESR commonly increases significantly in widespread inflammatory disorders; elevations may be prolonged in localized inflammation and malignancy.

Purpose
• To monitor inflammatory or malignant disease
• To aid detection and diagnosis of occult disease, such as tuberculosis, tissue necrosis, or connective tissue disease

Patient preparation
• Explain to the patient that this test is used to evaluate the condition of red blood cells.
• Tell him that a blood sample will be taken. Explain who will perform the venipuncture and when.
• Reassure him that drawing a blood sample will take less than 3 minutes.
• Explain that there may be slight discomfort from the tourniquet pressure and the needle puncture.
• Inform the patient that food or fluids need not be restricted before the test.

Procedure and posttest care
• Perform a venipuncture, and collect the sample in a 7-ml *lavender-top*, 4.5-ml *black-top*, or 4.5-ml *blue-top* tube. Check with the laboratory to determine its preference.
• If a hematoma develops at the venipuncture site, apply warm soaks.

Precautions
• Completely fill the collection tube, and invert it gently several times to thoroughly mix the sample and the anticoagulant.
• Because prolonged standing decreases the ESR, examine the sample for clots or clumps and send it to the laboratory immediately. It must be tested within 2 hours.
• Handle the sample gently to prevent hemolysis.

Reference values
Normal sedimentation rates range from 0 to 20 mm/hour; rates gradually increase with age.

Abnormal findings
The ESR rises in pregnancy, anemia, acute or chronic inflammation, tuberculosis, paraproteinemias (especially multiple myeloma and Waldenström's macroglobulinemia), rheumatic fever, rheumatoid arthritis, and some malignancies.

Polycythemia, sickle cell anemia, hyperviscosity, and low plasma fibrinogen or globulin levels tend to depress ESR.

RETICULOCYTE COUNT

Reticulocytes are nonnucleated, immature red blood cells (RBCs) that remain in the peripheral blood for 24 to 48 hours while maturing. They're generally larger than mature RBCs. In this test, reticulocytes in a whole blood sample are counted and expressed as a percentage of the total red cell count. Because the manual method of reticulocyte counting uses only a small sample, values may be imprecise and should be compared with RBC count or hematocrit.

Purpose
• To aid in distinguishing between hypoproliferative and hyperproliferative anemias
• To help assess blood loss, bone marrow response to anemia, and therapy for anemia

Patient preparation

• Explain to the patient that this test is used to detect anemia or to monitor its treatment.

• Tell him that a blood sample will be taken. Explain who will perform the venipuncture and when.

• Reassure him that drawing a blood sample will take less than 3 minutes.

• Explain that there may be slight discomfort from the tourniquet pressure and the needle puncture.

• If the patient is an infant or child, explain to the parents that a small amount of blood will be taken from the finger or earlobe.

• Withhold antimalarials, antipyretics, azathioprine, chloramphenicol, corticotropin, dactinomycin, furazolidone (from infants), levodopa, methotrexate, phenacetin, and sulfonamides, as needed. If such medications must be continued, note this on the laboratory slip.

• Inform the patient that food or fluids need not be restricted before the test.

Procedure and posttest care

• Perform a venipuncture, and collect the sample in a 7-ml *lavender-top* tube.

• If a hematoma develops at the venipuncture site, apply warm soaks.

• Resume administration of medications withheld before the test.

• Monitor a patient with an abnormal reticulocyte count for trends or significant changes in repeated tests.

Precautions

• Completely fill the collection tube and invert it gently several times to mix the sample and the anticoagulant.

• Handle the sample gently to prevent hemolysis.

Reference values

Reticulocytes compose 0.5% to 2% of the total RBC count. In infants the normal reticulocyte count ranges from 2% to 6% at birth, decreasing to adult levels in 1 to 2 weeks.

Abnormal findings

A low reticulocyte count indicates hypoproliferative bone marrow (hypoplastic anemia) or ineffective erythropoiesis (pernicious anemia).

A high reticulocyte count indicates a bone marrow response to anemia caused by hemolysis or blood loss. The reticulocyte count may also increase after therapy for iron deficiency anemia or pernicious anemia.

OSMOTIC FRAGILITY

Osmotic fragility measures red cell resistance to hemolysis when exposed to a series of increasingly dilute saline solutions. The sooner hemolysis occurs, the greater the osmotic fragility of the cells.

Purpose

• To aid diagnosis of hereditary spherocytosis

• To supplement a stained cell examination to detect morphologic red cell abnormalities

Patient preparation

• Explain to the patient that this test is used to identify the cause of anemia.

• Tell him that a blood sample will be taken, who will perform the venipuncture, and when.

• Reassure him that drawing a blood sample will take less than 3 minutes.

• Explain that there may be slight discomfort from the tourniquet pressure and the needle puncture.

• Inform him that food or fluids need not be restricted before the test.

Procedure and posttest care
• Perform a venipuncture, collecting the sample in a 7-ml *green-top* (heparinized) tube, or secure a special heparinized tube for collecting defibrinated blood.
• If a hematoma develops at the venipuncture site, apply warm soaks.

Precautions
• Because this test isn't routinely performed, notify the laboratory before drawing the sample.
• Completely fill the collection tube and invert it gently several times to mix the sample and anticoagulant thoroughly.
• Handle the sample gently to prevent accidental hemolysis.
• In some cases, red cells don't hemolyze immediately; incubation in solution for 24 hours improves test sensitivity.

Reference values
Osmotic fragility values (percent of red blood cells hemolyzed) are plotted against decreasing saline tonicities to produce an S-shaped curve that's compared with characteristic curves for various disorders.

Abnormal findings
Low osmotic fragility (increased resistance to hemolysis) is characteristic of thalassemia, iron deficiency anemia, sickle cell anemia, and other red cell disorders in which codocytes (target cells) and leptocytes are found. Low osmotic fragility also occurs after splenectomy.

High osmotic fragility (increased tendency to hemolysis) occurs in hereditary spherocytosis, in spherocytosis associated with autoimmune hemolytic anemia, severe burns, or chemical poisoning, or in hemolytic disease of the newborn (erythroblastosis fetalis).

HEMOGLOBIN

TOTAL HEMOGLOBIN

This test is used to measure the amount of hemoglobin (Hb) found in a deciliter (100 ml) of whole blood. It is usually part of a complete blood count. Hb concentration correlates closely with the red blood cell (RBC) count.

Purpose
• To measure the severity of anemia or polycythemia and to monitor response to therapy
• To obtain data for calculating mean corpuscular hemoglobin and mean corpuscular hemoglobin concentration

Patient preparation
• Explain to the patient that this test is used to detect anemia or polycythemia, or to assess his response to treatment.
• Tell him that a blood sample will be taken. Explain who will perform the venipuncture and when.
• Reassure him that drawing a blood sample will take less than 3 minutes.
• Explain that there may be slight discomfort from the tourniquet pressure and the needle puncture.
• If the patient is an infant or child, explain to the parents that a small amount of blood will be taken from the finger or earlobe.
• Inform him that food or fluids need not be restricted before the test.

Procedure and posttest care
• For adults and older children, perform a venipuncture, and collect the sample in a 7-ml *lavender-top* tube.
• For younger children and infants, collect capillary blood in a pipette.

• If a hematoma develops at the venipuncture site, apply warm soaks.

Precautions
• Completely fill the collection tube and invert it gently several times to thoroughly mix the sample and the anticoagulant.
• Handle the sample gently to prevent hemolysis.

Reference values
Hb concentration varies, depending on the type of sample drawn (capillary blood samples for infants and venous blood samples for all others) and on the patient's age and sex, as follows:
• Newborns: 17 to 22 g/dl
• 1 week old: 15 to 20 g/dl
• 1 month old: 11 to 15 g/dl
• Children: 11 to 13 g/dl
• Men: 14 to 18 g/dl
• Men after middle age: 12.4 to 14.9 g/dl
• Women: 12 to 16 g/dl
• Women after middle age: 11.7 to 13.8 g/dl.

Abnormal findings
Low Hb concentration may indicate anemia, recent hemorrhage, or fluid retention, causing hemodilution.

Elevated Hb suggests hemoconcentration from polycythemia or dehydration.

HEMOGLOBIN ELECTROPHORESIS

Hemoglobin (Hb) electrophoresis is probably the most useful laboratory method for separating and measuring normal and some abnormal hemoglobins. Through electrophoresis, different types of Hb are separated to form a series of distinctly pigmented bands in a medium (cellulose acetate or starch gel). Results are then compared with those of a normal sample.

Hemoglobins A, A_2, S, and C are routinely checked, but the laboratory may change the medium or its pH to expand the range of this test.

Purpose
• To measure the amount of Hb A and to detect abnormal hemoglobins
• To aid diagnosis of thalassemia

Patient preparation
• Explain to the patient that this test is used to evaluate hemoglobin.
• Tell him that a blood sample will be taken, who will perform the venipuncture, and when.
• Reassure him that drawing a blood sample will take less than 3 minutes.
• Explain that there may be slight discomfort from the tourniquet pressure and the needle puncture.
• If the patient is an infant or child, explain to the parents that a small amount of blood will be taken from the finger or earlobe.
• Check for blood transfusion within the past 4 months.
• Inform the patient that food or fluids need not be restricted before the test.

Procedure and posttest care
• Perform a venipuncture, and collect the sample in a 7-ml *lavender-top* tube.
• For very young children, collect capillary blood in a microcollection device.
• If a hematoma develops at the venipuncture site, apply warm soaks.

Precautions
• Completely fill the collection tube, and invert it gently several times to mix the sample and the anticoagulant. Do not shake the tube vigorously.
• Handle the sample gently to prevent hemolysis.

VARIATIONS OF HEMOGLOBIN TYPE AND DISTRIBUTION

HEMOGLOBIN	PERCENTAGE OF TOTAL HEMOGLOBIN	CLINICAL IMPLICATIONS
Hb A	95% to 100%	Normal
Hb A$_2$	4% to 5.8%	ß-thalassemia minor
	2% to 3%	Normal
	Under 2%	Hb H disease
Hb F	Under 1%	Normal
	2% to 5%	ß-thalassemia minor
	10% to 90%	ß-thalassemia major
	5% to 15%	ß-δ-thalassemia minor
	5% to 35%	Heterozygous hereditary persistence of fetal hemoglobin (HPFH)
	100%	Homozygous HPFH
	15%	Homozygous Hb S
Homozygous Hb S	70% to 98%	Sickle cell disease
Homozygous Hb C	90% to 98%	Hb C disease

Reference values

In adults, Hb A accounts for more than 95% of all hemoglobins; Hb A$_2$, 2% to 3%; and Hb F, less than 1%. In neonates, Hb F normally accounts for half the total. Hemoglobins A and C are normally absent.

Abnormal findings

Hemoglobin electrophoresis allows identification of various types of hemoglobin. Certain types may indicate a hemolytic disease. The above chart shows some possible results and their associated conditions. The chart above shows some possible results and their associated conditions. (See *Variations of hemoglobin type and distribution*.)

SICKLE CELL TEST

This test, also known as the Hemoglobin S Test, is used to detect sickle cells, which are severely deformed, rigid erythrocytes that may slow blood flow. Sickle cell trait (Hb S) is found almost exclusively in people of African ancestry, affecting 0.2% of African Americans.

Although this test is useful as a rapid screening procedure, it may produce erroneous results. Hemoglobin electrophoresis should be performed to confirm the diagnosis if Hb S is strongly suspected.

Purpose
- To identify sickle cell disease and sickle cell trait

Patient preparation
- Explain to the patient that this test is used to detect sickle cell disease.
- Tell him that a blood sample will be taken. Explain who will perform the venipuncture and when.
- Reassure him that drawing a blood sample will take less than 3 minutes.
- Explain that there may be slight discomfort from the tourniquet pressure and the needle puncture.
- If the patient is an infant or child, explain to his parents that a small amount of blood will be taken from the finger or earlobe.
- Check patient history for blood transfusion within the past 3 months.
- Inform him that food or fluids need not be restricted before the test.

Procedure and posttest care
- Perform a venipuncture, and collect the sample in a 7-ml *lavender-top* tube.
- For very young children, collect capillary blood in a microcollection device.
- If a hematoma develops at the venipuncture site, apply warm soaks.

Precautions
- Completely fill the collection tube and invert it gently several times to thoroughly mix the sample and the anticoagulant.
- Do not shake the tube vigorously.

Reference values
Results of this test are reported as positive or negative. A negative result suggests the absence of Hb S.

Abnormal findings
A positive result may indicate the presence of sickle cells, but hemoglobin electrophoresis is needed to further diagnose the sickling tendency of cells.

Rarely, in the absence of Hb S, other abnormal hemoglobins may cause sickling.

UNSTABLE HEMOGLOBINS

Unstable hemoglobins are rare, congenital defects caused by amino acid substitutions in the structure of hemoglobin. The presence of unstable hemoglobins may lead to the formation of small masses called Heinz bodies, which accumulate on red blood cell membranes. Although Heinz bodies are usually removed by the spleen or liver, they may cause mild to severe hemolysis. Unstable hemoglobins are best detected by precipitation tests (heat stability or isopropanol solubility).

Purpose
- To detect unstable hemoglobins

Patient preparation
- Explain to the patient that this test is used to detect abnormal hemoglobin in the blood.
- Tell him that a blood sample will be taken. Explain who will perform the venipuncture and when.
- Reassure him that drawing a blood sample will take less than 3 minutes.
- Explain that there may be slight discomfort from the tourniquet pressure and the needle puncture.
- As necessary, withhold antimalarials, furazolidone (from infants), nitrofurantoin, phenacetin, procarbazine, or sulfonamides before the test, since these drugs may induce hemolysis. If these medications must be continued, note this on the laboratory slip.
- Inform the patient that food or fluids need not be restricted before the test.

Procedure and posttest care
• Perform a venipuncture, and collect the sample in a 7-ml *lavender-top* tube.
• If a hematoma develops at the venipuncture site, apply warm soaks.
• Resume administration of medications withheld before the test.
• If a hematoma develops at the venipuncture site, apply warm soaks.

Precautions
• Completely fill the collection tube, and invert it gently several times to mix the sample and the anticoagulant thoroughly.
• To avoid hemolysis, do not shake the tube vigorously.

Reference values
When no unstable hemoglobins appear in the sample, the heat stability test result is negative; the isopropanol solubility test result is reported as stable.

Abnormal findings
A positive heat stability test result or unstable solubility test result, especially with hemolysis, strongly suggests the presence of unstable hemoglobins.

HEINZ BODIES

Heinz bodies are particles of denatured hemoglobin that precipitate from the cytoplasm of red blood cells and accumulate on red blood cell membranes. Although Heinz bodies are removed from red cells by the spleen, they are a major cause of hemolytic anemias.

Heinz bodies can be detected in a whole blood sample using phase microscopy or supravital stains; when they do not form spontaneously, various oxidant drugs may be added to the sample to induce their formation.

Purpose
• To help detect causes of hemolytic anemia

Patient preparation
• Explain to the patient that this test is used to determine the cause of anemia.
• Tell him that a blood sample will be taken, who will perform the venipuncture, and when.
• Reassure him that drawing a blood sample will take less than 3 minutes.
• Explain that there may be slight discomfort from the tourniquet pressure and the needle puncture.
• Review the patient's drug history for medications that may interfere with accurate determination of test results; withhold antimalarials, furazolidone, nitrofurantoin, phenacetin, procarbazine, and sulfonamides. If medications must be continued, note this on the laboratory slip.
• Inform the patient that food or fluids need not be restricted before the test.

Procedure and posttest care
• Perform a venipuncture, collecting the sample in a 7-ml *lavender-top* tube.
• If a hematoma develops at the venipuncture site, apply warm soaks.
• Resume administration of medications withheld before the test.

Precautions
• Completely fill the sample collection tube and invert it gently several times to mix the sample and the anticoagulant; do not shake the tube vigorously.

Reference values
A negative test result indicates an absence of Heinz bodies.

Abnormal findings
The presence of Heinz bodies — a positive test result — may indicate an inherited red cell enzyme deficiency, the presence of unstable hemoglobins,

thalassemia, or drug-induced red cell injury. Heinz bodies may also be present after splenectomy.

IRON AND TOTAL IRON-BINDING CAPACITY

Iron is essential to the formation and function of hemoglobin, as well as many other heme and nonheme compounds. After iron is absorbed by the intestine, it is distributed to various body compartments for synthesis, storage, and transport.

An iron assay is used to measure the amount of iron bound to transferrin in blood plasma. Total iron-binding capacity (TIBC) measures the amount of iron that would appear in plasma if all the transferrin were saturated with iron.

Serum iron and TIBC are of greater diagnostic usefulness when performed with the serum ferritin assay, but together these tests may not accurately reflect the state of other iron compartments, such as myoglobin iron and the labile iron pool. Bone marrow or liver biopsy, and iron absorption or excretion studies may yield more information.

Purpose
- To estimate total iron storage
- To aid diagnosis of hemochromatosis
- To help distinguish iron deficiency anemia from anemia of chronic disease
- To help evaluate nutrition status

Patient preparation
- Explain to the patient that this test evaluates the body's capacity to store iron.
- Tell him that a blood sample will be taken, who will perform the venipuncture, and when.

- Reassure him that drawing a blood sample will take less than 3 minutes.
- Explain that there may be slight discomfort from the tourniquet pressure and the needle puncture.
- Review the patient's drug history for medications that may interfere with test results; withhold chloramphenicol, corticotropin, iron supplements, and oral contraceptives. If such medications must be continued, note this on the laboratory slip.
- Inform the patient that food or fluids need not be restricted before the test.

Procedure and posttest care
- Perform a venipuncture, collecting the sample in a 7-ml *red-top* tube.
- If a hematoma develops at the venipuncture site, apply warm soaks.
- Resume administration of medications withheld before the test.

Precautions
- Handle the sample gently to prevent hemolysis; send it to the laboratory immediately.

Reference values
Normal serum iron and TIBC values are as follows.

	SERUM IRON (mcg/dl)	TIBC (mcg/dl)	SATURATION (%)
Men	70 to 150	300 to 400	20 to 50
Women	80 to 150	300 to 450	20 to 50

Abnormal findings
In iron deficiency, serum iron levels decrease and TIBC increases, which decreases saturation. In cases of chronic inflammation (such as in rheumatoid arthritis), serum iron may be low in the presence of adequate body stores, but TIBC may be unchanged or may decrease to preserve normal saturation.

SIDEROCYTE STAIN

Siderocytes are red blood cells (RBCs) containing particles of non-hemoglobin iron known as siderocytic granules. In newborn infants, siderocytic granules are normally present in normoblasts and reticulocytes during hemoglobin synthesis. However, the spleen removes most of these granules from normal RBCs, and they disappear rapidly with age. In adults, an elevated siderocyte level usually indicates abnormal erythropoiesis, which may occur in congenital spherocytic anemia, chronic hemolytic anemias (such as the thalassemias), pernicious anemia, hemochromatosis, toxicities (such as lead poisoning), infection, or severe burns. Elevated levels may also follow splenectomy, because the spleen normally removes siderocytic granules.

Performing the test

The siderocyte stain test measures the number of circulating siderocytes. Venous blood is drawn into a 7-ml *lavender-top* tube or, for infants and children, collected in a Microtainer or a pipette and smeared directly on a 3" by 1" glass slide. When the blood smear is stained, siderocytic granules appear as purple-blue specks clustered around the periphery of mature erythrocytes. Cells containing these granules are counted as a percentage of total RBCs. The results aid differential diagnosis of the anemias and hemochromatosis and help detect toxicities.

Interpreting results

Normally, newborn infants have a slightly elevated siderocyte level that reaches the normal adult value of 0.5% of total RBCs in 7 to 10 days. In patients with pernicious anemia, the siderocyte level is 8% to 14%; in chronic hemolytic anemia, 20% to 100%; in lead poisoning, 10% to 30%; and in hemochromatosis, 3% to 7%. A high siderocyte level mandates additional testing — including bone marrow examination — to determine the cause of abnormal erythropoiesis.

Iron overload may not alter serum levels until relatively late, but in general, serum iron increases and TIBC remains the same, which increases the saturation. (See *Siderocyte stain*.)

FERRITIN

Ferritin, a major iron-storage protein, normally appears in small quantities in serum. In healthy adults, serum ferritin levels are directly related to the amount of available iron stored in the body and can be measured accurately by radioimmunoassay.

Purpose

• To screen for iron deficiency and iron overload
• To measure iron storage
• To distinguish between iron deficiency (a condition of low iron storage) and chronic inflammation (a condition of normal storage)

Patient preparation

• Explain to the patient that this test is used to assess the available iron stored in the body.

- Tell him that a blood sample will be taken, who will perform the venipuncture, and when.
- Reassure him that drawing a blood sample will take less than 3 minutes.
- Explain that there may be slight discomfort from the tourniquet pressure and the needle puncture.
- Review the patient's history for transfusion within the last 4 months.
- Inform the patient that food or fluids need not be restricted before the test.

Procedure and posttest care
- Perform a venipuncture, collecting the sample in a 10-ml *red-top* tube.
- If a hematoma develops at the venipuncture site, apply warm soaks.

Reference values
Normal serum ferritin values vary with age. According to the Mayo Medical Laboratories, serum ferritin levels range as follows:
- Neonates: 25 to 200 ng/ml
- 1 month: 200 to 600 ng/ml
- 2 to 5 months: 50 to 200 ng/ml
- 6 months to 15 years: 7 to 140 ng/ml
- Men: 20 to 300 ng/ml
- Women: 20 to 120 ng/ml.

Abnormal findings
High serum ferritin levels may indicate acute or chronic hepatic disease, iron overload, leukemia, acute or chronic infection or inflammation, Hodgkin's disease, or chronic hemolytic anemias; in these disorders, iron stores in the bone marrow may be normal or significantly increased. Serum ferritin levels are characteristically normal or slightly elevated in patients with chronic renal disease.

Low serum ferritin levels indicate chronic iron deficiency.

WHITE BLOOD CELLS

WHITE BLOOD CELL COUNT

A white blood cell (WBC) count, also called a leukocyte count, is part of a complete blood count. It indicates the number of white cells in a microliter (cubic millimeter) of whole blood.

WBC counts may vary by as much as 2,000 on any given day, due to strenuous exercise, stress, or digestion. The WBC count may increase or decrease significantly in certain diseases, but is diagnostically useful only when the patient's white cell differential and clinical status are considered.

Purpose
- To determine infection or inflammation
- To determine the need for further tests, such as the WBC differential or bone marrow biopsy
- To monitor response to chemotherapy or radiation therapy

Patient preparation
- Explain to the patient that the test is used to detect an infection or inflammation.
- Tell him that a blood sample will be taken. Explain who will perform the venipuncture and when.
- Reassure him that drawing a blood sample will take less than 3 minutes.
- Explain that there may be slight discomfort from the tourniquet pressure and the needle puncture.
- Inform the patient that he should avoid strenuous exercise for 24 hours

before the test. Also tell him that he should avoid ingesting a heavy meal before the test.

• If the patient is being treated for an infection, advise him that this test will be repeated to monitor his progress.

• Review the patient's medication history for drugs that may interfere with accurate determination of test results, including anti-infectives, anticonvulsants, thyroid hormone antagonists, and nonsteroidal anti-inflammatory agents. Note use of such medications on the laboratory slip.

Procedure and posttest care

• Perform a venipuncture, and collect the sample in a 7-ml *lavender-top* tube.

• If a hematoma develops at the venipuncture site, apply warm soaks.

• Tell the patient that he may resume normal activity that was discontinued before the test.

• A patient with severe leukopenia may have little or no resistance to infection and requires protective isolation.

Precautions

• Completely fill the sample collection tube, and invert it gently several times to mix the sample and the anticoagulant.

Reference values

The WBC count ranges from 4,000 to 10,000/mm^3.

Abnormal findings

An elevated WBC count (leukocytosis) often signals infection, such as an abscess, meningitis, appendicitis, or tonsillitis. A high count may also result from leukemia and tissue necrosis due to burns, myocardial infarction, or gangrene.

A low WBC count (leukopenia) indicates bone marrow depression that may result from viral infections or from toxic reactions, such as those following treatment with antineoplastics, ingestion of mercury or other heavy metals, or exposure to benzene or arsenicals. Leukopenia characteristically accompanies influenza, typhoid fever, measles, infectious hepatitis, mononucleosis, and rubella.

WHITE BLOOD CELL DIFFERENTIAL

The white blood cell (WBC) differential is used to evaluate the distribution and morphology of white cells, providing more specific information about a patient's immune system than the WBC count alone.

White blood cells are classified according to five major types of leukocytes — neutrophils, eosinophils, basophils, lymphocytes, and monocytes — and the percentage of each type is determined. The differential count is the percentage value of each type of white cell in the blood. The absolute number of each type of white cell is obtained by multiplying the percentage value of each type by the total WBC count.

High levels of these leukocytes are associated with various allergic diseases and reactions to parasites. An eosinophil count is sometimes ordered as a follow-up test when an elevated or depressed eosinophil level is reported.

Purpose

• To evaluate the body's capacity to resist and overcome infection

• To detect and identify various types of leukemia

• To determine the stage and severity of an infection

• To detect allergic reactions

• To assess the severity of allergic reactions (eosinophil count)

Reference Values for White Blood Cell Differential

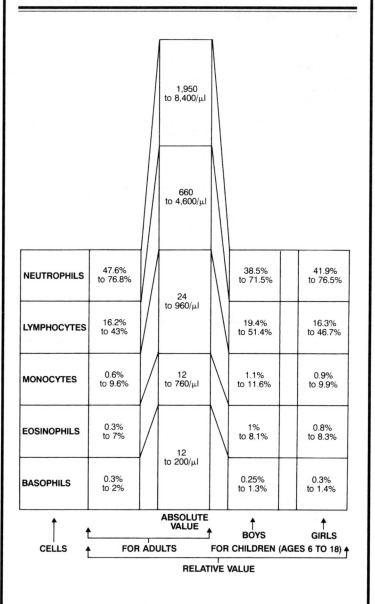

CELLS	FOR ADULTS (RELATIVE VALUE)	ABSOLUTE VALUE	FOR CHILDREN (AGES 6 TO 18) BOYS	FOR CHILDREN (AGES 6 TO 18) GIRLS
NEUTROPHILS	47.6% to 76.8%	1,950 to 8,400/μl	38.5% to 71.5%	41.9% to 76.5%
LYMPHOCYTES	16.2% to 43%	660 to 4,600/μl	19.4% to 51.4%	16.3% to 46.7%
MONOCYTES	0.6% to 9.6%	24 to 960/μl · 12 to 760/μl	1.1% to 11.6%	0.9% to 9.9%
EOSINOPHILS	0.3% to 7%	12 to 200/μl	1% to 8.1%	0.8% to 8.3%
BASOPHILS	0.3% to 2%		0.25% to 1.3%	0.3% to 1.4%

INFLUENCE OF DISEASE ON BLOOD CELL COUNT

CELL TYPE	HOW AFFECTED
Neutrophils	*Increased by:* • Infections: osteomyelitis, otitis media, salpingitis, septicemia, gonorrhea, endocarditis, smallpox, chicken pox, herpes, Rocky Mountain spotted fever • Ischemic necrosis due to myocardial infarction, burns, carcinoma • Metabolic disorders: diabetic acidosis, eclampsia, uremia, thyrotoxicosis • Stress response due to acute hemorrhage, surgery, excessive exercise, emotional distress, third trimester of pregnancy, childbirth • Inflammatory disease: rheumatic fever, rheumatoid arthritis, acute gout, vasculitis and myositis *Decreased by:* • Bone marrow depression due to radiation or cytotoxic drugs • Infections: typhoid, tularemia, brucellosis, hepatitis, influenza, measles, mumps, rubella, infectious mononucleosis • Hypersplenism: hepatic disease and storage diseases • Collagen vascular disease, such as systemic lupus erythematosus • Deficiency of folic acid or vitamin B_{12}
Eosinophils	*Increased by:* • Allergic disorders: asthma, hay fever, food or drug sensitivity, serum sickness, angioneurotic edema • Parasitic infections: trichinosis, hookworm, roundworm, amebiasis • Skin diseases: eczema, pemphigus, psoriasis, dermatitis herpes • Neoplastic diseases: chronic myelocytic leukemia, Hodgkin's disease, metastases and necrosis of solid tumors • Miscellaneous: collagen vascular disease, adrenocortical hypofunction, ulcerative colitis, polyarteritis nodosa, post-splenectomy, pernicious anemia, scarlet fever, excessive exercise *Decreased by:* • Stress response due to trauma, shock, burns, surgery, mental distress • Cushing's syndrome
Basophils	*Increased by:* • Chronic myelocytic leukemia, polycythemia vera, some chronic hemolytic anemias, Hodgkin's disease, systemic mastocytosis, myxedema, ulcerative colitis, chronic hypersensitivity states, and nephrosis *Decreased by:* • Hyperthyroidism • Ovulation, pregnancy • Stress

INFLUENCE OF DISEASE ON BLOOD CELL COUNT *(continued)*

Lymphocytes

Increased by:
• Infections: pertussis, brucellosis, syphilis, tuberculosis, hepatitis, infectious mononucleosis, mumps, rubella, cytomegalovirus
• Other: thyrotoxicosis, hypoadrenalism, ulcerative colitis, immune diseases, lymphocytic leukemia
Decreased by:
• Severe debilitating illness, such as congestive heart failure, renal failure, advanced tuberculosis
• Defective lymphatic circulation, high levels of adrenal corticosteroids, immunodeficiency due to immunosuppressives

Monocytes

Increased by:
• Infections: subacute bacterial endocarditis, tuberculosis, hepatitis, malaria, Rocky Mountain spotted fever
• Collagen vascular disease: systemic lupus erythematosus, rheumatoid arthritis, polyarteritis nodosa
• Carcinomas
• Monocytic leukemia
• Lymphomas

• To detect parasitic infections

Patient preparation
• Explain to the patient that this test is used to evaluate the immune system.
• Review the patient's history for use of medications that may interfere with test results, including methysergide, desipramine, indomethacin, procainamide, anticonvulsants, capreomycin, cephalosporins, D-penicillamine, gold compounds, isoniazid, nalidixic acid, novobiocin, para-aminosalicylic acid, paromomycin, penicillins, phenothiazines, rifampin, streptomycin, sulfonamides, and tetracyclines.
• Tell the patient that a blood sample will be taken. Explain who will perform the venipuncture and when.
• Inform the patient that he needn't restrict food or fluids but should refrain from strenuous exercise for 24 hours before the test.

• Reassure the patient that drawing a blood sample will take less than 3 minutes.
• Explain that there may be slight discomfort from the tourniquet pressure and the needle puncture.

Procedure and posttest care
• Perform a venipuncture, collecting the sample in a 7-ml *lavender-top* tube.
• If a hematoma develops at the venipuncture site, apply warm soaks.

Precautions
• Completely fill the collection tube; invert it gently several times to thoroughly mix the sample and the anticoagulant; to prevent hemolysis, do not shake the tube.

Reference values
For normal values for the five types of WBCs classified in the differential for adults and children, see *Reference values for white blood cell count differen-*

tial, page 101. For an accurate diagnosis, differential test results must always be interpreted in relation to the total white blood cell count.

Abnormal findings
Abnormal differential patterns provide evidence for a wide range of disease states and other conditions. (See *Influence of disease on blood cell count,* pages 102 and 103.)

PLATELET ACTIVITY

BLEEDING TIME

This test is used to measure the duration of bleeding after a measured skin incision. Bleeding time may be measured by one of four methods: Duke, Ivy, template, or modified template. The template methods are used most frequently and are the most accurate because the incision size is standardized. Bleeding time depends on the elasticity of the blood vessel wall and on the number and functional capacity of platelets. Although this test is usually performed on patients with personal or family histories of bleeding disorders, it is also useful for preoperative screening, along with a platelet count. It is usually not recommended for a patient whose platelet count is less than 75,000/mm³.

Purpose
• To assess overall hemostatic function (platelet response to injury and functional capacity of vasoconstriction)
• To detect congenital and acquired platelet function disorders

Patient preparation
• Explain to the patient this test is used to measure the time required to form a clot and stop bleeding.
• Tell him who will perform the test and when it will take place.
• Inform him that he need not restrict food or fluids before the test.
• Reassure the patient that, although he may feel some discomfort from the incisions, the antiseptic, and the tightness of the blood pressure cuff, the test takes only 10 to 20 minutes to perform. Advise the patient that the incisions will leave two small, hairline scars that should be barely visible when healed.
• Check patient history for recent use of drugs that prolong bleeding time, including sulfonamides, thiazides, antineoplastics, anticoagulants, nonsteroidal anti-inflammatory drugs, aspirin and aspirin compounds, and some nonnarcotic analgesics. If the patient has taken such drugs, check with the laboratory for special instructions. If the test is being used to identify a suspected bleeding disorder, it should be postponed and the drugs discontinued. If it is being used preoperatively, to assess hemostatic function, it should proceed as scheduled.

Equipment
Blood pressure cuff, disposable lancet, template with 9-mm slits (template method) or 5-mm slits (modified template method), spring-loaded blade (modified template method), 70% alcohol or povidone-iodine solution, filter paper, small pressure bandage, stopwatch.

Procedure and posttest care
• Template and modified template methods: Wrap the pressure cuff around the upper arm and inflate the cuff to 40 mm Hg. Select an area on the forearm free of superficial veins, and clean it with antiseptic. Allow the skin

to dry completely before making the incision. Apply the appropriate template lengthwise to the forearm. For the template method, use the lancet to make two incisions, 1 mm deep and 9 mm long. For the modified template method, use the spring-loaded blade to make two incisions, 1 mm deep and 5 mm long. Start the stopwatch. Without touching the cuts, gently blot the drops of blood with filter paper every 30 seconds, until the bleeding stops in both cuts. Average the time of the two cuts, and record the result.

• Ivy method: After applying the pressure cuff and preparing the test site, make three small punctures with a disposable lancet. Start the stopwatch immediately. Taking care not to touch the punctures, blot each site with filter paper every 30 seconds, until the bleeding stops. Average the bleeding time of the three punctures, and record the result.

• Duke method: Drape the patient's shoulder with a towel. Clean the earlobe, and let the skin air-dry. Then, make a puncture wound 2 to 4 mm deep on the earlobe, with a disposable lancet. Start the stopwatch. Being careful not to touch the ear, blot the site with filter paper every 30 seconds, until bleeding stops. Record bleeding time.

• In a patient with a bleeding tendency (hemophilia, for example), maintain a pressure bandage over the incision for 24 to 48 hours to prevent further bleeding; check the test area frequently; keep the edges of the cuts aligned to minimize scarring.

• In other patients, a piece of gauze held in place by an adhesive bandage is sufficient.

• Resume administration of medications discontinued before the test.

Precautions
• Maintain a pressure of 40 mm Hg throughout the test.

• If the bleeding does not diminish after 15 minutes, discontinue the test.

Reference values
The normal range of bleeding time is from 2 to 8 minutes in the template method; from 2 to 10 minutes in the modified template method; from 1 to 7 minutes in the Ivy method; and from 1 to 3 minutes in the Duke method.

Abnormal findings
Prolonged bleeding time may indicate the presence of disorders associated with thrombocytopenia, such as Hodgkin's disease, acute leukemia, disseminated intravascular coagulation, hemolytic disease of the newborn, Schönlein-Henoch purpura, severe hepatic disease (cirrhosis, for example), or severe deficiency of Factors I, II, V, VII, VIII, IX, and XI. Prolonged bleeding time in a person with a normal platelet count suggests a platelet function disorder (thrombasthenia, thrombocytopathia) and requires further investigation with clot retraction, prothrombin consumption, and platelet aggregation tests.

PLATELET COUNT

Platelets, or thrombocytes, are the smallest formed elements in blood. They promote coagulation and the formation of a hemostatic plug in vascular injury.

Platelet count is one of the most important screening tests of platelet function. Accurate counts are vital.

Purpose
• To evaluate platelet production
• To assess effects of chemotherapy or radiation therapy on platelet production

• To diagnose and monitor severe thrombocytosis or thrombocytopenia
• To confirm a visual estimate of platelet number and morphology from a stained blood film

Patient preparation
• Explain to the patient that this test is used to determine if the patient's blood clots normally.
• Tell him that a blood sample will be taken and explain who will perform the venipuncture and when.
• Inform the patient that food or fluids need not be restricted before the test.
• Reassure the patient that drawing a blood sample will take less than 3 minutes.
• Explain that there may be slight discomfort from the tourniquet pressure and the needle puncture.
• Check patient history for use of medications that may affect test results, including acetazolamide, acetohexamide, antimony, antineoplastics, brompheniramine maleate, carbamazepine, chloramphenicol, ethacrynic acid, furosemide, gold salts, hydroxychloroquine, indomethacin, isoniazid, mephenytoin, mefenamic acid, methazolamide, methimazole, methyldopa, oral diazoxide, oxyphenbutazone, penicillamine, penicillin, phenylbutazone, phenytoin, pyrimethamine, quinidine sulfate, quinine, salicylates, streptomycin, sulfonamides, thiazide and thiazide-like diuretics, and tricyclic antidepressants. Heparin causes transient, reversible thrombocytopenia. Notify the laboratory if such drugs have been used.

Procedure and posttest care
• Perform a venipuncture and collect the sample in a 7-ml *lavender-top* tube.
• If a hematoma develops at the venipuncture site, apply warm soaks.

Precautions
• To prevent hemolysis, avoid excessive probing at the venipuncture site and handle the sample gently.
• Completely fill the collection tube, and invert it gently several times to mix the sample and the anticoagulant thoroughly.

Reference values
Normal platelet counts range from 130,000 to 370,000/mm^3.

Abnormal findings
A decreased platelet count (thrombocytopenia) can result from aplastic or hypoplastic bone marrow; infiltrative bone marrow disease, such as carcinoma, leukemia, or disseminated infection; megakaryocytic hypoplasia; ineffective thrombopoiesis due to folic acid or vitamin B_{12} deficiency; pooling of platelets in an enlarged spleen; increased platelet destruction due to drugs or immune disorders; disseminated intravascular coagulation; Bernard-Soulier syndrome; or mechanical injury to platelets.

A platelet count that falls below 50,000 can cause spontaneous bleeding; when it drops below 5,000, fatal central nervous system bleeding or massive gastrointestinal hemorrhage is possible.

An increased platelet count (thrombocytosis) can result from hemorrhage; infectious disorders; malignancies; iron deficiency anemia; recent surgery, pregnancy, or splenectomy; and inflammatory disorders, such as collagen vascular disease. In such cases, the platelet count returns to normal after the patient recovers from the primary disorder. However, the count remains elevated in primary thrombocythemia, myelofibrosis with myeloid metaplasia, polycythemia vera, and chronic myelogenous leukemia.

When the platelet count is abnormal, diagnosis usually requires further studies, such as complete blood count, bone marrow biopsy, direct antiglobulin test (direct Coombs' test), and serum protein electrophoresis.

CAPILLARY FRAGILITY

Also called the tourniquet test, the capillary fragility test is a nonspecific method for evaluating bleeding tendencies. A positive-pressure test, it is used to measure the capillaries' ability to remain intact under increased intracapillary pressure, which is controlled by a blood pressure cuff around the patient's upper arm.

Purpose
• To assess the fragility of capillary walls
• To identify platelet deficiency (thrombocytopenia)

Patient preparation
• Explain to the patient that this test is used to identify abnormal bleeding tendencies.
• Tell him who will perform the procedure and when.
• Inform him that food or fluids need not be restricted.
• Explain that he may feel discomfort from the pressure of the blood pressure cuff.

Procedure and posttest care
• The patient's skin temperature and the room temperature should be normal to ensure accurate results.
• Select and mark a 2″ (5-cm) space on the patient's forearm. Ideally, the site should be free of petechiae; otherwise, record the number of petechiae present on the site before starting the test.

• Fasten the cuff around the arm, and raise the pressure to a point midway between the systolic and diastolic blood pressures. Maintain this pressure for 5 minutes; then release the cuff.
• Count the number of petechiae that appear in the 2″ (5-cm) space.
• Record test results.
• Encourage the patient to open and close his hand a few times to hasten return of blood to the forearm.

Precautions
• Do not repeat this test on the same arm within 1 week.
• This test is contraindicated in patients with disseminated intravascular coagulation (DIC) or other bleeding disorders, and in those with significant petechiae already present.

Reference values
A few petechiae may normally be present before the test. Less than 10 petechiae on the forearm 5 minutes after the test is considered normal, or negative; more than 10 petechiae is considered a positive result. The following scale may also be used to report test results:

NUMBER OF PETECHIAE/5 cm	SCORE
0 to 10	1+
11 to 20	2+
21 to 50	3+
51 or more	4+

Abnormal findings
A positive finding (more than 10 petechiae, or a score of 2+ to 4+) indicates weakness of the capillary walls (vascular purpura) or a platelet defect. It may occur in such conditions as thrombocytopenia, thrombasthenia, purpura senilis, scurvy, DIC, von Willebrand disease, vitamin K deficiency, dysproteinemia, polycythemia vera, and in severe deficiencies of Factor VII, fi-

brinogen, or prothrombin. Conditions unrelated to bleeding defects, such as scarlet fever, measles, influenza, chronic renal disease, hypertension, and diabetes with coexistent vascular disease, may also increase capillary fragility. An abnormal number of petechiae sometimes appears before menstruation and at other times in some healthy persons, especially in women over age 40.

PLATELET AGGREGATION

After vascular injury, platelets gather at the injury site and clump together to form an aggregate or plug that helps maintain hemostasis and promotes healing. The platelet aggregation test, an in vitro procedure, is used to measure the rate at which the platelets in a plasma sample form a clump after the addition of an aggregating reagent.

Purpose
• To assess platelet aggregation
• To detect congenital and acquired platelet bleeding disorders

Patient preparation
• Explain to the patient that this test is used to determine if blood clots properly.
• Tell him that the test requires a blood sample, who will perform the venipuncture, and when.
• Reassure him that drawing a blood sample will take less than 3 minutes.
• Explain that there may be slight discomfort from the tourniquet pressure and the needle puncture.
• Instruct the patient to fast or to maintain a nonfat diet for 8 hours before the test, because lipemia can affect test findings.

• Withhold aspirin and aspirin compounds for 14 days, and phenylbutazone, sulfinpyrazone, phenothiazines, antihistamines, anti-inflammatory drugs, and tricyclic antidepressants for 48 hours. If these medications must be continued, note this on the laboratory slip.

Procedure and posttest care
• Perform a venipuncture, and collect the sample in a 7-ml *blue-top* siliconized tube.
• Completely fill the collection tube, and invert it gently several times to mix the sample and the anticoagulant thoroughly.
• Maintain the sample at 71.6° F (22° C) to 98.6° F (37° C) to prevent aggregation.
• Apply pressure to the venipuncture site for 5 minutes, or until bleeding stops.
• Resume diet and administration of medications withheld before the test.
• If a hematoma develops at the venipuncture site, apply warm soaks.

Precautions
• Because the list of medications known to alter the results of this test is long and continually growing, the patient should be as free of drugs as possible before the test.
• If the patient has taken aspirin within the past 14 days and the test cannot be postponed, ask the laboratory to verify the presence of aspirin in the plasma. If test results are abnormal for such a sample, the use of aspirin must be discontinued and the test repeated in 2 weeks.
• Avoid excessive probing at the venipuncture site.
• Remove the tourniquet promptly to avoid bruising.
• Handle the sample gently to prevent hemolysis.

Reference values
Normal aggregation occurs in 3 to 5 minutes, but findings are temperature-dependent and vary with the laboratory. Aggregation curves obtained by using different reagents help to distinguish various qualitative platelet defects.

Abnormal findings
Abnormal findings may indicate von Willebrand disease, Bernard-Soulier syndrome, storage pool disease, Glanzmann's thrombasthenia, or polycythemia vera.

COAGULATION

ACTIVATED PARTIAL THROMBOPLASTIN TIME

The activated partial thromboplastin time (APTT) test is used to evaluate all the clotting factors of the intrinsic pathway — except platelets — by measuring the time required for formation of a fibrin clot after the addition of calcium and phospholipid emulsion to a plasma sample. An activator, such as kaolin, is used to shorten clotting time.

Purpose
• To aid preoperative screening for bleeding tendencies
• To screen for congenital coagulation deficiencies of the clotting factors
• To monitor heparin therapy

Patient preparation
• Explain to the patient that this test is used to determine if blood clots normally.

• Tell him that a blood sample will be taken, who will perform the venipuncture, and when.
• Reassure him that drawing a blood sample will take less than 3 minutes.
• Explain that there may be slight discomfort from the tourniquet pressure and the needle puncture.
• When appropriate, tell the patient receiving heparin therapy that this test may be repeated at regular intervals to assess the response to treatment.
• Inform the patient that food or fluids need not be restricted before the test.

Procedure and posttest care
• Perform a venipuncture, and collect the sample in a 7-ml *blue-top* tube.
• If a hematoma develops at the venipuncture site, apply warm soaks.

Precautions
• Completely fill the collection tube, invert it gently several times, and send it to the laboratory on ice.
• To prevent hemolysis, avoid excessive probing at the venipuncture site and handle the sample gently.
• For a patient on anticoagulant therapy, additional pressure may be needed at the venipuncture site to control bleeding.

Reference values
Normally, a fibrin clot forms 25 to 36 seconds after addition of reagents. For a patient on anticoagulant therapy, ask the attending doctor to specify the reference values for the therapy being delivered.

Abnormal findings
Prolonged APTT may indicate a deficiency of certain plasma clotting factors, the presence of heparin, or the presence of fibrin split products, fibrinolysins, or circulating anticoagulants that are antibodies to specific clotting factors.

PROTHROMBIN TIME

The prothrombin time (PT) test measures the time required for a fibrin clot to form in a citrated plasma sample after addition of calcium ions and tissue thromboplastin (Factor III).

Purpose
• To provide an overall evaluation of extrinsic coagulation Factors V, VII, and X and of prothrombin and fibrinogen
• To monitor response to oral anticoagulant therapy

Patient preparation
• Explain to the patient that this test is used to determine if the blood clots normally.
• Check patient history for use of medications that may interfere with accurate determination of test results, including antihistamines, chloral hydrate, digitalis glycosides, diuretics, glutethimide, griseofulvin, progestin-estrogen combinations, pyrazinamide, vitamin K, and xanthines.
• Tell the patient that a blood sample will be taken, who will perform the venipuncture, and when.
• Reassure him that drawing a blood sample will take less than 3 minutes.
• Explain that there may be slight discomfort from the tourniquet pressure and the needle puncture.
• When appropriate, explain that this test is used to monitor the effects of oral anticoagulants; the test will be performed daily when therapy begins and will be repeated at longer intervals when medication levels stabilize.
• Inform the patient that food or fluids need not be restricted before the test.

Procedure and posttest care
• Perform a venipuncture, and collect the sample in a 7-ml *blue-top* tube.
• If a hematoma develops at the venipuncture site, apply warm soaks.

Precautions
• Completely fill the collection tube, and invert it gently several times to mix the sample and the anticoagulant thoroughly. If the tube is not filled to the correct volume, an excess of citrate appears in the sample.
• To prevent hemolysis, avoid excessive probing during venipuncture and handle the sample gently.
• Promptly send the sample on ice to the laboratory.

Reference values
Normally, PT values range from 10 to 14 seconds. Values vary, however, depending on the source of tissue thromboplastin and the type of sensing devices used to measure clot formation. In a patient receiving oral anticoagulants, PT is usually maintained between one and a half and two times the normal control value.

Abnormal findings
Prolonged PT may indicate deficiencies in fibrinogen; prothrombin; Factors V, VII, or X (specific assays can pinpoint such deficiencies); or vitamin K; and hepatic disease. Or it may result from ongoing oral anticoagulant therapy. Prolonged PT that exceeds two and a half times the control value is commonly associated with abnormal bleeding.

Prolonged PT can result from the use of corticotropin, anabolic steroids, cholestyramine resin, heparin I.V. (within 5 hours of collection), indomethacin, mefenamic acid, para-aminosalicylic acid, methimazole, oxyphenbutazone, phenylbutazone, phenytoin, propylthiouracil, quinidine, quinine, thyroid hor-

mones, or vitamin A or overuse of alcohol.

Prolonged or shortened PT results
can follow ingestion of antibiotics, barbiturates, hydroxyzine, sulfonamides,
salicylates (more than 1 g/day prolongs
PT), mineral oil, or clofibrate.

ACTIVATED CLOTTING TIME

Activated clotting time (ACT) measures whole blood clotting time. This
test is commonly performed during
procedures that require extracorporeal
circulation, such as cardiopulmonary
bypass, ultrafiltration, hemodialysis,
and extracorporeal membrane oxygenation (ECMO).

Purpose
• To monitor the effect of heparin
• To monitor the effect of protamine
sulfate in heparin neutralization
• To detect severe deficiencies in clot-
ting factors (except Factor VII)

Patient preparation
• Explain to the patient that this test is
used to monitor the effect of heparin on
the blood's ability to coagulate.
• Tell him that the test requires a blood
sample, which is usually drawn from an
existing vascular access site; therefore
no venipuncture will be needed.
• Explain who will perform the test and
that the test is usually done at the bedside.
• Explain that two blood samples will
be drawn. The first one will be discarded so that any heparin in the tubing
doesn't interfere with the results.
• If the sample is drawn from a line
with a continuous infusion, stop the infusion prior to drawing the sample.

Procedure and posttest care
• Withdraw 5 to 10 ml of blood from
the line and discard it.
• Withdraw a clean sample of blood
into the special tube containing celite
provided with the ACT unit.
• Activate the ACT unit and wait for the
signal to insert the tube.
• Flush the vascular access site according to your facility's protocol.

Precautions
• Guard against contamination with
heparin if drawn from an access site
containing heparin.

Reference values
In a non-anticoagulated patient, normal
ACT is 107 seconds plus or minus 13
seconds. During cardiopulmonary bypass, heparin is titrated to maintain an
ACT between 400 and 600 seconds.
During ECMO, heparin is titrated to
maintain the ACT between 220 and 260
seconds.

ONE-STAGE FACTOR ASSAY: EXTRINSIC COAGULATION SYSTEM

When the prothrombin time (PT) and
activated partial thromboplastin time
(APTT) are prolonged, a one-stage assay is used to detect a deficiency of Factor II, Factor V, or Factor X. If the PT is
abnormal but APTT is normal, Factor
VII may be deficient.

Purpose
• To identify a specific factor deficien-
cy in persons with prolonged PT or
APTT
• To study patients with congenital or
acquired coagulation defects

- To monitor the effects of blood component therapy in factor-deficient patients

Patient preparation
- Explain to the patient that this test is used to assess the function of the blood coagulation mechanism.
- Tell him that a blood sample will be taken, who will perform the venipuncture, and when.
- Reassure him that drawing a blood sample will take less than 3 minutes.
- Explain that there may be slight discomfort from the tourniquet pressure and the needle puncture.
- When the patient is factor deficient and receiving blood component therapy, tell him that he may need a series of tests.
- Withhold oral anticoagulants before the test. If they must be continued, note this on the laboratory slip.
- Inform the patient that food or fluids need not be restricted before the test.

Procedure and posttest care
- Perform a venipuncture, and collect the sample in a 7-ml *blue-top* tube.
- If a hematoma develops at the venipuncture site, apply warm soaks.
- A patient with a bleeding disorder may require a pressure bandage to stop bleeding at the venipuncture site.

Precautions
- If the patient has a suspected coagulation defect, avoid excessive probing during venipuncture; don't leave the tourniquet on too long (it will cause bruising); and apply pressure to the puncture site for 5 minutes, or until the bleeding stops.
- Completely fill the collection tube, and invert it gently several times to mix the sample and the anticoagulant.
- Handle the sample gently to prevent hemolysis, and send it to the laboratory immediately, or place it on ice.

Reference values
Diluted samples of the patient's plasma are added to a substrate plasma deficient in a single factor. The activity of this mixture is compared with normal activity. The reference range for most factors is approximately 50% to 150% of normal activity.

Abnormal findings
If the clotting time for the substrate mixture is prolonged compared to normal, the patient my be deficient in the factor being tested. Deficiency of Factor II, Factor VII, or Factor X may indicate hepatic disease or vitamin K deficiency. Deficiency of Factor X may also indicate disseminated intravascular coagulation (DIC). Factor V deficiency suggests severe hepatic disease, DIC, or fibrinogenolysis. Deficiencies of all four factors may be congenital, although absence of Factor II is lethal.

ONE-STAGE FACTOR ASSAY: INTRINSIC COAGULATION SYSTEM

When prothrombin time (PT) is normal but activated partial thromboplastin time (APTT) is abnormal, a one-stage assay is used to identify a deficiency in the intrinsic coagulation system: Factor VIII, Factor IX, Factor XI, or Factor XII.

Purpose
- To identify a specific factor deficiency
- To study patients with congenital or acquired coagulation defects
- To monitor the effects of blood component therapy in factor-deficient patients

Patient preparation
• Explain to the patient that this test is used to assess the function of the blood coagulation mechanism.
• Tell him that a blood sample will be taken, who will perform the venipuncture, and when.
• Reassure him that drawing a blood sample will take less than 3 minutes.
• Explain that there may be slight discomfort from the tourniquet pressure and the needle puncture.
• Withhold oral anticoagulants before the test. If such medications must be continued, note this on the laboratory slip.
• When the patient is factor deficient and receiving blood component therapy, tell him that a series of tests may be needed to monitor therapeutic progress.
• Inform the patient that food or fluids need not be restricted before the test.

Procedure and posttest care
• Perform a venipuncture, and collect the sample in a 7-ml *blue-top* tube.
• If a hematoma develops at the venipuncture site, apply warm soaks.
• A patient with a bleeding disorder may require a pressure bandage to stop bleeding at the venipuncture site.
• Resume administration of medications discontinued before the test.

Precautions
• If a coagulation defect is suspected, avoid excessive probing during venipuncture, don't leave the tourniquet on too long (it will cause bruising), and apply pressure to the puncture site for 5 minutes, or until the bleeding stops.
• Completely fill the collection tube, and invert it gently several times to mix the sample and the anticoagulant thoroughly.
• Handle the sample gently to prevent hemolysis, and send it to the laboratory immediately, or place it on ice.

Reference values
Diluted samples of the patient's plasma are added to a substrate plasma deficient in a single factor. The activity of this mixture is compared with normal activity. The reference range for most factors is approximately 50% to 150% of normal activity.

Abnormal findings
If the clotting time for the substrate mixture is prolonged compared to normal, the patient my be deficient in the factor being tested. Factor VIII deficiency may indicate hemophilia A, von Willebrand disease, or Factor VIII inhibitor. An acquired deficiency of Factor VIII may result from disseminated intravascular coagulation or fibrinolysis. Factor VIII antigen and ristocetin cofactor tests distinguish between hemophilia A (and its carrier state) and von Willebrand disease.

Factor IX deficiency may suggest hemophilia B, or it may be acquired as a result of hepatic disease, Factor IX inhibitor, vitamin K deficiency, or coumarin therapy. Factors VIII and IX inhibitors occur after transfusions in patients deficient in either factor and are antibodies specific to each factor.

Factor XI deficiency may appear after the stress of trauma or surgery, or transiently in neonates. Factor XII deficiency may be inherited or acquired (as in nephrosis) and may also appear transiently in neonates.

PLASMA THROMBIN TIME

The thrombin time (or thrombin clotting time) test measures how quickly a clot forms when a standard amount of bovine thrombin is added to a platelet-poor plasma sample from the patient and to a normal plasma control sample. After thrombin is added, the clotting time for each sample is compared and recorded. This test allows a quick but imprecise estimation of plasma fibrinogen levels.

Purpose
• To detect fibrinogen deficiency or defect
• To aid diagnosis of disseminated intravascular coagulation (DIC) and hepatic disease
• To monitor the effectiveness of treatment with heparin or thrombolytic agents

Patient preparation
• Explain to the patient that this test is used to determine if blood clots normally.
• If possible, withhold heparin therapy before the test. If heparin must be continued, note this on the laboratory slip.
• Tell the patient that a blood sample will be taken, who will perform the venipuncture, and when.
• Reassure him that drawing a blood sample will take less than 3 minutes.
• Explain that there may be slight discomfort from the tourniquet pressure and the needle puncture.
• Inform the patient that food or fluids need not be restricted before the test.

Procedure and posttest care
• Perform a venipuncture, and collect the sample in a 7-ml *blue-top* tube.
• If a hematoma develops at the venipuncture site, apply warm soaks.

Precautions
• If the tube isn't filled to the correct volume, an excess of citrate appears in the sample. Completely fill the collection tube, and invert it gently several times to mix the sample and the anticoagulant thoroughly.

• To prevent hemolysis, avoid excessive probing during venipuncture and rough handling of the sample.
• Immediately send the sample on ice to the laboratory.

Reference values
Normal thrombin times range from 10 to 15 seconds. Test results are usually reported with a normal control value.

Abnormal findings
A prolonged thrombin time may indicate heparin therapy, hepatic disease, DIC, hypofibrinogenemia, or dysfibrinogenemia. Patients with prolonged thrombin times may require measurement of fibrinogen levels; in suspected DIC, the test for fibrin split products is also necessary.

PLASMA FIBRINOGEN

Fibrinogen (Factor I) originates in the liver and is converted to fibrin during clotting. Because fibrin is necessary for clot formation, fibrinogen deficiency can produce mild-to-severe bleeding disorders.

This test is used to determine the amount of fibrinogen present in a blood sample. Note that fibrinogen deficiency may also be indicated by prolonged activated partial thromboplastin time, prothrombin time, and thrombin time.

Purpose
• To aid the diagnosis of suspected clotting or bleeding disorders caused by fibrinogen abnormalities

Patient preparation
• Explain to the patient that this test is used to determine if blood clots normally.

• Tell him that a blood sample will be taken. Explain who will perform the venipuncture and when.

• Reassure him that drawing a blood sample will take less than 3 minutes.

• Explain that there may be slight discomfort from the tourniquet pressure and the needle puncture.

• Check patient history for use of heparin or oral contraceptives and notify the laboratory if these drugs are in use.

• Inform the patient that food or fluids need not be restricted before the test.

Procedure and posttest care

• Perform a venipuncture, and collect the sample in a 7-ml *blue-top* tube.

• Completely fill the collection tube, invert it gently several times, and send it to the laboratory immediately, or place it on ice.

• Avoid excessive probing during venipuncture, and handle the sample gently.

• If a hematoma develops at the venipuncture site, apply warm soaks.

Precautions

• This test is contraindicated in patients with active bleeding and acute infection or illness, and in those who have received blood transfusions within 4 weeks.

Reference values

Fibrinogen levels normally range from 195 to 365 mg/dl.

Abnormal findings

Depressed fibrinogen levels may indicate congenital afibrinogenemia; hypofibrinogenemia or dysfibrinogenemia; disseminated intravascular coagulation; fibrinolysis; severe hepatic disease; cancer of the prostate, pancreas, or lung; or bone marrow lesions. Obstetric complications or trauma may cause low levels.

Fibrinogen levels below 100 mg/dl impede the accurate interpretation of coagulation tests that have a fibrin clot as an end point.

Elevated levels may indicate cancer of the stomach, breast, or kidney, or inflammatory disorders, such as pneumonia or membranoproliferative glomerulonephritis.

FIBRIN SPLIT PRODUCTS

After a fibrin clot forms in response to vascular injury, the clot is eventually degraded by plasmin, a fibrin-dissolving enzyme. The resulting fragments are known as fibrin split products (FSP), or fibrinogen degradation products. In this test, FSP are detected in the diluted serum that is left in a blood sample after clotting.

Purpose

• To detect FSP in the circulation

• To help determine the presence and approximate severity of a hyperfibrinolytic state (such as disseminated intravascular coagulation [DIC]) that may result in primary fibrinogenolysis or hypercoagulability

Patient preparation

• Explain to the patient that this test is used to determine if blood clots normally.

• Tell him that a blood sample will be taken. Explain who will perform the venipuncture and when.

• Reassure him that drawing a blood sample will take less than 3 minutes.

• Explain that there may be slight discomfort from the tourniquet pressure and the needle puncture.

• Check patient history for use of any medications (especially heparin) that

may interfere with accurate determination of test results.
• Inform the patient that food or fluids need not be restricted before the test.

Procedure and posttest care
• Perform a venipuncture, and then draw 2 ml of blood into a plastic syringe.
• Transfer the sample to the tube provided by the laboratory, which contains a soybean trypsin inhibitor and bovine thrombin.
• If a hematoma develops at the venipuncture site, apply warm soaks.

Precautions
• Draw the sample before administering heparin to avoid false-positive test results.
• Gently invert the collection tube several times to mix the contents thoroughly.
• The blood clots within 2 seconds and must then be immediately sent to the laboratory, to be incubated at 98.6° F (37° C) for 30 minutes before testing proceeds.

Reference values
Serum contains less than 10 mcg/ml of FSP. A quantitative assay shows levels of less than 3 mcg/ml.

Abnormal findings
FSP levels increase in primary fibrinolytic states, due to increased levels of circulating profibrinolysin; in secondary states, due to DIC and subsequent fibrinolysis; and in alcoholic cirrhosis, preeclampsia, abruptio placentae, congenital heart disease, sunstroke, burns, intrauterine death, pulmonary embolus, deep-vein thrombosis (transient increase), and myocardial infarction (after 1 or 2 days). FSP levels usually exceed 100 mcg/ml in active renal disease or renal transplant rejection.

PLASMA PLASMINOGEN

This test is used to assess plasminogen levels in a plasma sample. During fibrinolysis, plasmin dissolves fibrin clots to prevent excessive coagulation and impaired blood flow. Plasmin does not circulate in active form, however, so it cannot be directly measured. Its circulating precursor, plasminogen, can be measured and used to evaluate the fibrinolytic system.

Purpose
• To assess fibrinolysis
• To detect congenital and acquired fibrinolytic disorders

Patient preparation
• Explain to the patient that this test is used to evaluate blood clotting.
• Tell him that a blood sample will be taken, who will perform the venipuncture, and when.
• Reassure him that drawing a blood sample will take less than 3 minutes.
• Explain that there may be slight discomfort from the tourniquet pressure and the needle puncture.
• Check patient history for use of thrombolytic drugs, such as streptokinase or urokinase, and oral contraceptives that may cause inaccurate test results. If these drugs must be continued, note this on the laboratory slip.
• Inform the patient that food or fluids need not be restricted before the test.

Procedure and posttest care
• Perform a venipuncture and collect the sample in a 7-ml *blue-top* tube.
• If a hematoma develops at the venipuncture site, apply warm soaks.
• Resume medications withheld before the test.

Precautions

• Collect the sample as quickly as possible to prevent stasis, which can slow blood flow, causing coagulation and plasminogen activation.
• To prevent hemolysis, avoid excessive probing during venipuncture and rough handling of the sample.
• Immediately after collection, invert the tube gently several times and send the sample to the laboratory. If testing must be delayed, plasma must be separated and frozen at −94° F (−70° C).

Reference values

Normal plasminogen levels are 10 to 20 mg/dl by immunologic methods and 80 to 120 U/dl by functional methods.

Abnormal findings

Diminished plasminogen levels can result from disseminated intravascular coagulation, tumors, preeclampsia, and eclampsia, which accelerate plasminogen conversion to plasmin and increase fibrinolysis. Some liver diseases prevent formation of sufficient plasminogen, decreasing fibrinolysis.

PROTEIN C

Vitamin K-dependent, protein C is produced in the liver and circulates in the plasma. It acts as a potent anticoagulant by suppressing activated Factors V and VIII. Deficiencies of protein C may be acquired or congenital.

If a deficiency of protein C is identified, further immunologic tests may be needed to determine the type of deficiency. Identifying the role of protein C deficiency in idiopathic venous thrombosis may help prevent thromboembolism.

Purpose

• To investigate the cause of otherwise unexplained thrombosis and to establish inheritance patterns

Patient preparation

• Explain to the patient that this test evaluates blood clotting.
• Tell him that a blood sample will be taken, who will perform the venipuncture, and when.
• Reassure him that drawing a blood sample will take less than 3 minutes.
• Explain that there may be slight discomfort from the tourniquet pressure and the needle puncture.
• Inform the patient that food or fluids need not be restricted before the test.
• If the patient is receiving anticoagulant therapy, note this on the laboratory slip.

Procedure and posttest care

• Perform a venipuncture. Collect a 3-ml sample in a *blue-top* vacuum specimen tube or in a special syringe with anticoagulant provided by the laboratory.
• If a hematoma develops at the venipuncture site, apply warm soaks.

Precautions

• Avoid excessive probing during venipuncture.
• Completely fill the collection tube, and invert it several times to mix the sample and anticoagulant thoroughly; handle the sample gently.
• Send the sample to the laboratory immediately.

Reference values

The normal range is 70% to 140% of the population mean, depending on the test method.

Abnormal findings

Rare, homozygous protein C deficiency is characterized by rapidly fatal thrombosis in the perinatal period, a condition known as purpura fulminans.

The more common heterozygous deficiency is associated with genetic susceptibility to venous thromboembolism before age 30 and continuing throughout life. The patient may require long-term treatment with warfarin therapy or protein C supplements from plasma fractions.

EUGLOBULIN LYSIS TIME

This test measures the interval between clot formation and clot dissolution in plasma. A precipitated plasma extract is clotted with thrombin, and the time required for the clot to lyse is measured.

Purpose
• To assess the fibrinolytic system
• To help detect abnormal fibrinolytic states

Patient preparation
• Explain to the patient that this test is used to evaluate the blood clotting mechanism.
• Tell him that a blood sample will be taken, who will perform the venipuncture, and when.
• Reassure him that drawing a blood sample will take less than 3 minutes.
• Explain that there may be slight discomfort from the tourniquet pressure and the needle puncture.
• Inform the patient that food or fluids need not be restricted before the test.

Procedure and posttest care
• Perform a venipuncture. Collect a 4.5-ml sample in a *blue-top* tube or in a chilled tube with 0.5 ml sodium oxalate.

• If a hematoma develops at the venipuncture site, apply warm soaks.

Precautions
• When drawing the sample, be careful not to rub the area over the vein too vigorously, to pump the fist excessively, or to leave the tourniquet in place too long.
• Avoid excessive probing during venipuncture, and handle the sample gently.
• If a *blue-top* tube is used, mix the sample and anticoagulant thoroughly. If a chilled tube containing 0.5 ml sodium oxalate is used, mix the sample and preservative thoroughly, pack the sample in ice, and send it to the laboratory immediately.

Reference values
Normal lysis time is at least 2 hours.

Abnormal findings
Clot lysis within 1 hour indicates increased plasminogen activator activity. In pathologic fibrinolysis, lysis time may be as brief as 5 to 10 minutes.

CHAPTER 2

Blood Chemistry Tests

ARTERIAL BLOOD GASES

ELECTROLYTES

CARDIAC ENZYMES

HEPATIC ENZYMES

PANCREATIC ENZYMES

SPECIAL ENZYMES

LIPIDS AND LIPOPROTEINS

PROTEINS AND PROTEIN METABOLITES

PIGMENTS

CARBOHYDRATES

ARTERIAL BLOOD GASES

ARTERIAL BLOOD GAS ANALYSIS

Arterial blood gas (ABG) analysis is used to measure the partial pressures of oxygen (PaO_2) and carbon dioxide ($PaCO_2$), and the pH of an arterial sample. Oxygen content (O_2CT), oxygen saturation (SaO_2), and bicarbonate (HCO_3^-) values are also measured. A blood sample for ABG analysis may be drawn by percutaneous arterial puncture or from an arterial line.

Purpose
• To evaluate gas exchange in the lungs
• To assess integrity of the ventilatory control system
• To determine the acid-base level of the blood
• To monitor respiratory therapy

Patient preparation
• Explain to the patient that this test is used to evaluate how well the lungs are delivering oxygen to blood and eliminating carbon dioxide.
• Tell him that the test requires a blood sample. Explain who will perform the arterial puncture and when and which site — radial, brachial, or femoral artery — has been selected for the puncture.
• Inform him that he need not restrict food or fluids.
• Instruct the patient to breathe normally during the test, and warn him that he may experience a brief cramping or throbbing pain at the puncture site.

Procedure and posttest care
• Perform an arterial puncture.
• After applying pressure for 3 to 5 minutes to the puncture site, tape a gauze pad firmly over it. (If the puncture site is on the arm, do not tape the entire circumference; this may restrict circulation.)
• If the patient is receiving anticoagulants or has a coagulopathy, hold the puncture site longer than 5 minutes if necessary.
• Monitor vital signs, and observe for signs of circulatory impairment, such as swelling, discoloration, pain, numbness, or tingling in the bandaged arm or leg.
• Watch for bleeding from the puncture site.

Precautions
• Wait at least 15 minutes before drawing arterial blood if a change in oxygen therapy has been made or when starting or removing oxygen therapy.
• Before sending the sample to the laboratory, note whether the patient was breathing room air or receiving oxygen therapy when the sample was drawn and include this information on the laboratory slip.
• If the patient was receiving oxygen therapy, note the flow rate. If he is on a ventilator, note the fraction of inspired oxygen and tidal volume.
• Note the patient's rectal temperature and respiratory rate.

Reference values
Normal ABG values fall within the following ranges:
• PaO_2: 75 to 100 mm Hg
• $PaCO_2$: 35 to 45 mm Hg
• pH: 7.35 to 7.42
• O_2CT: 15% to 23%
• SaO_2: 94% to 100%
• HCO_3^-: 22 to 26 mEq/liter.

Acid-Base Disorders

DISORDERS AND A.B.G. FINDINGS	POSSIBLE CAUSES	SIGNS AND SYMPTOMS
Respiratory acidosis (excess CO_2 retention) pH < 7.35 HCO_3^- > 26 mEq/liter (if compensating) $PaCO_2$ > 45 mm Hg	• CNS depression from drugs, injury, or disease • Asphyxia • Hypoventilation due to pulmonary, cardiac, musculoskeletal, or neuromuscular disease	• Diaphoresis, headache, tachycardia, confusion, restlessness, apprehension
Respiratory alkalosis (excess CO_2 excretion) pH > 7.42 HCO_3^- < 22 mEq/liter (if compensating) $PaCO_2$ < 35 mm Hg	• Hyperventilation due to anxiety, pain, or improper ventilator settings • Respiratory stimulation by drugs, disease, hypoxia, fever, or high room temperature • Gram-negative bacteremia	• Rapid, deep respirations; paresthesia; lightheadedness; twitching; anxiety; fear
Metabolic acidosis (HCO_3^- loss, acid retention) pH < 7.35 HCO_3^- < 22 mEq/liter $PaCO_2$ < 35 mm Hg (if compensating)	• HCO_3^- depletion due to renal disease, diarrhea, or small bowel fistulas • Excessive production of organic acids due to hepatic disease; endocrine disorders, including diabetes mellitus; hypoxia; shock; or drug intoxication • Inadequate excretion of acids due to renal disease	• Rapid, deep breathing; fruity breath; fatigue; headache; lethargy; drowsiness; nausea; vomiting; coma (if severe)
Metabolic alkalosis (HCO_3^- retention, acid loss) pH > 7.42 HCO_3^- > 26 mEq/liter $PaCO_2$ > 45 mm Hg (if compensating)	• Loss of hydrochloric acid from prolonged vomiting, gastric suctioning • Loss of potassium due to increased renal excretion (as in diuretic therapy), steroid overdose • Excessive alkali ingestion	• Slow, shallow breathing; hypertonic muscles; restlessness; twitching; confusion; irritability; apathy; tetany; seizures; coma (if severe)

Abnormal findings

Low PaO_2, O_2CT, and SaO_2 levels, in combination with a high $PaCO_2$ value, may result from conditions that impair respiratory function, such as respiratory muscle weakness or paralysis, respiratory center inhibition (from head injury, brain tumor, or drug abuse, for example), and airway obstruction (possibly from mucous plugs or a tumor). Similarly, low readings may result from bronchiole obstruction caused by asthma or emphysema, from an abnormal ventilation-perfusion ratio due to partially blocked alveoli or pulmonary capillaries, or from alveoli that are damaged or filled with fluid because of disease, hemorrhage, or near-drowning.

When inspired air contains insufficient oxygen, PaO_2, O_2CT, and SaO_2 also decrease, but $PaCO_2$ may be normal. Such findings are common in pneumothorax, impaired diffusion between alveoli and blood (due to interstitial fibrosis, for example), or in an arteriovenous shunt that permits blood to bypass the lungs.

Low O_2CT — with normal PaO_2, SaO_2 and, possibly, $PaCO_2$ values — may result from severe anemia, decreased blood volume, and reduced hemoglobin oxygen-carrying capacity.

In addition to clarifying blood oxygen disorders, ABG values can give considerable information about acid-base disorders. (See *Acid-base disorders*.)

TOTAL CARBON DIOXIDE CONTENT

When carbon dioxide (CO_2) pressure in red blood cells exceeds 40 mm Hg, CO_2 spills out of the cells and dissolves in plasma. There it may combine with water to form carbonic acid, which in turn may dissociate into hydrogen and bicarbonate ions.

This test is used to measure the total concentration of all forms of CO_2 in serum, plasma, or whole blood samples. It is commonly ordered for patients with respiratory insufficiency and is usually included in any assessment of electrolyte balance. Test results are most significant when considered with pH and arterial blood gas values.

Purpose
• To help evaluate acid-base balance

Patient preparation
• Explain to the patient that this test is performed to measure the amount of CO_2 in the blood.
• Tell him that the test requires a blood sample. Explain who will perform the venipuncture and when.
• Explain that he may experience discomfort from the needle puncture and the tourniquet, but that collecting the sample usually takes less than 3 minutes.
• Inform the patient that he need not restrict food or fluids before the test.
• Check the patient's history for use of medications that may affect test results, including ACTH, cortisone, thiazide diuretics, salicylates, paraldehyde, methicillin, dimercaprol, ammonium chloride, or acetazolamide. Also note excessive ingestion of alkalis or licorice or accidental ingestion of ethylene glycol or methyl alcohol.

Procedure and posttest care
• Perform a venipuncture.
• When CO_2 content is measured along with electrolytes, a 7-ml *red-marble-top* tube may be used.
• When this test is performed alone, a *green-top* (heparinized) tube is appropriate.
• If a hematoma develops at the venipuncture site, apply warm soaks.

Precautions
• Completely fill the tube to prevent diffusion of CO_2 into the vacuum.

Reference values
Normally, total CO_2 levels range from 22 to 34 mEq/liter.

Abnormal findings
High CO_2 levels may occur in metabolic alkalosis, respiratory acidosis, prima-

ry aldosteronism, and Cushing's syndrome. CO_2 levels may also increase after excessive loss of acids, as in severe vomiting and continuous gastric drainage.

Decreased CO_2 levels are common in metabolic acidosis. Decreased total CO_2 levels in metabolic acidosis also result from loss of bicarbonate. Levels may decrease in respiratory alkalosis.

ELECTROLYTES

CALCIUM

This test is used to measure serum levels of calcium. More than 98% of the body's calcium is in bones and teeth, but relative concentrations in those structures may vary as the body maintains calcium balance. For example, when calcium concentrations in the blood fall below normal, calcium ions move out of the bones and teeth to restore the blood's calcium level. Because the body excretes calcium daily, regular ingestion of calcium in food (at least 1 g/day) is necessary for normal calcium balance.

Purpose
• To aid diagnosis of neuromuscular, skeletal, and endocrine disorders; arrhythmias; blood-clotting deficiencies; and acid-base imbalance

Patient preparation
• Explain to the patient that this test is used to determine blood calcium levels.
• Tell him that the test requires a blood sample, who will perform the venipuncture, and when.

• Explain that he may experience slight discomfort from the needle puncture and the tourniquet, but that collecting the sample usually takes less than 3 minutes.
• Inform him that he need not restrict food or fluids before the test.

Procedure and posttest care
• Perform a venipuncture (without a tourniquet if possible), and collect the sample in a 7-ml *red-top* or *red-marble-top* tube.
• If a hematoma develops at the venipuncture site, apply warm soaks.

Reference values
Normally, serum calcium levels range from 8.9 to 10.1 mg/dl (atomic absorption), or from 4.5 to 5.5 mEq/liter. In children, serum calcium levels are higher than in adults. Calcium levels can rise as high as 12 mg/dl or 6 mEq/liter during phases of rapid bone growth.

Abnormal findings
Abnormally high serum calcium levels (hypercalcemia) may occur in hyperparathyroidism and parathyroid tumors, Paget's disease of the bone, multiple myeloma, metastatic carcinoma, multiple fractures, or prolonged immobilization. Elevated levels may also result from inadequate excretion of calcium, as in adrenal insufficiency and renal disease; from excessive calcium ingestion; or from overuse of antacids such as calcium carbonate.

Observe the patient with hypercalcemia for deep bone pain, flank pain due to renal calculi, and muscle hypotonicity. Hypercalcemic crisis begins with nausea, vomiting, and dehydration, leading to stupor and coma, and can end in cardiac arrest.

Low calcium levels (hypocalcemia) may result from hypoparathyroidism, total parathyroidectomy, or malabsorption. Decreased serum calcium levels may also occur with Cushing's syndrome, renal failure, acute pancreatitis, and peritonitis.

In a patient with hypocalcemia, be alert for circumoral and peripheral numbness and tingling, muscle twitching, Chvostek's sign (facial muscle spasm), tetany, muscle cramping, Trousseau's sign (carpopedal spasm), seizures, and arrhythmias.

CHLORIDE

This test is used to measure serum levels of chloride, the major extracellular fluid anion. Chloride helps maintain osmotic pressure of blood and therefore helps regulate blood volume and arterial pressure. Chloride levels also affect acid-base balance. It is absorbed from the intestines and is excreted primarily by the kidneys.

Purpose
• To detect acid-base imbalance (acidosis or alkalosis) and to aid evaluation of fluid status and extracellular cation-anion balance

Patient preparation
• Explain to the patient that the test is used to evaluate the chloride content of blood.
• Tell him that the test requires a blood sample. Explain who will perform the venipuncture and when.
• Explain that he may experience slight discomfort from the needle puncture and the tourniquet, but that collecting the sample usually takes less than 3 minutes.
• Inform him that he need not restrict food or fluids before the test.
• Check his history for treatment with drugs that may elevate chloride levels such as ammonium chloride, choles-

tyramine, boric acid, oxyphenbutazone, phenylbutazone, or excessive I.V. infusion of sodium chloride. Serum chloride levels are decreased by thiazides, furosemide, ethacrynic acid, bicarbonates, or prolonged I.V. infusion of dextrose 5% in water.

Procedure and posttest care
• Perform a venipuncture, and collect the sample in a 7-ml *red-top* or *red-marble-top* tube.
• If a hematoma develops at the venipuncture site, apply warm soaks.

Precautions
• Handle the sample gently to prevent hemolysis.

Reference values
Normally, serum chloride levels range from 100 to 108 mEq/liter.

Abnormal findings
Chloride levels are inversely related to bicarbonate levels, reflecting acid-base balance. Excessive loss of gastric juices or other secretions containing chloride may cause hypochloremic metabolic alkalosis; excessive chloride retention or ingestion may lead to hyperchloremic metabolic acidosis.

Elevated serum chloride levels (hyperchloremia) may result from severe dehydration, complete renal shutdown, head injury (producing neurogenic hyperventilation), and primary aldosteronism.

Low chloride levels (hypochloremia) are usually associated with low sodium and potassium levels. Possible underlying causes include prolonged vomiting, gastric suctioning, intestinal fistula, chronic renal failure, and Addison's disease. Congestive heart failure or edema resulting in excess extracellular fluid can cause dilutional hypochloremia.

Observe a patient with hypochloremia for hypertonicity of muscles, tetany, and depressed respirations. In a patient with hyperchloremia, be alert for signs of developing stupor, rapid deep breathing, and weakness that may lead to coma.

MAGNESIUM

This test is used to measure serum levels of magnesium, an electrolyte that is vital to neuromuscular function. Most magnesium is in bone and intracellular fluid; a small amount is in extracellular fluid. Magnesium is absorbed by the small intestine and excreted in the urine and feces.

Purpose
• To evaluate electrolyte status
• To assess neuromuscular or renal function

Patient preparation
• Explain to the patient that this test is used to determine the magnesium content of the blood.
• Instruct him not to use magnesium salts (such as milk of magnesia or Epsom salt) for at least 3 days before the test, but tell him that he need not restrict food or fluids.
• Tell the patient that the test requires a blood sample. Explain who will perform the venipuncture and when.
• Explain that he may feel transient discomfort from the needle puncture, but reassure him that collecting the sample takes only a few minutes.

Procedure and posttest care
• Perform a venipuncture, without a tourniquet if possible, and collect the sample in a 7-ml *red-top* or *red-marble-top* tube.

• If a hematoma develops at the venipuncture site, apply warm soaks.

Precautions
• Handle the sample gently to prevent hemolysis.

Reference values
Normally, serum magnesium levels range from 1.7 to 2.1 mg/dl (atomic absorption) or from 1.5 to 2.5 mEq/liter.

Abnormal findings
Elevated serum magnesium levels (hypermagnesemia) most commonly occur in renal failure, when the kidneys excrete inadequate amounts of magnesium. Adrenal insufficiency (Addison's disease) can also elevate serum magnesium.

In suspected or confirmed hypermagnesemia, observe the patient for lethargy; flushing; diaphoresis; decreased blood pressure; slow, weak pulse; diminished deep tendon reflexes; muscle weakness; and slow, shallow respirations.

Suppressed serum magnesium levels (hypomagnesemia) most commonly result from chronic alcoholism. Other causes include malabsorption syndrome, diarrhea, faulty absorption following bowel resection, prolonged bowel or gastric aspiration, acute pancreatitis, primary aldosteronism, severe burns, hypercalcemic conditions (including hyperparathyroidism), and certain diuretic therapy.

In hypomagnesemia, watch for leg and foot cramps, hyperactive deep tendon reflexes, cardiac arrhythmias, muscle weakness, seizures, twitching, tetany, and tremors.

PHOSPHATES

This test is used to measure serum levels of phosphates, the primary anion in intracellular fluid. About 85% of the body's phosphates are found in bone. The intestine absorbs most phosphates from dietary sources; the kidneys excrete phosphates and serve as a regulatory mechanism. Abnormal concentrations of serum phosphates usually result from improper excretion rather than faulty ingestion or absorption from dietary sources.

Normally, calcium and phosphates have an inverse relationship; if one is elevated, the other is decreased.

Purpose
• To aid diagnosis of renal disorders and acid-base imbalance
• To detect endocrine, skeletal, and calcium disorders

Patient preparation
• Explain to the patient that this test is used to measure phosphate levels in the blood.
• Tell him that the test requires a blood sample. Explain who will perform the venipuncture and when.
• Explain that he may experience slight discomfort from the needle puncture and the tourniquet, but that collecting the sample usually takes less than 3 minutes.
• Inform him that he need not restrict food or fluids before the test.
• Check the patient's medication history for drugs that alter phosphate levels, such as vitamin D, anabolic steroids, androgens, phosphate-binding antacids, acetazolamide, insulin, and epinephrine.

Procedure and posttest care
• Perform a venipuncture, without using a tourniquet if possible, and collect the sample in a 7-ml *red-top* or *red-marble-top* tube.
• If a hematoma develops at the venipuncture site, apply warm soaks.

Precautions
• Handle the sample gently to prevent hemolysis.

Reference values
Normally, serum phosphate levels range from 2.5 to 4.5 mg/dl (atomic absorption), or from 1.8 to 2.6 mEq/liter. Children have higher serum phosphate levels than adults. Phosphate levels can rise as high as 7 mg/dl or 4.1 mEq/liter during periods of increased bone growth.

Abnormal findings
Serum phosphate values alone are of limited diagnostic use (only a few rare conditions directly affect phosphate metabolism), so they should be interpreted in light of serum calcium results.

Depressed phosphate levels (hypophosphatemia) may result from malnutrition, malabsorption syndromes, hyperparathyroidism, renal tubular acidosis, or treatment of diabetic acidosis. In children, hypophosphatemia can suppress normal growth.

Elevated levels (hyperphosphatemia) may result from skeletal disease, healing fractures, hypoparathyroidism, acromegaly, diabetic acidosis, high intestinal obstruction, or renal failure. Hyperphosphatemia is rarely clinically significant, but it can alter bone metabolism in prolonged cases.

POTASSIUM

This test is used to measure serum levels of potassium, the major intracellular cation. Potassium functions to maintain cellular osmotic equilibrium and to regulate muscle activity, enzyme activity, and acid-base balance. It also influences kidney function. The body has no efficient method for conserving potassium; the kidneys excrete nearly all ingested potassium, even when the body's supply is depleted. Potassium deficiency can develop rapidly and is quite common. Dietary intake of at least 40 mEq/day is essential.

Purpose
• To evaluate clinical signs of potassium excess (hyperkalemia) or potassium depletion (hypokalemia)
• To monitor renal function, acid-base balance, and glucose metabolism
• To evaluate neuromuscular and endocrine disorders
• To detect the origin of arrhythmias

Patient preparation
• Explain to the patient that this test is used to determine the potassium content of blood.
• Tell him that the test requires a blood sample. Explain who will perform the venipuncture and when.
• Explain that he may experience slight discomfort from the needle puncture and the tourniquet, but that collecting the sample usually takes less than 3 minutes.
• Inform him that he need not restrict food or fluids before the test.
• Check the patient's history for use of drugs that may influence test results. These include diuretics, penicillin G potassium, amphotericin B, methicillin, tetracycline, insulin, or glucose. If these

medications must be continued, note this on the laboratory slip.

Procedure and posttest care
• Perform a venipuncture, and collect the sample in a 7-ml *red-top* or *red-marble-top* tube.
• If a hematoma develops at the venipuncture site, apply warm soaks.

Precautions
• Draw the sample immediately after applying the tourniquet, as a delay may elevate the potassium level by allowing intracellular potassium to leak into the serum.
• Handle the sample gently to avoid hemolysis.

Reference values
Normally, serum potassium levels range from 3.5 to 5.0 mEq/liter.

Abnormal findings
Abnormally high serum potassium levels are common under conditions in which excess cellular potassium enters the blood, such as in patients with burns, crushing injuries, diabetic ketoacidosis, or myocardial infarction. Hyperkalemia may also indicate reduced sodium excretion, possibly due to renal failure (preventing normal exchange of sodium and potassium) or Addison's disease (due to potassium buildup and sodium depletion).

Observe a patient with hyperkalemia for weakness, malaise, nausea, diarrhea, colicky pain, muscle irritability progressing to flaccid paralysis, oliguria, and bradycardia. Electrocardiography (ECG) reveals a prolonged PR interval; wide QRS complex; tall, tented T wave; and ST depression.

Below-normal potassium values often result from aldosteronism or Cushing's syndrome, loss of body fluids (as in long-term diuretic therapy), or excessive licorice ingestion. Although serum values and clinical symptoms can indicate a potassium imbalance, an ECG allows a definitive diagnosis.

Observe a patient with hypokalemia for decreased reflexes; rapid, weak, irregular pulse; mental confusion; hypotension; anorexia; muscle weakness; and paresthesia. ECG shows a flattened T wave, ST depression, and U wave elevation. In severe cases, ventricular fibrillation, respiratory paralysis, and cardiac arrest can develop.

SODIUM

This test is used to measure serum levels of sodium in relation to the amount of water in the body. Sodium, the major extracellular cation, affects body water distribution, maintains osmotic pressure of extracellular fluid, and helps promote neuromuscular function. It also helps maintain acid-base balance and influences chloride and potassium levels.

Purpose
• To evaluate fluid-electrolyte and acid-base balance, and related neuromuscular, renal, and adrenal functions

Patient preparation
• Explain to the patient that this test is used to determine the sodium content of blood.
• Tell him that the test requires a blood sample. Explain who will perform the venipuncture and when.
• Explain that he may experience slight discomfort from the needle puncture and the tourniquet, but that collecting the sample usually takes less than 3 minutes.
• Inform him that he need not restrict food or fluids before the test.

• Check the patient's medication history for use of drugs that influence sodium levels, including most diuretics, lithium, chlorpropamide, vasopressin, corticosteroids, and antihypertensives such as methyldopa, hydralazine, and reserpine. If these medications must be continued, note this on the laboratory slip.

Procedure and posttest care
• Perform a venipuncture, and collect the sample in a 7-ml *red-top* or *red-marble-top* tube.
• If a hematoma develops at the venipuncture site, apply warm soaks.

Precautions
• Handle the sample gently to prevent hemolysis.

Reference values
Normally, serum sodium levels range from 135 to 145 mEq/liter.

Abnormal findings
Sodium imbalance can result from a loss or gain of sodium, or from a change in the patient's state of hydration. Elevated serum sodium levels (hypernatremia) may be due to inadequate water intake, water loss in excess of sodium (as in diabetes insipidus, impaired renal function, prolonged hyperventilation, and occasionally, severe vomiting or diarrhea), and sodium retention (as in aldosteronism). Hypernatremia can also result from excessive sodium intake.

In a patient with hypernatremia and associated loss of water, observe for signs of thirst, restlessness, dry and sticky mucous membranes, flushed skin, oliguria, and diminished reflexes. However, if increased total body sodium causes water retention, observe for hypertension, dyspnea, and edema.

Abnormally low serum sodium levels (hyponatremia) may result from inadequate sodium intake or excessive sodium loss due to profuse sweating, gastrointestinal suctioning, diuretic therapy, diarrhea, vomiting, adrenal insufficiency, burns, or chronic renal insufficiency with acidosis. Urine sodium determinations are frequently more sensitive to early changes in sodium balance and should always be evaluated simultaneously with serum sodium findings.

In a patient with hyponatremia, watch for apprehension, lassitude, headache, decreased skin turgor, abdominal cramps, and tremors that may progress to seizures.

ANION GAP

Total concentrations of cations and anions are normally equal, making serum electrically neutral. Measuring the gap between measured cation and anion levels provides information about the level of anions (including sulfate, phosphate, organic acids such as ketone bodies and lactic acid, and proteins) that are not routinely measured in laboratory tests. In metabolic acidosis, measuring the anion gap helps to understand the type of acidosis and possible causes. Further tests are usually needed to determine the specific cause of metabolic acidosis.

Purpose
• To distinguish types of metabolic acidosis
• To monitor renal function and total parenteral nutrition

Patient preparation
• Explain to the patient that this test is used to determine the cause of acidosis.

• Tell him that the test requires a blood sample. Explain who will perform the venipuncture and when.
• Explain that he may experience slight discomfort from the needle puncture and the tourniquet, but that collecting the sample usually takes less than 3 minutes.
• Inform him that he need not restrict food or fluids before the test.
• Check the history for use of drugs (such as diuretics, corticosteroids, and antihypertensives) that may influence sodium, chloride, or bicarbonate blood levels. If these drugs must be continued, note this on the laboratory slip.

Procedure and posttest care
• Perform a venipuncture, and collect the sample in a 7-ml *red-top* or *red-marble-top* tube.
• If a hematoma develops at the venipuncture site, apply warm soaks.
• Instruct the patient to resume use of any drugs discontinued before the test.

Precautions
• Handle the sample gently to prevent hemolysis.

Reference values
Normally, the anion gap ranges from 8 to 14 mEq/liter.

Abnormal findings
A normal anion gap does not rule out metabolic acidosis. It may occur in hyperchloremic acidoses, renal tubular acidosis, and severe bicarbonate-wasting conditions, such as biliary or pancreatic fistulas and poorly functioning ileal loops.

When acidosis results from loss of bicarbonate in the urine or other body fluids, the anion gap remains unchanged. This is known as a *normal anion gap acidosis.*

An increased anion gap indicates an increase in one or more of the unmeasured anions (sulfate, phosphates, organic acids such as ketone bodies and lactic acid, and proteins). This may occur with acidoses that are characterized by excessive organic or inorganic acids, such as lactic acidosis or ketoacidosis.

When acidosis results from accumulation of metabolic acids — as occurs in lactic acidosis, for example — the anion gap increases (above 14 mEq/liter) with the increase in unmeasured anions. Metabolic acidosis caused by such accumulation is known as a *high anion gap acidosis.*

A decreased anion gap (below 8 mEq/liter) is rare, but may occur with hypermagnesemia and with paraproteinemic states, such as multiple myeloma and Waldenström's macroglobulinemia.

CARDIAC ENZYMES

CREATINE KINASE

Creatine kinase (CK) is an enzyme that catalyzes the creatine-creatinine metabolic pathway in muscle cells and brain tissue. Because of its intimate role in energy production, CK reflects normal tissue catabolism; an increase above normal serum levels indicates trauma to cells with high CK content.

Fractionation and measurement of three distinct CK isoenzymes — CK-BB (CK_1), CK-MB (CK_2), and CK-MM (CK_3) — has replaced use of total CK levels to accurately localize the site of increased tissue destruction in acute myocardial infarction (MI). In addition, subunits of CK-MM and CK-MB, called isoforms, can be assayed to increase the sensitivity of the test.

Purpose
• To detect and diagnose acute MI and reinfarction (CK-MB primarily used)
• To evaluate possible causes of chest pain and to monitor the severity of myocardial ischemia after cardiac surgery, cardiac catheterization, or cardioversion (CK-MB primarily used)
• To detect skeletal muscle disorders that are not neurogenic in origin, such as Duchenne muscular dystrophy (total CK primarily used), and early dermatomyositis

Patient preparation
• Explain to the patient that this test is used to assess myocardial and skeletal muscle function, and that multiple blood samples are required to detect fluctuations in serum levels.
• Tell him who will perform the venipunctures and when, and that he may feel some discomfort from the needle or the tourniquet, but that collecting the sample usually takes less than 3 minutes.
• Inform him that he need not restrict food or most fluids before the test.
• If the patient is being evaluated for skeletal muscle disorders, advise him to avoid exercising for 24 hours before the test.
• Before the test, withhold alcohol, aminocaproic acid, and lithium. If these substances must be continued, note this on the laboratory slip.

Procedure and posttest care
• Perform a venipuncture, and collect the sample in a 7-ml *red-top* tube.
• If a hematoma develops at the venipuncture site, apply warm soaks.
• Resume medications discontinued before the test.

Precautions
• Draw the sample before or within 1 hour of giving intramuscular injec-

SERUM ENZYME AND ISOENZYME LEVELS AFTER MYOCARDIAL INFARCTION

Because they're released by damaged tissue, serum enzymes and isoenzymes (catalytic proteins that vary in concentration in specific organs) can help identify the compromised organ and assess the extent of damage. The serum enzyme and isoenzyme determinations listed below are most significant in myocardial infarction.

Isoenzymes
• Creatine kinase-MB (CK-MB): in the heart muscle and a small amount in skeletal muscle
• Lactate dehydrogenase 1 and 2 (LD_1, LD_2): in the heart, brain, kidneys, liver, skeletal muscles, and red blood cells (RBCs)

Enzymes
• Hydroxybutyric dehydrogenase (HBD): an indirect measurement of LD_1, LD_2
• Aspartate aminotransferase (AST): heart muscle and liver and less extensively in skeletal muscles, kidneys, pancreas, and RBCs

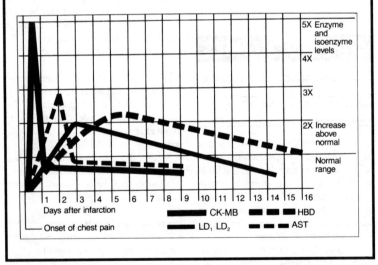

tions, as muscle trauma increases total CK level.
• Obtain the sample on schedule. Note, on the laboratory slip, the time the sample was drawn and the hours elapsed since onset of chest pain.

• Handle the collection tube gently to prevent hemolysis.
• Send the sample to the laboratory immediately because CK activity diminishes significantly after 2 hours at room temperature.

Reference values

Total CK values determined by ultraviolet or kinetic measurement range from 25 to 130 U/L for men, and from 10 to 150 U/L for women. CK levels may be significantly higher in very muscular people. Infants up to age 1 have levels two to four times higher than adult levels, possibly reflecting birth trauma and striated muscle development. Normal ranges for isoenzyme levels are as follows: CK-BB, undetectable; CK-MB, undetectable to 7 U/L; CK-MM, 5 to 70 U/L.

Abnormal findings

CK-MM makes up 99% of total CK normally present in serum. Detectable CK-BB isoenzyme may indicate (but does not confirm a diagnosis of) brain tissue injury, widespread malignant tumors, severe shock, or renal failure.

CK-MB isoenzyme greater than 5% of total CK (or more than 10 U/L) indicates MI, especially if the LD_1/LD_2 isoenzyme ratio is greater than 1 (flipped LD). In acute MI and following cardiac surgery, CK-MB begins to increase in 2 to 4 hours, peaks in 12 to 24 hours, and usually returns to normal in 24 to 48 hours; persistent elevations or increasing levels indicate ongoing myocardial damage. Total CK follows roughly the same pattern but increases slightly later. CK-MB levels may not increase in congestive heart failure or during angina pectoris not accompanied by myocardial cell necrosis. Serious skeletal muscle injury that occurs in certain muscular dystrophies, polymyositis, and severe myoglobinuria may produce mild CK-MB elevation, because a small amount of this isoenzyme is present in some skeletal muscles.

Rising CK-MM values follow skeletal muscle damage from trauma, such as surgery and I.M. injections, or from diseases, such as dermatomyositis and muscular dystrophy (values may be 50 to 100 times normal). A moderate rise in CK-MM levels develops in patients with hypothyroidism; sharp elevations occur with muscular activity caused by agitation, such as in an acute psychotic episode.

Total CK levels may be elevated in patients with severe hypokalemia, carbon monoxide poisoning, malignant hyperthermia, or alcoholic cardiomyopathy. They may also be elevated following seizures and, occasionally, in patients who have suffered pulmonary or cerebral infarctions. (See *Serum enzyme and isoenzyme levels after myocardial infarction.*)

CREATINE KINASE ISOFORMS

Creatine kinase, an enzyme found in muscle tissue, has three isoenzymes: CK-BB (CK_1), CK-MB (CK_2), and CK-MM (CK_3). CK-BB, not usually seen in serum, is most prevalent in brain tissue. CK-MM and CK-MB are found primarily in skeletal and heart muscle.

Cardiac muscle damage releases CK-MM, CK-MB, and lactate dehydrogenase (LD) isoenzymes into serum. Isoforms, or subforms, of CK-MM and CK-MB isoenzymes are called $CK-MM_1$, $CK-MM_2$, $CK-MB_1$, and $CK-MB_2$. Isoforms are determined by high-voltage electrophoresis or isoelectric focusing.

Purpose

• To detect or provide early confirmation of myocardial infarction (MI)
• To evaluate reperfusion therapy

Patient preparation

• Explain to the patient that the test will help to confirm or rule out MI.

• Tell him that it will require a blood test, with samples drawn at timed intervals.
• Tell him who will perform the venipuncture and when, and that he may feel discomfort from the tourniquet and the needle.

Procedure and posttest care
• Perform a venipuncture and collect blood in a 7-ml *lavender-top* tube.
• Record the time the sample was drawn. Obtain samples every 2 hours as indicated and note the times.
• Place each sample in ice and deliver it to the laboratory immediately.
• If a hematoma develops at the venipuncture site, apply warm soaks.

Precautions
• Obtain each sample on schedule and note the collection time on each.
• Handle samples gently.

Reference values
CK-MB$_2$ concentrations are less than 1.0. The CK-MB$_2$/CK-MB$_1$ ratio is less than 1.5.

Abnormal findings
An increase in CK-MB indicates MI. Within 2 to 4 hours after MI, more than 50% of patients will have a ratio of CK-MB$_2$ (tissue form) to CK-MB$_1$ greater than 1.5. By 6 hours after MI, more than 90% of patients will have a ratio of 1.5 or greater.

LACTATE DEHYDROGENASE

Lactate dehydrogenase (LD) catalyzes the reversible conversion of muscle lactic acid into pyruvic acid, an essential step in the metabolic processes ulti-mately producing cellular energy. Because LD is present in almost all body tissues, cellular damage causes an elevation of total serum LD, limiting the diagnostic usefulness of LD. Five tissue-specific isoenzymes can be identified and measured: LD$_1$ and LD$_2$ appear primarily in the heart, red blood cells (RBCs), and kidneys; LD$_3$ is primarily in the lungs; and LD$_4$ and LD$_5$ are in the liver and the skeletal muscles.

Purpose
• To aid differential diagnosis of MI, pulmonary infarction, anemias, and hepatic disease
• To support CK isoenzyme test results in diagnosing myocardial infarction (MI), or to provide diagnosis when CK-MB samples are drawn too late to display elevation
• To monitor patient response to some forms of chemotherapy

Patient preparation
• Explain to the patient that this test is used primarily to detect tissue alterations.
• Tell him that the test requires a blood sample. Explain who will perform the venipuncture and when.
• Explain that he may experience slight discomfort from the needle puncture and the tourniquet, but that collecting the sample usually takes less than 3 minutes.
• Inform him that he need not restrict food or fluids before the test.
• If MI is suspected, tell him that the test will be repeated on the next two mornings to monitor progressive changes.

Procedure and posttest care
• Perform a venipuncture, and collect the sample in a 7-ml *red-top* tube.
• If a hematoma develops at the venipuncture site, apply warm soaks.

Precautions

• Draw the samples on schedule to avoid missing peak levels, and mark the collection time on the laboratory slip.

• Handle the sample gently to prevent artifact blood sample hemolysis because RBCs contain LD_1.

• Send the sample to the laboratory immediately or, if transport is delayed, keep the sample at room temperature. Changes in temperature reportedly inactivate LD_5, thus altering isoenzyme patterns.

Reference values

Total LD levels normally range from 45 to 90 U/L. Normal distribution is as follows:

• LD_1: 14% to 26% of total
• LD_2: 29% to 39% of total
• LD_3: 20% to 26% of total
• LD_4: 8% to 16% of total
• LD_5: 6% to 16% of total.

Abnormal findings

Because many common diseases cause elevations in total LD levels, isoenzyme electrophoresis is usually necessary for diagnosis. In some disorders, total LD may be within normal limits, but abnormal proportions of each enzyme indicate specific organ tissue damage. For instance, in acute MI, the LD_1/LD_2 isoenzyme ratio is typically greater than 1 within 12 to 48 hours after onset of symptoms (known as flipped LD).

Midzone fractions (LD_2, LD_3, LD_4) can be elevated in granulocytic leukemia, lymphomas, and platelet disorders.

HEPATIC ENZYMES

ASPARTATE AMINOTRANSFERASE

Aspartate aminotransferase (AST), formerly called serum glutamic-oxaloacetic transaminase, is one of two enzymes that catalyze the conversion of the nitrogenous portion of an amino acid to an amino acid residue. It is essential to energy production in the Krebs cycle. AST is found in the cytoplasm and mitochondria of many cells, primarily in the liver, heart, skeletal muscles, kidneys, pancreas, and red blood cells. It is released into serum in proportion to cellular damage. The change in AST values over time is a reliable monitoring mechanism.

Purpose

• To aid detection and differential diagnosis of acute hepatic disease

• To monitor patient progress and prognosis in cardiac and hepatic diseases

• To aid in diagnosing myocardial infarction in correlation with creatine kinase and lactate dehydrogenase levels

Patient preparation

• Explain to the patient that this test is used to assess heart and liver function.

• Inform him that the test usually requires three venipunctures on three consecutive days.

• Tell the patient that he need not restrict food or fluids.

• Reassure him that discomfort from the needle and the tourniquet is transient and that collecting each sample takes less than 3 minutes.

• Withhold morphine, codeine, meperidine, chlorpropamide, methyldopa, phenazopyridine, and antitubercular drugs (isoniazid, para-aminosalicylates and pyrazinamide). If any of these medications must be continued, note this on the laboratory slip.

Procedure and posttest care
• Perform a venipuncture, and collect the sample in a 7-ml *red-top* tube.
• If a hematoma develops, apply warm soaks.
• Resume medications discontinued before the test.

Precautions
• To avoid missing peak AST levels, draw serum samples at the same time each day.
• Handle the collection tube gently to prevent hemolysis, and send the sample to the laboratory immediately.

Reference values
AST levels range from 8 to 20 U/L. Normal values for infants are as high as four times those of adults.

Abnormal findings
AST levels fluctuate in response to the extent of cellular necrosis, being transiently and minimally elevated early in the disease process and extremely elevated during the most acute phase. Depending on when the initial sample is drawn, AST levels may increase, indicating increasing disease severity and tissue damage, or decrease, indicating disease resolution and tissue repair.

Maximum elevations (more than 20 times normal) may indicate acute viral hepatitis, severe skeletal muscle trauma, extensive surgery, drug-induced hepatic injury, or severe passive liver congestion.

High levels (10 to 20 times greater than normal) may indicate severe myocardial infarction, severe infectious mononucleosis, or alcoholic cirrhosis. High levels also occur during the pro-

dromal or resolving stages of conditions that cause maximum elevations.

Moderate-to-high levels (5 to 10 times greater than normal) may indicate Duchenne muscular dystrophy, dermatomyositis, or chronic hepatitis. Moderate-to-high levels also occur during prodromal and resolving stages of diseases that cause high elevations.

Low-to-moderate levels (2 to 5 times normal) occur at some time during any of the preceding conditions or diseases, or may indicate hemolytic anemia, metastatic hepatic tumors, acute pancreatitis, pulmonary emboli, delirium tremens, or fatty liver. AST levels rise slightly after the first few days of biliary duct obstruction.

ALANINE AMINOTRANSFERASE

Formerly called serum glutamic-pyruvic transaminase, alanine aminotransferase (ALT) is necessary for tissue energy production. It is one of two enzymes that catalyzes a reversible amino group transfer reaction in the Krebs cycle. ALT primarily appears in hepatocellular cytoplasm, with lesser amounts in the kidneys, heart, and skeletal muscles, and is an indicator of acute hepatocellular damage. This test is used to measure serum ALT levels. Abnormally high serum levels may remain elevated for days or weeks.

Purpose
• To detect and evaluate treatment of acute hepatic disease, especially hepatitis or cirrhosis without jaundice
• To distinguish between myocardial and hepatic tissue damage (used with AST)

• To assess hepatotoxicity of some drugs

Patient preparation
• Explain to the patient that this test is used to assess liver function.
• Tell him that the test requires a blood sample. Explain who will perform the venipuncture and when.
• Explain that he may experience slight discomfort from the needle puncture and the tourniquet, but that collecting the sample usually takes less than 3 minutes.
• Inform him that he need not restrict food or fluids before the test.
• Withhold hepatotoxic or cholestatic drugs such as methotrexate, chlorprom-azine, salicylates, and narcotics. If these medications must be continued, note this on the laboratory slip.

Procedure and posttest care
• Perform a venipuncture, and collect the sample in a 7-ml *red-top* tube.
• If a hematoma develops at the veni-puncture site, apply warm soaks.
• Resume administration of drugs that were withheld before the test.

Precautions
• Handle the sample gently to prevent hemolysis.
• ALT activity is stable in serum for up to 3 days at room temperature.

Reference values
Serum ALT levels range from 8 to 20 U/L.

Abnormal findings
Very high ALT levels (up to 50 times normal) suggest viral or severe drug-in-duced hepatitis, or other hepatic disease with extensive necrosis. Moderate-to-high levels may indicate infectious mononucleosis, chronic hepatitis, in-trahepatic cholestasis or cholecystitis, early or improving acute viral hepatitis,

or severe hepatic congestion due to heart failure. Slight-to-moderate eleva-tions of ALT may appear in any condi-tion that produces acute hepatocellular injury — such as active cirrhosis and drug-induced or alcoholic hepatitis. Marginal elevations occasionally occur in acute myocardial infarction, reflect-ing secondary hepatic congestion or the release of small amounts of ALT from myocardial tissue.

ALKALINE PHOSPHATASE

This test is used to measure serum lev-els of alkaline phosphatase (ALP). ALP influences bone calcification and lipid and metabolite transport. ALP measure-ments reflect the combined activity of several ALP isoenzymes found in the liver, bones, kidneys, intestinal lining, and placenta. Bone and liver ALP are always present in adult serum, with liv-er ALP most prominent except during the third trimester of pregnancy (when the placenta originates about half of all ALP). The intestinal variant of ALP can be a normal component (in less than 10% of normal patterns; almost exclu-sively in the sera of blood groups B and O), or it can be an abnormal finding as-sociated with hepatic disease.

Purpose
• To detect and identify skeletal diseases, primarily characterized by marked ost-eoblastic activity
• To detect focal hepatic lesions caus-ing biliary obstruction, such as tumor or abscess
• To assess response to vitamin D in the treatment of rickets
• To supplement information from oth-er liver function studies and gastroin-

testinal enzyme tests; additional liver function studies are usually required to identify hepatobiliary disorders

Patient preparation
• Explain to the patient that this test is used to assess liver or bone function.
• Instruct him to fast for at least 8 hours before the test, because fat intake stimulates intestinal ALP secretion.
• Tell him that this test requires a blood sample. Explain who will perform the venipuncture and when, and that he may experience discomfort from the needle puncture and the pressure of the tourniquet.
• Reassure him that collecting the sample usually takes less than 3 minutes.

Procedure and posttest care
• Perform a venipuncture, and collect the sample in a 7-ml *red-top* tube.
• If a hematoma develops at the venipuncture site, apply warm soaks.
• Tell the patient he may resume his usual diet.

Precautions
• Handle the collection tube gently to prevent hemolysis.
• Send the sample to the laboratory immediately; ALP activity increases at room temperature due to a rise in pH.

Reference values
Total ALP levels, when measured by chemical inhibition, range from 90 to 239 U/L for males. For females under age 45, total ALP levels range from 76 to 196 U/L; for women over age 45, the range widens to 87 to 250 U/L.

Abnormal findings
Although significant ALP elevations are possible with diseases that affect many organs, they are most likely to indicate skeletal disease, or extra- or intrahepatic biliary obstruction causing cholestasis. Many acute hepatic dis-

eases cause ALP elevations before they affect serum bilirubin levels.

Moderate increases in ALP levels may reflect acute biliary obstruction from hepatocellular inflammation in active cirrhosis, mononucleosis, and viral hepatitis. Moderate increases are also seen in osteomalacia and deficiency-induced rickets.

Sharp elevations of ALP levels may indicate complete biliary obstruction by malignant or infectious infiltrations or fibrosis, most common in Paget's disease and, occasionally, in biliary obstruction, extensive bone metastases, or hyperparathyroidism. Metastatic bone tumors resulting from pancreatic cancer raise ALP levels without a concomitant rise in serum alanine aminotransferase levels.

Isoenzyme fractionation and additional enzyme tests — gamma glutamyl transferase, lactate dehydrogenase, 5'-nucleotidase, and leucine amino-peptidase — are sometimes performed when the cause of ALP elevations (skeletal or hepatic disease) is in doubt. Rarely, low levels of serum ALP are associated with hypophosphatasia and protein or magnesium deficiency.

GAMMA GLUTAMYL TRANSFERASE

Also called gamma glutamyl transpeptidase, gamma glutamyl transferase (GGT) participates in the transfer of amino acids across cellular membranes and, possibly, in glutathione metabolism. Highest concentrations of GGT exist in the renal tubules, but the enzyme also appears in the liver, biliary tract epithelium, pancreas, lymphocytes, brain, and testes. This test is used to measure serum GGT levels.

Purpose

• To provide information about hepatobiliary diseases, to assess liver function, and to detect alcohol ingestion

• To distinguish between skeletal disease and hepatic disease when serum alkaline phosphatase is elevated (a normal GGT level suggests such elevation stems from skeletal disease)

Patient preparation

• Explain to the patient that this test is used to evaluate liver function.

• Tell him that the test requires a blood sample. Explain who will perform the venipuncture and when.

• Explain that he may experience slight discomfort from the needle puncture and the tourniquet, but that collecting the sample usually takes less than 3 minutes.

• Inform him that he need not restrict food or fluids before the test.

Procedure and posttest care

• Perform a venipuncture, and collect the sample in a 7-ml *red-top* tube.

• If a hematoma develops, apply warm soaks.

Precautions

• Handle the collection tube gently to prevent hemolysis.

• GGT activity is stable in serum at room temperature for 2 days.

Reference values

Serum GGT values vary with the assay method used (kinetic or end-point method). Normal levels range from 5 to 24 U/L in females; in males, levels range from 8 to 37 U/L.

Abnormal findings

Serum GGT rises in any acute hepatic disease, as enzyme production increases in response to hepatocellular injury. Moderate increases occur in acute pancreatitis, in renal disease, in prostat-

ic metastases, postoperatively, and in some patients, with epilepsy or brain tumors. Levels also increase due to enzyme induction after alcohol ingestion. The sharpest elevations occur in patients with obstructive jaundice and hepatic metastatic infiltrations. GGT may increase 5 to 10 days after acute myocardial infarction, either as a result of tissue granulation and healing, or as an indication of the effects of cardiac insufficiency on the liver.

5′-NUCLEOTIDASE

The enzyme 5′-nucleotidase (5′NT) is a phosphatase formed almost entirely in the hepatobiliary tract. Unlike alkaline phosphatase (ALP), it hydrolyzes nucleoside 5′-phosphate groups only. Measurement of serum 5′NT levels helps to determine whether ALP elevation originates from skeletal or hepatic disease. 5′NT remains normal in skeletal disease and pregnancy, and so is more specific for assessing hepatic dysfunction than ALP or leukocyte alkaline phosphatase.

Purpose

• To distinguish between hepatobiliary and skeletal disease when the source of elevated ALP levels is uncertain

• To help differentiate biliary obstruction from acute hepatocellular damage

• To detect hepatic metastasis in the absence of jaundice

Patient preparation

• Explain to the patient that this test is used to evaluate liver function.

• Tell him that the test requires a blood sample. Explain who will perform the venipuncture and when.

• Explain that he may experience slight discomfort from the needle puncture and the tourniquet, but that collecting the sample usually takes less than 3 minutes.

• Inform him that he need not restrict food or fluids before the test.

Procedure and posttest care

• Perform a venipuncture, and collect the sample in a 7-ml *red-top* tube.

• If a hematoma develops at the venipuncture site, apply warm soaks.

Precautions

• Handle the sample gently.

Reference values

Serum 5'NT values for adults range from 2 to 17 U/L; values for children may be lower.

Abnormal findings

Highest 5'NT elevations occur in common bile duct obstruction by calculi or tumors in diseases that cause severe intrahepatic cholestasis, such as neoplastic infiltrations of the liver. Slight-to-moderate increases may reflect acute hepatocellular damage or active cirrhosis.

Hemolysis may interfere with results.

Ingestion of cholestatic drugs, such as phenothiazines, morphine, meperidine, and codeine, elevates 5'NT levels.

PANCREATIC ENZYMES

AMYLASE

Amylase (alpha-amylase or AML), an enzyme that is synthesized primarily in the pancreas and the salivary glands, helps digest starch and glycogen in the mouth, stomach, and intestine. In cases of suspected acute pancreatic disease, measurement of serum or urine AML is the most important laboratory test.

Purpose

• To diagnose acute pancreatitis

• To distinguish between acute pancreatitis and other causes of abdominal pain that require immediate surgery

• To evaluate possible pancreatic injury caused by abdominal trauma or surgery

Patient preparation

• Explain to the patient that this test is used to assess pancreatic function.

• Inform him that he need not fast before the test, but must abstain from alcohol.

• Tell him that this test requires a blood sample. Explain who will perform the venipuncture and when and that he may experience transient discomfort from the needle puncture and the pressure of the tourniquet.

• Reassure him that collecting the sample takes less than 3 minutes.

• Withhold drugs that may elevate AML levels. These include ethyl alcohol in large amounts, aminosalicylic acid, asparaginase, azathioprine, corticosteroids, cyproheptadine, narcotic analgesics, oral contraceptives, rifampin, sulfasalazine, and thiazide or loop diuretics. If these drugs must be continued, note this on the laboratory slip.

Procedure and posttest care

• Perform a venipuncture, and collect the sample in a 7-ml *red-top* tube.

• If a hematoma develops at the venipuncture site, apply warm soaks.

• Resume administration of drugs discontinued before the test.

Precautions
• If the patient has severe abdominal pain, draw the sample before diagnostic or therapeutic intervention. For accurate results, it's important to obtain an early sample.
• Handle the sample gently to prevent hemolysis.

Reference values
Serum levels range from 30 to 220 U/L. A general average is less than 300 U/L. (More than 20 methods of measuring serum AML exist, with different ranges of normal values. Unfortunately, test values cannot always be converted to a standard measurement.)

Abnormal findings
After the onset of acute pancreatitis, AML levels begin to rise in 2 hours, peak at 12 to 48 hours, and return to normal in 3 to 4 days. Determination of urine levels should follow normal serum AML results to rule out pancreatitis. Moderate serum elevations may accompany obstruction of the common bile duct, the pancreatic duct, or the ampulla of Vater; pancreatic injury from perforated peptic ulcer; pancreatic cancer; and acute salivary gland disease. Impaired renal function may increase serum levels.

Levels may be slightly elevated in a patient who is asymptomatic or who is responding unusually to therapy. An AML fractionation test is used to determine the source of the AML and aids selection of additional tests.

Depressed levels can occur in chronic pancreatitis, pancreatic cancer, cirrhosis, hepatitis, and toxemia of pregnancy.

LIPASE

Lipase is produced in the pancreas and secreted into the duodenum, where it converts triglycerides and other fats into fatty acids and glycerol. Destruction of pancreatic cells, which occurs in acute pancreatitis, releases large amounts of lipase into the blood. This test is used to measure serum lipase levels; it's most useful when performed with a serum or urine amylase test.

Purpose
• To aid diagnosis of acute pancreatitis

Patient preparation
• Explain to the patient that this test is used to evaluate pancreatic function.
• Instruct him to fast overnight before the test.
• Tell him that the test requires a blood sample. Explain who will perform the venipuncture and when and also inform him that he may feel some transient discomfort, but that collecting the sample takes less than 3 minutes.
• Withhold cholinergics, codeine, meperidine, and morphine. If they must be continued, note this on the laboratory slip.

Procedure and posttest care
• Perform a venipuncture, and collect the sample in a 7-ml *red-top* tube.
• If a hematoma develops at the venipuncture site, apply warm soaks.
• Resume administration of drugs discontinued before the test.

Precautions
• Handle the collection tube gently.

Reference values
Serum levels are method dependent and are generally less than 300 U/L.

Abnormal findings
High lipase levels suggest acute pancreatitis or pancreatic duct obstruction. After an acute attack, levels remain elevated up to 14 days. Lipase levels may also increase in other pancreatic injuries, such as perforated peptic ulcer with chemical pancreatitis due to gastric juices, and in patients with high intestinal obstruction, pancreatic cancer, or renal disease with impaired excretion.

SPECIAL ENZYMES

ACID PHOSPHATASE

Acid phosphatase (ACP) — a group of phosphatase enzymes most active at a pH of about 5.0 — is found primarily in the prostate gland and semen and, to a lesser extent, in the liver, spleen, red blood cells, bone marrow, and platelets. This test is used to measure total ACP and the prostatic fraction in serum.

Purpose
• To detect prostatic cancer
• To monitor response to therapy for prostatic cancer; successful treatment decreases ACP levels

Patient preparation
• Explain to the patient that this test is used to evaluate prostate function.
• Tell him that the test requires a blood sample. Explain who will perform the venipuncture and when.
• Explain that he may experience discomfort from the needle puncture and the tourniquet, but that collecting the sample usually takes less than 3 minutes.

• Inform him that he need not restrict food or fluids before the test.
• Withhold fluorides, phosphates, and clofibrate. If they must be continued, note this on the laboratory slip.

Procedure and posttest care
• Perform a venipuncture, and collect the sample in a 7-ml *red-top* tube.
• If a hematoma develops at the venipuncture site, apply warm soaks.
• Resume administration of any medications discontinued before the test.

Precautions
• Do not draw the sample within 48 hours of prostate manipulation (rectal exam).
• Handle the collection tube gently.
• Send the sample to the laboratory immediately. Acid phosphatase levels decrease by 50% within 1 hour if the sample remains at room temperature without a preservative or if it is not packed in ice.

Reference values
Serum values for total ACP depend on the assay method, ranging from approximately 0.5 to 1.9 U/L.

Abnormal findings
High prostatic ACP levels generally indicate a tumor that has spread beyond the prostatic capsule. If the tumor has metastasized to bone, high ACP levels are accompanied by high ALP levels, reflecting increased osteoblastic activity.

ACP levels rise moderately in prostatic infarction, Paget's disease (some patients), Gaucher's disease, and occasionally in other conditions, such as multiple myeloma. False results may occur if ALP levels are high, because ACP and ALP are similar, differing mainly in their optimum pH ranges.

PROSTATE-SPECIFIC ANTIGEN

Prostate-specific antigen (PSA) appears in normal, benign hyperplastic, and malignant prostatic tissue, as well as in metastatic prostatic carcinoma. Serum PSA levels are used to monitor the spread of recurrence of prostate cancer and to evaluate the patient's response to treatment. This test is not a suitable screening procedure for prostate cancer.

Purpose
• To monitor the course of prostate cancer and aid evaluation of treatment

Patient preparation
• Explain to the patient that this test is used to monitor prostate cancer and the patient's response to treatment.
• Tell him that the test requires a blood sample. Explain who will perform the venipuncture and when.
• Explain that he may experience slight discomfort from the needle puncture and the tourniquet, but that collecting the sample usually takes less than 3 minutes.
• Inform him that he need not restrict food or fluids before the test.

Procedure and posttest care
• Perform a venipuncture, and collect the sample in a 7-ml *red-top* tube.
• Send the specimen, on ice, to the laboratory immediately.
• If a hematoma develops at the venipuncture site, apply warm soaks.

Precautions
• Collect the sample either before digital prostate examination or at least 48 hours after examination to avoid falsely elevated PSA levels.

• Handle the sample gently to prevent hemolysis.
• Excessive doses of chemotherapeutic drugs such as cyclophosphamide, diethylstilbestrol, and methotrexate, may alter test results.

Reference values
Normal serum values for PSA should not exceed 2.7 ng/ml in males under age 40 and 4 ng/ml in males age 40 or older.

Abnormal findings
About 80% of patients with prostate cancer have pretreatment PSA values greater than 4 ng/ml. PSA results alone do not confirm diagnosis of prostate cancer. Approximately 20% of patients with benign prostatic hypertrophy also have levels greater than 4 ng/ml. Further assessment and testing, including tissue biopsy, are needed to confirm cancer.

PLASMA RENIN ACTIVITY

Renin secretion from the kidneys is the first stage of the renin-angiotensin-aldosterone cycle that controls the body's sodium-potassium balance, fluid volume, and blood pressure. Renin is released into the renal veins in response to sodium depletion and blood loss.

The plasma renin activity test is a screening procedure for renovascular hypertension but does not unequivocally confirm it.

Purpose
• To screen for renal origin of hypertension
• To help plan treatment of essential hypertension, a genetic disease often aggravated by excess sodium intake

• To help identify hypertension linked to unilateral (sometimes bilateral) reno-vascular disease by renal vein catheterization
• To help identify primary aldosteronism (Conn's syndrome) resulting from aldosterone-secreting adrenal adenoma
• To confirm primary aldosteronism (sodium-depleted plasma renin test)

Patient preparation
• Explain to the patient that this test is used to determine the cause of hypertension.
• Tell the patient to discontinue use of diuretics, antihypertensives, vasodilators, oral contraceptives, and licorice for 2 to 4 weeks before the test and to maintain a normal-sodium diet (3 g/day) during this period.
• For the sodium-depleted renin test, tell the patient that he'll receive furosemide or, if he has angina or cerebrovascular insufficiency, that he'll receive chlorthiazide and follow a specific low-sodium diet for 3 days.
• The patient should not receive radioactive treatments for several days prior to the test.
• Tell him to collect his urine for 24 hours.
• Tell him that the test requires a blood sample. Explain who will perform the venipuncture and when.
• Explain that he may experience slight discomfort from the needle puncture and the tourniquet, but that collecting the sample usually takes less than 3 minutes. Collect a morning specimen if possible.
• If a recumbent sample is ordered, instruct the patient to remain in bed at least 2 hours before the sample is obtained. (Posture influences renin secretion.) If an upright sample is ordered, instruct him to stand or sit upright for 2 hours before the test is performed.
• If renal vein catheterization is ordered, make sure the patient has signed an informed consent form. Tell him that the procedure will be done in the X-ray department and that a local anesthetic will be given.

Procedure and posttest care
Peripheral vein sample:
• Perform a venipuncture, and collect the sample in a 7-ml *lavender-top* tube.
• Note on the laboratory slip if the patient was fasting and whether he was upright or supine during specimen collection.
• If a hematoma develops at the peripheral venipuncture site, apply warm soaks.
Renal vein catheterization:
• A catheter is advanced to the kidneys through the femoral vein, under fluoroscopic control, and samples are obtained from both renal veins and the vena cava.
• After renal vein catheterization, apply pressure to the catheterization site for 10 to 20 minutes to prevent extravasation.
• Monitor vital signs, and check the catheterization site every half hour for 2 hours, then every hour for 4 hours, to ensure that the bleeding has stopped. Check distal pulse for signs of thrombus formation and arterial occlusion (cyanosis, loss of pulse, coolness of skin).
Both methods:
• Tell the patient he may resume his usual diet.
• Resume administration of any medications that were discontinued before the test.

Precautions
• Because renin is very unstable, the sample must be drawn into a chilled syringe and collection tube, placed on ice, and sent to the laboratory immediately.
• Completely fill the collection tube, and invert it gently several times to mix the sample and the anticoagulant.

Reference values

Levels of plasma renin activity and of aldosterone decrease with advancing age.

Sodium-depleted, upright, peripheral vein: For ages 18 to 39, the range is from 2.9 to 24 ng/ml/hour; mean, 10.8 ng/ml/hour. For age 40 and over, range is from 2.9 to 10.8 ng/ml/hour; mean, 5.9 ng/ml/hour.

Sodium-replete, upright, peripheral vein: For ages 18 to 39, range is from 0.6 to 4.3 ng/ml/hour; mean, 1.9 ng/ml/hour. For age 40 and over, the range is from 1.0 to 3.0 ng/ml/hour; the mean is 1.0 ng/ml/hour.

In renal vein catheterization, the renal venous renin ratio (the renin level in the renal vein compared to the level in the inferior vena cava) is less than 1.5:1.0.

Abnormal findings

Elevated renin levels may occur in essential hypertension (uncommon), malignant and renovascular hypertension, cirrhosis, hypokalemia, hypovolemia due to hemorrhage, renin-producing renal tumors (Bartter's syndrome), and adrenal hypofunction (Addison's disease). High renin levels may also be found in chronic renal failure with parenchymal disease, end-stage renal disease, and transplant rejection.

Decreased renin levels may indicate hypervolemia due to a high-sodium diet, salt-retaining steroids, primary aldosteronism, Cushing's syndrome, licorice ingestion syndrome, or essential hypertension with low renin levels.

High serum and urine aldosterone levels, with low plasma renin activity, help identify primary aldosteronism: in the sodium-depleted renin test, low plasma renin confirms this and differentiates it from secondary aldosteronism (characterized by increased renin).

CHOLINESTERASE

The cholinesterase test is used to measure the amounts of two similar enzymes that hydrolyze acetylcholine: acetylcholinesterase and pseudocholinesterase. Acetylcholinesterase is present in nerve tissue, red cells of the spleen, and the gray matter of the brain. Pseudocholinesterase is produced primarily in the liver and appears in small amounts in the pancreas, intestine, heart, and white matter of the brain.

When poisoning by an organophosphate (used by the military in nerve gases and common in many insecticides) is suspected, either cholinesterase may be measured. For technical reasons, pseudocholinesterase is generally tested, although this analysis is less sensitive than the one for acetylcholinesterase.

In suspected poisoning by muscle relaxant, the patient lacks adequate pseudocholinesterase, which normally inactivates the muscle relaxant. In this case, measurement of pseudocholinesterase is required.

Purpose

• To evaluate, before surgery or electroconvulsive therapy, the patient's potential response to succinylcholine, which is hydrolyzed by cholinesterase
• To detect patients who may have adverse reactions to muscle relaxants
• To assess overexposure to insecticides containing organophosphate compounds
• To assess liver function and aid diagnosis of liver disease (a rare purpose)

Patient preparation

• Explain to the patient that this test is used to assess muscle function or the extent of poisoning.

• Tell him that the test requires a blood sample. Explain who will perform the venipuncture and when.

• Explain that he may experience slight discomfort from the needle puncture and the tourniquet, but that collecting the sample usually takes less than 3 minutes.

• Inform him that he need not restrict food or fluids before the test.

• Withhold substances that affect serum cholinesterase levels, such as cyclophosphamide, echothiophate iodide, MAO inhibitors, succinylcholine, neostigmine, quinine, quinidine, chloroquine, caffeine, theophylline, epinephrine, ether, barbiturates, atropine, morphine, codeine, phenothiazines, vitamin K, and folic acid. If such substances must be continued, note this on the laboratory slip.

Procedure and posttest care

• Perform a venipuncture, and collect the sample in a 7-ml *red-top* tube.

• If a hematoma develops at the venipuncture site, apply warm soaks.

• Resume administration of medications that were discontinued before the test.

Precautions

• Handle the collection tube gently because excessive agitation can cause hemolysis.

• If the sample cannot be sent to the laboratory within 6 hours after being drawn, refrigerate it.

Reference values

Pseudocholinesterase levels range from 8 to 18 U/ml (when determined by kinetic colorimetric technique).

Abnormal findings

Severely depressed pseudocholinesterase levels suggest a congenital deficiency or organophosphate insecticide poisoning; levels near zero necessitate emergency treatment.

Pseudocholinesterase levels are usually normal in early extrahepatic obstruction and are variably decreased in hepatocellular damage, such as hepatitis or cirrhosis (especially cirrhosis with ascites and jaundice). Levels also decline in acute infections, chronic malnutrition, anemia, myocardial infarction, obstructive jaundice, and metastasis.

GLUCOSE-6-PHOSPHATE DEHYDROGENASE

Glucose-6-phosphate dehydrogenase (G6PD), an enzyme found in most body cells, is involved in metabolizing glucose. This test is used to detect G6PD deficiency, which is a hereditary, sex-linked condition that impairs stability of the red cell membrane and allows red cells to be destroyed by strong oxidizing agents.

About 10% of all African American males in the United States inherit mild G6PD deficiencies; some people of Mediterranean origin inherit severe deficiencies. In some whites, fava beans may produce hemolytic episodes. Although deficiency of G6PD provides partial immunity to falciparum malaria, it precipitates an adverse reaction to antimalarials.

Purpose

• To detect hemolytic anemia caused by G6PD deficiency

• To aid differential diagnosis of hemolytic anemia

Patient preparation

• Explain to the patient that this test is used to detect an inherited enzyme deficiency that may affect red blood cells.

- Tell him that the test requires a blood sample. Explain who will perform the venipuncture and when.
- Explain that he may experience slight discomfort from the needle puncture and the tourniquet, but that collecting the sample usually takes less than 3 minutes.
- Inform him that he need not restrict food or fluids before the test.
- Check patient history, and report recent blood transfusion or ingestion of aspirin, sulfonamides, phenacetin, nitrofurantoin, vitamin K derivatives, antimalarials, or fava beans, which cause hemolysis in people who are G6PD-deficient.

Procedure and posttest care
- Perform a venipuncture, and collect the sample in a 7-ml *lavender-top* tube.
- If a hematoma develops at the venipuncture site, apply warm soaks.

Precautions
- Completely fill the collection tube, and invert it gently several times to mix the sample and the anticoagulant.
- Handle the sample gently to prevent hemolysis.
- Send the sample to the laboratory immediately. If delayed, refrigerate the specimen.

Reference values
Serum values of G6PD vary with the measurement method used and may be reported as normal or abnormal.

Abnormal findings
Fluorescent spot testing or staining for Heinz bodies or erythrocytes can test for G6PD deficiency. If results are positive, the kinetic quantitative assay for G6PD may be performed. Electrophoretic techniques assess genetic variants of deficiencies (which may cause lifelong, mild, or asymptomatic anemia). Some variants are symptomatic only when the patient has stress, illness, or exposure to drugs or agents that elicit hemolytic episodes.

PYRUVATE KINASE

An erythrocyte enzyme, pyruvate kinase (PK) takes part in the anaerobic metabolism of glucose. An abnormally low PK level is an inherited autosomal recessive trait that may cause a red cell membrane defect associated with congenital hemolytic anemia. PK assay confirms PK deficiency when red cell enzyme deficiency is the suspected cause of anemia.

Purpose
- To differentiate PK-deficient hemolytic anemia from other congenital hemolytic anemias, or from acquired hemolytic anemia
- To detect PK deficiency in asymptomatic, heterozygous inheritance

Patient preparation
- Explain to the patient that this test is used to detect inherited enzyme deficiencies.
- Tell him that the test requires a blood sample. Explain who will perform the venipuncture and when.
- Explain that he may experience slight discomfort from the needle puncture and the tourniquet, but that collecting the sample usually takes less than 3 minutes.
- Inform him that he need not restrict food or fluids before the test.
- Check history for recent blood transfusion, and note it on the laboratory slip.

Procedure and posttest care
- Perform a venipuncture, and collect the sample in a 7-ml *lavender-top* tube.

• If a hematoma develops at the venipuncture site, apply warm soaks.

Precautions
• Completely fill the collection tube, and invert it *gently* several times to mix the sample and the anticoagulant without causing hemolysis.
• Refrigerate the specimen if you cannot send it to the laboratory immediately.

Reference values
In a routine assay (ultraviolet), serum PK levels range from 2.0 to 8.8 U/g of hemoglobin; in the low substrate assay, 0.9 to 3.9 U/g of hemoglobin.

Abnormal findings
Low serum PK levels confirm diagnosis of PK deficiency and allow differentiation between the PK-deficient hemolytic anemia and other inherited disorders.

HEXOSAMINIDASE A AND B

Hexosaminidase is a group of enzymes necessary for metabolism of gangliosides, water-soluble glycolipids found primarily in brain tissue. This test is used to measure the hexosaminidase A and B content of serum or amniotic fluid.

Deficiency of hexosaminidase A indicates Tay-Sachs disease, a disorder that affects people of Ashkenazic Jewish ancestry about 100 times more often than the general population. Both parents must carry the defective gene to transmit Tay-Sachs disease to their children. Sandhoff's disease, which results from deficiency of both hexosaminidase A and B, is uncommon and not prevalent in any ethnic group.

Purpose
• To confirm or rule out Tay-Sachs disease in neonates
• To screen for Tay-Sachs carriers
• To establish prenatal diagnosis of hexosaminidase A deficiency

Patient preparation
• Explain to the patient that this test is used to identify carriers of Tay-Sachs disease.
• Tell him that the test requires a blood sample. Explain who will perform the venipuncture and when.
• Explain that slight discomfort may result from the needle puncture and the tourniquet, but that collecting the sample usually takes less than 3 minutes.
• Inform the patient that food or fluids need not be restricted before the test.
• When testing a neonate, explain to the parents that this test is used to detect Tay-Sachs disease. Tell them blood will be drawn from the baby's arm, neck, or umbilical cord, and explain that the procedure is safe and quickly performed. Inform the parents that no pretest restrictions of food or fluid are necessary. Tell them the infant will have a small bandage on the site of venipuncture.
• If the test is being performed prenatally, advise the patient of preparations for amniocentesis.

Procedure and posttest care
• Perform a venipuncture, collect cord blood, or assist with amniocentesis, as appropriate. Collect the sample in a 7-ml *red-top* tube.
• If a hematoma develops at the venipuncture site, apply warm soaks.
• If both partners are carriers of Tay-Sachs disease, refer them for genetic counseling.
• When testing a neonate, follow laboratory procedure for collecting serum samples.

Precautions
• Handle the collection tube gently.
• This test cannot be done on a pregnant woman's serum (but her leukocytes or amniotic fluid may be tested if necessary); if the father's blood test result is negative, the child will not get Tay-Sachs disease.

Reference values
Total serum levels of hexosaminidase range from 5 to 12.9 U/L; hexosaminidase A accounts for 55% to 76% of total.

Abnormal findings
Absence of hexosaminidase A indicates Tay-Sachs disease (total hexosaminidase levels can be normal). Absence of both hexosaminidase A and B indicates Sandhoff's disease, an uncommon, virulent variant of Tay-Sachs disease that causes faster deterioration.

UROPORPHYRINOGEN I SYNTHASE

This test is used to measure blood levels of uroporphyrinogen I synthase, an enzyme involved in heme biosynthesis. This enzyme is normally present in erythrocytes, fibroblasts, lymphocytes, liver cells, and amniotic fluid cells. A hereditary deficiency that can reduce uroporphyrinogen I synthase levels by 50% or more results in acute intermittent porphyria (AIP). This disorder can be latent indefinitely, until certain factors (some sex hormones and drugs, a low-carbohydrate diet, or an infection) precipitate active disease.

Purpose
• To aid diagnosis of latent or active AIP

• To differentiate AIP from other types of porphyria

Patient preparation
• Explain to the patient that this test is used to detect a red blood cell disorder.
• Inform him that he will need to fast for 12 to 14 hours before the test, and to abstain from alcohol for 24 hours, but that he may drink water.
• Tell him that the test requires a blood sample. Explain who will perform the venipuncture and when.
• Explain that he may experience slight discomfort from the needle puncture and the tourniquet, but that collecting the sample usually takes less than 3 minutes.
• If the patient's hematocrit is available, record this on the laboratory slip.
• Check the patient's medication history. Withhold any drugs that may decrease uroporphyrinogen I synthase levels. These may include steroid hormones, estrogens, barbiturates, sulfonamides, phenytoin, griseofulvin, chlordiazepoxide, meprobamate, glutethimide, methyprylon, and ergot alkaloids. If they must be continued, note this on the laboratory slip.

Procedure and posttest care
• Perform a venipuncture and collect the sample in a 10-ml *green-top* tube.
• If a hematoma develops at the venipuncture site, apply warm soaks.
• Instruct the patient to resume usual diet and medications.
• If AIP is present, refer the patient for nutrition and genetic counseling. Advise him to avoid low-carbohydrate diets, alcohol, and drugs which may trigger an acute episode. Remind him to seek care promptly for all infections to avoid precipitating an acute episode.

Precautions
• Handle the sample gently.

• Send the specimen, on ice, to the laboratory immediately.

Reference values

Normal values for uroporphyrinogen I synthase are greater than or equal to 7.0 nmol/sec/L.

Abnormal findings

Decreased levels generally indicate latent or active AIP; symptoms differentiate these phases. Levels that are below 6.0 nmol/sec/L confirm AIP. Levels between 6.0 and 6.9 nmol/sec/L are indeterminate, in which case urine and stool tests for the porphyrin precursors aminolevulinic acid and porphobilinogen may be ordered to support the diagnosis.

GALACTOSE-1-PHOSPHATE URIDYL TRANSFERASE

This enzyme is involved in the conversion of galactose to glucose during lactose metabolism. Deficiency may lead to galactosemia, a hereditary disorder marked by elevated serum galactose and decreased serum glucose. Unless detected and treated soon after birth, galactosemia can impair eye, brain, and liver development, causing irreversible cataracts, mental retardation, and cirrhosis.

The qualitative test, a simple screening test for deficiency of galactose-1-phosphate uridyl transferase, is required in some hospitals for all neonates. Prenatal testing of amniotic fluid can also detect transferase deficiency, but is rarely performed.

Purpose

• To screen infants for galactosemia

• To detect heterozygous carriers of galactosemia

Patient preparation

• When testing a neonate, explain to the parents that the test screens for galactosemia, a potentially dangerous enzyme deficiency.

• If a blood sample was not taken from the umbilical cord at birth, tell the parents that a small amount of blood will be drawn from their infant's heel. Explain that the procedure is safe and quickly performed.

• When testing an adult, explain that the test is used to identify a carrier state of galactosemia, a genetic disorder that may be transmitted to his children.

• Tell him that the test requires a blood sample. Explain who will perform the venipuncture and when.

• Explain that he may experience slight discomfort from the needle puncture and the tourniquet, but that collecting the sample usually takes less than 3 minutes.

• Inform him that he need not restrict food or fluids before the test.

Procedure and posttest care

• For a qualitative (screening) test, collect cord blood or blood from a heel stick on special filter paper, saturating all three circles.

• For a quantitative test, perform a venipuncture and collect a 4-ml sample in a *green-top* or *lavender-top* tube, depending on the laboratory method used.

• Indicate the patient's age on the laboratory slip.

• Check his history for a recent exchange transfusion. Note this on the laboratory slip or postpone the test.

• If a hematoma develops at the venipuncture site, apply warm soaks.

• If test results indicate galactosemia, refer parents for nutrition counseling, and provide a galactose- and lactose-free diet for their infant. A soybean or meat-based formula may be substituted for milk.

Precautions
• Handle the collection tube gently to prevent hemolysis.
• Send the collection tube to the laboratory on wet ice.

Reference values
Normally, the qualitative test is negative. The normal range for the quantitative test is 18.5 to 28.5 U/g of hemoglobin; however, confirm the normal range with the laboratory in case a different method is used.

Abnormal findings
A positive qualitative test may indicate a transferase deficiency. A follow-up quantitative test should be performed as soon as possible. Quantitative test results less than 5 U/g of hemoglobin indicate galactosemia. Levels between 5 and 18.5 U/g of hemoglobin may indicate a carrier state.

ANGIOTENSIN-CONVERTING ENZYME

This test is used to measure serum levels of angiotensin-converting enzyme (ACE), which is found in lung capillaries and, in lesser concentrations, in blood vessels and kidney tissue. Its primary function is to help regulate arterial pressure by converting angiotensin I to angiotensin II. However, measurement of ACE is of little use in diagnosing hypertension.

Purpose
• To aid diagnosis of sarcoidosis, especially pulmonary sarcoidosis

• To monitor response to therapy in sarcoidosis
• To help confirm Gaucher's disease or leprosy

Patient preparation
• Explain to the patient that this test is used to diagnose sarcoidosis, Gaucher's disease, or leprosy, or to check his response to treatment for sarcoidosis.
• Tell him that the test requires a blood sample. Explain who will perform the venipuncture and when.
• Explain that he may experience slight discomfort from the needle puncture and the tourniquet, but that collecting the sample usually takes less than 3 minutes.
• Inform the patient that he must fast for 12 hours before the test.
• Note the patient's age on the laboratory slip. Because patients under age 20 have variable ACE levels, the test may need to be postponed if the patient is under age 20.

Procedure and posttest care
• Perform a venipuncture, and collect the sample in a 7-ml *red-top* tube.
• If a hematoma develops at the venipuncture site, apply warm soaks.

Precautions
• Avoid using a *lavender-top* tube or contaminating the sample with ethylenediaminetetraacetic acid because this can decrease ACE levels, thereby altering test results.
• Handle the collection tube gently to prevent hemolysis.
• Send the sample to the laboratory immediately, or freeze the sample and place it on dry ice until the test can be performed.

Reference values
In the colorimetric assay, normal values for serum ACE for patients over age 20 range from 6.1 to 21.1 U/L.

Abnormal findings

Elevated serum ACE levels may indicate sarcoidosis, Gaucher's disease, or leprosy, but results must be correlated with the patient's clinical condition. In some patients, elevated ACE levels may result from hyperthyroidism, diabetic retinopathy, or liver diseases.

Serum ACE levels decline as the patient responds to steroid or prednisone therapy for sarcoidosis.

LIPIDS AND LIPOPROTEINS

TRIGLYCERIDES

Serum triglyceride analysis provides quantitative analysis of triglycerides — the main storage form of lipids — which constitute about 95% of fatty tissue. Although not in itself diagnostic, it permits early identification of hyperlipemia and risk of coronary artery disease (CAD).

Purpose

• To screen for hyperlipemia
• To help identify nephrotic syndrome
• To determine the risk of CAD

Patient preparation

• Explain to the patient that this test is used to detect disorders of fat metabolism.
• Tell him that the test requires a blood sample. Explain who will perform the venipuncture and when.
• Explain that he may experience slight discomfort from the needle puncture and the tourniquet, but not collecting

the sample usually takes less than 3 minutes.
• Advise him to abstain from food for 10 to 14 hours before the test and to abstain from alcohol for 24 hours. Tell him it is not necessary to abstain from water.
• Withhold medications that may interfere with the accuracy of test results, including antilipemics, corticosteroids, estrogen, and some diuretics.

Procedure and posttest care

• Perform a venipuncture, and collect a serum sample in a 7-ml *lavender-top* tube that contains the anticoagulant ethylenediaminetetraacetic acid.
• If a hematoma develops at the venipuncture site, apply warm soaks.
• Tell the patient he may resume his usual diet.
• Resume the administration of any medications discontinued before the test.

Precautions

• Send the sample to the laboratory immediately.
• Some redistribution may occur among lipids.

Reference values

Triglyceride values are age- and sex-related. There is some controversy about the most appropriate normal ranges. Nonetheless, serum values of 40 to 160 mg/dl for men and 35 to 135 mg/dl for women are widely accepted.

Abnormal findings

Increased or decreased serum triglyceride levels suggest a clinical abnormality; additional tests are required for definitive diagnosis.

Mild-to-moderate increase in serum triglyceride levels indicates biliary obstruction, diabetes, nephrotic syndrome, endocrinopathies, or overconsumption of alcohol. Markedly increased levels without an identifiable cause reflect congenital hyperlipoproteinemia and necessitate lipoprotein phenotyping to confirm diagnosis.

Decreased serum levels are rare, occurring mainly in malnutrition or abetalipoproteinemia.

TOTAL CHOLESTEROL

This test, the quantitative analysis of serum cholesterol, is used to measure the circulating levels of free cholesterol and cholesterol esters; it reflects the level of the two forms in which this biochemical compound appears in the body. High serum cholesterol levels may be associated with an increased risk of coronary artery disease (CAD).

Purpose
• To assess the risk of CAD
• To evaluate fat metabolism
• To aid diagnosis of nephrotic syndrome, pancreatitis, hepatic disease, and hypo- and hyperthyroidism

Patient preparation
• Explain to the patient that this test is used to assess the body's fat metabolism.
• Tell him that the test requires a blood sample. Explain who will perform the venipuncture and when.
• Explain that he may experience slight discomfort from the needle puncture and the tourniquet, but that collecting the sample usually takes less than 3 minutes.
• Advise the patient not to eat or drink for 12 hours before the test.
• Withhold drugs that influence cholesterol levels. These may include cholestyramine, clofibrate, colestipol, dextrothyroxine, haloperidol, neomycin, niacin, chlortetracycline, epinephrine, chlorpromazine, trifluoperazine, oral

contraceptives, trimethadione, and androgens.

Procedure and posttest care
• Perform a venipuncture, and collect the sample in a 7-ml *lavender-top* tube containing ethylenediaminetetraacetic acid anticoagulant.
• If a hematoma develops at the venipuncture site, apply warm soaks.
• Tell the patient he may resume his usual diet.
• Resume administration of medications discontinued before the test.

Precautions
• Send the sample to the laboratory immediately.

Reference values
Total cholesterol concentrations vary with age and sex. The normal range is 170 to 200 mg/dl. Levels of 280 to 320 mg/dl are considered elevated.

Abnormal findings
Elevated serum cholesterol (hypercholesterolemia) may indicate risk of CAD, as well as incipient hepatitis, lipid disorders, bile duct blockage, nephrotic syndrome, obstructive jaundice, pancreatitis, and hypothyroidism.

Low serum cholesterol (hypocholesterolemia) is commonly associated with malnutrition, cellular necrosis of the liver, and hyperthyroidism. Abnormal cholesterol levels frequently necessitate further testing to pinpoint the cause.

PHOSPHOLIPIDS

This test is a quantitative analysis of phospholipid levels. Phospholipids are involved in cellular membrane composition and permeability, and in controlling enzyme activity within the membrane. They aid transport of fatty acids and lipids across the intestinal barrier, and from the liver and other fat depots to other body tissues, and they are essential for pulmonary gas exchange.

Purpose
• To aid in the evaluation of fat metabolism
• To aid diagnosis of hypothyroidism, diabetes mellitus, nephrotic syndrome, chronic pancreatitis, obstructive jaundice, and hypolipoproteinemia

Patient preparation
• Explain to the patient that this test is used to determine how the body metabolizes fats.
• Tell him that the test requires a blood sample. Explain who will perform the venipuncture and when.
• Explain that he may experience slight discomfort from the needle puncture and the tourniquet, but that collecting the sample usually takes less than 3 minutes.
• Instruct him to abstain from drinking alcohol for 24 hours before the test, and from food and fluids after midnight before the test.

Procedure and posttest care
• Perform a venipuncture, and collect the sample in a 10- to 15-ml *red-top* tube.
• If a hematoma develops at the venipuncture site, apply warm soaks.
• Tell the patient he may resume his usual diet.
• Resume administration of medications discontinued before the test.

Precautions
• Send the sample to the laboratory immediately, as spontaneous redistribution may occur among plasma lipids.

Reference values
Normal levels range from 180 to 320 mg/dl. Although men usually have higher levels than women, values in pregnant women exceed those of men.

Abnormal findings
Elevated levels may indicate hypothyroidism, diabetes mellitus, nephrotic syndrome, chronic pancreatitis, or obstructive jaundice. Decreased levels may indicate primary hypolipoproteinemia.

Lack of phospholipids in premature infants leads to neonatal respiratory distress syndrome.

LIPOPROTEIN-CHOLESTEROL FRACTIONATION

Cholesterol fractionation tests are used to isolate and measure the type of cholesterol in serum, low-density lipoproteins (LDL) and high-density lipoproteins (HDL). The HDL level is inversely related to the incidence of coronary artery disease (CAD); the higher the HDL level, the lower the incidence of CAD. Conversely, the higher the LDL level, the higher the incidence of CAD.

Purpose
• To assess the risk of CAD

Patient preparation
• Tell the patient that this test is used to determine the risk of CAD.
• Tell him that the test requires a blood sample. Explain who will perform the venipuncture and when.
• Explain that he may experience slight discomfort from the needle puncture and the tourniquet, but that collecting

the sample usually takes less than 3 minutes.

• Instruct him to maintain his normal diet for 2 weeks before the test, to abstain from alcohol for 24 hours before the test, and to fast and avoid exercise for 12 to 14 hours before the test.

• Withhold thyroid hormones, oral contraceptives, and antilipemics.

Procedure and posttest care

• Perform a venipuncture, and collect the sample in a 7-ml *red-top* or *red-marble-top* tube.

• If a hematoma develops at the venipuncture site, apply warm soaks.

• Tell the patient he may resume his usual diet.

• Resume administration of medications discontinued before the test.

Precautions

• Send the sample to the laboratory immediately, to avoid spontaneous redistribution among the lipoproteins.

• If the sample cannot be transported immediately, refrigerate, but do not freeze, it.

Reference values

Normal cholesterol values vary according to age, sex, geographic region, and ethnic group; check the laboratory for reference values. Normal HDL-cholesterol levels range from 29 to 77 mg/dl and normal LDL-cholesterol levels range from 62 to 185 mg/dl.

Abnormal findings

High LDL levels increase the risk of CAD. Elevated HDL levels generally reflect a healthy state but can also indicate chronic hepatitis, early-stage primary biliary cirrhosis, or alcohol consumption. Rarely, a sharp rise (to as high as 100 mg/dl) in a second type of HDL (alpha$_2$-HDL) may signal CAD.

LIPOPROTEIN PHENOTYPING

Lipoprotein phenotyping is used to determine levels of the four major lipoproteins: chylomicrons, very low-density (prebeta) lipoproteins (VLDL), low-density (beta) lipoproteins (LDL), and high-density (alpha) lipoproteins (HDL). Detecting altered lipoprotein patterns is key to identifying hyper- or hypolipoproteinemia.

Purpose

• To determine classification of hyper- or hypolipoproteinemia

Patient preparation

• Explain to the patient that this test is used to determine how the body metabolizes fats.

• Tell him that the test requires a blood sample. Explain who will perform the venipuncture and when. Explain that he may experience slight discomfort from the needle puncture and the tourniquet, but that collecting the sample usually takes less than 3 minutes.

• Instruct him to abstain from alcohol for 24 hours before the test and to fast after midnight before the test. Provide a low-fat meal the night before the test.

• Check the patient's drug history for use of heparin. Withhold antilipemics, such as cholestyramine, about 2 weeks before the test.

• Notify the laboratory if the patient is hospitalized for any other condition that might significantly alter lipoprotein metabolism, such as diabetes mellitus, nephrosis, or hypothyroidism.

Procedure and posttest care

• Perform a venipuncture, and collect the sample in a 7-ml *lavender-top* tube.

FAMILIAL HYPERLIPOPROTEINEMIAS

TYPE	CAUSES AND INCIDENCE	CLINICAL SIGNS	LABORATORY FINDINGS
I	• Deficient lipoprotein lipase, resulting in increased chylomicrons • May be induced by alcoholism • Incidence: rare	• Eruptive xanthomas • Lipemia retinalis • Abdominal pain	• Increased chylomicron, total cholesterol, and triglyceride levels • Normal or slightly increased VLDL • Normal or decreased LDL and HDL • Cholesterol-triglyceride ratio under 0.2
IIa	• Deficient cell receptor, resulting in increased LDL and excessive cholesterol synthesis • May be induced by hypothyroidism • Incidence: common	• Premature coronary artery disease (CAD) • Arcus cornea • Xanthelasma • Tendinous and tuberous xanthomas	• Increased LDL • Normal VLDL • Cholesterol-triglyceride ratio over 2.0
IIb	• Deficient cell receptor resulting in increased LDL and excessive cholesterol synthesis • May be induced by dysgammaglobulinemia, hypothyroidism, uncontrolled diabetes mellitus, and nephrotic syndrome • Incidence: common	• Premature CAD • Obesity • Possible xanthelasmas	• Increased LDL, VLDL, total cholesterol, and triglycerides
III	• Unknown cause, resulting in deficient VLDL-to-LDL conversion • May be induced by hypothyroidism, uncontrolled diabetes mellitus, and paraproteinemia • Incidence: rare	• Premature CAD • Arcus cornea • Eruptive tuberous xanthomas	• Increased total cholesterol, VLDL, and triglycerides • Normal or decreased LDL • Cholesterol-triglyceride ratio of VLDL over 0.4 • Broad beta band observed on electrophoresis
IV	• Unknown cause, resulting in decreased levels of lipoprotein lipase (LPL) • May be induced by uncontrolled diabetes mellitus, alcoholism, pregnancy, steroid or estrogen therapy, dysgammaglobulinemia, and hyperthyroidism • Incidence: common	• Possible premature CAD • Obesity • Hypertension • Peripheral neuropathy	• Increased VLDL and triglycerides • Normal LDL • Cholesterol-triglyceride ratio of VLDL under 0.25

(continued)

Familial Hyperlipoproteinemias *(continued)*

TYPE	CAUSES AND INCIDENCE	CLINICAL SIGNS	LABORATORY FINDINGS
V	• Unknown cause, resulting in defective triglyceride clearance • May be induced by alcoholism, dysgamma-globulinemia, uncontrolled diabetes mellitus, neph-rotic syndrome, pancre-atitis, and steroid therapy • Incidence: rare	• Premature CAD • Abdominal pain • Lipemia retinalis • Eruptive xantho-mas • Hepatospleno-megaly	• Increased VLDL, total cholesterol, and triglycer-ides • Chylomicrons present • Cholesterol-triglyceride ratio under 0.6

• If a hematoma develops at the veni-puncture site, apply warm soaks.
• Instruct the patient to resume his diet.
• Resume administration of medica-tions withheld before the test.

Precautions
• When drawing multiple samples, col-lect the sample for lipoprotein pheno-typing first, as venous obstruction for 2 minutes can affect test results.
• Fill the collection tube completely, and invert it gently several times to mix the sample and the anticoagulant.
• Handle the sample gently to prevent hemolysis, which can alter test results.

Findings
The types of hyperlipoproteinemias or hypolipoproteinemias are identified by characteristic electrophoretic patterns. (See *Familial hyperlipoproteinemias*.)

Familial lipoprotein disorders are classified as either hyper- or hypo-lipoproteinemias. There are six types of hyperlipoproteinemias: I, IIa, IIb, III, IV, and V. Types IIa, IIb, and IV are relative-ly common. All hypolipoproteinemias are rare, including hypobetalipoprotein-emia, abetalipoproteinemia , and alpha-lipoprotein deficiency.

PROTEINS AND PROTEIN METABOLITES

PROTEIN ELECTROPHORESIS

This test is used to measure serum albu-min and globulins, the major blood pro-teins, by separating the proteins into five distinct fractions: albumin and al-pha$_1$, alpha$_2$, beta, and gamma proteins.

Purpose
• To aid diagnosis of hepatic disease, protein deficiency, renal disorders, and gastrointestinal and neoplastic diseases

Patient preparation
• Explain to the patient that this test is used to determine the protein content of blood.

• Tell him that the test requires a blood sample. Explain who will perform the venipuncture and when.

• Explain that he may experience slight discomfort from the needle puncture and the tourniquet, but that collecting the sample usually takes less than 3 minutes.

• Inform him that he need not restrict food or fluids before the test.

• Check the patient's medication history for drugs that may influence serum protein levels such as alkalating agents, antimetabolites, antibiotic antineoplastic agents, and antineoplastics that alter hormone balance. If they must be continued, note this on the laboratory slip.

Procedure and posttest care

• Perform a venipuncture, and collect the sample in a 7-ml *red-top* or *red-marble-top* tube.

• If a hematoma develops at the venipuncture site, apply warm soaks.

Precautions

• This test must be performed on a serum sample to avoid measuring the fibrinogen fraction.

• Pretest administration of a contrast dye (such as sulfobromophthalein) falsely elevates total protein test results.

• Pregnancy and the use of cytotoxic agents may lower serum albumin.

Reference values

Normally, total serum protein levels range from 6.6 to 7.9 g/dl. The albumin fraction ranges from 3.3 to 4.5 g/dl. The alpha$_1$-globulin fraction ranges from 0.1 to 0.4 g/dl; alpha$_2$-globulin ranges from 0.5 to 1 g/dl. Beta globulin ranges from 0.7 to 1.2 g/dl; gamma globulin ranges from 0.5 to 1.6 g/dl.

Abnormal findings

For common findings, see *Clinical implications of abnormal protein levels.*

CERULOPLASMIN

This test is used to measure serum levels of ceruloplasmin, an alpha$_2$-globulin that binds about 95% of serum copper, usually in the liver. Ceruloplasmin is thought to regulate iron uptake by transferrin, making iron available to reticulocytes for heme synthesis.

Purpose

• To aid diagnosis of Wilson's disease, Menkes' kinky hair syndrome, and copper deficiency from total parenteral nutrition

Patient preparation

• Explain to the patient that this test is used to determine the copper content of blood.

• Tell him that the test requires a blood sample. Explain who will perform the venipuncture and when.

• Explain that he may experience slight discomfort from the needle puncture and the tourniquet, but that collecting the sample usually takes less than 3 minutes.

• Check his history for drugs that may influence ceruloplasmin levels, such as estrogen, methadone, and phenytoin.

Procedure and posttest care

• Perform a venipuncture, and collect the sample in a 7-ml *red-top* or *red-marble-top* tube.

• If a hematoma develops at the venipuncture site, apply warm soaks.

Precautions

• Send the sample to the laboratory immediately.

Reference values

Serum ceruloplasmin levels for adults normally range from 22.9 to 43.1 mg/dl.

CLINICAL IMPLICATIONS OF ABNORMAL PROTEIN LEVELS

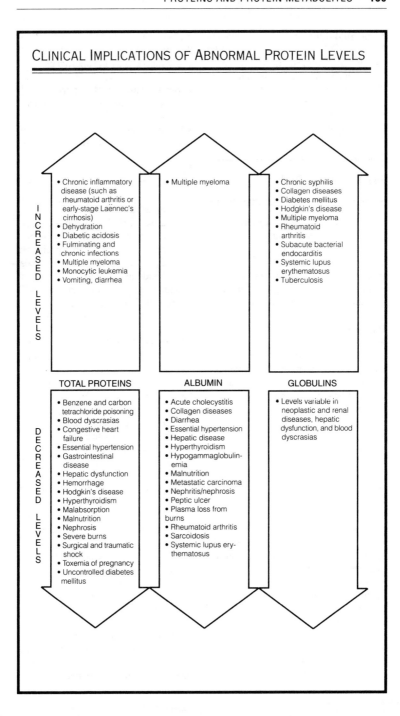

INCREASED LEVELS

TOTAL PROTEINS

- Chronic inflammatory disease (such as rheumatoid arthritis or early-stage Laënnec's cirrhosis)
- Dehydration
- Diabetic acidosis
- Fulminating and chronic infections
- Multiple myeloma
- Monocytic leukemia
- Vomiting, diarrhea

ALBUMIN

- Multiple myeloma

GLOBULINS

- Chronic syphilis
- Collagen diseases
- Diabetes mellitus
- Hodgkin's disease
- Multiple myeloma
- Rheumatoid arthritis
- Subacute bacterial endocarditis
- Systemic lupus erythematosus
- Tuberculosis

DECREASED LEVELS

TOTAL PROTEINS

- Benzene and carbon tetrachloride poisoning
- Blood dyscrasias
- Congestive heart failure
- Essential hypertension
- Gastrointestinal disease
- Hepatic dysfunction
- Hemorrhage
- Hodgkin's disease
- Hyperthyroidism
- Malabsorption
- Malnutrition
- Nephrosis
- Severe burns
- Surgical and traumatic shock
- Toxemia of pregnancy
- Uncontrolled diabetes mellitus

ALBUMIN

- Acute cholecystitis
- Collagen diseases
- Diarrhea
- Essential hypertension
- Hepatic disease
- Hyperthyroidism
- Hypogammaglobulin-emia
- Malnutrition
- Metastatic carcinoma
- Nephritis/nephrosis
- Peptic ulcer
- Plasma loss from burns
- Rheumatoid arthritis
- Sarcoidosis
- Systemic lupus erythematosus

GLOBULINS

- Levels variable in neoplastic and renal diseases, hepatic dysfunction, and blood dyscrasias

Abnormal findings

Low ceruloplasmin levels usually indicate Wilson's disease. Low levels may also occur in Menkes' kinky hair syndrome, nephrotic syndrome, and hypocupremia caused by total parenteral nutrition. Elevated levels may indicate certain hepatic diseases and infections.

HAPTOGLOBIN

This test is used to measure serum levels of haptoglobin — a glycoprotein produced in the liver. In acute intravascular hemolysis, haptoglobin concentration decreases rapidly and may remain so for 5 to 7 days, until the liver synthesizes more glycoprotein.

Purpose

• To serve as an index of hemolysis
• To distinguish between hemoglobin and myoglobin in plasma, as haptoglobin binds with free hemoglobin but does not bind with myoglobin
• To investigate hemolytic transfusion reactions
• To establish proof of paternity, using genetic (phenotypic) variations in haptoglobin structure

Patient preparation

• Explain to the patient that this test is used to determine the condition of red blood cells.
• Tell him that the test requires a blood sample. Explain who will perform the venipuncture and when.
• Explain that he may experience slight discomfort from the needle puncture and the tourniquet, but that collecting the sample usually takes less than 3 minutes.
• Inform him that he need not restrict food or fluids before the test.

• Check the patient's history for drugs that may influence haptoglobin levels, including steroids and androgens.

Procedure and posttest care

• Draw a venous blood sample into a 7-ml *red-top* or *red-marble-top* tube.
• If a hematoma develops at the venipuncture site, apply warm soaks.

Precautions

• Handle the sample gently.

Reference values

Normally, serum haptoglobin concentrations, measured in terms of the protein's hemoglobin-binding capacity, are 38 to 270 mg/dl. Nephelometric procedures yield lower results.

Although haptoglobin is absent in 90% of neonates, in most cases levels gradually increase to normal by age 4 months.

Abnormal findings

Markedly depressed serum haptoglobin levels are characteristic in acute and chronic hemolysis, severe hepatocellular disease, infectious mononucleosis, and transfusion reactions. Hepatocellular disease inhibits the synthesis of haptoglobin. In hemolytic transfusion reactions, haptoglobin levels begin decreasing after 6 to 8 hours and drop to 40% of pretransfusion levels after 24 hours.

If serum haptoglobin values are very low, watch for symptoms of hemolysis: chills, fever, back pain, flushing, distended neck veins, tachycardia, tachypnea, and hypotension.

In about 1% of the population — including 4% of African Americans — haptoglobin is permanently absent; this disorder is known as congenital ahaptoglobinemia.

Strikingly elevated serum haptoglobin levels occur in diseases marked by chronic inflammatory reactions or tissue destruction, such as rheumatoid arthritis and malignant neoplasms.

TRANSFERRIN

A quantitative analysis of serum transferrin (siderophilin) levels is used to evaluate iron metabolism. Transferrin, a glycoprotein that is formed in the liver, transports circulating iron, obtained from dietary sources or the breakdown of red blood cells by reticuloendothelial cells, to bone marrow for use in hemoglobin synthesis or to the liver, spleen, and bone marrow for storage. A serum iron level is usually obtained simultaneously.

Purpose
• To determine the iron-transporting capacity of the blood
• To evaluate iron metabolism in iron deficiency anemia

Patient preparation
• Explain to the patient that this test is used to determine the cause of anemia.
• Tell him that the test requires a blood sample. Explain who will perform the venipuncture and when.
• Explain that he may experience slight discomfort from the needle puncture and the tourniquet, but that collecting the sample usually takes less than 3 minutes.
• Inform him that he need not restrict food or fluids before the test.
• Check the patient's history for drugs that may influence transferrin levels.

Procedure and posttest care
• Perform a venipuncture, and collect the sample in a 7-ml *red-top* or *red-marble-top* tube.
• If a hematoma develops at the venipuncture site, apply warm soaks.

Precautions
• Handle the sample gently, and send it to the laboratory immediately.

Reference values
Normal serum transferrin values range from 220 to 400 mcg/dl, of which 65 to 170 mcg/dl are usually bound to iron.

Abnormal findings
Inadequate transferrin levels may lead to impaired hemoglobin synthesis and, possibly, anemia. Depressed serum levels may indicate inadequate production of transferrin due to hepatic damage or excessive protein loss from renal disease. Decreased transferrin levels may also result from acute or chronic infection or from cancer.

Elevated serum transferrin levels may indicate severe iron deficiency.

PLASMA AMINO ACID SCREENING

This test is a qualitative screen for inborn errors of amino acid metabolism. Amino acids are the chief component of all proteins and polypeptides. The body contains at least 20 amino acids, the chief components of all proteins and polypeptides. There are 10 amino acids which aren't formed in the body and must be acquired by diet. Certain congenital enzymatic deficiencies interfere with normal metabolism of these amino acids and cause accumulation or deficiency of them.

Purpose
• To screen for inborn errors of amino acid metabolism

Patient preparation
• Explain to the parents that this test is used to determine how well their infant metabolizes amino acids.
• The infant must fast for 4 hours before the test.
• Tell the parents that a small amount of blood will be drawn from the infant's heel, but that collecting the sample only takes a few minutes.

Procedure and posttest care
• Perform a heelstick, and collect 0.1 ml of blood in a heparinized capillary tube.
• If a hematoma develops at the heelstick site, apply warm soaks.
• Tell parents to resume their infant's usual diet.

Precautions
• Handle the sample gently to prevent hemolysis.

Reference values
Chromatography shows a normal plasma amino acid pattern.

Abnormal findings
Excessive accumulation of amino acids typically produces overflow aminoacidurias. Congenital abnormalities of the amino acid transport system in the kidneys produce a second group of disorders called renal aminoacidurias. Comparisons of blood and urine chromatography can help distinguish between the two types of aminoacidurias. The plasma amino acid pattern is normal in renal aminoacidurias and abnormal in overflow aminoacidurias.

PHENYLALANINE SCREENING

Also called the Guthrie screening test, this test is used to screen infants for elevated serum phenylalanine, a possible indication of phenylketonuria (PKU). Phenylalanine is a naturally occurring amino acid essential to growth and nitrogen balance; accumulation of this amino acid may indicate a serious enzyme deficiency. This test detects abnormal phenylalanine levels through the growth rate of *Bacillus subtilis*, an organism that needs phenylalanine to thrive. To ensure accurate results, the test must be performed after 3 full days (preferably 4 days) of milk or formula feeding.

Purpose
• To screen infants for possible PKU

Patient preparation
• Explain to the parents of the infant that the test is a routine screening measure for possible PKU and is a required test in many states.
• Tell them the test requires a blood sample and that a small amount of blood will be drawn from the infant's heel.

Procedure and posttest care
• Perform a heelstick, and collect three drops of blood — one in each circle — on the filter paper.
• Reassure the parents of a child who may have PKU that although this disease is a common cause of congenital mental deficiency, early detection and continuous treatment with a low-phenylalanine diet can prevent permanent mental retardation.

Precautions
• Note the infant's name and birth date, and the date of the first milk or formula feeding on the laboratory slip, and send the sample to the laboratory immediately.

Reference values
A negative test indicates normal phenylalanine levels (less than 2 mg/dl) and no appreciable danger of PKU.

Abnormal findings
At birth, an infant with PKU usually has normal phenylalanine levels, but after milk or formula feeding begins, levels gradually increase due to deficiency of the liver enzyme that converts phenylalanine to tyrosine. A positive test result suggests *a possibility* of PKU. Diagnosis requires exact serum phenylalanine measurement and urine testing. A positive test may also result from hepatic disease, galactosemia, or delayed development of certain enzyme systems. (See *Confirming PKU.*)

PLASMA AMMONIA

This test measures plasma levels of ammonia, a nonprotein nitrogen compound that helps maintain acid-base balance.

In diseases such as cirrhosis of the liver, ammonia can bypass the liver and accumulate in the blood. Plasma ammonia levels may help indicate the severity of hepatocellular damage.

Purpose
• To help monitor the progression of severe hepatic disease and the effectiveness of therapy
• To recognize impending or established hepatic coma

CONFIRMING PKU

After the Guthrie screening test detects the possible presence of PKU, serum phenylalanine and tyrosine levels are measured to confirm diagnosis. Phenylalanine hydroxylase is the enzyme that converts phenylalanine to tyrosine. If this enzyme is absent, increasing phenylalanine levels and falling tyrosine levels indicate PKU. Samples are obtained by venipuncture (femoral or external jugular) and measured by fluorometry. Elevated serum phenylalanine (more than 4 mg/dl) and decreased tyrosine (less than 0.6mg/dl) — with urinary excretion of phenylpyruvic acid — confirm diagnosis of PKU.

Patient preparation
• Explain to the patient (or to a family member if the patient is comatose) that this test is used to evaluate liver function.
• Inform the patient to fast overnight before the test.
• Tell him that the test requires a blood sample. Explain who will perform the venipuncture and when and that he may feel transient discomfort from the needle puncture.
• Reassure him that collecting the sample takes only a few minutes.
• Check the patient's history for drugs that influence plasma ammonia levels. These include acetazolamide, thiazides, ammonium salts, or furosemide, which raise ammonia levels, and lactulose, neomycin, and kanamycin, which depress ammonia levels.

Procedure and posttest care
• Perform a venipuncture, and collect the sample in a 10-ml *green-marble-top* (heparinized) tube.
• Make sure bleeding has stopped before removing pressure from the venipuncture site.
• If a hematoma develops, apply warm soaks.
• Watch for signs of impending or established hepatic coma if plasma ammonia levels are high.

Precautions
• Notify the laboratory before performing the venipuncture, so that preliminary preparations can begin.
• Handle the sample gently, pack it in ice, and send it to the laboratory immediately.
• *Do not* use a chilled container.

Reference values
Normally, plasma ammonia levels are less than 50 µg/dl

Abnormal findings
Elevated plasma ammonia levels are common in severe hepatic disease — such as cirrhosis and acute hepatic necrosis — and may lead to hepatic coma. Elevated ammonia levels are also possible in Reye's syndrome, severe congestive heart failure, gastrointestinal hemorrhage, and erythroblastosis fetalis.

BLOOD UREA NITROGEN

This test is used to measure the nitrogen fraction of urea, the chief end product of protein metabolism. Formed in the liver from ammonia and excreted by the kidneys, urea constitutes 40% to 50% of the blood's nonprotein nitrogen. The blood urea nitrogen (BUN) level reflects protein intake and renal excretory capacity, but is a less reliable indicator of uremia than the serum creatinine level.

Purpose
• To evaluate renal function and aid diagnosis of renal disease
• To aid assessment of hydration

Patient preparation
• Tell the patient his test is used to evaluate kidney function.
• Inform him that he need not restrict food or fluids, but he should avoid a diet high in meat.
• Tell him that the test requires a blood sample. Explain who will perform the venipuncture and when.
• Explain that he may experience slight discomfort from the needle puncture and the tourniquet.
• Reassure him that collecting the sample takes only a few minutes and that test results should be available the next day.
• Check the patient's history for drugs that influence BUN levels, including chloramphenicol and nephrotoxic drugs, such as aminoglycosides, amphotericin B, and methicillin.

Procedure and posttest care
• Perform a venipuncture, and collect the sample in a 7-ml *red-top* or *red-marble-top* tube.
• If a hematoma develops at the venipuncture site, apply warm soaks.

Precautions
• Handle the sample gently to prevent hemolysis.

Reference values
BUN values normally range from 8 to 20 mg/dl, with slightly higher values in elderly patients.

Abnormal findings

Elevated BUN levels occur in renal disease, reduced renal blood flow (due to dehydration, for example), urinary tract obstruction, and in increased protein catabolism (as in burns).

Depressed BUN levels occur in severe hepatic damage, malnutrition, and overhydration.

CREATININE

Analysis of serum creatinine levels provides a more sensitive measure of renal damage than blood urea nitrogen levels. Creatinine is a nonprotein end product of creatine metabolism that appears in serum in amounts proportional to the body's muscle mass.

Purpose
• To assess renal glomerular filtration
• To screen for renal damage

Patient preparation
• Explain to the patient that this test is used to evaluate kidney function.
• Tell him that the test requires a blood sample. Explain who will perform the venipuncture and when.
• Explain that he may experience slight discomfort from the needle puncture and the tourniquet, but that collecting the sample usually takes less than 3 minutes.
• Instruct him to restrict food and fluids for about 8 hours before the test.
• Check whether he has received ascorbic acid, barbiturates, or diuretics within the past 24 hours.

Procedure and posttest care
• Perform a venipuncture, and collect the sample in a 7-ml *red-top* or *red-marble-top* tube.

• If a hematoma develops at the venipuncture site, apply warm soaks.

Precautions
• Handle the specimen gently, and send it to the laboratory immediately.

Reference values
Creatinine concentrations in males normally range from 0.8 to 1.2 mg/dl; in females, from 0.6 to 0.9 mg/dl.

Abnormal findings
Elevated levels generally indicate renal disease that has seriously damaged 50% or more of the nephrons. Elevated levels may also be associated with gigantism and acromegaly.

URIC ACID

This test is used to measure serum levels of uric acid, the major end metabolite of purine. Disorders of purine metabolism, rapid destruction of nucleic acids, and conditions marked by impaired renal excretion characteristically raise serum uric acid levels.

Purpose
• To confirm diagnosis of gout
• To help detect kidney dysfunction

Patient preparation
• Explain to the patient that this test is used to detect gout or kidney dysfunction.
• Tell him that the test requires a blood sample. Explain who will perform the venipuncture and when.
• Explain that he may experience slight discomfort from the needle puncture and the tourniquet. Reassure him that collecting the sample takes only a few minutes.
• Inform him that he must fast for 8 hours before the test.

• Check his medication history for loop diuretics, ethambutol, vincristine, pyrazinamide, thiazides, aspirin (low doses), acetaminophen, ascorbic acid, levodopa, or phenacetin.

Procedure and posttest care
• Perform a venipuncture, and collect the sample in a 7-ml *red-top* or *red-marble-top* tube.
• If a hematoma develops at the venipuncture site, apply warm soaks.

Precautions
• Handle the sample gently to prevent hemolysis.

Reference values
Uric acid concentrations in men normally range from 4.3 to 8.0 mg/dl; in women, from 2.3 to 6.0 mg/dl.

Abnormal findings
Increased levels may indicate gout or impaired renal function. Levels may also rise in congestive heart failure, glycogen storage disease, infections, hemolytic or sickle cell anemia, polycythemia, neoplasms, and psoriasis.

Depressed levels may indicate defective tubular absorption (as in Fanconi's syndrome) or acute hepatic atrophy.

PIGMENTS

BILIRUBIN

This test is used to measure serum levels of bilirubin, the predominant pigment in bile. Bilirubin is the major product of hemoglobin catabolism. Serum bilirubin measurements are especially significant in newborns, as elevated un-

conjugated bilirubin can accumulate in the brain, causing irreparable damage.

Purpose
• To evaluate hepatobiliary and erythropoietic functions
• To aid differential diagnosis of jaundice and monitor its progress.
• To aid diagnosis of biliary obstruction and hemolytic anemia
• To determine whether a newborn requires an exchange transfusion or phototherapy because of dangerously high unconjugated bilirubin levels

Patient preparation
• Explain to the patient that this test is used to evaluate liver function and the condition of red blood cells.
• Tell him that the test requires a blood sample. Explain who will perform the venipuncture and when.
• Explain that he may experience slight discomfort from the needle puncture and the tourniquet, but that collecting the sample usually takes less than 3 minutes.
• Inform the adult patient that he need not restrict fluids but should fast for at least 4 hours before the test. (Fasting is not necessary for newborns.)
• If the patient is an infant, tell the parents that a small amount of blood will be drawn from his heel, and who will perform the heelstick and when.
• Check the patient's medication history for use of drugs that are known to interfere with serum bilirubin levels.

Procedure and posttest care
• If the patient is an adult, perform a venipuncture, and collect the sample in a 7-ml *red-top* or *red-marble-top* tube.
• If the patient is an infant, perform a heelstick, and fill the microcapillary tube to the designated level with blood.
• If a hematoma develops at the venipuncture or heelstick site, apply warm soaks.

Precautions
• Protect the sample from strong sunlight and ultraviolet light.
• Handle the sample gently, and send it to the laboratory immediately.

Reference values
Normally in an adult, indirect serum bilirubin measures 1.1 mg/dl or less; direct serum bilirubin, less than 0.5 mg/dl. Total serum bilirubin in the newborn measures 1.0 to 12.0 mg/dl.

Abnormal findings
Elevated indirect serum bilirubin levels often indicate hepatic damage. High levels of indirect bilirubin are also likely in severe hemolytic anemia. If hemolysis continues, both direct and indirect bilirubin may rise. Other causes of elevated indirect bilirubin levels include congenital enzyme deficiencies, such as Gilbert's disease

Elevated direct serum bilirubin levels usually indicate biliary obstruction. If obstruction continues, both direct and indirect bilirubin may become elevated. In severe chronic hepatic damage, direct bilirubin concentrations may return to normal or near-normal levels, but elevated indirect bilirubin levels persist.

In newborns, total bilirubin levels that reach or exceed 18.0 mg/dl indicate the need for exchange transfusion.

FRACTIONATED ERYTHROCYTE PORPHYRINS

This test is used to measure erythrocyte porphyrins (also called erythropoietic porphyrins): protoporphyrin, coproporphyrin and uroporphyrin. Porphyrins are present in all protoplasm and are significant in energy storage and use. They are produced during heme biosynthesis and normally appear in small amounts in blood, urine, and feces. Production and excretion of porphyrins or their precursors increase in porphyria.

Purpose
• To aid diagnosis of congenital or acquired erythropoietic porphyrias
• To help confirm diagnosis of disorders affecting red blood cell activity

Patient preparation
• Explain to the patient that this test is used to detect red blood cell disorders.
• Tell him that the test requires a blood sample. Explain who will perform the venipuncture and when.
• Explain that he may experience slight discomfort from the needle puncture and the tourniquet, but that collecting the sample usually takes less than 3 minutes.

Procedure and posttest care
• Perform a venipuncture and collect the sample in a 5-ml or larger *green-top* tube.
• Label the sample, place it on ice, and send it to the laboratory.
• If a hematoma develops at the venipuncture site, apply warm soaks.

Precautions
• Handle the sample gently to prevent hemolysis.
• Promptly send the sample to the laboratory.

Reference values
Total porphyrin levels range from 16 to 60 µg/dl of packed red blood cells. Protoporphyrin levels range from 16 to 60 µg/dl. Coproporphyrins and uroporphyrins each have levels below 2 µg/dl.

Abnormal findings
Elevated levels suggest the need for further enzyme testing to identify the specific porphyria. Elevated protoporphyrin levels may indicate erythropoietic protoporphyria, infection, increased erythropoiesis, thalassemia, sideroblastic anemia, iron deficiency anemia, or lead poisoning.

Increased coproporphyrin levels may indicate congenital erythropoietic porphyria, erythropoietic protoporphyria or coproporphyria, and sideroblastic anemia.

Elevated uroporphyrin levels may indicate congenital erythropoietic porphyria or erythropoietic protoporphyria.

CARBOHYDRATES

FASTING PLASMA GLUCOSE

The fasting plasma glucose (or fasting blood sugar) test is used to measure plasma glucose levels following a 12- to 14-hour fast. It is commonly used to screen for diabetes mellitus, in which absence or deficiency of insulin allows persistently high glucose levels.

Purpose
• To screen for diabetes mellitus
• To monitor drug or dietary therapy in patients with diabetes mellitus

Patient preparation
• Explain to the patient that this test is used to detect disorders of glucose metabolism and aids diagnosis of diabetes.

• Tell him that the test requires a blood sample. Explain who will perform the venipuncture and when.
• Explain that he may experience slight discomfort from the needle puncture and the tourniquet, but that collecting the sample usually takes less than 3 minutes.
• Advise him to fast for 12 to 14 hours before the test.
• Withhold drugs that may affect test results, such as acetaminophen, chlorthalidone, thiazide diuretics, furosemide, triamterene, oral contraceptives (estrogen-progestogen combination), benzodiazepines, phenytoin, phenothiazines, lithium, epinephrine, arginine, phenolphthalein, dextrothyroxine, diazoxide, nicotinic acid (large doses), corticosteroids, I.V. glucose (note recent infusions), beta-adrenergic blockers, ethanol, clofibrate, insulin, oral antidiabetic agents, monamine oxidase inhibitors, and ethacrynic acid. If these medications must be continued, note this on the laboratory slip. Advise the patient with diabetes that he will receive his medication after the test.
• Alert the patient to the symptoms of hypoglycemia — weakness, restlessness, nervousness, hunger, and sweating — and tell him to report such symptoms immediately.

Procedure and posttest care
• Perform a venipuncture, and collect the sample in a 5-ml *gray-top* tube.
• If a hematoma develops at the venipuncture site, apply warm soaks.
• Provide a balanced meal or a snack.
• Resume administration of medications withheld before the test.

Precautions
• Send the sample to the laboratory immediately. If transport is delayed, refrigerate the sample.
• Specify on the laboratory slip the time when the patient last ate, the sample

collection time, and the time the last pretest insulin or oral hypoglycemic dose (if applicable) was given.

Reference values

Normal range for fasting plasma glucose varies according to the laboratory procedure. Generally, normal values after a 12- to 14-hour fast are 70 to 100 mg of "true glucose"/dl of blood when measured by the glucose oxidase and hexokinase methods.

Abnormal findings

Confirmation of diabetes mellitus requires fasting plasma glucose levels of 140 mg/dl or more obtained on two or more occasions. In patients with borderline or transient elevated levels, a 2-hour postprandial plasma glucose test or the oral glucose tolerance test may be performed to confirm diagnosis.

Increased fasting plasma glucose levels can also result from pancreatitis, recent acute illness (such as myocardial infarction), Cushing's syndrome, acromegaly, and pheochromocytoma. Hyperglycemia may also stem from hyperlipoproteinemia (especially type III, type IV, or type V), chronic hepatic disease, nephrotic syndrome, brain tumor, sepsis, or gastrectomy with dumping syndrome, and is typical in eclampsia, anoxia, and seizure disorder.

Depressed plasma glucose levels can result from hyperinsulinism, insulinoma, von Gierke's disease, functional or reactive hypoglycemia, myxedema, adrenal insufficiency, congenital adrenal hyperplasia, hypopituitarism, malabsorption syndrome, and some cases of hepatic insufficiency.

TWO-HOUR POSTPRANDIAL PLASMA GLUCOSE

Also called the 2-hour postprandial blood sugar test, this procedure is a valuable screening tool for detecting diabetes mellitus. This procedure is performed when the patient demonstrates symptoms of diabetes (polydipsia and polyuria) or when results of the fasting plasma glucose test suggest diabetes.

Purpose

• To aid diagnosis of diabetes mellitus
• To monitor drug or diet therapy in patients with diabetes mellitus

Patient preparation

• Explain to the patient that this test is used to evaluate glucose metabolism and to detect diabetes.
• Tell him that the test requires a blood sample. Explain who will perform the venipuncture and when.
• Explain that he may experience slight discomfort from the needle puncture and the tourniquet, but that collecting the sample usually takes less than 3 minutes.
• Tell him to eat a balanced meal or one containing 100 g of carbohydrate before the test and then to fast for 2 hours. Instruct him to avoid smoking and strenuous exercise after the meal.

Procedure and posttest care

• Perform a venipuncture, and collect the sample in a 5-ml *gray-top* tube.
• If a hematoma develops at the venipuncture site, apply warm soaks.
• Tell the patient to resume his usual diet and normal activity.

TWO-HOUR POSTPRANDIAL PLASMA GLUCOSE LEVELS BY AGE

The greatest difference in normal and diabetic insulin responses, and thus in plasma glucose concentration, occurs about 2 hours after a glucose challenge. Values of this test, however, can fluctuate according to the patient's age. After age 50, for example, normal levels rise markedly and steadily, sometimes reaching 160 mg/dl or higher. In younger patients, glucose concentration over 145 mg/dl suggests incipient diabetes and requires further evaluation.

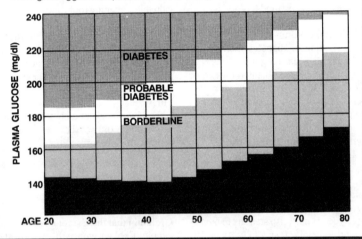

• Resume administration of medications discontinued before the test.

Precautions
• Send the sample to the laboratory immediately or refrigerate it.
• Specify on the laboratory slip the time when the patient last ate, the sample collection time, and the time the last pretest insulin or hypoglycemic dose was given.
• If the sample is to be drawn by a technician, tell him the exact time the venipuncture must be performed.

Reference values
In a person who doesn't have diabetes, postprandial glucose values are less than 145 mg/dl by the glucose oxidase or hexokinase method; levels are slightly elevated in persons over age 87. (See *Two-hour postprandial plasma glucose levels by age*.)

Abnormal findings
Two 2-hour postprandial blood glucose values of 200 mg/dl or above indicate diabetes mellitus. High levels may also occur with pancreatitis, Cushing's syndrome, acromegaly, and pheochromocytoma. Hyperglycemia may also be caused by hyperlipoproteinemia (especially type III, type IV, or type V), chronic hepatic disease, nephrotic syndrome, brain tumor, sepsis, gastrectomy with dumping syndrome, eclampsia, anoxia, or seizure disorders.

Depressed glucose levels occur in hyperinsulinism, insulinoma, von Gierke's disease, functional or reactive hypoglycemia, myxedema, adrenal insufficiency, congenital adrenal hyperplasia, hypopituitarism, malabsorption syndrome, and some cases of hepatic insufficiency.

ORAL GLUCOSE TOLERANCE TEST

The oral glucose tolerance test is the most sensitive method of evaluating borderline cases of diabetes mellitus. Plasma and urine glucose levels are monitored for 3 hours after ingestion of a challenge dose of glucose to assess insulin secretion and the body's ability to metabolize glucose.

The oral glucose tolerance test is not generally used in patients with fasting plasma glucose values greater than 140 mg/dl or postprandial plasma glucose values greater than 200 mg/dl.

Purpose
• To confirm diabetes mellitus in selected patients
• To aid diagnosis of hypoglycemia and malabsorption syndrome (requires monitoring for an additional 2 to 3 hours to aid diagnosis, which is contraindicated when insulinoma is strongly suspected because prolonged fasting may lead to fainting and coma)

Patient preparation
• Explain to the patient that this test is used to evaluate glucose metabolism.
• Instruct him to maintain a high-carbohydrate diet for 3 days and then to fast for 10 to 16 hours before the test.

• Advise him not to smoke, drink coffee or alcohol, or exercise strenuously for 8 hours before or during the test.
• Tell him this test requires five blood samples and usually five urine specimens. Explain who will perform the venipunctures and when, and that he may experience transient discomfort from the needle punctures and the pressure of the tourniquet.
• Suggest that he bring a book or other quiet diversions with him to the test, since the procedure usually takes 3 hours but can last as long as 6 hours.
• Withhold drugs that may affect test results. These may include chlorthalidone, thiazide diuretics, furosemide, triamterene, and contraceptives (estrogen-progestogen combination), benzodiazepines, phenytoin, phenothiazines, lithium, epinephrine, phenolphthalein, caffeine, arginine, dextrothyroxine, diazoxide, nicotinic acid (recent infusions), corticosteroids, I.V. glucose (note recent infusions), beta-adrenergic blockers, amphetamines, ethanol, clofibrate, insulin, oral antidiabetic drugs, and monamine oxidase inhibitors. If these drugs must be continued, note this on the laboratory slip.
• Alert the patient to the symptoms of hypoglycemia — weakness, restlessness, nervousness, hunger, and sweating — and tell him to report such symptoms immediately.

Procedure and posttest care
• Between 7 a.m. and 9 a.m., perform a venipuncture to obtain a fasting blood sample. Draw this sample into a 7-ml *gray-top* tube.
• Collect a urine specimen at the same time, if your institution includes this as part of the test.
• After collecting these samples, administer the test load of oral glucose, and record the time of ingestion. Encourage the patient to drink the entire glucose solution within 5 minutes.

INTERPRETING RESULTS OF THE ORAL GLUCOSE TOLERANCE TEST

Because various methods are used to measure serum glucose levels, inconsistent results or misinterpretations are common. Keep in mind that age, activity level, weight, and other factors may affect glucose levels. The American Diabetes Association recommends using the following diagnostic values obtained with the Wilkerson point system, the Fajans-Conn method, or the NIH method.

METHOD	HOUR	WHOLE BLOOD	PLASMA	POINTS
Wilkerson point system	Fasting	≥ 110 mg/dl	≥ 130 mg/dl	1
	1	≥ 170 mg/dl	≥ 195 mg/dl	1½
	2	≥ 120 mg/dl	≥ 140 mg/dl	1½
	3	≥ 110 mg/dl	≥ 130 mg/dl	1
Two or more total points confirm diagnosis of diabetes.				
Fajans-Conn	1	≥ 160 mg/dl	≥ 185 mg/dl	
	1½	≥ 140 mg/dl	≥ 165 mg/dl	
	2	≥ 120 mg/dl	≥ 140 mg/dl	
If all levels exceed or equal established values, diagnosis of diabetes is confirmed.				
National Institutes of Health (NIH)	Fasting		> 140 mg/dl	
	2		> 200 mg/dl	
If all levels exceed established values, diagnosis of diabetes is confirmed.				

- Draw blood samples 30 minutes, 1 hour, 2 hours, and 3 hours after giving the loading dose, using 7-ml *gray-top* tubes.
- Collect urine specimens at the same intervals.
- Tell the patient to lie down if he feels faint from the numerous venipunctures.
- Encourage him to drink water throughout the test to promote adequate urine excretion.
- If a hematoma develops at the venipuncture site, apply warm soaks.
- Provide a balanced meal or a snack, but observe for hypoglycemic reaction.
- Resume administration of medications withheld before the test.

Precautions
- Send blood and urine samples to the laboratory immediately, or refrigerate them.
- Specify when the patient last ate, and the blood and urine sample collection times.
- As appropriate, record the time the patient received his last pretest insulin or oral antidiabetic dose.
- If the patient develops severe hypoglycemia, notify the doctor. Draw a blood sample, record the time on the laboratory slip, and discontinue the test. Have the patient drink a glass of orange juice with sugar added, or administer glucose I.V. to reverse the reaction.

Reference values

Normal plasma glucose levels peak at 160 to 180 mg/dl within 30 minutes to 1 hour after administration of an oral glucose test dose and return to fasting levels or lower within 2 to 3 hours. Urine glucose tests remain negative throughout. (See *Interpreting results of the oral glucose tolerance test.*)

Abnormal findings

Depressed glucose tolerance, in which levels peak sharply before falling slowly to fasting levels, may confirm diabetes mellitus, or may result from Cushing's disease, hemochromatosis, pheochromocytoma, or central nervous system lesions.

Increased glucose tolerance, in which levels may peak at less than normal, may indicate insulinoma, malabsorption syndrome, adrenocortical insufficiency (Addison's disease), hypothyroidism, or hypopituitarism.

β-HYDROXYBUTYRATE

This test is used to measure serum levels of β-hydroxybutyric acid (β-hydroxybutyrate), which is one of three ketone bodies. The other two ketone bodies are acetoacetate and acetone. An accumulation of all three ketone bodies is referred to as ketosis: excessive formation of ketone bodies in the blood is called ketonemia.

Purpose

• To diagnose carbohydrate deprivation, which may result from starvation, digestive disturbances, dietary imbalances, or frequent vomiting
• To aid diagnosis of diabetes mellitus resulting from decreased utilization of carbohydrates

• To aid diagnosis of glycogen storage diseases, specifically von Gierke's disease
• To monitor the effect of insulin therapy during treatment of diabetic ketoacidosis
• To monitor patient status during emergency management of hypoglycemia, acidosis, excessive alcohol ingestion, or an unexplained increase in the anion gap

Patient preparation

• Explain to the patient that this test is used to evaluate ketones in the blood.
• Tell him that the test requires a blood sample. Explain who will perform the venipuncture and when.
• Explain that he may experience slight discomfort from the needle puncture and the tourniquet, but that collecting the sample usually takes less than 3 minutes.
• Inform him that he need not restrict food or fluids before the test.

Procedure and posttest care

• Perform a venipuncture and collect the sample in a 5-ml *red-top* tube.
• Allow the specimen to clot.
• Centrifuge and remove the serum.
• If an acetone level is requested, have this analysis performed first.
• Serum β-hydroxybutyrate remains stable for at least 1 week at 35.6° to 46.4° F (2° to 8° C). Plasma is also an acceptable specimen for analysis of β-hydroxybutyrate.
• If a hematoma develops at the venipuncture site, apply warm soaks.

Precautions

• Send the specimen to the laboratory immediately.

Reference values

The normal value for serum or plasma β-hydroxybutyrate levels is less than 0.4 mmol/L.

Abnormal findings

Elevated levels may suggest worsening of ketosis. Reference values greater than 2 mmol/L require immediate notification of the patient's doctor.

GLYCOSYLATED HEMOGLOBIN

Also called total fasting hemoglobin (Hb), this test is a tool for monitoring diabetes therapy. Three minor hemoglobins are measured in this test: Hb A_{1a}, Hb A_{1b}, and Hb A_{1c}. These minor hemoglobins are variants of Hb A, a hemoglobin formed by glycosylation, a molecular process in which glucose becomes incorporated in Hb A. Measurement of glycosylated hemoglobin levels provides information about the average blood glucose level during the preceding 2 to 3 months. This test requires only one venipuncture every 6 to 8 weeks and can therefore be used for evaluating long-term effectiveness of diabetes therapy.

Purpose

• To assess control of diabetes mellitus

Patient preparation

• Explain to the patient that this test is used to evaluate diabetes therapy.

• Tell him that the test requires a blood sample. Explain who will perform the venipuncture and when. Explain that he may experience slight discomfort from the needle puncture and the tourniquet, but that collecting the sample usually takes less than 3 minutes.

• Advise him that he need not restrict food or fluids, and instruct him to maintain his prescribed medication or diet regimen.

Procedure and posttest care

• Perform a venipuncture, and collect the sample in a 5-ml *lavender-top* tube.

• If a hematoma develops at the venipuncture site, apply warm soaks.

• Schedule the patient for an appointment in 6 to 8 weeks for appropriate follow-up testing.

Precautions

• Completely fill the collection tube, and invert it gently several times to mix the sample and anticoagulant adequately.

Reference values

Glycosylated hemoglobin values are reported as a percentage of the total hemoglobin within an erythrocyte. Because Hb A_{1c} is present in a larger quantity than the other minor hemoglobins, it's commonly measured and reported separately. Hbs A_{1a} and A_{1b} account for about 1.6% and 0.8%, respectively; Hb A_{1c} accounts for approximately 5%; and total glycosylated hemoglobin accounts for 5.5% to 9%.

Abnormal findings

In diabetes, Hbs A_{1a} and A_{1b} constitute approximately 2.5% to 3.9% of total hemoglobin; Hb A_{1c} constitutes 8% to 11.9%; and total glycosylated hemoglobin, 10.9% to 15.5%. As effective therapy brings diabetes under control, levels approach normal range.

ORAL LACTOSE TOLERANCE TEST

This test is used to measure plasma glucose levels after ingestion of a challenge dose of lactose. It's used to screen for lactose intolerance due to lactase deficiency.

Absence or deficiency of lactase causes undigested lactose to remain in the intestinal lumen, producing such symptoms as abdominal cramps and watery diarrhea. True congenital lactase deficiency is rare. Usually, lactose intolerance is acquired, as lactase levels generally decrease with age.

Purpose
• To detect lactose intolerance

Patient preparation
• Explain to the patient that this test is used to determine if his symptoms are due to an inability to digest lactose.
• Instruct him to fast and to avoid strenuous activity for 8 hours before the test.
• Tell him this test may require a stool sample.
• Also tell him this test requires four blood samples, who will perform the venipunctures and when, and that he may feel transient discomfort from the needle punctures and the pressure of the tourniquet.
• Reassure him that collecting each blood sample takes less than 3 minutes, but explain that the entire procedure may take as long as 2 hours.
• Withhold drugs that may affect plasma glucose levels including thiazide diuretics, oral contraceptives, benzodiazepines, propranolol, and insulin. If these drugs must be continued, note this on the laboratory slip.

Procedure and posttest care
• After the patient has fasted for 8 hours, perform a venipuncture and collect a blood sample in a 7-ml *gray-top* tube.
• Administer the test load of lactose: for an adult, 50 g of lactose dissolved in 400 ml of water; for a child, 50 g/m^2 of body surface area.
• Record the time of ingestion.
• Draw a blood sample 30, 60, and 120 minutes after giving the loading dose, using 7-ml *gray-top* tubes.

• Collect a stool sample 5 hours after the loading dose.
• If a hematoma develops at the venipuncture site, apply warm soaks.
• Instruct the patient to resume his usual diet and activity.
• Resume administration of medications withheld before the test.

Precautions
• Send blood and stool samples to the laboratory immediately, or refrigerate them if transport is delayed.
• Specify the time of collection on the laboratory slips.
• Watch for symptoms of lactose intolerance — abdominal cramps, nausea, bloating, flatulence, and watery diarrhea — caused by the loading dose.

Reference values
Normally, plasma glucose levels rise more than 20 mg/dl over fasting levels within 15 to 60 minutes after ingestion of the lactose loading dose. Stool sample analysis shows normal pH (7 to 8) and low glucose content (less than 1+ on a glucose-indicating dipstick).

Abnormal findings
A rise in plasma glucose of less than 20 mg/dl indicates lactose intolerance, as does stool acidity (pH of 5.5 or less) and high glucose content (greater than 1+ on the dipstick). Accompanying signs and symptoms provoked by the test also suggest but do not confirm the diagnosis as such symptoms may appear in patients with normal lactase activity after a loading dose of lactose. Small-bowel biopsy with lactase assay may be performed to confirm the diagnosis.

LACTIC ACID AND PYRUVIC ACID

Lactic acid, present in blood as lactate ion, is derived primarily from muscle cells and erythrocytes. It is an intermediate product of carbohydrate metabolism and is normally metabolized by the liver. Blood lactate concentration depends on the rates of production and metabolism; levels may increase significantly during exercise.

Lactate and pyruvate together form a reversible reaction that's regulated by oxygen supply. When oxygen levels are deficient, pyruvate converts to lactate; when they are adequate, lactate converts to pyruvate. When the hepatic system fails to metabolize lactose sufficiently or when excess pyruvate converts to lactate, lactic acidosis may result. Measurement of blood lactate levels is recommended for all patients with symptoms of lactic acidosis, such as Kussmaul's respiration.

Comparison of pyruvate and lactate levels provides reliable information about tissue oxidation, but measurement of pyruvate is technically difficult and infrequently performed.

Purpose
• To assess tissue oxidation
• To help determine the cause of lactic acidosis

Patient preparation
• Explain to the patient that this blood test is used to evaluate the oxygen level in tissues.
• Tell him that the test requires a blood sample. Explain who will perform the venipuncture and when.
• Explain that he may experience slight discomfort from the needle puncture and the tourniquet, but that collecting the sample usually takes less than 3 minutes.
• Withhold food overnight, and make sure the patient rests for at least 1 hour before the test.

Procedure and posttest care
• Perform a venipuncture, and collect the sample in a 5-ml *gray-top* tube.
• If a hematoma develops at the venipuncture site, apply warm soaks.
• Tell the patient he may resume his normal diet.

Precautions
• Because venostasis may raise blood lactate levels, tell the patient he must not clench his fist during the venipuncture.
• Because lactate and pyruvate are extremely unstable, place the sample container in an ice-filled cup, and send it to the laboratory immediately.

Reference values
Blood lactate values range from 0.93 to 1.65 mEq/liter; pyruvate levels, from 0.08 to 0.16 mEq/liter. Normally, the lactate-pyruvate ratio is less than 10:1.

Abnormal findings
Elevated blood lactate levels associated with hypoxia may result from strenuous muscle exercise, shock, hemorrhage, septicemia, myocardial infarction, pulmonary embolism, and cardiac arrest. When no reason for diminished tissue perfusion is apparent, increased lactate levels may result from systemic disorders — such as diabetes mellitus, leukemias and lymphomas, hepatic disease, or renal failure — and from enzymatic defects — such as in von Gierke's disease (glycogen storage disease) and fructose 1,6-diphosphatase deficiency.

Lactic acidosis can follow ingestion of large doses of acetaminophen and ethanol, and I.V. infusion of epinephrine, glucagon, fructose, or sorbitol.

Hormone Tests

PITUITARY HORMONES

CORTICOTROPIN

This test measures the plasma levels of corticotropin (also known as adrenocorticotropic hormone or ACTH) by radioimmunoassay. Corticotropin stimulates the adrenal cortex to secrete cortisol and, to a lesser degree, androgens and aldosterone. It also has some melanocyte-stimulating activity and increases the uptake of amino acids by muscle cells, promotes lipolysis by fat cells, stimulates pancreatic beta cells to secrete insulin, and may contribute to the release of growth hormone. Corticotropin levels vary diurnally, peaking between 6 a.m. and 8 a.m. and ebbing between 6 p.m. and 11 p.m.

The corticotropin test may be ordered for patients with signs of adrenal hypofunction (insufficiency) or hyperfunction (Cushing's syndrome). However, corticotropin suppression or stimulation testing is usually necessary to confirm diagnosis. The instability and unavailability of corticotropin greatly limit its diagnostic significance and reliability.

Purpose
• To facilitate differential diagnosis of primary and secondary adrenal hypofunction
• To aid differential diagnosis of Cushing's syndrome

Patient preparation
• Explain to the patient that this test helps determine if his hormonal secretion is normal.

• Advise him that he must fast and limit his physical activity for 10 to 12 hours before the test.
• Tell him that the test requires a blood sample, and explain who will perform the venipuncture and when.
• Inform him that he may experience some transient discomfort from the needle puncture and the pressure of the tourniquet.
• Reassure him that collecting the sample takes only a few minutes, although the laboratory requires up to 4 days to complete the analysis.
• Check the patient's drug history for the use of any medications that may affect accurate determination of test results, such as corticosteroids, and drugs that affect cortisol levels: estrogens, amphetamines, spironolactone, calcium gluconate, or alcohol (ethanol). Withhold these drugs for 48 hours or longer before the test. If these medications must be continued, note this on the laboratory slip.
• Arrange with the dietary department to provide a low-carbohydrate diet for 2 days before the test. This requirement may vary, depending on the laboratory.

Procedure and posttest care
• For a patient with suspected adrenal hypofunction, perform the venipuncture for a baseline level between 6 a.m. and 8 a.m. (peak secretion).
• For a patient with suspected Cushing's syndrome, perform the venipuncture between 6 p.m. and 11 p.m. (low secretion).
• Collect the sample in a plastic tube, because corticotropin may adhere to glass, or in a *lavender-top* tube. The tube must be full because excess anticoagulant will affect results.
• Pack the sample in ice, and send it to the laboratory immediately, where plasma must be rapidly separated from blood cells at 39.2° F (4° C). The col-

lection technique may vary, depending on the laboratory.

• If a hematoma develops at the puncture site, apply warm soaks.

• Resume diet and administration of medications that were discontinued before the test.

Precautions

• Because proteolytic enzymes in the plasma degrade corticotropin, a temperature of 39.2° F (4° C) is necessary to retard enzyme activity. Immediate transfer of the sample, packed in ice, to the laboratory is essential for reliable test results.

Reference values

The Mayo Clinic sets baseline values at less than 60 pg/ml, but these values may vary, depending on the laboratory.

Abnormal findings

A higher-than-normal corticotropin level may indicate primary adrenal hypofunction (Addison's disease), in which the pituitary gland attempts to compensate for the unresponsiveness of the target organ by releasing excessive corticotropin. The underlying cause of adrenocortical hypofunction may be idiopathic atrophy of the adrenal cortex, or partial destruction of the gland by granuloma, neoplasm, amyloidosis, or inflammatory necrosis.

A low-normal corticotropin level suggests secondary adrenal hypofunction resulting from pituitary or hypothalamic dysfunction. The primary determinant may be panhypopituitarism, absence of corticotropin-releasing hormone in the hypothalamus, or chronic blunting of corticotropin levels by long-term corticosteroid therapy.

In suspected Cushing's syndrome, an elevated corticotropin level suggests Cushing's disease, in which pituitary dysfunction (due to adenoma) causes continuous hypersecretion of corticotropin and, consequently, continuously elevated cortisol levels, without diurnal variations. Moderately elevated corticotropin levels suggest pituitary-dependent adrenal hyperplasia, and nonadrenal tumors, such as oat cell carcinoma of the lungs.

A low-normal corticotropin level implies adrenal hyperfunction due to adrenocortical tumor or hyperplasia.

RAPID CORTICOTROPIN TEST

The rapid corticotropin test (also known as the rapid ACTH test or cosyntropin test) is gradually replacing the 8-hour corticotropin stimulation test as the most effective diagnostic tool for evaluating adrenal hypofunction. Using cosyntropin, the rapid corticotropin test provides faster results and causes fewer allergic reactions than the 8-hour test, which uses natural corticotropin from animal sources.

This test requires prior determination of baseline cortisol levels to evaluate the effect of cosyntropin administration on cortisol secretion. An unequivocally high morning cortisol level rules out adrenal hypofunction and makes further testing unnecessary.

Purpose

• To aid in identification of primary and secondary adrenal hypofunction

Patient preparation

• Explain to the patient that this test helps determine if his condition is due to a hormonal deficiency.

• Inform him that he may be required to fast for 10 to 12 hours before the test, and must be relaxed and resting quietly for 30 minutes before the test.

• Tell him the test takes at least 1 hour to perform and requires three venipunctures and an injection.

• If the patient is hospitalized, withhold corticotropin and all steroid medications before the test. If the test is given on an outpatient basis, instruct the patient to refrain from taking them. If they must be continued, note this on the laboratory slip.

Procedure and posttest care

• Draw 5 ml of blood for a baseline value. Collect the sample in a 5-ml *green-top* (heparinized) tube. Label this sample "preinjection," and send it to the laboratory.

• Inject 250 mcg (0.25 mg) cosyntropin I.V. or I.M. (I.V. administration provides more accurate results because ineffective absorption following I.M. administration may cause wide variations in response.) Direct I.V. injection should take 2 minutes.

• Draw another 5 ml of blood 30 and 60 minutes following the cosyntropin injection. Collect the samples in 5-ml *green-top* (heparinized) tubes. Label the samples "30 minutes postinjection" and "60 minutes postinjection," then send them to the laboratory. Include the actual collection times on the laboratory slip.

• If a hematoma develops at the venipuncture sites, apply warm soaks.

• Observe the patient for signs of a rare allergic reaction to cosyntropin, such as hives and itching, or tachycardia.

• Allow patient to resume diet.

• Resume administration of medications that were discontinued before the test.

Precautions

• Handle the samples gently to prevent hemolysis. These samples require no special precautions other than avoiding stasis.

Reference values

Normally, cortisol levels rise 7mcg/dl or more above the baseline value to a peak of 18 mcg/dl or more 60 minutes after the cosyntropin injection. Generally, a doubling of the baseline value indicates a normal response.

Abnormal findings

A normal result excludes adrenal hypofunction (insufficiency). In patients with primary adrenal hypofunction (Addison's disease), cortisol levels remain low. Thus, the rapid corticotropin test provides an effective method of screening for adrenal hypofunction. However, if test results show subnormal increases in cortisol levels, prolonged stimulation of the adrenal cortex may be required to differentiate between primary and secondary adrenal hypofunction.

GROWTH HORMONE

Human growth hormone (hGH), also called somatotrophic hormone, is a protein secreted by acidophils of the anterior pituitary. It is the primary regulator of human growth. Unlike other pituitary hormones, hGH has no easily defined feedback mechanism or single target gland — it affects many body tissues. Like insulin, hGH promotes protein synthesis and stimulates amino acid uptake by cells. Hypo- or hypersecretion of this hormone may induce pathologic states (such as dwarfism or gigantism). Altered hGH levels are common in patients with pituitary dysfunction.

This test, a quantitative analysis of plasma hGH levels, is usually performed as part of an anterior pituitary stimulation or suppression test. Such testing is crucial, since clinical manifestations of an hGH deficiency can rarely be reversed by therapy.

Purpose

• To aid differential diagnosis of dwarfism, since retarded growth in children can result from pituitary or thyroid hypofunction

• To confirm diagnosis of acromegaly and gigantism

• To aid diagnosis of pituitary or hypothalamic tumors

• To help evaluate hGH therapy

Patient preparation

• Explain to the patient, or to his parents if the patient is a child, that this test measures hormone levels and helps determine the cause of abnormal growth.

• Instruct him to fast and limit physical activity for 10 to 12 hours before the test.

• Tell him the test requires a blood sample, and explain who will perform the venipuncture and when. Reassure him that although he may feel some discomfort from the needle puncture, collecting the sample takes less than 3 minutes.

• Inform him that another sample may have to be drawn the following day for comparison. The laboratory requires at least 2 days for analysis.

• Withhold all medications that affect hGH levels, such as pituitary-based steroids. If these medications must be continued, note this on the laboratory slip.

• Make sure the patient is relaxed and recumbent for 30 minutes before the test, since stress and physical activity elevate hGH levels.

Procedure and posttest care

• Between 6 a.m. and 8 a.m. on 2 consecutive days, or as ordered, draw at least 7 ml of venous blood into a 10-ml *red-top* tube.

• If a hematoma develops at the venipuncture site, apply warm soaks.

• Allow the patient to resume his normal diet and any medications that were discontinued before the test.

Precautions

• Handle the sample gently to prevent hemolysis.

• Send it to the laboratory immediately because hGH has a half-life of only 20 to 25 minutes.

Reference values

Normal hGH levels for men range from undetectable to 5 ng/ml; for women, from undetectable to 10 ng/ml. Higher values in women are due to estrogen effects. Children generally have higher hGH levels; nevertheless, they may range from undetectable to 16 ng/ml.

Abnormal findings

Increased hGH levels may indicate a pituitary or hypothalamic tumor, frequently an adenoma, which causes gigantism in children and acromegaly in adults and adolescents. Patients with diabetes mellitus sometimes have elevated hGH levels, without acromegaly. Suppression testing is necessary to confirm diagnosis.

Pituitary infarction, metastatic disease, or tumors may reduce hGH levels. Dwarfism may be due to low hGH levels, although only 15% of all cases of growth failure relate to endocrine dysfunction. Confirmation of diagnosis requires stimulation testing with arginine or insulin.

GROWTH HORMONE SUPPRESSION TEST

Also called glucose loading, this test evaluates excessive baseline levels of human growth hormone (hGH) from the anterior pituitary. Normally, a glucose load should suppress hGH secretion. In a patient with excessive hGH levels, failure of suppression indicates anterior pituitary dysfunction and confirms diagnosis of acromegaly and gigantism.

Purpose
• To assess elevated baseline hGH levels
• To confirm diagnosis of gigantism in children and acromegaly in adults

Patient preparation
• Explain to the patient, or to his family if the patient is a child, that this test helps determine the cause of his abnormal growth.
• Instruct him to fast and limit physical activity for 10 to 12 hours before the test.
• Tell him two blood samples will be drawn and warn that he may experience nausea after drinking the glucose solution and feel some discomfort from the needle punctures. Inform him that the test takes 1 hour, but that the laboratory requires at least another 2 days to complete this analysis.
• Before the test, you should withhold all steroids — including estrogens and progestogens — and other pituitary-based hormones. If these or other medications must be continued, note this on the laboratory slip.
• Because hGH levels rise after exercise or excitement, make sure the patient is relaxed and recumbent for 30 minutes before the test.

Procedure and posttest care
• Between 6 a.m. and 8 a.m., draw 6 ml of venous blood (basal sample) into a 10- to 15-ml *red-top* tube.
• Administer 100 g of glucose solution by mouth. To prevent nausea, advise the patient to drink the glucose slowly.

• After about 2 hours, draw another 6 ml of venous blood into a second 10- to 15-ml *red-top* tube. Label the tubes appropriately, and send them to the laboratory.
• If a hematoma develops at the puncture sites, apply warm soaks.
• Allow the patient to resume diet and medications discontinued before the test.

Precautions
• Handle the samples gently to prevent hemolysis.
• Send each sample to the laboratory immediately because hGH has a half-life of only 20 to 25 minutes.

Reference values
Normally, glucose suppresses hGH to levels ranging from undetectable to 3 ng/ml in 30 minutes to 2 hours. In children, rebound stimulation may occur after 2 to 5 hours.

Abnormal findings
In a patient with active acromegaly, basal levels are elevated (75 ng/ml) and are not suppressed to less than 5 ng/ml during the test. Unchanged or rising hGH levels in response to glucose loading indicate hGH hypersecretion and may confirm suspected acromegaly or gigantism. This response may be verified by repeating the test after a 1-day rest.

INSULIN TOLERANCE TEST

This test measures serum levels of human growth hormone (hGH) and corticotropin after administration of a loading dose of insulin, and is more reliable than direct measurement of hGH and corticotropin. Insulin-induced hypo-glycemia stimulates hGH and cortico-tropin secretion. Failure of stimulation indicates anterior pituitary or adrenal hypofunction and helps confirm an hGH or corticotropin insufficiency.

This test is not recommended for patients with cardiovascular or cerebro-vascular disorders, epilepsy, or low basal cortisol levels.

Purpose
• To aid diagnosis of hGH or cortico-tropin deficiency
• To identify pituitary dysfunction
• To aid differential diagnosis of primary and secondary adrenal hypofunction

Patient preparation
• Explain to the patient, or to his family if the patient is a child, that this test evaluates hormonal secretion.
• Instruct him to fast and to restrict physical activity for 10 to 12 hours before the test.
• Explain that the test involves I.V. infusion of insulin and the collection of multiple blood samples.
• Warn him that he may experience an increased heart rate, diaphoresis, hunger, and anxiety after administration of insulin. Reassure him that these symptoms are transient, but that if they become severe the test will be discontinued.
• Inform him that the test takes about 2 hours and that results are usually available in 2 days.
• Because physical activity and excitement increase hGH and corticotropin levels, make sure the patient is relaxed and recumbent for 90 minutes before the test.

Procedure and posttest care
• Between 6 a.m. and 8 a.m., collect three 5-ml samples of venous blood for basal levels — one in a *gray-top* tube

(for blood glucose) and two in *green-top* tubes (for hGH and corticotropin).
• Administer an I.V. bolus of U-100 regular insulin (0.15 U/kg, or as ordered) over a 1- to 2-minute period.
• Draw additional blood samples 15, 30, 45, 60, 90, and 120 minutes after administration of insulin. Use an indwelling venous catheter to avoid repeated venipunctures.
• At each interval, collect three samples: one in a *gray-top* tube and two in *green-top* tubes. Label the tubes appropriately and send them to the laboratory immediately.
• If a hematoma develops at the I.V. or venipuncture site, apply warm soaks.
• Instruct the patient to resume diet, activity, and medications.

Precautions
• Be sure to have concentrated glucose solution readily available in the event that the patient has a severe hypoglycemic reaction to insulin.
• Label the tubes appropriately, including the time of collection on the laboratory slip, and send all samples to the laboratory immediately.
• Handle the samples gently to prevent hemolysis.

Reference values
Normally, blood glucose falls to 50% of the fasting level 20 to 30 minutes after insulin administration. This stimulates a 10 to 20 ng/dl increase over baseline values in both hGH and corticotropin, with peak levels occurring 60 to 90 minutes after insulin administration.

Abnormal findings
Failure of stimulation or a blunted response suggests dysfunction of the hypothalamic-pituitary-adrenal axis. An increase in hGH levels below 10 ng/dl above basal suggests hGH deficiency. However, definitive diagnosis of hGH deficiency requires a supplementary

stimulation test, such as the arginine test. Additional testing is necessary to determine the site of the abnormality.

An increase in corticotropin levels below 10 ng/dl above basal suggests adrenal insufficiency. The metyrapone or corticotropin stimulation test then confirms the diagnosis and determines whether insufficiency is primary or secondary.

ARGININE TEST

This test, also known as the human growth hormone stimulation test, measures growth hormone (hGH) levels after I.V. administration of arginine, an amino acid that normally stimulates hGH secretion. It is commonly used to identify pituitary dysfunction in infants and children with growth retardation and to confirm hGH deficiency. This test may be performed concomitantly with an insulin tolerance test or after administration of other hGH stimulants, such as glucagon, vasopressin, and levodopa.

Purpose
• To aid diagnosis of pituitary tumors
• To confirm hGH deficiency in infants and children with low baseline levels

Patient preparation
• Explain to the patient, or to his parents if the patient is a child, that this test identifies hGH deficiency.
• Instruct him to fast and limit physical activity for 10 to 12 hours before the test.
• Explain that this test requires venous infusion of a drug and collection of several blood samples. Tell him the test takes at least 2 hours to perform; results are available in 2 days.

• Before the test, withhold all steroid medications, including pituitary-based hormones. If these medications must be continued, record this on the laboratory slip.
• Because hGH levels may rise after exercise or excitement, make sure the patient is relaxed and recumbent for at least 90 minutes before the test.

Procedure and posttest care
• Between 6 a.m. and 8 a.m., draw 6 ml of venous blood (basal sample) into a *red-top* tube.
• Start I.V. infusion of arginine (0.5 g/kg of body weight) in 0.9% sodium chloride solution, and continue for 30 minutes. Use of an indwelling venous catheter avoids repeated venipunctures and minimizes stress and anxiety.
• Discontinue I.V. infusion, then draw a total of three 6-ml samples at 30-minute intervals. Collect each sample in a *red-top* tube, and label it appropriately.
• If a hematoma develops at the venipuncture site, apply warm soaks.
• Allow the patient to resume diet and medications discontinued before the test.

Precautions
• Draw each sample at the scheduled time, and specify the collection time on the laboratory slip.
• Send each sample to the laboratory immediately, because hGH has a half-life of 20 to 25 minutes.
• Handle the samples gently to prevent hemolysis.

Reference values
Arginine should raise hGH levels to more than 10 ng/ml in men, 15 ng/ml in women, and 48 ng/ml in children. Such an increase may appear in the first sample drawn 30 minutes after arginine infusion is discontinued, or in the samples drawn 60 and 90 minutes afterward.

Abnormal findings
Elevated fasting levels and rises during sleep help to rule out hGH deficiency. Failure of hGH levels to rise after arginine infusion indicates decreased anterior pituitary hGH reserve. In children, this deficiency causes dwarfism; in adults, it can indicate panhypopituitarism. When hGH levels fail to reach 10 ng/ml, retesting is required at the same time of day as the original test.

FOLLICLE-STIMULATING HORMONE

This test of gonadal function, performed more often on women than on men, measures follicle-stimulating hormone (FSH) levels. It is vital to infertility studies. Plasma levels fluctuate widely in females: to obtain a true baseline level, daily testing may be necessary (for 3 to 5 days). Alternatively, multiple samples can be drawn on the same day.

Purpose
• To aid in the diagnosis of infertility and disorders of menstruation, such as amenorrhea
• To aid in the diagnosis of precocious puberty in girls (before age 9) and in boys (before age 10)
• To aid in the differential diagnosis of hypogonadism

Patient preparation
• Explain to the patient, or to her parents if she's a minor, that this test helps determine if her hormonal secretion is normal.
• Inform her that she needn't fast or limit physical activity before the test.

• Tell her a blood sample will be drawn and that she may feel some discomfort from the needle puncture.
• Although collecting the sample takes only a few minutes, advise the patient that the laboratory requires at least 3 days to complete the analysis.
• Withhold medications, such as estrogens or progestogen, that may interfere with accurate determination of test results for 48 hours before the test. If these medications must be continued, note this on the laboratory slip.
• Make sure the patient is relaxed and recumbent for 30 minutes before the test.

Procedure and posttest care
• Perform a venipuncture, preferably between 6 a.m. and 8 a.m., using a 7-ml *red-top* tube, and send the sample to the laboratory immediately.
• If a hematoma develops at the venipuncture site, apply warm soaks.
• Resume administration of medications discontinued before the test.

Precautions
• Handle the sample gently to prevent hemolysis.
• If the patient is female, indicate the phase of her menstrual cycle on the laboratory slip. If she is menopausal, note this on the laboratory slip.

Reference values
Reference values vary greatly, depending on the patient's age and stage of sexual development, and — for a female — the phase of her menstrual cycle. For menstruating females, approximate values are as follows:
• Follicular phase: 5 to 20 mIU/ml
• Midcycle peak: 15 to 30 mIU/ml
• Luteal phase: 5 to 15 mIU/ml.
    Approximate values for adult males are 5 to 20 mIU/ml; for menopausal women, 50 to 100 mIU/ml.

Abnormal findings

Decreased FSH levels may cause male or female infertility: aspermatogenesis in men and anovulation in women. Low FSH levels may indicate secondary hypogonadotropic states, which can result from anorexia nervosa, panhypopituitarism, or hypothalamic lesions.

High FSH levels in women may indicate ovarian failure associated with Turner's syndrome (primary hypogonadism) or Stein-Leventhal syndrome (polycystic ovary syndrome). Elevated levels may occur in patients with precocious puberty (idiopathic or with central nervous system lesions) and in postmenopausal women. In men, abnormally high FSH levels may indicate destruction of the testes (from mumps orchitis or X-ray exposure), testicular failure, seminoma, or male climacteric. Congenital absence of the gonads and early-stage acromegaly may cause FSH levels to rise in both sexes.

PLASMA LUTEINIZING HORMONE

This test, usually ordered for anovulation and infertility studies and performed most often on women, is a quantitative analysis of plasma luteinizing hormone (LH) or interstitial-cell-stimulating hormone (ICSH) levels. In women, cyclic LH secretion (with follicle-stimulating hormone [FSH]) causes ovulation and transforms the ovarian follicle into the corpus luteum, which, in turn, secretes progesterone. (See *LH secretion peaks at ovulation*.) In males, continuous LH secretion stimulates the interstitial (Leydig) cells of the testes to release testosterone, which stimulates and maintains spermatogenesis (with FSH).

Purpose
• To detect ovulation
• To assess male or female infertility
• To evaluate amenorrhea
• To monitor therapy designed to induce ovulation

Patient preparation
• Explain to the patient that this test helps determine if her secretion of female hormones is normal.
• Because there is no evidence that LH levels are affected by fasting, eating, or exercise, such pretest restrictions may be unnecessary.
• Tell the patient that this test requires a blood sample.
• Explain to her who will perform the venipuncture and when. Let her know that she may feel some discomfort from the needle puncture.
• Inform her that collecting the sample takes only a few minutes, but the laboratory requires at least 3 days to complete the analysis.
• Withhold drugs, such as steroids (including estrogens or progesterone), that may interfere with plasma LH levels, for 48 hours before the test. If these medications must be continued, note this on the laboratory slip.

Procedure and posttest care
• Perform a venipuncture, and collect the sample in a 7-ml *red-top* tube.
• If a hematoma develops at the venipuncture site, apply warm soaks.
• Resume administration of medications discontinued before the test.

Precautions
• Handle the sample gently to prevent hemolysis.
• If the patient is a female, indicate the phase of her menstrual cycle on the laboratory slip. Make a note if the patient is menopausal.

LH Secretion Peaks at Ovulation

The menstrual cycle is divided into three distinct phases: the menstrual phase (days 1 to 5); the proliferative, or follicular, phase (days 6 to 13); and, after ovulation on day 14, the secretory, or luteal, phase (days 15 to 28).

The menstrual phase
This phase of the normal cycle is characterized by endometrial sloughing, corpus luteum degeneration, and new follicle growth. During this stage, the concentration of both estrogen and progesterone is low, triggering increased follicle-stimulating hormone (FSH) and luteinizing hormone (LH) secretion.

The follicular phase
During the follicular phase, the follicle stimulated by FSH reaches full size and increases its secretion of estrogen. Simultaneously with increased estrogen,

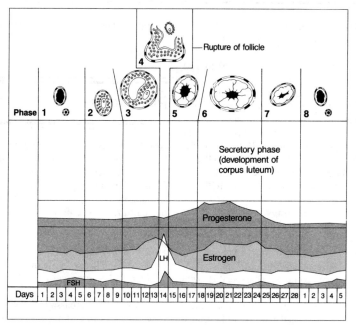

1. Menstrual phase (degeneration of corpus luteum)
2. Early follicular phase (development of follicle)
3. Late follicular phase (development of follicle)
4. Ovulation at midcycle (rupture of follicle)

5. Early luteal phase (development of corpus luteum)
6. Midluteal phase (development of corpus luteum)
7. Late luteal phase (development of corpus luteum)
8. Menstrual phase (degeneration of corpus luteum)

(continued)

> ## LH SECRETION PEAKS AT OVULATION (continued)
>
> FSH decreases while LH increases slowly but steadily. During the late follicular phase, LH rises sharply and FSH rises slightly. At about the 14th day, within hours of this abrupt surge in LH, estrogen levels in the plasma drop and ovulation occurs. After ovulation, the concentration of both LH and FSH falls rapidly.
>
> ### The secretory phase
> During the final, or luteal, phase, the follicle reorganizes as the corpus luteum secretes progesterone and estrogen. Within 7 or 8 days following ovulation, if fertilization has not occurred, the corpus luteum regresses while progesterone and estrogen levels decrease. The endometrium sloughs, and the menstrual cycle begins again.

Reference values
Normal values may have a wide range:
- Adult men: 1 to 10 IU/L
- Postmenopausal women: 20 to 100 IU/L
- Adult women: reference values vary, depending on the phase of the patient's menstrual cycle. During the follicular phase, values are 1 to 20 IU/L; during midcycle (ovulation), 25 to 100 IU/L; during the luteal phase, 0.2 to 20 IU/L
- Males (prepuberty): < 0.5 IU/L
- Females (prepuberty): < 0.2 IU/L

Abnormal findings
In women, absence of a midcycle peak in LH secretion may indicate anovulation. Decreased or low-normal levels may indicate hypogonadotropism; these findings are commonly associated with amenorrhea. High LH levels may indicate congenital absence of ovaries or ovarian failure associated with Stein-Leventhal syndrome (polycystic ovary syndrome), Turner's syndrome (ovarian dysgenesis), menopause, or early-stage acromegaly. Infertility can result from either primary or secondary gonadal dysfunction.

In men, low values may indicate secondary gonadal dysfunction (of hypothalamic or pituitary origin); high values may indicate testicular failure (primary hypogonadism) or destruction or congenital absence of testes.

PROLACTIN

Also known as lactogenic hormone or lactogen, prolactin is essential for the development of the mammary glands for lactation during pregnancy, and for stimulating and maintaining lactation postpartum. Prolactin is secreted in men and nonpregnant women, but its function is unknown. Like human growth hormone, prolactin acts directly on tissues, and its levels rise in response to sleep and to physical or emotional stress.

This radioimmunoassay is a quantitative analysis of serum prolactin levels, which normally rise ten- to twentyfold during pregnancy, corresponding to concomitant elevations in human placental lactogen levels. After delivery, prolactin secretion falls to basal levels in mothers who don't breastfeed. However, prolactin secretion increases during breast-feeding, apparently as a result of a stimulus triggered by suckling that curtails the release of prolactin-inhibiting factor by the hypothalamus. This, in turn, allows transient elevations of prolactin secretion by the pituitary. This test is considered useful in patients suspected of having pituitary tumors, which are known to secrete prolactin in excessive amounts.

Purpose
• To facilitate diagnosis of pituitary dysfunction, possibly due to pituitary adenoma
• To aid in the diagnosis of hypothalamic dysfunction regardless of cause
• To evaluate secondary amenorrhea and galactorrhea

Patient preparation
• Tell the patient that this test helps evaluate hormonal secretion.
• Advise her that she need not restrict food or fluids, or limit physical activity. But encourage her to relax for about 30 minutes before the test.
• Tell her who will draw the blood sample and when and that she may experience some discomfort from the needle puncture.
• Advise her that collecting the sample takes only a few minutes, but the laboratory requires at least 4 days to complete the analysis.
• Withhold drugs that may interfere with test results, such as ethanol, morphine, methyldopa, estrogens, apomorphine, ergot alkaloids, and levodopa. If the drug must be continued, note this on the laboratory slip.

Procedure and posttest care
• Perform a venipuncture at least 2 hours after the patient wakes; samples drawn earlier are likely to show sleep-induced peak levels. Collect the sample in a 7-ml *red-top* tube.

• If a hematoma develops at the venipuncture site, apply warm soaks.
• Resume administration of medications discontinued before the test.

Precautions
• Handle the sample gently to prevent hemolysis.

Reference values
Normal values range from undetectable to 23 ng/dl in nonlactating women.

Abnormal findings
Abnormally high prolactin levels (100 to 300 ng/ml) suggest autonomous prolactin production by a pituitary adenoma, especially when amenorrhea or galactorrhea is present (Forbes-Albright syndrome). Rarely, hyperprolactinemia may also result from severe endocrine disorders, such as hypothyroidism. Idiopathic hyperprolactinemia may be associated with anovulatory infertility. Confirm slight elevations with repeat measurements on two other occasions.

Decreased prolactin levels in a lactating mother cause failure of lactation and may be associated with postpartum pituitary infarction (Sheehan's syndrome). Abnormally low prolactin levels have also been found in a few patients with empty-sella syndrome. In these patients, a flattened pituitary gland makes the pituitary fossa look empty.

THYROID-STIMULATING HORMONE

Thyroid-stimulating hormone (TSH) or thyrotropin promotes increases in the size, number, and activity of thyroid cells and stimulates the release of triio-

TRH STIMULATION TEST

This test evaluates hypothalmic dysfunction and pituitary tumors by stimulating the release of prolactin. The procedure is as follows: perform a venipuncture in the basal state to obtain a baseline prolactin level, then place the patient supine. Administer an I.V. bolus of synthetic thyrotropin-releasing hormone (TRH) in a dose of 500 mcg over 15 to 30 seconds. Blood samples are taken at 15- and 30-minute intervals for measurement of prolactin.

A baseline prolactin reading greater than 200 ng/ml indicates a pituitary tumor, yet levels between 30 and 200 ng/ml are also consistent with this condition. Normally, patients show at least a twofold increase in prolactin after injection with TRH. If the prolactin level fails to rise, hypothalmic dysfunction or adenoma of the pituitary gland is likely.

dothyronine (T_3) and thyroxine (T_4). These hormones affect total body metabolism and are essential for normal growth and development.

This test measures serum TSH levels by radioimmunoassay. It can detect primary hypothyroidism and can determine whether it results from thyroid gland failure, or from pituitary or hypothalamic dysfunction. Normal serum TSH levels rule out primary hypothyroidism. This test may not distinguish between low-normal and subnormal levels, especially in secondary hypothyroidism.

Purpose
• To confirm or rule out primary hypothyroidism and distinguish it from secondary hypothyroidism

• To monitor drug therapy in patients with primary hypothyroidism

Patient preparation
• Explain to the patient that this test helps assess thyroid gland function.
• Tell him that the test requires a blood sample, inform him who will perform the venipuncture and when, and explain that he may feel a few minutes' discomfort from the needle puncture.
• Explain that the laboratory requires up to 2 days to complete the analysis.
• Withhold steroids, thyroid hormones, aspirin, and other drugs that may influence test results. If these medications must be continued, note this on the laboratory slip.
• Keep the patient relaxed and recumbent for 30 minutes before the test.

Procedure and posttest care
• Between 6 a.m. and 8 a.m., perform a venipuncture. Collect the sample in a 5-ml *red-top* tube.
• If a hematoma develops at the venipuncture site, apply warm soaks.
• Resume administration of drugs discontinued before the test.

Precautions
• Handle the sample gently to prevent hemolysis.

Reference values
Normal values for adults and children range from undetectable to 15 μU/ml.

Abnormal findings
TSH levels that exceed 20 μU/ml suggest primary hypothyroidism or, possibly, an endemic goiter due to dietary iodine deficiency. TSH levels may be slightly elevated in euthyroid patients with thyroid cancer.

Low or undetectable TSH levels may be normal but may occasionally indicate secondary hypothyroidism (with inadequate secretion of TSH or thyro-

TRH CHALLENGE TEST

This test, which evaluates thyroid function and is the first direct test of pituitary reserve, is a reliable diagnostic tool in thyrotoxicosis (Graves' disease). The challenge test requires an injection of thyrotropin-releasing hormone (TRH).

One commonly accepted procedure is the following: After a venipuncture is performed to obtain a baseline thyroid-stimulating hormone (TSH) reading, synthetic TRH (protirelin) is administered by I.V. bolus in a dosage of 200 to 500 µg. As many as five samples (5 ml each) are then drawn at 5-,

10-, 15-, 20-, and 60-minute intervals to assess thyroid response. To facilitate blood collection, an indwelling catheter can be used to obtain the required samples.

A sudden spike above the baseline TSH reading indicates a normally functioning pituitary but suggests hypothalamic dysfunction. If the TSH level fails to rise or remains undetectable, pituitary failure is likely. In thyrotoxicosis or thyroiditis, TSH levels fail to rise when challenged by TRH.

---

tropin-releasing hormone [TRH]). Low TSH levels may also result from hyperthyroidism (Graves' disease) or thyroiditis; both are marked by hypersecretion of thyroid hormones, which suppresses TSH release. Provocative testing with TRH is necessary to confirm diagnosis. (See *TRH stimulation test,* opposite, and *TRH challenge test.*)

NEONATAL THYROID-STIMULATING HORMONE

This immunoassay confirms congenital hypothyroidism after an initial screening test detects low thyroxine (T_4) levels. Normally, thyroid-stimulating hormone (TSH) levels surge after birth, triggering a rise in thyroid hormone that's essential for neurologic development. In primary congenital hypothyroidism, the thyroid gland doesn't respond to TSH stimulation, resulting in

diminished thyroid hormone levels and elevated TSH levels. Early detection and treatment of congenital hypothyroidism is critical to prevent mental retardation and cretinism.

Purpose
• To confirm diagnosis of congenital hypothyroidism

Patient preparation
• Explain to the infant's parents that this test helps confirm the diagnosis of congenital hypothyroidism. Emphasize the test's importance in detecting the disorder early, so that prompt therapy can prevent irreversible brain damage.

Equipment
For a filter paper sample: alcohol or povidone-iodine swabs, sterile lancet, specially marked filter paper, 2" × 2" sterile gauze pads, adhesive bandage, labels, gloves.

For a serum sample: venipuncture equipment.

Procedure and posttest care

For a filter paper sample:
• Assemble the necessary equipment, wash your hands thoroughly, and put on gloves.
• Wipe the infant's heel with an alcohol or povidone-iodine swab, then dry it thoroughly with a gauze pad.
• Perform a heelstick.
• Squeezing the infant's heel gently, fill the circles on the filter paper with blood. Make sure the blood saturates the paper.
• Gently apply pressure with a gauze pad to ensure hemostasis at the puncture site.
• Allow the filter paper to dry, label it appropriately, and send it to the laboratory.
    For a serum sample:
• Perform a venipuncture and collect the sample in a 5-ml *red-top* tube. Label the sample and send it to the laboratory immediately.
• If a hematoma develops at the venipuncture site, apply warm soaks. Heelsticks require no special care.

Precautions
• Handle serum samples carefully.

Reference values
At age 1 to 2 days, TSH levels are normally 25 to 30 μU/ml. Thereafter, levels are normally less than 25 μU/ml.

Abnormal findings
Neonatal TSH levels must be interpreted in light of T_4 concentrations. Elevated TSH accompanied by decreased T_4 indicates primary congenital hypothyroidism (thyroid gland dysfunction). Depressed TSH and T_4 may be present in secondary congenital hypothyroidism (pituitary or hypothalamic dysfunction). Normal TSH accompanied by depressed T_4 may indicate hypothyroidism due to a congenital defect in thyroxine-binding globulin or may in-

dicate transient congenital hypothyroidism due to prematurity or prenatal hypoxia. A complete thyroid workup must be done to confirm the cause of hypothyroidism before treatment can begin.

ANTIDIURETIC HORMONE

Antidiuretic hormone (ADH), also called vasopressin, promotes water reabsorption in response to increased osmolality (water deficiency with high concentration of sodium and other solutes). In response to decreased osmolality (water excess), reduced secretion of ADH allows increased excretion of water to maintain fluid balance. Along with aldosterone, ADH helps regulate sodium, potassium, and fluid balance. It also stimulates vascular smooth-muscle contraction, causing an increase in arterial blood pressure.

This relatively rare test, a quantitative analysis of serum ADH level, may identify diabetes insipidus and other causes of severe homeostatic imbalance. It may be ordered as part of dehydration or hypertonic saline infusion testing, which determines the body's response to states of hyperosmolality.

Purpose
• To aid in the differential diagnosis of pituitary diabetes insipidus, nephrogenic diabetes insipidus (congenital or familial), and syndrome of inappropriate antidiuretic hormone (SIADH)

Patient preparation
• Explain to the patient that this test to measure hormonal secretion levels may aid in identifying the cause of his symptoms.

• Instruct him to fast and limit physical activity for 10 to 12 hours before the test.

• Tell him a blood sample will be drawn, and reassure him that although he may feel some discomfort from the needle puncture, collecting the sample takes only a few minutes.

• Inform him that the laboratory requires at least 5 days to complete the analysis.

• Withhold conjugated estrogens, morphine, tranquilizers, hypnotics, oxytocin, anesthetics (such as ether), lithium carbonate, vincristine, carbamazepine, cyclophosphamide, and chlorothiazide; these drugs and others may cause SIADH. If these medications must be continued, note this on the laboratory slip.

• Make sure the patient is relaxed and recumbent for 30 minutes before the test.

Procedure and posttest care

• Perform a venipuncture, and collect the sample in a *red-top,* plastic collection tube.

• Immediately send the sample to the laboratory, where serum must be separated from the clot within 10 minutes.

• Do serum osmolality test at the same time to facilitate interpretation of results.

• If a hematoma develops at the venipuncture site, apply warm soaks.

• Allow the patient to resume diet and medications discontinued before the test.

Precautions

• The syringe and the collection tube must be plastic because the fragile ADH degrades upon contact with glass.

Reference values

ADH values range from 1 to 5 pg/ml, but they can be evaluated in light of the serum osmolality. If serum osmolality is less than 285 mOsm/kg, the ADH is normally less than 2 pg/ml. If serum osmolality is greater than 290 mOsm/kg, the ADH may range from 2 to 12 pg/ml.

Abnormal findings

Absent or below-normal ADH levels indicate pituitary diabetes insipidus, resulting from a neurohypophyseal or hypothalamic tumor, viral infection, metastatic disease, sarcoidosis, tuberculosis, Hand-Schüller-Christian disease, syphilis, neurosurgical procedures, or head trauma.

Normal ADH levels, in the presence of signs of diabetes insipidus (such as polydipsia, polyuria, and hypotonic urine), may indicate the nephrogenic form of the disease, marked by renal tubular resistance to ADH; however, levels may rise if the pituitary tries to compensate.

Elevated ADH levels may also indicate SIADH, possibly as a result of bronchogenic carcinoma, acute porphyria, hypothyroidism, Addison's disease, cirrhosis of the liver, infectious hepatitis, severe hemorrhage, or circulatory shock.

ALPHA-SUBUNIT OF PITUITARY GLYCO- PROTEIN HORMONES

Using radioimmunoassay, this test measures the alpha-subunit of the pituitary glycoprotein hormones (alpha-PGH). These hormones — follicle-stimulating hormone (FSH), luteinizing hormone (LH), and thyroid-stimulating hormone (TSH) — comprise similar alpha-subunits but differ in their beta-subunits. Alpha-PGH measurement assesses total pituitary production of these hormones.

Purpose
• To aid in the diagnosis of pituitary hypofunction related to reduced production of FSH, LH, and TSH
• To aid in the diagnosis of recurrent pituitary tumors

Patient preparation
• Explain to the patient that this test helps assess pituitary function.
• Inform him that he needn't fast.
• Tell him that this test requires a blood sample, and inform him who will perform the venipuncture and when.
• Explain that he may feel discomfort from the needle puncture, but that the procedure takes only a few minutes.
• Tell the patient the laboratory needs up to 4 days to do the analysis.

Procedure and posttest care
• Perform a venipuncture, and collect the sample in a 5-ml *red-top* tube. Send the sample to the laboratory immediately.
• If a hematoma develops at the venipuncture site, apply warm soaks.

Precautions
• Handle the specimen gently.
• Indicate the sex of the patient on the laboratory slip.

Reference values
Normal values are up to 1.2 ng/ml.

Abnormal findings
Low levels of alpha-PGH appear in patients with inadequate pituitary hormone production. Hypopituitarism results in reduced FSH, LH, and TSH levels.

Elevated levels indicate recurrent pituitary tumors or ineffective treatment.

THYROID AND PARATHYROID HORMONES

THYROXINE

Thyroxine (T_4) is an amine secreted by the thyroid gland in response to thyroid-stimulating hormone (TSH) and, indirectly, to thyrotropin-releasing hormone (TRH). The rate of secretion is normally regulated by a complex system of negative and positive feedback systems.

Only a fraction of T_4 (about 0.3%) circulates freely in the blood; the rest binds strongly to plasma proteins, primarily thyroxine-binding globulin (TBG). This minute fraction is responsible for the clinical effects of thyroid hormone. TBG binds so tenaciously that T_4 survives in the plasma for a relatively long time, with a half-life of about 6 days. This immunoassay, one of the most common thyroid diagnostic tools, measures the total circulating T_4 level when TBG is normal. An alternative test is the Murphy-Pattee or T_4(D), based on competitive protein binding.

Purpose
• To evaluate thyroid function
• To aid diagnosis of hyperthyroidism and hypothyroidism
• To monitor response to antithyroid medication in hyperthyroidism or to thyroid replacement therapy in hypothyroidism (TSH estimates are needed to confirm hypothyroidism)

Patient preparation
• Explain to the patient that this test helps evaluate thyroid gland function.

• Inform him that he needn't fast or restrict activity.
• Tell him a blood sample is needed, and that the procedure, which takes a few minutes, may cause some discomfort.
• Inform him who will perform the venipuncture and when.
• Withhold any medications that may interfere with test results. Estrogens, progestins, levothyroxins, and methadone increase T_4 levels. Free fatty acids, heparin, iodides, liothyronine sodium, lithium, phenylbutazone, phenytoin, salicylates (high doses), propylthiouracil, steroids, sulfonamides, and sulfonylureas all decrease T_4. If these medications must be continued, note this on the laboratory slip. If this test is being performed to monitor thyroid therapy, the patient continues to receive daily thyroid supplements.

Procedure and posttest care
• Perform a venipuncture, and collect the sample in a 7-ml *red-top* tube. Send the sample to the laboratory immediately so the serum may be separated.
• If a hematoma develops at the venipuncture site, apply warm soaks.
• Resume administration of medications discontinued before the test.

Precautions
• Handle the sample gently to prevent hemolysis.

Reference values
Normally, total T_4 levels range from 5 to 13.5 μg/dl.

Abnormal findings
Abnormally elevated levels of T_4 are consistent with primary and secondary hyperthyroidism, including excessive T_4 (L-thyroxine) replacement therapy (factitious or iatrogenic hyperthyroidism). Subnormal levels suggest primary or secondary hypothyroidism, or may

be due to T_4 suppression by normal, elevated, or replacement levels of triiodothyronine (T_3). In doubtful cases of hypothyroidism, TSH levels or TRH test may be indicated. Normal T_4 levels don't guarantee euthyroidism; for example, normal readings occur in T_3 toxicosis. Overt signs of hyperthyroidism require further testing.

TRIIODOTHYRONINE

This highly specific radioimmunoassay measures total (bound and free) serum content of triiodothyronine (T_3) to investigate clinical indications of thyroid dysfunction. Like thyroxine (T_4) secretion, T_3 secretion occurs in response to thyroid-stimulating hormone (TSH) and, secondarily, to thyrotropin-releasing hormone.

Although T_3 is present in the bloodstream in minute quantities and is metabolically active for only a short time, its impact on body metabolism dominates that of T_4. Another significant difference between the two major thyroid hormones is that T_3 binds less firmly to thyroxine-binding globulin. Consequently, T_3 persists in the bloodstream for a short time; half disappears in about 1 day, while half of T_4 disappears in 6 days.

Purpose
• To aid diagnosis of T_3 toxicosis
• To aid diagnosis of hypothyroidism and hyperthyroidism
• To monitor clinical response to thyroid replacement therapy in hypothyroidism

Patient preparation
• Explain to the patient that this test helps to evaluate thyroid gland function

and to determine the cause of his symptoms.

• Withhold medications, such as steroids, propranolol, and cholestyramine, that may influence thyroid function. If such medications must be continued, record this information on the laboratory slip.

Procedure and posttest care

• Draw venous blood into a 7-ml *red-top* tube. Send the sample to the laboratory as soon as possible to avoid stasis and to allow early separation of serum from the clotted blood.

• If a hematoma develops at the venipuncture site, apply warm soaks.

• Resume administration of drugs discontinued before the test.

Precautions

• Handle the sample gently to prevent hemolysis.

• If a patient must receive thyroid preparations such as T_3 (liothyronine), note the time of administration of the drug on the laboratory slip. Otherwise, T_3 levels are not reliable.

Reference values

Serum T_3 levels normally range from 90 to 230 ng/dl. These values may vary with the laboratory performing this test.

Abnormal findings

Serum T_3 and serum T_4 levels usually rise and fall in tandem. However, in T_3 toxicosis, only T_3 levels rise, while total and free T_4 levels remain normal. T_3 toxicosis occurs in patients with Graves' disease, toxic adenoma, or toxic nodular goiter. T_3 levels also surpass T_4 levels in patients receiving thyroid replacement containing more T_3 than T_4. In iodine-deficient areas, the thyroid may produce larger amounts of the more cellularly active T_3 than of T_4 in an effort to maintain the euthyroid state.

Generally, T_3 levels appear to be a more accurate diagnostic indicator of hyperthyroidism. Although hyperthyroidism increases both T_3 and T_4 levels in about 90% of patients, it causes a disproportionate increase in T_3. In some patients with hypothyroidism, T_3 levels may fall within the normal range and may not be diagnostically significant.

A rise in serum T_3 levels normally occurs during pregnancy. Low T_3 levels may appear in euthyroid patients with systemic illness (especially hepatic or renal disease), during severe acute illness, or following trauma or major surgery; in such patients, however, TSH levels are within normal limits. Low serum T_3 levels are sometimes found in euthyroid patients with malnutrition.

THYROXINE-BINDING GLOBULIN

This test measures the serum level of thyroxine-binding globulin (TBG), the predominant protein carrier for circulating thyroxine (T_4) and triiodothyronine (T_3).

Any condition that affects TBG levels and subsequent binding capacity also affects the amount of free T_4 (FT_4) and free T_3 (FT_3) in circulation. This can be clinically significant because only FT_4 and FT_3 are metabolically active. An underlying TBG abnormality renders tests for total T_3 and T_4 inaccurate but does not alter tests for FT_3 and FT_4.

Purpose

• To evaluate abnormal thyrometabolic states that do not correlate with thyroid hormone (T_3 or T_4) values; an example is a patient with overt signs of hypothyroidism and a low FT_4 level with a high

total T_4 level due to a marked increase of TBG secondary to oral contraceptives
• To identify TBG abnormalities

Patient preparation
• Explain to the patient that this test helps evaluate thyroid function.
• Tell him a blood sample is needed, and that the procedure, which takes a few minutes, may cause some discomfort.
• Inform him who will perform the venipuncture and when.
• Withhold medications that may interfere with accurate determination of test results, such as estrogens, anabolic steroids, phenytoin, salicylates, or thyroid preparations. If these medications must be continued, note this on the laboratory slip. (They may be continued to determine if prescribed drugs are affecting TBG levels.)

Procedure and posttest care
• Draw venous blood into a 10-ml *red-top* tube.
• If a hematoma develops at the venipuncture site, apply warm soaks.
• Resume administration of medications discontinued before the test.

Precautions
• Be sure to handle the sample gently because excessive agitation may cause hemolysis.

Reference values
Normal values for serum TBG by electrophoresis range from 10 to 26 mcg T_4 (binding capacity) per 100 ml. Values for serum TBG by radioimmunoassay range from 1.3 to 2 mg/dl.

Abnormal findings
Elevated TBG levels may indicate hypothyroidism or congenital (genetic) excess, some forms of hepatic disease, or acute intermittent porphyria. TBG

levels normally rise during pregnancy and are high in neonates. Suppressed levels may indicate hyperthyroidism or congenital deficiency, and can occur in active acromegaly, nephrotic syndrome, and malnutrition with hypoproteinemia, acute illness, or surgical stress.
Patients with TBG abnormalities require additional testing, such as the serum FT_3 and serum FT_4 tests, to evaluate thyroid function more precisely.

T_3 RESIN UPTAKE

Also called T_3 RU, resin triiodothyronine uptake or T_3 uptake ratio (T_3UR), this test indirectly measures free thyroxine (FT_4) levels by demonstrating the availability of serum protein–binding sites for T_4.
The results of T_3 resin uptake are frequently combined with a T_4 radioimmunoassay or T_4(D) (competitive protein-binding test) to determine the free thyroxine index, a mathematical calculation that is thought to reflect FT_4 by correcting for thyroxine-binding globulin (TBG) abnormalities. The T_3 resin uptake has become less popular because rapid tests for T_3, T_4, and thyroid-stimulating hormone are readily available.

Purpose
• To aid diagnosis of hypothyroidism and hyperthyroidism when TBG is normal
• To aid diagnosis of primary disorders of TBG levels

Patient preparation
• Explain to the patient that this test helps evaluate thyroid function.
• Tell him a blood sample is needed, and that the procedure, which takes a

few minutes, may cause some discomfort.
• Inform him who will perform the venipuncture and when.
• Tell him the laboratory requires several days to complete the analysis.
• Withhold medications, such as estrogens, androgens, phenytoin, salicylates or thyroid preparations, that may interfere with test results. If these medications must be continued, note this on the laboratory slip.

Procedure and posttest care
• Draw venous blood into a 7-ml *red-top* tube.
• If a hematoma develops at the venipuncture site, apply warm soaks.
• Resume administration of medications discontinued before the test.

Precautions
• Handle the collection tube gently to prevent hemolysis.

Reference values
Normally, 25% to 35% of T_3 binds to the resin.

Abnormal findings
A high resin uptake percentage in the presence of elevated T_4 levels indicates hyperthyroidism (implying few TBG free binding sites and high FT_4 levels). However, a low resin uptake percentage, together with low T_4 levels, indicates hypothyroidism (implying more TBG free binding sites and low FT_4 levels). Thus, in primary disease of thyroid function, measured T_4 and T_3 RU vary in the same direction; availability of binding sites varies inversely.

Discordant variance in T_4 and T_3 RU suggests abnormality of TBG. For example, a high resin uptake percentage and a low or normal FT_4 suggest decreased TBG levels. Such decreased levels may result from protein loss (as in nephrotic syndrome), decreased production (due to androgen excess, or genetic or idiopathic causes), or competition for T_4 binding sites by certain drugs (salicylates, phenylbutazone, or phenytoin). Conversely, a low resin uptake percentage and a high or normal FT_4 suggest increased TBG levels. Such increased levels may be due to exogenous or endogenous estrogen (pregnancy), or may result from idiopathic causes. Thus, in primary disorders of TBG levels, measured T_4 and free sites change in the same direction.

FREE THYROXINE AND FREE TRIIODOTHYRONINE

These tests, often done simultaneously, measure serum levels of free thyroxine (FT_4) and free triiodothyronine (FT_3), the minute portions of T_4 and T_3 not bound to thyroxine-binding globulin (TBG) and other serum proteins. These unbound hormones are responsible for the thyroid's effects on cellular metabolism. Measurement of free hormone levels is the best indicator of thyroid function.

Disagreement exists as to whether FT_4 or FT_3 is the better indicator; therefore, laboratories commonly measure both. The disadvantages of these tests include a cumbersome and difficult laboratory method, inaccessibility, and cost. This test may be useful in the 5% of patients in whom the standard T_3 or T_4 tests fail to produce diagnostic results.

Purpose
• To measure the metabolically active form of the thyroid hormones

• To aid diagnosis of hyperthyroidism or hypothyroidism when TBG levels are abnormal

Patient preparation
• Explain to the patient that this special test helps evaluate thyroid function.
• Tell him a blood sample is needed, and that the procedure, which takes a few minutes, may cause some discomfort.
• Inform him who will perform the venipuncture and when.
• Tell him the laboratory requires several days to complete the analysis.

Procedure and posttest care
• Draw venous blood into a 7-ml *red-top* tube.
• If a hematoma develops at the venipuncture site, apply warm soaks.

Precautions
• Handle the sample gently to prevent hemolysis.

Reference values
Normal range for FT_4 is from 0.8 to 3.3 ng/dl; for FT_3, from 0.2 to 0.6 ng/dl. Values vary, depending on the laboratory.

Abnormal findings
Elevated FT_4 and FT_3 levels indicate hyperthyroidism, unless peripheral resistance to thyroid hormone is present. T_3 toxicosis, a distinct form of hyperthyroidism, yields high FT_3 levels, with normal or low FT_4 values. Low FT_4 levels usually indicate hypothyroidism, except in patients receiving replacement therapy with T_3. Patients on thyroid therapy may have varying levels of FT_4 and FT_3, depending on the preparation used and the time of sample collection.

LONG-ACTING THYROID STIMULATOR

In this test, the McKenzie mouse bioassay method is used to determine whether a patient's serum contains long-acting thyroid stimulator (LATS). LATS is an abnormal immunoglobulin (called 75 IgG) that mimics the action of thyroid-stimulating hormone (TSH) but has more prolonged effects. LATS stimulates the thyroid gland to produce and secrete thyroid hormones in excessive amounts, inhibiting TSH secretion.

Some authorities believe that the thyroid gland hyperplasia seen in Graves' disease may be due to LATS or other circulating antibodies. Others consider the clinical significance of this test questionable.

Purpose
• To confirm diagnosis of Graves' disease (this test is not done routinely to diagnose thyroid disorders)

Patient preparation
• Explain to the patient (or the parents of an infant) that this test helps evaluate thyroid function.
• Tell him this test requires a blood sample, and inform him who will perform the venipuncture and when.
• Inform him that he may feel transient discomfort from the needle puncture. Reassure him that collecting the sample takes only a few minutes, although the laboratory requires several days to complete the analysis.

Procedure and posttest care
• Draw venous blood into a 5-ml *red-top* tube.
• If a hematoma develops at the venipuncture site, apply warm soaks.

Precautions
• Handle the sample gently to prevent hemolysis.
• Note on the laboratory slip if the patient had an ^{131}I radioactive scan within 48 hours before the test.

Reference values
Normally, LATS does not appear in serum.

Abnormal findings
LATS in serum indicates Graves' disease, whether or not overt signs of hyperthyroidism are present. About 80% of patients with Graves' disease have detectable LATS in their sera.

SCREENING TEST FOR CONGENITAL HYPOTHYROIDISM

This test measures serum thyroxine (T_4) levels in the neonate to detect congenital hypothyroidism. Characterized by low or absent levels of T_4, congenital hypothyroidism affects roughly 1 in 5,000 neonates, occurring in girls three times more often than in boys. This disorder can result from thyroid dysgenesis or hypoplasia, congenital goiter, or maternal use of thyroid inhibitors during pregnancy. If untreated, it can lead to irreversible brain damage by age 3 months.

Because clinical signs are few, in the past, most cases of congenital hypothyroidism went undetected until cretinism became apparent or death followed respiratory distress. Recently, however, radioimmunoassays for T_4 and thyroid-stimulating hormone (TSH) have been used effectively to screen neonates for congenital hypothyroidism. This test is now mandatory in some states.

Purpose
• To screen neonates for congenital hypothyroidism

Patient preparation
• Explain to the parents that although hypothyroidism is uncommon in infants, this screening test detects the disorder early enough to begin therapy before irreversible brain damage occurs.
• Tell the parents the test will be performed before the infant is discharged from the hospital and again 4 to 6 weeks later.
• Emphasize the importance of the screening and the need for following the test protocol.
• Because false-positive findings can result from variations in the test procedure or from a congenital thyroxine-binding globulin (TBG) defect, inform the parents that a second test may be done before the infant is discharged.

Equipment
Gloves, alcohol or povidone-iodine swabs, sterile lancet, specially marked filter paper, 2" × 2" sterile gauze pads, small adhesive bandage strip, labels for infant's and mother's names, doctor's name, room number, and date.

Procedure and posttest care
• After assembling the necessary equipment and washing your hands, put on gloves.
• Wipe the infant's heel with an alcohol or povidone-iodine swab, and then dry it thoroughly with a gauze pad.
• Perform a heelstick.
• Squeezing the heel gently, fill the circles on the filter paper with blood. Make sure the blood saturates the paper. Apply gentle pressure with a gauze pad to ensure hemostasis at the puncture site.

• When the filter paper is dry, label it appropriately and send it to the laboratory.

• Heelsticks heal readily and require no special care.

• If results of the screening test indicate congenital hypothyroidism, tell the parents additional testing is necessary to determine the cause of the disorder.

• If diagnosis is confirmed, inform the parents that replacement therapy can restore normal thyroid gland function. Also tell them that such therapy is lifelong and that dosage will increase until adult requirement is reached.

• If the sample is not processed in the hospital laboratory, be sure parents are notified when test results are available.

Reference values

Immediately after birth, neonatal T_4 levels are considerably higher than normal adult levels. By the end of the first week, however, T_4 values decrease markedly:

• 1 to 5 days: 4.9 mcg/dl
• 6 to 8 days: ≤ 4.0 mcg/dl
• 9 to 11 days: ≤ 3.5 mcg/dl
• 12 to 120 days: ≤ 3.0 mcg/dl.

Abnormal findings

Low serum T_4 levels in the neonate require TSH testing for clarification of the diagnosis. Decreased T_4 levels accompanied by elevated TSH readings (more than 25 µU/ml) indicate primary congenital hypothyroidism (thyroid gland dysfunction). If T_4 and TSH levels are depressed, secondary congenital hypothyroidism (resulting from pituitary or hypothalamic dysfunction) should be suspected.

If T_4 levels are subnormal in the presence of normal TSH readings, further testing is required. Serum TBG levels must be analyzed to identify infants with hypothyroidism resulting from congenital defects in TBG. This low T_4–normal TSH pattern also occurs in a transient form of congenital hypothyroidism, which may accompany prematurity, or prenatal hypoxia.

A complete thyroid workup — including serum T_3, TBG, and free T_4 levels — is necessary for unequivocal diagnosis of congenital hypothyroidism before treatment begins.

PLASMA CALCITONIN

This radioimmunoassay measures plasma levels of calcitonin (thyrocalcitonin). The exact role of calcitonin in normal human physiology has not been fully defined. However, calcitonin is known to act as an antagonist to parathyroid hormone and lower serum calcium levels. The usual clinical indication for this test is suspected medullary carcinoma of the thyroid, which causes hypersecretion of calcitonin (without associated hypocalcemia). Equivocal results require provocative testing with I.V. pentagastrin or calcium to rule out disease.

Purpose

• To aid diagnosis of thyroid medullary carcinoma or ectopic calcitonin-producing tumors (rare)

Patient preparation

• Explain to the patient that this test helps evaluate thyroid function.

• Instruct him to fast overnight, because food may interfere with calcium homeostasis and, subsequently, calcitonin levels.

• Tell him this test requires a blood sample, and advise him who will perform the venipuncture and when.

• Inform him that although he may feel transient discomfort from the needle puncture, collecting the sample takes only a few minutes.

• Explain that the laboratory requires several days to complete the analysis.

Procedure and posttest care
• Draw venous blood into a 10-ml *green-top* (heparinized) tube.
• If a hematoma develops at the venipuncture site, apply warm soaks.

Precautions
• Handle the sample gently to prevent hemolysis, and send it to the laboratory immediately.

Reference values
Serum calcitonin levels (basal) normally are ≤ 0.155 ng/ml in men; in women, ≤ 0.105 ng/ml.

Reference values after provocative testing with 4-hour calcium infusion are:
• Men: 0.265 ng/ml
• Women: 0.120 ng/ml.

Values after provocative testing with pentagastrin infusion are:
• Men: 0.210 ng/ml
• Women: 0.105 ng/ml.

The detection limit of assay is 0.030 ng/ml.

Abnormal findings
Elevated serum calcitonin levels, in the absence of hypocalcemia, usually indicate medullary carcinoma of the thyroid. Transmitted as an autosomal dominant trait, thyroid medullary carcinoma may occur as part of multiple endocrine neoplasia. Occasionally, increased calcitonin levels may be due to ectopic calcitonin production by oat cell carcinoma of the lung or by breast carcinoma.

PARATHYROID HORMONE

Parathyroid hormone (PTH) regulates plasma concentration of calcium and phosphorus. The overall effect of PTH is to raise plasma levels of calcium while lowering phosphorus levels.

Circulating PTH exists in three distinct molecular forms: the intact PTH molecule, which originates in the parathyroids, and two smaller circulating forms: N-terminal fragments and C-terminal fragments. Currently, two radioimmunoassays are available to detect intact PTH and the N- and C-terminal fragments. Both tests can be used to confirm diagnosis of hyperparathyroidism and hypoparathyroidism.

Each test has other specific applications as well. The C-terminal PTH assay is more useful in diagnosing chronic disturbances in PTH metabolism, such as secondary and tertiary hyperparathyroidism; it also better differentiates ectopic from primary hyperparathyroidism. The assay for intact PTH and the N-terminal fragment (both forms are measured concomitantly) more accurately reflects acute changes in PTH metabolism, and thus is useful in monitoring a patient's response to PTH therapy.

The clinical and diagnostic effects of PTH excess or deficiency are directly related to the effects of PTH on bone and on the renal tubules and to its interaction with ionized calcium and biologically active vitamin D. Therefore, measuring serum calcium, phosphorus, and creatinine levels with serum PTH is helpful when trying to understand the causes and effects of pathologic parathyroid function. Suppression or stimu-

Clinical Implications of Abnormal Parathyroid Secretion

CONDITIONS	CAUSES	P.T.H. LEVELS	IONIZED CALCIUM LEVELS
Primary hyperparathyroidism	• Parathyroid adenoma or carcinoma • Parathyroid hyperplasia	High	High to Normal
Secondary hyperparathyroidism	• Parathyroid hyperplasia • Chronic renal disease • Severe vitamin D deficiency • Calcium malabsorption • Pregnancy and lactation	High	Low
Tertiary hyperparathyroidism	• Progressive secondary hyperparathyroidism leading to autonomous hyperparathyroidism	High	High to Normal
Hypoparathyroidism	• Usually, accidental removal of the parathyroid glands during surgery • Occasionally, in association with autoimmune disease	Low	Low
Malignant tumors	• Squamous cell carcinoma of the lung • Renal, pancreatic, or ovarian carcinoma	High to Normal	High

KEY
High ●   Normal ◓   Low ○

lation tests may help to confirm findings.

Purpose
• To aid the differential diagnosis of parathyroid disorders

Patient preparation
• Explain to the patient that this test helps evaluate parathyroid function.
• Instruct him to observe an overnight fast because food may affect PTH levels and interfere with the test results.

• Tell the patient that this test requires a blood sample and who will perform the venipuncture and when.
• Explain that although he may experience transient discomfort from the needle puncture, collecting the sample takes only a few minutes.
• Inform him that the laboratory requires several days to complete the analysis.

Procedure and posttest care
• Draw 3 ml of venous blood into two separate 7-ml *red-top* tubes.

• If a hematoma develops at the venipuncture site, apply warm soaks.
• Allow the patient to resume diet.

Precautions
• Handle the sample gently to prevent hemolysis. Send it to the laboratory immediately so the serum can be separated and frozen for assay.

Reference values
Normal serum PTH levels vary, depending on the laboratory, and must be interpreted in association with serum calcium levels. Typical values are as follows:
• Intact PTH: 210 to 310 pg/ml
• N-terminal fraction: 230 to 630 pg/ml
• C-terminal fraction: 410 to 1,760 pg/ml.

Abnormal findings
Measured concomitantly with serum calcium levels, abnormally elevated PTH values may indicate primary, secondary, or tertiary hyperparathyroidism. Abnormally low PTH levels may result from hypoparathyroidism and from certain malignant diseases. (See *Clinical implications of abnormal parathyroid secretion,* page 203.)

ADRENAL AND RENAL HORMONES

ALDOSTERONE

This test measures serum aldosterone levels by quantitative analysis and radioimmunoassay. Aldosterone regulates ion transport across cell membranes to promote reabsorption of sodium and chloride in exchange for potassium and hydrogen ions. Consequently, it helps to maintain blood pressure and blood volume and to regulate fluid and electrolyte balance.

This test identifies aldosteronism and, when supported by plasma renin levels, distinguishes between the primary and secondary forms of this disorder.

Purpose
• To aid diagnosis of primary aldosteronism and potential causes of the disorder, including adrenal adenoma and adrenal hyperplasia
• To aid diagnosis of secondary hypoaldosteronism and commonly related conditions, such as salt-losing syndrome, potassium excess, congestive heart failure with ascites, or other conditions that characteristically increase activity of the renin-angiotensin system

Patient preparation
• Explain to the patient that this test helps determine if symptoms are due to improper hormonal secretion.
• Instruct him to maintain a low-carbohydrate, normal-sodium diet (135 mEq or 3 g/day) for at least 2 weeks or, preferably, for 30 days before the test.
• Tell him that the test requires a blood sample and that he may feel some discomfort from the needle puncture. Tell him who will perform the venipuncture and when.
• Explain that collecting the sample takes only a few minutes, but the laboratory requires at least 10 days to complete the multistage analysis.
• Withhold all drugs that alter fluid, sodium, and potassium balance — especially diuretics, antihypertensives, steroids, cyclic progestational agents, and estrogens — for at least 2 weeks or, preferably, for 30 days before the test.
• Withhold all renin inhibitors (such as propranolol) for 1 week before the test.

If these medications must be continued, note this on the laboratory slip.

• Tell the patient to avoid licorice for at least 2 weeks before the test because it produces an aldosterone-like effect.

Procedure and posttest care

• Perform a venipuncture while the patient is still supine after a night's rest.

• Collect the sample in a 7-ml *red-top* tube, and send it to the laboratory.

• Draw another sample 4 hours later, while the patient is standing and after he has been up and about, to evaluate the effect of postural change.

• Collect the second sample in a 7-ml *red-top* tube, and send it to the laboratory.

• If a hematoma develops at the venipuncture site, apply warm soaks.

• Allow the patient to resume diet and medications discontinued before the test.

Precautions

• Handle the sample gently to prevent hemolysis.

• Record on the laboratory slip whether the patient was supine or standing during the venipuncture.

• If the patient is a premenopausal female, specify the phase of her menstrual cycle because aldosterone levels may fluctuate during the menstrual cycle.

• Send the specimen to the laboratory immediately.

Reference values

Normally, serum aldosterone levels (in a standing, nonpregnant patient) range from 1 to 16 ng/dl. However, the range for an adult man or woman who has been standing for at least 2 hours is 4 to 31 ng/dl. Values for female patients are variable.

Abnormal findings

Excessive aldosterone secretion may indicate a primary or secondary disease. Primary aldosteronism (Conn's syndrome) may result from adrenocortical adenoma or carcinoma, or bilateral adrenal hyperplasia. Secondary aldosteronism can result from renovascular hypertension, congestive heart failure, cirrhosis of the liver, nephrotic syndrome, idiopathic cyclic edema, or the third trimester of pregnancy.

Depressed serum aldosterone levels may indicate primary hypoaldosteronism, salt-losing syndrome, toxemia of pregnancy, or Addison's disease.

PLASMA CORTISOL

Cortisol — the principal glucocorticoid secreted by the zona fasciculata of the adrenal cortex — helps metabolize nutrients, mediate physiologic stress, and regulate the immune system. Cortisol secretion normally follows a diurnal pattern: Levels rise during the early morning hours and peak around 8 a.m., then decline to very low levels in the evening and during the early phase of sleep. Intense heat or cold, infection, trauma, exercise, obesity, and debilitating disease influence cortisol secretion.

This radioimmunoassay, a quantitative analysis of plasma cortisol levels, is usually ordered for patients with signs of adrenal dysfunction. However, dynamic tests, suppression tests for hyperfunction, and stimulation tests for hypofunction are generally required for confirmation of diagnoses.

Purpose

• To aid in the diagnosis of Cushing's disease, Cushing's syndrome, Addison's disease, and secondary adrenal insufficiency

Patient preparation
• Explain to the patient that this test helps determine if his symptoms are due to improper hormonal secretion.
• Instruct him to maintain a normal salt diet (2 to 3 g/day) for 3 days before the test and to fast and limit physical activity for 10 to 12 hours before the test.
• Tell him a blood sample is required and who will perform the venipuncture and when.
• Explain that there may be some discomfort from the needle puncture, but that collecting the sample takes only a few minutes.
• Inform him that the laboratory requires at least 2 days to complete the analysis.
• Withhold all medications that may interfere with plasma cortisol levels, such as estrogens, androgens, and phenytoin, for 48 hours before the test. If the patient is receiving replacement therapy and is dependent on exogenous steroids for survival, note this on the laboratory slip, as well as any other medications that must be continued.
• Make sure the patient is relaxed and recumbent for at least 30 minutes before the test.

Procedure and posttest care
• Perform a venipuncture between 6 a.m. and 8 a.m.
• Collect the sample in a *green-top* tube, label appropriately, and send to the laboratory immediately.
• For diurnal variation testing, draw another sample between 4 p.m. and 6 p.m.
• Collect the second sample in a *green-top* tube, label appropriately, and send to the laboratory immediately.
• If a hematoma develops at the venipuncture site, apply warm soaks.
• Allow the patient to resume diet and administration of medications discontinued before the test.

Precautions
• Handle the sample gently to prevent hemolysis.
• Record the collection time on the laboratory slip.

Reference values
Normally, plasma cortisol levels range from 7 to 28 mcg/dl in the morning and from 2 to 18 mcg/dl in the afternoon. The afternoon level is usually half the morning level.

Abnormal findings
Increased plasma cortisol levels may indicate adrenocortical hyperfunction in Cushing's disease (a rare disease due to basophilic adenoma of the pituitary gland) or in Cushing's syndrome (glucocorticoid excess from any cause). In most patients with Cushing's syndrome, the adrenal cortex tends to secrete independently of any natural rhythm. Thus, absence of diurnal variation in cortisol secretion is a significant finding in almost all patients with Cushing's syndrome; in these patients, little difference in values, if any, is found between morning samples and those taken in the afternoon. Diurnal variations may also be absent in otherwise healthy people who are under considerable emotional or physical stress.

Decreased cortisol levels may indicate primary adrenal hypofunction (Addison's disease), most often due to idiopathic glandular atrophy (a presumed autoimmune process). Tuberculosis, fungal invasion, and hemorrhage can cause adrenocortical destruction. Low cortisol levels resulting from secondary adrenal insufficiency may occur in conditions of impaired corticotropin secretion, such as hypophysectomy, postpartum pituitary necrosis, craniopharyngioma, or chromophobe adenoma.

PLASMA CATECHOLAMINES

This test, a quantitative (total or fractionated) analysis of plasma catecholamines, has clinical importance in patients with hypertension and signs of adrenal medullary tumor, and in patients with neural tumors that affect endocrine function. Elevated plasma catecholamine levels necessitate supportive confirmation by urinalysis.

Major catecholamines include the hormones epinephrine, norepinephrine, and dopamine. When secreted into the bloodstream, catecholamines produced in the adrenal medulla prepare the body for the fight-or-flight reaction. They increase heart rate and contractility, constrict blood vessels and redistribute circulating blood toward the skeletal and coronary muscles, mobilize carbohydrate and lipid reserves, and sharpen alertness. Excessive catecholamine secretion by tumors causes hypertension, weight loss, episodic sweating, headache, palpitations, and anxiety.

Plasma levels commonly fluctuate in response to temperature, stress, postural change, diet, smoking, anoxia, volume depletion, renal failure, obesity, and many drugs.

Purpose

• To rule out pheochromocytoma (adrenal medullary or extra-adrenal) in patients with hypertension
• To help identify neuroblastoma, ganglioneuroblastoma, and ganglioneuroma
• To distinguish between adrenal medullary tumors and other catecholamine-producing tumors, through fractional analysis; urinalysis for catecholamine degradation products is recommended to support diagnosis
• To aid diagnosis of autonomic nervous system dysfunction, such as idiopathic orthostatic hypotension

Patient preparation

• Explain to the patient that this test helps determine if hypertension or other symptoms are related to improper hormonal secretion. Advise the patient to strictly follow pretest instructions for a reliable test result. Instruct him to refrain from using self-prescribed medications, especially cold or allergy remedies that may contain sympathomimetics, for 2 weeks before the test.
• Tell him to exclude amine-rich foods and beverages, such as bananas, avocados, cheese, coffee, tea, cocoa, beer, and Chianti, from his diet for 48 hours; to maintain vitamin C intake, which is necessary for formation of catecholamines; to abstain from smoking for 24 hours; and to fast for 10 to 12 hours.
• Tell the patient that this test requires one or two blood samples and who will perform the venipunctures and when.
• Explain that he may feel some discomfort from the needle punctures, but that collecting the samples takes less than 20 minutes.
• Inform him that the laboratory requires up to 1 week to complete the analysis.
• If the patient is hospitalized, withhold medications that affect catecholamine levels, such as amphetamines, phenothiazines (chlorpromazine), sympathomimetics, and tricyclic antidepressants.
• Insert an indwelling venous catheter (heparin lock) 24 hours before the test, because the stress of the venipuncture itself may significantly raise catecholamine levels.
• Make sure the patient is relaxed and recumbent for 45 to 60 minutes before the test.

• If necessary, provide blankets to keep him warm; low temperatures stimulate catecholamine secretion.

Procedure and posttest care
• Perform a venipuncture between 6 a.m. and 8 a.m.
• Collect the sample in a 10-ml chilled tube containing EDTA (sodium metabisulfite solution), which can be obtained from the laboratory on request.
• If a second sample is requested, have the patient stand for 10 minutes, and draw the sample into another tube, exactly like the first.
• If a heparin lock is used, it may be necessary to discard the first 1 or 2 ml of blood. Check with the laboratory for the preferred procedure.
• If a hematoma develops at the venipuncture site, apply warm soaks.
• Allow the patient to resume normal diet and any medications discontinued before the test.

Precautions
• After collecting each sample, roll the tube slowly between your palms to distribute the EDTA without agitating the blood.
• Pack the tube in crushed ice to minimize deactivation of catecholamines, and send it to the laboratory immediately.
• Indicate on the laboratory slip whether the patient was supine or standing and the time the sample was drawn.

Reference values
In fractional analysis, catecholamine levels range as follows:
• Supine: epinephrine, undetectable to 110 pg/ml; norepinephrine, 70 to 750 pg/ml; dopamine, undetectable to 30 pg/ml
• Standing: epinephrine, undetectable to 140 pg/ml; norepinephrine, 200 to 1,700 pg/ml; dopamine, undetectable to 30 pg/ml.

Abnormal findings
High catecholamine levels may indicate pheochromocytoma, neuroblastoma, ganglioneuroblastoma, or ganglioneuroma. Elevations are possible with, but do not directly confirm thyroid disorders, hypoglycemia, or cardiac disease. Electroshock therapy, shock resulting from hemorrhage, endotoxins, or anaphylaxis also raises catecholamine levels.

In the patient with normal or low baseline catecholamine levels, failure to show an increase in the sample taken after standing suggests autonomic nervous system dysfunction.

Fractional analysis helps identify the cause of elevated catecholamine levels. For example, adrenal medullary tumors secrete epinephrine, whereas ganglioneuromas, ganglioblastomas, and neuroblastomas secrete norepinephrine.

ANDROSTENEDIONE

This test identifies the causes of disorders related to altered estrogen levels. Androstenedione is converted to estrone, an estrogen of relatively low biological activity. In premenopausal women, the amount of estrogen derived from androstenedione is relatively small. In obesity, increased levels of estrone may lead to menstrual irregularities.

In children and postmenopausal women, estrone is a major source of estrogen. Increased androstenedione production may induce premature sexual development in children. It may produce renewed ovarian stimulation, endometriosis, bleeding, and polycystic ovaries in postmenopausal women. In men, overproduction of androstenedione may cause feminizing signs, such as gynecomastia.

Purpose

• To aid in determining the cause of gonadal dysfunction, menstrual or menopausal irregularities, and premature sexual development

Patient preparation

• Explain to the patient that this test determines the cause of her symptoms.

• Tell her that the test requires a blood sample and who will perform the venipuncture and when.

• Explain that she may experience transient discomfort from the needle puncture.

• If appropriate, explain that the test should be done 1 week before or after her menstrual period and that it may be repeated.

• Withhold steroid and pituitary-based hormones. If these must be continued, note this on the laboratory slip.

Procedure and posttest care

• Perform a venipuncture, and collect a serum sample in a 10-ml *red-top* tube or collect a plasma sample in a *green-top* tube. (If a plasma sample is taken, refrigerate it or place it on ice.)

• Label it appropriately and send it to the laboratory immediately.

• If a hematoma develops at the venipuncture site, apply warm soaks.

• Resume administration of medications discontinued before the test.

Precautions

• Handle the sample gently to prevent hemolysis.

• Refrigerate or place plasma samples on ice.

• Record the patient's age, sex, and (if appropriate) phase of menstrual cycle on the laboratory slip.

Reference values

• Females: premenopausal, 0.6 to 3 ng/ml; postmenopausal, 0.3 to 8 ng/ml

• Males: 0.9 to 1.7 ng/ml.

Abnormal findings

Elevated androstenedione levels are associated with Stein-Levanthal syndrome; Cushing's syndrome; ovarian, testicular, or adrenocortical tumors; ectopic corticotropin-producing tumors; late-onset congenital adrenal hyperplasia; and ovarian stromal hyperplasia. Elevated levels result in increased estrone levels, causing premature sexual development in children; menstrual irregularities in premenopausal women; bleeding, endometriosis, or polycystic ovaries in postmenopausal women; or feminizing signs, such as gynecomastia in men. Decreased levels occur in hypogonadism.

ERYTHROPOIETIN

This test of renal hormone production measures erythropoietin (EPO) by immunoassay. It's used to evaluate anemia, polycythemia, and kidney tumors. It's also used to evaluate abuse of commercially prepared erythropoietin by athletes who believe the drug enhances performance.

Purpose

• To aid diagnosis of anemia and polycythemia

• To aid diagnosis of kidney tumors

• To detect abuse of erythropoietin by athletes

Patient preparation

• Explain to the patient that this test determines if hormonal secretion is causing changes in his red blood cells.

• Instruct him to fast for 8 to 10 hours before the test.

• Tell him that this test requires a blood sample and who will perform the venipuncture and when.

• Explain that although he may feel transient discomfort from the puncture, collection takes only a few minutes.

• Tell him the laboratory requires up to 4 days to complete the analysis.

• Keep the patient relaxed and recumbent for 30 minutes before the test.

Procedure and posttest care

• Perform a venipuncture, and collect the sample in a 5-ml *red-top* tube.

• If requested, a hematocrit may be performed at the same time by collecting an additional sample in a 2-ml *lavender-top* tube.

• If a hematoma develops at the venipuncture site, apply warm soaks.

Precautions

• Handle the specimen gently to prevent hemolysis.

Reference values

The reference range is up to 24 mU/ml. When the values are interpreted in light of the hematocrit, the range is up to 19 mU/ml or greater than 19 mU/ml when the hematocrit falls below 30.

Abnormal findings

Low levels of EPO appear in anemic patients with inadequate or absent hormone production. Congenital absence of EPO can occur. Severe renal disease may decrease production of EPO.

Elevated levels occur in anemias as a compensatory mechanism in the reestablishment of homeostasis. Inappropriate elevations (when the hematocrit level is normal to high) are seen in polycythemia and erythropoietin-secreting tumors.

Some athletes use EPO to enhance performance. The increased red cell volume conveys additional oxygen-carrying capacity to the blood. Adverse reactions may include clotting abnormalities, headache, seizures, hypertension, nausea, vomiting, diarrhea, and rash.

PLASMA ATRIAL NATRIURETIC FACTOR

This radioimmunoassay measures the plasma level of atrial natriuretic factor (ANF), also known as atrionatriuretic peptides or atriopeptins. An extremely potent natriuretic agent and vasodilator, ANF rapidly produces diuresis and increases glomerular filtration rate. ANF's role in regulating extracellular fluid volume, blood pressure, and sodium metabolism appears critical.

Patients with overt congestive heart failure (CHF) have highly elevated plasma levels of ANF. Patients with cardiovascular disease and elevated cardiac filling pressure, but without CHF, also have markedly elevated ANF. ANF may provide a marker for early asymptomatic left ventricular dysfunction and increased cardiac volume.

Purpose

• To confirm CHF

• To identify asymptomatic cardiac volume overload

Patient preparation

• As appropriate, explain the purpose of the test to the patient.

• Inform him that he must fast before the test.

• Tell him that this test requires a blood sample and who will perform the venipuncture and when.

• Reassure him that although he may feel some transient discomfort from the needle puncture, collecting the sample takes less than 3 minutes.

• Explain that the laboratory needs up to 4 days for analysis.

• Check patient history for use of medications that can influence test results.

• Withhold beta-blocking agents, calcium antagonists, diuretics, vasodilators and digitalis glycosides for 24 hours before collection.

Procedure and posttest care

• Perform a venipuncture, and collect the sample in a prechilled potassium-EDTA tube.

• After chilled centrifugation, the EDTA plasma should be promptly frozen and sent to the laboratory to be analyzed.

• If a hematoma develops at the venipuncture site, apply warm soaks.

• Tell the patient that he may resume normal diet and any discontinued medications.

Precautions

• Handle the specimen gently to prevent hemolysis.

• Place the specimen on ice, and send it to the laboratory immediately.

Reference values

Normal ANF levels range from 20 to 77 pg/ml.

Abnormal findings

Markedly elevated levels of ANF are found in patients with frank CHF and significantly elevated cardiac filling pressure.

PANCREATIC AND GASTRIC HORMONES

INSULIN

This radioimmunoassay is a quantitative analysis of serum insulin levels. These are usually measured concomitantly with glucose levels, because glucose is the primary stimulus for insulin release.

Insulin regulates the metabolism and transport or mobilization of carbohydrates, amino acids, proteins, and lipids. Stimulated by increased plasma levels of glucose, insulin secretion reaches peak levels after meals, when metabolism and food storage are greatest.

Purpose

• To aid diagnosis of hyperinsulinemia or hypoglycemia resulting from tumor or hyperplasia of pancreatic islet cells, glucocorticoid deficiency, or severe hepatic disease

• To aid diagnosis of diabetes mellitus and insulin-resistant states

Patient preparation

• Explain to the patient that this test helps determine if the pancreas is functioning normally.

• Instruct the patient to fast for 10 to 12 hours before the test.

• Explain that questionable results may need a repeat test or, frequently, a simultaneous glucose tolerance test, which requires the patient to drink glucose solution.

CONNECTING PEPTIDE ASSAY

Connecting peptide (C-peptide) is a biologically inactive peptide chain formed during the proteolytic conversion of proinsulin to insulin in the pancreatic beta cells. It has no insulin effect, either biologically or immunologically. This is important, because circulating insulin is measured by immunologic assay. As insulin is released into the bloodstream, the C-peptide chain splits off from the hormone. Except in patients with islet cell tumors and, possibly, in obese patients, serum C-peptide levels generally parallel those of insulin: normal values range between 0.9 and 4.2 ng/ml.

Purpose
A C-peptide assay may help to:
• determine the cause of hypoglyce-mia by distinguishing between endogenous hyperinsulinism or insulinoma (elevated C-peptide levels) or surreptitious insulin injection (decreased C-peptide levels).
• determine beta cell function in patients with diabetes mellitus. Absence of C-peptide indicates no beta cell function; presence indicates residual beta cell function.
• indirectly measure insulin secretion in the presence of circulating insulin antibodies, which interfere with insulin assays but not with C-peptide assays.
• detect residual tissue (some C-peptide present) after total pancreatectomy for carcinoma.
• indicate the remission phase (some C-peptide present) of diabetes mellitus.

• Inform the patient that the test requires blood samples and who will perform the venipuncture and when.
• Explain that he may feel discomfort from the needle, but that collecting the samples takes only a few minutes.
• Withhold corticotropin, steroids (including oral contraceptives), thyroid supplements, epinephrine, or other medications that may interfere with test results. If they must be continued, note this on the laboratory slip.
• Make sure the patient is relaxed and recumbent for 30 minutes before the test.

Procedure and posttest care
• Perform a venipuncture, and collect one sample for insulin level in a 7-ml *lavender-top* tube.
• Collect a sample for glucose in a *gray-top* tube, if requested.

• If a hematoma develops at the venipuncture site, apply warm soaks.
• Allow the patient to resume diet and medications discontinued before the test.

Precautions
• Agitation or stress may affect insulin levels.
• Pack the sample for insulin in ice, and immediately send it, along with the glucose sample, to the laboratory.
• In the patient with an insulinoma, fasting for this test may precipitate dangerously severe hypoglycemia. Keep glucose I.V. (50%) available to combat possible hypoglycemia.
• Handle the sample gently.

Reference values
Serum insulin levels normally range from 2 to 25 µU/ml.

Abnormal findings

Insulin levels are interpreted in light of the prevailing glucose concentration. A normal insulin level may be inappropriate for the glucose results. High insulin and low glucose levels after a significant fast suggest an insulinoma. Prolonged fasting or stimulation testing may be required to confirm diagnosis. (See *Connecting peptide assay.*) In insulin-resistant diabetic states, insulin levels are elevated; in non-insulin-resistant diabetes, they are low.

GASTRIN

Gastrin is a polypeptide hormone produced and stored primarily in the antrum of the stomach and, to a lesser degree, in the islets of Langerhans. The main function of gastrin is to facilitate digestion of food by triggering gastric acid secretion. Gastrin also stimulates the release of pancreatic enzymes and the gastric enzyme pepsin, increases gastric and intestinal motility, and stimulates bile flow from the liver. Abnormal secretion of gastrin can result from tumors (gastrinomas) and from pathologic disorders affecting the stomach, pancreas, and less commonly, the esophagus and the small bowel.

This radioimmunoassay, a quantitative analysis of gastrin levels, is especially useful in patients suspected of having gastrinomas (Zollinger-Ellison syndrome). In doubtful situations, provocative testing may be necessary.

Purpose

• To confirm diagnosis of gastrinoma, the gastrin-secreting tumor in Zollinger-Ellison syndrome

• To aid differential diagnosis of gastric and duodenal ulcers and pernicious anemia (gastrin estimation has limited value in patients with duodenal ulcer)

Patient preparation

• Explain to the patient that this test helps determine the cause of gastrointestinal symptoms.

• Instruct him to abstain from alcohol for at least 24 hours before the test and to fast for 12 hours before the test, although he may drink water.

• Tell him the test requires a blood sample and who will perform the venipuncture and when.

• Reassure him that although he may feel some transient discomfort from the needle puncture, collecting the sample takes only a few minutes.

• Withhold all medications that may interfere with test results, especially insulin or anticholinergics such as atropine and belladonna. If these medications must be continued, note this on the laboratory slip.

• Because stress can increase gastrin levels, make sure the patient is relaxed and recumbent for at least 30 minutes before the test.

Procedure and posttest care

• Perform a venipuncture, and collect the sample in a 10- to 15-ml *red-top* tube.

• If a hematoma develops at the venipuncture site, apply warm soaks.

• Allow the patient to resume normal diet and medications discontinued before the test.

Precautions

• Handle the sample gently to avoid hemolysis.

• To prevent destruction of serum gastrin by proteolytic enzymes, immediately send the sample to the laboratory to have the serum separated and frozen.

Reference values
Serum gastrin levels are less than 300 pg/ml.

Abnormal findings
Strikingly high serum gastrin levels (more than 1,000 pg/ml) confirm Zollinger-Ellison syndrome. (Levels as high as 450,000 pg/ml have been reported.)

Increased serum levels of gastrin may occur in a few patients with duodenal ulceration (less than 1%) and in patients with achlorhydria (with or without pernicious anemia) or with extensive stomach carcinoma (because of hyposecretion of gastric juices and hydrochloric acid).

GONADAL HORMONES

ESTROGENS

Estrogens (and progesterone) are secreted by the ovaries and are responsible for the development of secondary female sexual characteristics and for normal menstruation. Levels are usually undetectable in children. These hormones are secreted by ovarian follicular cells during the first half of the menstrual cycle and by the corpus luteum during the luteal phase and during pregnancy. In menopause, estrogen secretion drops to a constant, low level.

This radioimmunoassay measures serum levels of estradiol, estrone, and estriol — the only estrogens that appear in serum in measurable amounts — and has diagnostic significance in evaluating female gonadal dysfunction. Tests of hypothalamic-pituitary function may be required to confirm diagnosis.

Purpose
● To determine sexual maturation and fertility
● To aid diagnosis of gonadal dysfunction: precocious or delayed puberty, menstrual disorders (especially amenorrhea), or infertility
● To determine fetal well-being
● To aid diagnosis of tumors known to secrete estrogen

Patient preparation
● Explain to the patient that this test helps determine if secretion of female hormones is normal, and that the test may be repeated during the various phases of the menstrual cycle.
● Tell her she needn't restrict food or fluids.
● Inform her that the test requires a blood sample and who will perform the venipuncture and when.
● Explain that she may experience transient discomfort from the needle puncture, but that collecting the sample takes only a few minutes.
● Withhold all steroid and pituitary-based hormones (including estrogens and progestogen). If these medications must be continued, note this on the laboratory slip.

Procedure and posttest care
Procedure and posttest care may vary slightly, depending on choice of plasma or serum assay.
● Perform a venipuncture, and collect the sample in a 10-ml *red-top* tube.
● If the patient is premenopausal, indicate the phase of her menstrual cycle on the laboratory slip.
● If a hematoma develops at the venipuncture site, apply warm soaks.
● Resume administration of medications discontinued before the test.

Precautions
• To prevent hemolysis, handle the sample gently.
• Send it to the laboratory immediately for centrifugation.

Reference values
Normal serum estrogen levels for premenopausal women vary widely during the menstrual cycle:
• 1 to 10 days: 24 to 68 pg/ml
• 11 to 20 days: 50 to 186 pg/ml
• 21 to 30 days: 73 to 149 pg/ml.

Serum estrogen levels in men range from 12 to 34 pg/ml. In children under age 6, the normal range of serum estrogen is 3 to 10 pg/ml.

Abnormal findings
Decreased estrogen levels may indicate primary hypogonadism, or ovarian failure, as in Turner's syndrome or ovarian agenesis; secondary hypogonadism, as in hypopituitarism; or menopause.

Abnormally high levels may occur with estrogen-producing tumors, in precocious puberty, or in severe hepatic disease, such as cirrhosis, that prevents clearance of plasma estrogens. High levels may also result from congenital adrenal hyperplasia (increased conversion of androgens to estrogen).

PLASMA PROGESTERONE

Progesterone, an ovarian steroid hormone secreted by the corpus luteum, causes thickening and secretory development of the endometrium in preparation for implantation of the fertilized ovum. Progesterone levels, therefore, peak during the midluteal phase of the menstrual cycle. If implantation doesn't occur, progesterone (and estrogen) lev-els drop sharply and menstruation begins about 2 days later.

During pregnancy, the placenta releases about 10 times the normal monthly amount of progesterone to maintain the pregnancy. Increased secretion begins toward the end of the first trimester and continues until delivery. Progesterone causes thickening of the endometrium, which contains large amounts of stored nutrients for the developing ovum (blastocyst). Progesterone also prevents abortion by decreasing uterine contractions. Along with estrogen, progesterone helps prepare the breasts for lactation.

This radioimmunoassay is a quantitative analysis of plasma progesterone levels and provides reliable information about corpus luteum function in fertility studies or placental function in pregnancy. Serial determinations are recommended. Although plasma levels provide accurate information, progesterone can also be monitored by measuring urine pregnanediol, a catabolite of progesterone.

Purpose
• To assess corpus luteum function as part of infertility studies
• To evaluate placental function during pregnancy
• To aid in confirming ovulation; test results support basal body temperature readings

Patient preparation
• Explain to the patient that this test helps determine if her female sex hormone secretion is normal.
• Inform her that she needn't restrict food or fluids.
• Tell her the test requires a blood sample, and who will perform the venipuncture and when.
• Reassure her that although she may experience some transient discomfort

from the needle puncture, collecting the blood sample takes only a few minutes.

• Inform her that the test may be repeated at specific times coinciding with phases of her menstrual cycle or with each prenatal visit

• Check the patient's medication history to determine if she is taking any drugs, including progesterone or estrogen therapy, that may interfere with test results. Note your findings on the laboratory slip.

Procedure and posttest care

• Perform a venipuncture, and collect the sample in a 7-ml *green-top* (heparinized) tube.

• If a hematoma develops at the venipuncture site, apply warm soaks.

Precautions

• Handle the sample gently to prevent hemolysis.

• Completely fill the collection tube; then invert it gently at least 10 times to mix sample and anticoagulant adequately.

• Indicate the date of the patient's last menstrual period and the phase of her cycle on the laboratory slip. If the patient is pregnant, also indicate the month of gestation.

• Send the sample to the laboratory immediately.

Reference values

During menstruation, normal values are as follows:

• Follicular phase: less than 150 ng/dl

• Luteal phase: about 300 ng/dl (rises daily during periovulation)

• Midluteal phase: 2,000 ng/dl.

During pregnancy, normal values are as follows:

• First trimester: 1,500 to 5,000 ng/dl

• Second and third trimesters: 8,000 to 20,000 ng/dl.

Abnormal findings

Elevated progesterone levels may indicate ovulation, luteinizing tumors, ovarian cysts that produce progesterone, or adrenocortical hyperplasias and tumors that produce progesterone along with other steroidal hormones.

Low progesterone levels are associated with amenorrhea due to several causes (such as panhypopituitarism or gonadal dysfunction), toxemia of pregnancy, threatened abortion, and fetal death.

TESTOSTERONE

The principal androgen secreted by the interstitial cells of the testes (Leydig cells), testosterone induces puberty in the male and maintains male secondary sex characteristics. Prepubertal levels of testosterone are low. Increased testosterone secretion during puberty stimulates growth of the seminiferous tubules and the production of sperm; it also contributes to the enlargement of external genitalia, accessory sex organs (such as prostate glands), and voluntary muscles, and to the growth of facial, pubic, and axillary hair.

Testosterone production begins to increase at onset of puberty and continues to rise during adulthood. Production begins to taper off at about age 40, eventually dropping to approximately one fifth the peak level by age 80. In women, the adrenal glands and the ovaries secrete small amounts of testosterone.

This competitive protein-binding test measures plasma or serum testosterone levels. When combined with measurement of plasma gonadotropin levels (follicle-stimulating hormone and luteinizing hormone), it is a reliable aid in the evaluation of gonadal dysfunction in men and women.

Purpose
• To facilitate differential diagnosis of male sexual precocity in boys under age 10 (true precocious puberty must be distinguished from pseudoprecocious puberty)
• To aid differential diagnosis of hypogonadism; primary hypogonadism must be distinguished from secondary hypogonadism
• To evaluate male infertility or other sexual dysfunction
• To evaluate hirsutism and virilization in women

Patient preparation
• Explain to the patient that this test helps determine if male sex hormone secretion is adequate.
• Inform him that he needn't restrict food or fluids.
• Tell him this test requires a blood sample and who will perform the venipuncture and when.
• Reassure him that he may experience some discomfort from the needle puncture, but that collecting the sample takes only a few minutes.

Procedure and posttest care
• Perform a venipuncture, and collect the sample in a 7-ml *red-top* tube.
• Use a *green-top* (heparinized) tube if plasma is to be collected.
• Indicate the patient's age, sex, and history of hormone therapy on the laboratory slip.
• If a hematoma develops at the venipuncture site, apply warm soaks.

Precautions
• Handle the sample gently to prevent hemolysis, and send it to the laboratory.
• Note that the sample is stable and requires no refrigeration or preservative for up to 1 week. Frozen samples are stable for at least 6 months.

Reference values
Normal levels of testosterone are as follows (laboratory values vary slightly):
• Men: 300 to 1,200 ng/dl
• Women: 30 to 95 ng/dl
• Prepubertal children: in boys, less than 100 ng/dl; in girls, less than 40 ng/dl.

Abnormal findings
Elevated testosterone levels in prepubertal boys may indicate true sexual precocity due to excessive gonadotropin secretion, or pseudoprecocious puberty due to male hormone production by a testicular tumor. They can also indicate congenital adrenal hyperplasia, which results in precocious puberty in boys (from ages 2 to 3), and pseudohermaphroditism and milder virilization in girls.

Increased levels can occur with a benign adrenal tumor or cancer, hyperthyroidism, or incipient puberty. In women with ovarian tumors or polycystic ovary syndrome, testosterone levels may rise, leading to hirsutism.

Depressed testosterone levels can indicate primary hypogonadism (as in Klinefelter's syndrome) or secondary hypogonadism (hypogonadotropic eunuchoidism) from hypothalamic-pituitary dysfunction. Depressed testosterone levels can also follow orchiectomy, testicular or prostatic cancer, delayed male puberty, estrogen therapy, or cirrhosis.

PLACENTAL HORMONES

HUMAN CHORIONIC GONADOTROPIN

Human chorionic gonadotropin (hCG) is a glycoprotein hormone produced in the placenta. If conception occurs, a specific assay for hCG — commonly called the beta-subunit assay — may detect this hormone in the blood 9 days after ovulation. This interval coincides with the implantation of the fertilized ovum into the uterine wall. Although the precise function of hCG is still unclear, it appears that hCG, with progesterone, maintains the corpus luteum during early pregnancy.

Production of hCG increases steadily during the first trimester, peaking around the 10th week of gestation. Levels then fall to less than 10% of first trimester peak levels during the remainder of the pregnancy. At approximately 2 weeks after delivery, the hormone may no longer be detectable.

This serum immunoassay, a quantitative analysis of hCG beta-subunit level, is more sensitive (and costly) than the routine pregnancy test using a urine specimen.

Purpose
• To detect early pregnancy
• To determine adequacy of hormonal production in high-risk pregnancies (for example, habitual abortion)
• To aid diagnosis of trophoblastic tumors, such as hydatidiform moles or choriocarcinoma, and of tumors that ectopically secrete hCG

• To monitor treatment for induction of ovulation and conception

Patient preparation
• Explain to the patient that this test determines if she is pregnant. If detection of pregnancy isn't the diagnostic objective, offer the appropriate explanation.
• Inform her she needn't restrict food or fluids.
• Tell her the test requires a blood sample and who will perform the venipuncture and when.
• Explain that she may feel transient discomfort from the needle puncture, but collecting the sample takes only a few minutes.

Procedure and posttest care
• Perform a venipuncture, and collect the sample in a 7-ml *red-top* tube.
• If a hematoma develops at the venipuncture site, apply warm soaks.

Precautions
• Handle the sample gently to prevent hemolysis, and send it to the laboratory immediately.

Reference values
Normal values for hCG are less than 5 IU/L. During pregnancy, hCG levels are quite variable and depend partially on the number of days after the last normal menstrual period.

Abnormal findings
Elevated hCG beta-subunit levels indicate pregnancy; significantly higher concentrations are present in a multiple pregnancy. Increased levels may also suggest hydatidiform mole, trophoblastic neoplasms of the placenta, or nontrophoblastic carcinomas that secrete hCG (including gastric, pancreatic, and ovarian adenocarcinomas). Low hCG beta-subunit levels can occur in ectopic pregnancy or pregnancy of less than 9 days. Beta-subunit levels cannot dif-

ferentiate between pregnancy and tumor recurrence because these levels are high in both conditions.

HUMAN PLACENTAL LACTOGEN

A polypeptide hormone, human placental lactogen (hPL) — also known as human chorionic somatomammotropin (hCS) — displays lactogenic and somatotropic (growth hormone) properties in a pregnant female. In combination with prolactin, hPL prepares the breasts for lactation. It also indirectly provides energy for maternal metabolism and fetal nutrition. It facilitates protein synthesis and mobilization essential to fetal growth. Secretion is autonomous, beginning about the fifth week of gestation and declining rapidly after delivery. According to some evidence, this hormone may not be essential for a successful pregnancy.

This radioimmunoassay measures plasma hPL levels, which are roughly proportional to placental mass. Such assays may be required in high-risk pregnancies (patients with diabetes mellitus, hypertension, or toxemia) or in suspected placental tissue dysfunction. Because values vary widely during the last half of pregnancy, serial determinations over several days provide the most reliable test results.

Purpose
• To assess placental function and fetal well-being (combined with measurement of estriol levels)
• To aid diagnosis of hydatidiform moles and choriocarcinoma (human chorionic gonadotropin levels may be more useful in diagnosing these conditions)

• To aid diagnosis and monitor treatment of nontrophoblastic tumors that ectopically secrete hPL

Patient preparation
• Explain to the patient that this test helps assess placental function and fetal well-being. (If assessing fetal well-being isn't the diagnostic objective, offer an appropriate explanation.)
• Tell her the test requires a blood sample and who will perform the venipuncture and when.
• Reassure her that although she may experience transient discomfort from the needle puncture, collecting the sample takes only a few minutes.
• Inform the pregnant patient that this test may be repeated during her pregnancy.

Procedure and posttest care
• Perform a venipuncture, and collect the sample in a 7-ml *red-top* tube.
• If a hematoma develops at the venipuncture site, apply warm soaks.

Precautions
• Handle the sample gently to prevent hemolysis, and send it to the laboratory without delay.

Reference values
For pregnant women, normal hPL levels are as listed in the chart below.

GESTATION PERIOD	hPL LEVELS
5 to 27 weeks	< 4.6 mcg/ml
28 to 31 weeks	2.4 to 6.1 mcg/ml
32 to 35 weeks	3.7 to 7.7 mcg/ml
36 weeks to term	5 to 8.6 mcg/ml

At term, patients with diabetes mellitus may have mean levels of 9 to 11 mcg/ml.

Normal levels for nonpregnant women are < 0.5 mcg/ml; normal levels for men, < 0.5 mcg/ml.

Abnormal findings

For reliable interpretation, hPL levels must be correlated with gestational age; for example, after 30 weeks' gestation, levels below 4 mcg/ml may indicate placental dysfunction. Low hPL concentrations are also characteristically associated with postmaturity syndrome, retardation of intrauterine growth, and toxemia of pregnancy. Declining concentrations may help differentiate incomplete abortion from threatened abortion.

Be aware that low hPL concentrations don't confirm fetal distress. Conversely, concentrations over 4 mcg/ml after 30 weeks' gestation don't guarantee fetal well-being because elevated levels have been reported after fetal death.

An hPL value above 6 mcg/ml after 30 weeks' gestation may suggest an unusually large placenta, commonly occurring in patients with diabetes mellitus, multiple pregnancy, or Rh isoimmunization. However, the usefulness of this test in predicting fetal death in a patient with diabetes mellitus or in managing Rh isoimmunization during pregnancy is limited.

Below normal concentrations of hPL may be associated with trophoblastic neoplastic disease, such as hydatidiform mole or choriocarcinoma. Abnormal concentrations of hPL have been found in the sera of patients with other malignancies, including bronchogenic carcinoma, hepatoma, lymphoma, and pheochromocytoma. In these patients, hPL levels are used as tumor markers for evaluation of chemotherapy, for monitoring tumor growth and recurrence, and for detection of residual tissue after excision.

Vitamin and Trace Element Tests

VITAMINS

VITAMIN A AND CAROTENE

This test measures serum levels of vitamin A (retinol) and its precursor, carotene. A fat-soluble vitamin normally supplied by diet, vitamin A is important for reproduction, vision (especially night vision), and epithelial tissue and bone growth. Vitamin A is found mostly in fruits, vegetables, eggs, poultry, meat, and fish. Carotene is present in leafy green vegetables and in yellow fruits and vegetables.

In this serum test, the color reactions produced by vitamin A and related compounds with various reagents provide both quantitative and qualitative information.

Purpose
- To investigate suspected vitamin A deficiency or toxicity
- To aid diagnosis of visual disturbances, especially night blindness and xerophthalmia
- To aid diagnosis of skin diseases, such as keratosis follicularis or ichthyosis
- To screen for malabsorption

Patient preparation
- Explain to the patient that this test measures the level of vitamin A in the blood.
- Instruct him to fast overnight, but that he needn't restrict water intake.
- Tell him this test requires a blood sample and who will perform the venipuncture and when.
- Reassure him that although he may feel some discomfort from the needle puncture and the pressure of the tourniquet, collecting the sample takes only a few minutes.

Procedure and posttest care
- Perform a venipuncture, and collect the sample in a 7-ml *red-top* or *royal-blue-top* tube.
- If a hematoma develops at the venipuncture site, apply warm soaks.
- Remove diet restrictions.

Precautions
- Protect the sample from light, because vitamin A characteristically absorbs light.
- Handle the sample gently, and send it to the laboratory immediately.

Reference values
Values differ according to age and gender. For children, the range of values is 30 to 80 µg/dl. For adults, it is 30 to 65 µg/dl (values for men are usually 20% higher).

Abnormal findings
Low serum levels of vitamin A (hypovitaminosis A) may indicate impaired fat absorption, as in celiac disease, infectious hepatitis, cystic fibrosis of the pancreas, or obstructive jaundice. Low levels are also associated with protein-calorie malnutrition (marasmic kwashiorkor). Similar decreases in vitamin A levels may also result from chronic nephritis.

Elevated vitamin A levels (hypervitaminosis A) usually indicate chronically excessive intake of vitamin A supplements or of foods high in vitamin A. Increased levels are also associated with hyperlipemia and hypercholesterolemia of uncontrolled diabetes mellitus.

Decreased serum carotene levels may indicate impaired fat absorption or, rarely, insufficient dietary intake of carotene. Carotene levels may also be suppressed during pregnancy. Elevated carotene levels indicate grossly excessive dietary intake.

VITAMIN B₂

This test evaluates serum levels of vitamin B_2 (riboflavin), a vitamin essential for growth and tissue function. The serum test is considered more reliable than the urine vitamin B_2 test, which can produce artificially high values in patients after surgery or prolonged fasting.

Purpose
• To detect vitamin B_2 deficiency

Patient preparation
• Explain to the patient that this test evaluates vitamin B_2 levels.
• Instruct him to maintain a normal diet before the test.
• Inform him that the test requires a blood sample and who will perform the venipuncture and when.
• Reassure him that although he may experience some discomfort from the needle puncture and the pressure of the tourniquet, collecting the sample takes only a few minutes.

Procedure and posttest care
• Perform a venipuncture, and collect the sample in a 7-ml *royal-blue-top* tube.
• If a hematoma develops at the venipuncture site, apply warm soaks.
• Inform the patient with vitamin B_2 deficiency that good dietary sources of vitamin B_2 are milk products, organ meats (liver and kidneys), fish, green leafy vegetables, and legumes.

Precautions
• Handle the sample gently to prevent hemolysis.

• Send the sample to the laboratory immediately.
• Do not refrigerate or freeze the sample.

Reference values
Normal test results are 3 to 5 μg/dl.

Abnormal findings
Test results below 3 μg/dl indicate vitamin B_2 deficiency. Such deficiency can result from insufficient dietary intake of vitamin B_2, malabsorption syndrome, or conditions that increase metabolic demands, such as stress.

VITAMIN B₁₂

This radioisotopic assay of competitive binding is a quantitative analysis of serum levels of vitamin B_{12} levels (also called cyanocobalamin, antipernicious anemia factor, or extrinsic factor). This test is usually performed concurrently with measurement of serum folic acid levels.

A water-soluble vitamin containing cobalt, vitamin B_{12} is essential to hematopoiesis, deoxyribonucleic acid synthesis and growth, and myelin synthesis and nervous system integrity. This vitamin is found almost exclusively in animal products, such as meat (also shellfish), milk, and eggs. (See *Cobalt: Critical trace element,* page 224.)

Purpose
• To aid differential diagnosis of megaloblastic anemia, which may be due to a deficiency of vitamin B_{12} or folic acid
• To aid differential diagnosis of central nervous system (CNS) disorders that are affecting peripheral and spinal myelinated nerves

COBALT: CRITICAL TRACE ELEMENT

A trace element found mainly in the liver, cobalt is an essential component of vitamin B_{12} and therefore is a critical factor in hematopoiesis. A balanced diet supplies sufficient cobalt to maintain hematopoiesis, primarily through foods containing vitamin B_{12}. However, excessive ingestion of cobalt may have toxic effects. Toxicity has occurred, for example, in individuals who consumed large quantities of beer containing cobalt as a stabilizer, resulting in congestive heart failure from cardiomyopathy. Since quantitative analysis of cobalt alone is difficult because of the minute amount found in the body, cobalt is often measured by bioassay as part of vitamin B_{12}.

The normal cobalt concentration of human plasma is about 60 to 80 pg/ml.

Patient preparation

• Explain to the patient that this test determines the amount of vitamin B_{12} in the blood.

• If folic acid level is also being measured, instruct the patient to observe an overnight fast before the test.

• Tell him this test requires a blood sample and who will perform the venipuncture and when.

• Reassure him that although he may feel some discomfort from the needle puncture and the pressure of the tourniquet, collecting the sample takes only a few minutes.

• Check patient history for the use of drugs — such as para-aminosalicylic acid, phenytoin, neomycin, and colchicine — that may alter test results.

Procedure and posttest care

• Perform a venipuncture, and collect the sample in a 7-ml *royal-blue-top* tube.

• If a hematoma develops at the venipuncture site, apply warm soaks.

• Remove diet restrictions.

Precautions

• Handle the sample gently to prevent hemolysis, and send it to the laboratory immediately.

Reference values

Normally, serum vitamin B_{12} values range from 100 to 700 pg/ml.

Abnormal findings

Decreased serum levels may indicate inadequate dietary intake, especially if the patient is a strict vegetarian. Low levels are also associated with malabsorption syndromes (such as celiac disease), isolated malabsorption of vitamin B_{12}, hypermetabolic states (such as hyperthyroidism), pregnancy, and CNS damage (posterolateral sclerosis or funicular degeneration, for example).

Elevated levels of serum vitamin B_{12} may result from excessive dietary intake; hepatic disease, such as cirrhosis, or acute or chronic hepatitis; and myeloproliferative disorders, such as myelocytic leukemia.

VITAMIN C

This chemical assay measures plasma levels of vitamin C (ascorbic acid), a water-soluble vitamin required for collagen synthesis, and cartilage and bone maintenance. Vitamin C also promotes iron absorption, influences folic acid metabolism, and may be necessary for withstanding the stresses of injury and infection.

This vitamin is present in generous amounts in citrus fruits, berries, tomatoes, raw cabbage, green peppers, and green leafy vegetables. Severe vitamin C deficiency, or scurvy, causes capillary fragility, joint abnormalities, and multiple systemic symptoms.

Purpose
• To aid diagnosis of scurvy, scurvy-like conditions, and metabolic disorders, such as malnutrition and malabsorption syndromes

Patient preparation
• Explain to the patient that this test detects the amount of vitamin C in the blood.
• Instruct him to observe an overnight fast before the test.
• Tell him that this test requires a blood sample and who will perform the venipuncture and when.
• Reassure him that although he may feel some discomfort from the needle puncture and the pressure of the tourniquet, collecting the sample takes only a few minutes.

Procedure and posttest care
• Perform a venipuncture, and collect the sample in a 7-ml *green-top* (heparinized) tube.
• If a hematoma develops at the venipuncture site, apply warm soaks.
• Remove diet restrictions.

Precautions
• Avoid rough handling or excessive agitation of the sample in order to prevent hemolysis.
• Send the sample to the laboratory immediately.

Reference values
Normally, plasma vitamin C values of 0.3 mg/dl or greater are acceptable.

Abnormal findings
Patients with values of 0.2 to 0.29 mg/dl are considered "at risk"; values under 0.2 mg/dl indicate deficiency. Vitamin C levels diminish during pregnancy to a low point immediately postpartum. Depressed levels occur with infection, fever, and anemia. Severe deficiencies result in scurvy.

High plasma levels can indicate increased ingestion of vitamin C. Excess vitamin C is converted to oxalate, which is excreted in the urine. Excessive concentration of oxalate can produce urinary calculi.

VITAMIN D_3

Vitamin D_3 (cholecalciferol), the major form of vitamin D, is endogenously produced in the skin by the sun's ultraviolet rays and occurs naturally in fish liver oils, egg yolks, liver, and butter.

This test, a competitive protein binding assay, determines serum levels of 25-hydroxycholecalciferol after chromatography has separated it from other vitamin D metabolites and contaminants. It is commonly combined with measurement of serum calcium and alkaline phosphatase levels.

Purpose
• To evaluate skeletal disease, such as rickets and osteomalacia
• To aid diagnosis of hypercalcemia
• To detect vitamin D toxicity
• To monitor therapy with vitamin D_3

Patient preparation
• Explain to the patient that this test measures vitamin D in the body.
• Tell the patient he needn't restrict food or fluids.

• Inform him that the test requires a blood sample and who will perform the venipuncture and when.

• Reassure him that although he may feel discomfort from the needle and the tourniquet, collecting the sample takes less than 3 minutes.

• Check for drugs that alter test results (corticosteroids or anticonvulsants). If they must be continued, note this on the laboratory slip.

Procedure and posttest care

• Perform a venipuncture, and collect the sample in a 7-ml *royal-blue-top* tube.

• If a hematoma develops at the venipuncture site, apply warm soaks.

Precautions

• Handle the sample carefully to prevent hemolysis.

Reference values

In summer, the range for serum 25-hydroxycholecalciferol values is from 15 to 80 ng/ml; in winter, it's 14 to 42 ng/ml.

Abnormal findings

Low or undetectable levels may result from vitamin D deficiency, which can cause rickets or osteomalacia. Such deficiency may stem from poor diet, decreased exposure to the sun, or impaired absorption of vitamin D (secondary to hepatobiliary disease, pancreatitis, celiac disease, cystic fibrosis, or gastric or small bowel resection). Low levels may also be related to various hepatic diseases that directly affect vitamin D metabolism.

Elevated levels (over 100 ng/ml) may indicate toxicity due to excessive self-medication or prolonged therapy. Elevated levels associated with hypercalcemia may be due to hypersensitivity to vitamin D, as in sarcoidosis.

FOLIC ACID

This test is a quantitative analysis of serum levels of folic acid (also called pteroylglutamic acid, folacin, or folate) by radioisotopic assay of competitive binding. It is often performed concomitantly with measurement of serum vitamin B_{12} levels. Like vitamin B_{12}, folic acid is a water-soluble vitamin that influences hematopoiesis, deoxyribonucleic acid synthesis, and overall body growth.

Normally, diet supplies folic acid in liver, kidney, yeast, fruits, leafy vegetables, eggs, and milk. Inadequate dietary intake may cause a deficiency, especially during pregnancy. Because of folic acid's vital role in hematopoiesis, the usual indication for this test is a suspected hematologic abnormality.

Purpose

• To aid differential diagnosis of megaloblastic anemia, which may result from deficiency of folic acid or vitamin B_{12}

• To assess folate stores in pregnancy

Patient preparation

• Explain to the patient that this test determines the folic acid level in the blood.

• Instruct him to observe an overnight fast before the test.

• Tell him the test requires a blood sample and who will perform the venipuncture and when.

• Reassure him that although he may experience some discomfort from the needle puncture and the pressure of the tourniquet, collecting the sample takes only a few minutes.

• Check the patient's medication history for drugs that may affect test results, such as phenytoin or pyrimethamine.

Procedure and posttest care
• Perform a venipuncture, and collect the sample in a 7-ml *royal-blue-top* tube.
• If a hematoma develops at the venipuncture site, apply warm soaks.
• Remove diet restrictions.

Precautions
• Handle the sample gently to prevent hemolysis.
• Protect it from light.
• Send it to the laboratory immediately.

Reference values
Normally, serum folic acid values range from 3 to 16 ng/ml.

Abnormal findings
Low serum levels (less than 2 ng/ml) may indicate hematologic abnormalities, such as anemia (especially megaloblastic anemia), leukopenia, and thrombocytopenia. The Schilling test is often performed to rule out vitamin B_{12} deficiency, which also causes megaloblastic anemia. Decreased folic acid levels can also result from hypermetabolic states (such as hyperthyroidism), inadequate dietary intake, chronic alcoholism, small-bowel malabsorption syndrome, or pregnancy.

Serum levels greater than 20 ng/ml may indicate excessive dietary intake of folic acid or folic acid supplements. Even when taken in large doses, this vitamin is nontoxic.

TRACE ELEMENTS

MANGANESE

This test, an analysis by atomic absorption spectroscopy, measures serum levels of manganese, a trace element. Although its function is only partially understood, manganese is known to activate several enzymes — including cholinesterase and arginase — that are essential to metabolism. Dietary sources of manganese include unrefined cereals, green leafy vegetables, and nuts.

Manganese toxicity may result from the inhalation of manganese dust or fumes — a hazard in the steel and dry-cell battery industries — or from ingestion of contaminated water.

Purpose
• To detect manganese toxicity

Patient preparation
• Explain to the patient that this test determines the level of manganese in the blood.
• Inform him he needn't restrict food or fluids.
• Tell him this test requires a blood sample and who will perform the venipuncture and when.
• Reassure him that although he may feel some transient discomfort from the needle puncture and the pressure of the tourniquet, collecting the sample takes only a few minutes.
• Check patient history for use of medications that may influence serum manganese levels, such as estrogens and glucocorticoids.

Procedure and posttest care
• Perform a venipuncture, and collect the sample in a metal-free collection tube. Laboratories will supply a special kit for this test on request.
• If a hematoma develops at the venipuncture site, apply warm soaks.

Precautions
• Handle the sample gently to prevent hemolysis, and send it to the laboratory immediately.

Reference values

Normally, serum manganese values range from 0.04 to 1.4 μg/dl.

Abnormal findings

Significantly elevated serum levels indicate manganese toxicity, which requires prompt medical attention to prevent central nervous system deterioration. Depressed serum manganese levels may indicate deficient dietary intake, although deficiency hasn't been linked to disease.

ZINC

This test, an analysis by atomic absorption spectroscopy, measures serum levels of zinc. An important trace element, zinc is an integral component of more than 80 enzymes and proteins, and plays a critical role in enzyme catalytic reactions.

Zinc occurs naturally in water and in most foods; high concentrations are found in meat, seafood, dairy products, whole grains, nuts, and legumes. Zinc deficiency (hypozincemia) can seriously impair body metabolism, growth, and development.

Purpose

• To detect zinc deficiency or toxicity

Patient preparation

• Explain to the patient that this test determines the concentration of zinc in the blood.
• Inform him he needn't restrict food or fluids.
• Tell him the test requires a blood sample and who will perform the venipuncture and when.
• Reassure him that although he may feel some discomfort from the needle and the pressure of the tourniquet, collecting the sample takes only a few minutes.
• Check the patient's recent drug history for medications, such as zinc-chelating agents and corticosteroids, that may interfere with the test results.

Procedure and posttest care

• Perform a venipuncture, and collect a 3-ml sample in a zinc-free collection tube.
• If a hematoma develops at the venipuncture site, apply warm soaks.

Precautions

• Handle the sample gently to prevent hemolysis, and send it to the laboratory immediately. Reliable analysis must begin before platelet disintegration can alter test results.

Reference values

Normally, plasma zinc values range from 70 to 150 μg/dl.

Abnormal findings

Values below 70 μg/dl indicate zinc deficiency. Decreased serum zinc levels may indicate an acquired deficiency (due to insufficient dietary intake or to an underlying disease) or a hereditary deficiency. Markedly depressed levels are common in leukemia and may be related to impaired zinc-dependent enzyme systems. Low serum zinc levels are commonly associated with alcoholic cirrhosis of the liver, myocardial infarction, ileitis, chronic renal failure, rheumatoid arthritis, and anemia (such as hemolytic or sickle cell anemia).

Elevated and potentially toxic serum zinc levels may result from accidental ingestion or industrial exposure.

Immunologic Tests

BACTERIA AND FUNGI

MISCELLANEOUS TESTS

IMMUNO-HEMATOLOGY

ABO BLOOD TYPING

This test classifies blood according to the presence of major antigens A and B on red cell surfaces and according to serum antibodies anti-A and anti-B. ABO blood typing, using both forward and reverse methods, is required before transfusion to prevent a lethal reaction.

In forward typing, the patient's red cells are mixed with anti-A serum, then with anti-B serum; the presence or absence of agglutination determines the blood group. In reverse typing, the results of the forward method are verified by mixing the patient's serum with known group A and group B cells. Blood group determination is confirmed when the results of forward and reverse typing match perfectly.

Purpose
• To establish blood group according to the ABO system
• To check compatibility of donor and recipient blood before transfusion

Patient preparation
• Tell the patient this test determines blood group.
• If he's scheduled for a transfusion, explain that once his blood group is known, it can be matched with the right donor blood.
• Inform him he needn't fast.
• Tell him the test requires a blood sample and who will perform the venipuncture and when.
• Reassure him that although he may feel transient discomfort from the needle puncture and the pressure of the tourniquet, collecting the sample takes only a few minutes.
• Check his history for recent administration of blood, dextran, or I.V. contrast media.
• Before the transfusion, compare current and past ABO typing and crossmatching to detect mistaken identification and prevent transfusion reaction.

Procedure and posttest care
• Perform a venipuncture, and collect the sample in a 10-ml *lavender-top* tube or *red-top* tube (one tube per three units of blood).
• If a hematoma develops at the venipuncture site, apply warm soaks.

Precautions
• Label the sample with the patient's name, hospital or blood bank number, date, and initials of phlebotomist.
• Handle the sample gently, and send it to the lab immediately, with a properly completed laboratory slip.

Findings
In forward typing, if agglutination occurs when the patient's red cells are mixed with anti-A serum, the A antigen is present and the blood is typed A. If agglutination occurs when the patient's red cells are mixed with anti-B serum, the B antigen is present and the blood is typed B. If agglutination occurs in both mixes, both A and B antigens are present and the blood is typed AB. If it does not occur in either mix, no antigens are present and the blood is typed O.

In reverse typing, if agglutination occurs when B cells are mixed with the patient's serum, anti-B is present and the blood is typed A. If agglutination occurs when A cells are mixed, anti-A is present and the blood is typed B. If agglutination occurs when both A and B cells are mixed, anti-A and anti-B are present and the blood is typed O. If agglutination does not occur when both A and B cells are mixed, neither anti-A nor anti-B is present and the blood is typed AB.

RH TYPING

The Rh system classifies blood by the presence or absence of the $Rh_o(D)$ antigen on the surface of red blood cells (RBCs). In this test, a patient's RBCs are mixed with serum containing anti-$Rh_o(D)$ antibodies and are observed for agglutination. If agglutination occurs, the $Rh_o(D)$ antigen is present, and the patient's blood is typed Rh-positive; if agglutination doesn't occur, the antigen is absent, and the patient's blood is typed Rh-negative.

Prospective blood donors are fully tested to exclude the D^u variant of the $Rh_o(D)$ antigen before being classified as having Rh-negative blood. People who have this antigen are considered Rh-positive donors but are generally transfused as Rh-negative recipients.

Purpose
• To establish blood type according to the Rh system
• To help determine the compatibility of donor and recipient before transfusion
• To determine if the patient will require an Rh immune globulin (RhIG) injection

Patient preparation
• Explain to the patient that the test determines or verifies blood group to ensure safe transfusion.
• Inform him he needn't fast before the test.
• Tell him the test requires a blood sample and who will perform the venipuncture and when.

• Reassure him that although he may experience transient discomfort from the needle puncture and the pressure of the tourniquet, collecting the sample takes only a few minutes.
• Check patient history for recent administration of dextran, I.V. contrast media, or drugs that may alter results.

Procedure and posttest care
• Perform a venipuncture, and collect the sample in a 10- to 15-ml *lavender-top* tube or *red-top* tube (one tube per three units of blood).
• If a hematoma develops at the venipuncture site, apply warm soaks.
• If necessary, give the pregnant patient a card identifying that she may need to receive RhIG.

Precautions
• Label the sample with the patient's name, hospital or blood bank number, date, and initials of the phlebotomist.
• Send it to the laboratory immediately, because the test must be performed within 48 hours.
• If a transfusion is ordered, a transfusion request form must accompany the sample to the laboratory.

Findings
Classified as Rh-positive, Rh-negative, or Rh-positive Du, donor blood may be transfused only if compatible with the recipient's blood. (See *Implications of $RH_o(D)$ typing test results.*)

If an Rh-negative woman delivers an Rh-positive baby or aborts a fetus whose Rh-type is unknown, she should receive an RhIG injection within 72 hours to prevent hemolytic disease of the newborn in future births.

IMPLICATIONS OF $Rh_o(D)$ TYPING TEST RESULTS

Classified as $Rh_o(D)$-positive, $Rh_o(D)$-negative, or $Rh(D^u)$-positive, donor blood may be transfused only if it's compatible with the recipient's blood.

$Rh_o(D)$ RECIPIENT TYPES	COMPATIBLE $Rh_o(D)$ DONOR TYPES	INCOMPATIBLE $Rh_o(D)$ DONOR TYPES
$Rh_o(D)$-positive	$Rh_o(D)$-positive or $Rh_o(D)$-negative	None
$Rh_o(D)$-negative	$Rh_o(D)$-negative	$Rh_o(D)$-positive
$Rh(D^u)$-positive	$Rh(D^u)$-positive, $Rh_o(D)$-negative, or $Rh_o(D)$-positive (the least desirable choice because it may cause a mild hemolytic reaction)	None

FETAL-MATERNAL ERYTHROCYTE DISTRIBUTION

Some transfer of red blood cells from fetal to maternal circulation occurs during most spontaneous or elective abortions and most normal deliveries. Usually, the amount of blood transferred is minimal and has no clinical significance. But transfer of significant amounts of blood from an Rh-positive fetus to an Rh-negative mother can result in maternal immunization to the $Rh_o(D)$ antigen and the development of anti-Rh-positive antibodies in maternal circulation.

During a subsequent pregnancy, the maternal immunization subjects an Rh-positive fetus to potentially fatal hemolysis and erythroblastosis. This test measures the number of fetal red blood cells in maternal circulation.

Purpose

• To detect and measure fetal-maternal blood transfer

• To determine the amount of Rh immune globulin (RhIG) needed to prevent maternal immunization to the $Rh_o(D)$ antigen

Patient preparation

• Explain to the patient that the test determines or verifies blood group — an important step in ensuring safe transfusion.

• Inform the patient that she needn't fast before the test.

• Tell her that the test requires a blood sample and who will perform the venipuncture and when.

• Reassure her that although she may feel transient discomfort from the needle and the tourniquet, collecting the sample takes only a few minutes.

• Check the patient's history for recent administration of dextran, I.V. contrast media, or drugs that may alter results.

Procedure and posttest care
• Perform a venipuncture, and collect the sample in a 10- to 15-ml *lavender-top* tube or *red-top* tube (one tube per three units of blood).
• If a hematoma develops at the venipuncture site, apply warm soaks.

Precautions
• Label the sample with the patient's name, hospital or blood bank number, date, and initials of the phlebotomist.
• Send the sample to the laboratory immediately with a properly completed laboratory slip.

Normal findings
Normal maternal whole blood contains no fetal red blood cells.

Abnormal findings
An elevated fetal red blood cell volume in maternal circulation necessitates administration of more than one dose of RhIG. The number of vials needed is determined by dividing the calculated fetomaternal hemorrhage by 30 (a single vial of RhIG will provide protection against a 30-ml fetomaternal hemorrhage).

Administration of RhIG to an unsensitized Rh-negative mother as soon as possible (no later than 72 hours) after the birth of an Rh-positive infant or after a spontaneous or elective abortion prevents complications in subsequent pregnancies. Most clinicians are now administering RhIG prophylactically at 28 weeks' gestation to women who are Rh-negative but have no detectable Rh antibodies.

The following patients should be screened for Rh isoimmunization or irregular antibodies: all Rh-negative mothers during their first prenatal visit and at 28 weeks' gestation and all Rh-positive mothers with histories of transfusion, a jaundiced infant, stillbirth, cesarean delivery, or induced or spontaneous abortion.

CROSSMATCHING

Crossmatching establishes compatibility or incompatibility of the donor's and the recipient's blood. It's the best antibody detection test available for avoiding lethal transfusion reactions. After the donor's and the recipient's ABO blood type and Rh factor type are determined, major crossmatching tests for compatibility between the donor's red blood cells (RBCs) and the recipient's serum. Minor crossmatching tests for compatibility between the donor's serum and the recipient's RBCs. Because the antibody-screening test is routinely performed on all blood donors, minor crossmatching is often omitted.

Because a complete crossmatch may take from 45 minutes to 2 hours, an incomplete (10-minute) crossmatch may be performed in an emergency, such as severe blood loss due to trauma. In an emergency, transfusion can begin with limited amounts of group O packed RBCs while crossmatching is completed. Incomplete typing and crossmatching increases the risk of complications. After crossmatching, compatible units of blood are labeled, and a compatibility record is completed.

Purpose
• To serve as the final check for compatibility between the donor's blood and the recipient's blood

Patient preparation
• Explain to the patient that this test ensures that the blood he receives correctly matches his own to prevent a transfusion reaction.

• Inform him that he needn't fast before the test.
• Tell him the test requires a blood sample and who will perform the venipuncture and when.
• Reassure him that although he may experience some transient discomfort from the needle puncture and the pressure of the tourniquet, collecting the sample takes only a few minutes.
• Check the patient's history for recent administration of blood, dextran, or I.V. contrast media.

Procedure and posttest care
• Perform a venipuncture, and collect the sample in a 10-ml *red-top* tube (one tube per three units of blood). ABO typing, Rh typing, and crossmatching are all done together.
• If a hematoma develops at the venipuncture site, apply warm soaks.
• Encourage the patient to carry an ABO group identification card. Such identification is helpful but doesn't replace crossmatching before a transfusion.

Precautions
• Handle the sample gently to prevent hemolysis, which can mask hemolysis of the donor RBCs.
• Label the sample with the patient's name, the hospital or blood bank number, date, and the initials of the phlebotomist.
• Indicate on the laboratory slip the amount and type of blood component needed.
• Send the sample to the laboratory immediately. Crossmatching must be performed on the sample within 72 hours.
• If more than 72 hours have elapsed since the previous transfusion, previously crossmatched donor blood must be recrossmatched with a new recipient serum sample to detect newly acquired incompatibilities before transfusion.

• If the patient is scheduled for surgery and has received blood during the previous three months, his blood will need to be crossmatched again if his surgery is rescheduled to detect recently acquired incompatibilities.

Normal findings
Absence of agglutination indicates compatibility between the donor's and the recipient's blood, which means that the transfusion of donor blood can proceed. Note, however, that this does not guarantee a safe transfusion.

Abnormal findings
A positive crossmatch indicates incompatibility between the donor's blood and the recipient's blood, which means the donor's blood can't be transfused to the recipient. The sign of a positive crossmatch is agglutination, or clumping, when the donor's red cells and the recipient's serum are correctly mixed and incubated. Agglutination indicates an undesirable antigen-antibody reaction. The donor's blood must be withheld and the crossmatch continued, to determine the cause of the incompatibility and to identify the antibody.

DIRECT ANTIGLOBULIN TEST

The direct antiglobulin test (or direct Coombs' test) detects immunoglobulins (antibodies) on the surfaces of red blood cells (RBCs). These immunoglobulins coat RBCs when they become sensitized to an antigen, such as the Rh factor.

In this test, antiglobulin (Coombs') serum added to saline-washed RBCs results in agglutination if immunoglobulins or complement is present. This test is "direct" because it requires only one step — the addition of Coombs' serum to washed cells.

Purpose
• To diagnose hemolytic disease of the newborn (HDN)
• To investigate hemolytic transfusion reactions
• To aid differential diagnosis of hemolytic anemias, which may result from an autoimmune reaction or drugs or may be congenital

Patient preparation
• If the patient is a newborn, explain to the parents that the test helps diagnose HDN.
• If the patient is suspected of having hemolytic anemia, explain that the test determines whether the condition results from an abnormality in the body's immune system, from the use of certain drugs, or from some unknown cause.
• Inform the adult patient he needn't fast.
• Tell the patient (or a neonate's parents) that the test requires a blood sample and who will collect the blood or perform the venipuncture and when.
• Provide assurance that although the procedure may cause transient discomfort, collecting the sample takes only a few minutes.
• Withhold medications that may interfere with test results, including quinidine, methyldopa, cephalosporins, sulfonamides, chlorpromazine, diphenylhydantoin, dipyrone, ethosuximide, hydralazine, levodopa, mefenamic acid, melphalan, penicillin, procainamide, rifampin, streptomycin, tetracyclines, and isoniazid.

Procedure and posttest care
• For an adult, perform a venipuncture and collect the sample in two 5-ml *red-top* tubes.

• For a neonate, draw 5 ml of cord blood into a *red-top* or *lavender-top* tube after the cord is clamped and cut.
• If a hematoma develops at the venipuncture site, apply warm soaks.
• Resume administration of medications withheld before the test.
• Tell the patient or the parents of an infant with HDN that further testing will be necessary to monitor anemia.

Precautions
• Handle the sample gently to prevent hemolysis.
• Send it to the laboratory immediately. The test must be performed within 24 hours.
• Label the sample with the patient's full name, hospital or blood bank number, date, and initials of phlebotomist.

Normal findings
A negative test, in which neither antibodies nor complement appears on the RBCs, is normal.

Abnormal findings
A positive test on umbilical cord blood indicates that maternal antibodies have crossed the placenta and have coated fetal RBCs, causing HDN. Transfusion of compatible blood lacking the antigens to these maternal antibodies may be necessary to prevent anemia.

In other patients, a positive test result may indicate hemolytic anemia and help differentiate between autoimmune and secondary hemolytic anemia, which can be drug-induced or associated with an underlying disease, such as lymphoma. A positive test can also indicate sepsis.

A weakly positive test may suggest a transfusion reaction in which the patient's antibodies react with transfused RBCs containing the corresponding antigen.

ANTIBODY SCREENING TEST

Also called the indirect Coombs' test, this test detects unexpected circulating antibodies in the patient's serum. After incubating the serum with group O red cells, which are unaffected by anti-A or anti-B antibodies, an antiglobulin (Coombs') serum is added. Agglutination occurs if the patient's serum contains an antibody to one or more antigens on the red cells.

The antibody screening test detects 95% to 99% of the circulating antibodies. After this screening procedure detects them, the antibody identification test can determine the specific identity of the antibodies present.

Purpose
• To detect unexpected circulating antibodies to red cell antigens in the recipient's or donor's serum before transfusion
• To determine the presence of anti-Rh_o(D) (Rh-positive) antibody in maternal blood
• To evaluate the need for Rh Immune Globulin administration
• To aid diagnosis of acquired hemolytic anemia

Patient preparation
• Explain to the prospective blood recipient that the antibody screening test helps evaluate the possibility of a transfusion reaction.
• If the test is being performed because the patient is anemic, explain to him that it helps identify the specific type of anemia.
• Inform the patient that he needn't fast before the test.

• Tell him that the test requires a blood sample and who will perform the venipuncture and when.
• Reassure him that although he may experience transient discomfort from the needle puncture and the pressure of the tourniquet, collecting the sample takes only a few minutes.
• Check patient history for recent administration of blood, dextran, or I.V. contrast media. Be sure to note any such administration on the laboratory slip to prevent spurious interpretation of test results.

Procedure and posttest care
• Perform a venipuncture, and collect the sample in two 10-ml *red-top* tubes. Some laboratories require 20 ml of clotted blood to perform this test.
• If a hematoma develops at the venipuncture site, apply warm soaks.

Precautions
• Handle the sample gently to prevent hemolysis.
• Label the sample with the patient's name, the hospital or blood bank number, date, and the initials of the phlebotomist. Be sure to include the patient's diagnosis, and any history of transfusions, pregnancy, and drug therapy on the laboratory slip.
• Send the sample to the laboratory immediately: The antibody screening must be done within 72 hours after the sample is drawn.

Normal findings
Normally, agglutination does not occur, indicating that the patient's serum contains no circulating antibodies other than anti-A and anti-B.

Abnormal findings
A positive result indicates the presence of unexpected circulating antibodies to red cell antigens. Such a reaction

demonstrates donor and recipient incompatibility.

A positive result in a pregnant patient with Rh-negative blood may indicate the presence of antibodies to the Rh factor from previous transfusion with incompatible blood or from a previous pregnancy with an Rh-positive fetus.

A positive result above a titer of 1:8 indicates that the fetus may develop hemolytic disease of the newborn. As a result, repeated testing throughout the patient's pregnancy is necessary for evaluating progressive development of circulating antibody levels.

LEUKOAGGLUTININ TEST

This test detects leukoagglutinins — antibodies that react with white blood cells (white cell antibodies) and may cause a transfusion reaction. These antibodies usually develop after exposure to foreign white cells through transfusions, pregnancies, or allografts.

If a blood recipient has these antibodies, a febrile nonhemolytic reaction may occur 1 to 4 hours after the start of whole blood, red blood cell, platelet, or granulocyte transfusion. This nonhemolytic reaction (marked by fever and severe chills, sometimes with nausea, headache, and transient hypertension) must be distinguished from a true hemolytic reaction before further transfusion can proceed.

Two methods can detect leukoagglutinins. The older method detects white cell agglutination by microscopic examination of the patient's serum. The newer, more sensitive method uses a special fluorescence microscope to detect antibodies attached to normal granulocytes that have been incubated with recipient or donor serum.

Purpose
• To detect leukoagglutinins in blood recipients who develop transfusion reactions, thus differentiating between hemolytic and febrile nonhemolytic transfusion reactions
• To detect leukoagglutinins in blood donors after transfusion of donor blood causes a reaction

Patient preparation
• Explain to the patient that this test helps determine the cause of his transfusion reaction.
• Tell him that the test requires a blood sample and who will perform the venipuncture and when.
• Reassure him that although he may feel some transient discomfort from the needle puncture and the pressure of the tourniquet, collecting the sample takes only a few minutes.
• Note recent administration of blood or dextran or testing with I.V. contrast media on the laboratory slip.

Procedure and posttest care
• Perform a venipuncture and collect a blood sample in a 10-ml *red-top* tube. The laboratory will require 3 to 4 ml of serum for testing.
• If a hematoma develops at the venipuncture site, apply warm soaks.
• If a transfusion recipient has a positive leukoagglutinin test, continued transfusions require premedication with acetaminophen 1 to 2 hours before the transfusion, specially prepared leukocyte-poor blood, or use of leukocyte removal blood filters to prevent further reactions.

Precautions
• Label the sample with the patient's name, hospital or blood bank number, date, and initials of phlebotomist.

• Be sure to include on the laboratory slip the patient's suspected diagnosis and any history of blood transfusions, pregnancies, and drug therapy.

• Note that tests for these antibodies are not useful in deciding which patients should receive leukocyte-poor blood components; the decision must be based on clinical experience.

Normal findings

Normally, test results are negative: Agglutination doesn't occur because serum contains no antibodies.

Abnormal findings

In a recipient's blood, a positive result indicates the presence of leukoagglutinins, identifying his transfusion reaction as a febrile nonhemolytic reaction to these antibodies.

In a donor's blood, a positive result indicates the presence of leukoagglutinins, identifying the cause of a recipient's reaction as an acute, noncardiogenic pulmonary edema.

GENERAL CELLULAR FUNCTION

T- AND B-LYMPHOCYTE ASSAYS

Lymphocytes — key cells in the immune system — have the capacity to recognize antigens through special receptors found on their surfaces.

Cell separation is used to isolate lymphocytes from other cellular blood elements. This procedure recovers approximately 80% of the lymphocytes but

doesn't differentiate between T cells and B cells. The percent of T cells and B cells is determined by attaching a label or marker and by using different identification techniques.

Null cells possess Fc receptors but no other detectable surface markers and currently have no diagnostic significance. Null cells are usually determined by subtracting the sum of T cells and B cells from total lymphocytes.

Purpose

• To aid diagnosis of primary and secondary immunodeficiency diseases

• To distinguish benign from malignant lymphocytic proliferative diseases

• To monitor response to therapy

Patient preparation

• Explain to the patient that this test measures certain white blood cells.

• Tell him the test requires a blood sample, and who will perform the venipuncture and when.

• Reassure him that although he may experience transient discomfort from the needle puncture and the pressure of the tourniquet, collecting the sample takes less than 3 minutes.

Procedure and posttest care

• Perform a venipuncture, and collect the sample in a 7-ml *green-top* tube.

• Because many patients with T-cell and B-cell changes have a compromised immune system, keep the venipuncture site clean and dry.

• If a hematoma develops at the venipuncture site, apply warm soaks.

Precautions

• Completely fill the collection tube, and invert it gently several times to mix the sample and anticoagulant adequately.

• Send the sample to the laboratory immediately to ensure viable lymphocytes.

- If antilymphocyte antibodies are suspected, as in autoimmune disease, notify the laboratory.

Reference values
Currently, T-cell and B-cell assays are being standardized, and values may differ from one laboratory to another, depending on test technique.
    Percent of total lymphocytes:
- T cells: 68% to 75%
- B cells: 10% to 20%
- Null cells: 5% to 20%
- Total lymphocyte count ranges from 1,500 to 3,000/mm³.
- T-cell count varies from 1,400 to 2,700/mm³.
- B-cell count ranges from 270 to 640/mm³.
These counts are higher in children.

    Normal T-cell and B-cell counts don't necessarily ensure a competent immune system. In autoimmune diseases, such as systemic lupus erythematosus and rheumatoid arthritis, T cells and B cells, though present in normal numbers, may not be functionally competent.

Abnormal findings
An abnormal T-cell or B-cell count suggests but doesn't confirm specific diseases. The B-cell count is elevated in chronic lymphocytic leukemia, multiple myeloma, Waldenström's macroglobulinemia, and DiGeorge's syndrome.

    B cells decrease in acute lymphocytic leukemia and in certain congenital or acquired immunoglobulin deficiency diseases. In other immunoglobulin deficiency diseases, especially if only one immunoglobulin class is deficient, the B-cell count remains normal.

    The T-cell count rises occasionally in infectious mononucleosis; it rises more often in multiple myeloma and acute lymphocytic leukemia.

    T-cell count decreases in congenital T-cell deficiency diseases, such as DiGeorge's, Nezelof's, and Wiskott-Aldrich syndromes, and in certain B-cell proliferative disorders, such as chronic lymphocytic leukemia, Waldenström's macroglobulinemia, and acquired immunodeficiency syndrome.

LYMPHOCYTE TRANSFORMATION TESTS

Transformation tests evaluate lymphocyte competency without injection of antigens into the patient's skin. These in vitro tests eliminate the risk of adverse effects but can still accurately assess the ability of lymphocytes to proliferate and to recognize and respond to antigens.

    The mitogen assay evaluates the mitotic response of T lymphocytes and B lymphocytes to a foreign antigen. The antigen assay uses specific antigens, such as purified protein derivative, *Candida*, mumps, tetanus toxoid, and streptokinase, to stimulate lymphocyte transformation. The mixed lymphocyte culture (MLC) assay is useful in matching transplant recipients and donors and in testing immunocompetence. (See *Lymphocyte marker assays*.)

Purpose
- To assess and monitor genetic and acquired immunodeficiency states
- To provide histocompatibility typing of both tissue transplant recipients and donors
- To detect if a patient has been exposed to various pathogens, such as those that cause malaria, hepatitis, and mycoplasmal pneumonia

LYMPHOCYTE MARKER ASSAYS

A normal immune response requires a balance between the regulatory activities of several interacting cell types — most notably, T-helper and T-suppressor cells. By using highly specific monoclonal antibodies, levels of lymphocyte differentiation can be defined, and both normal and malignant cell populations can be analyzed. Direct and indirect immunofluorescence, microcytotoxicity, and immunoperoxidase immunoassay techniques are used most frequently: These employ an anticoagulated blood sample combined with monoclonal antibodies that react with specific T- and B-cell markers. The chart below lists some commonly ordered lymphocyte marker assays and their indications.

LYMPHOCYTE MARKER ASSAY	PURPOSE
Pan T-cell marker	• To measure mature T cells in immune dysfunction
T-helper/inducer subset marker	• To identify and characterize the proportion of T-helper cells in autoimmune or immunoregulatory disorders • To detect immunodeficiency disorders, such as acquired immunodeficiency syndrome • To differentiate T-cell acute lymphoblastic leukemia from T-cell lymphomas and other lymphoproliferative disorders
T-suppressor/cytotoxic subset marker	• To identify and characterize the proportion of T-suppressor cells in autoimmune and immuno-regulatory disorders • To characterize lymphoproliferative disorders
T-cell/E-Rosette receptor	• To differentiate lymphoproliferative disorders of T-cell origin, such as T-cell lymphocytic leukemia and lymphoblastic lymphoma, from those of non-T-cell origin
Pan-B (B-1) marker	• To differentiate lymphoproliferative disorders of B-cell origin, such as B-cell chronic lymphocytic leukemia, from those of T-cell origin
Pan-B (BA-1) marker	• To identify B-cell lymphoproliferative disorders, such as B-cell chronic lymphocytic leukemia
CALLA (common acute lymphocytic leukemia antigen) marker	• To identify bone marrow regeneration • To identify non-T-cell acute lymphocytic leukemia
Lymphocyte subset panel (B, pan-T, T-helper/inducer, T-suppressor/cytotoxic, and T-helper/T-suppressor ratio)	• To evaluate immunodeficiencies • To identify immunoregulation associated with autoimmune disorders • To characterize lymphoid malignancies
Lymphocytic leukemia marker panel (T-cell markers [E-Rosette receptor and Leu-9], B-cell markers [B-1 and BA-1], and CALLA)	• To characterize lymphocytic leukemias as T, B, non-T, or non-B, regardless of the stage of differentiation of the malignant cells

Patient preparation

• Explain to the patient that this test evaluates lymphocyte function, which is crucial to the immune system.

• If appropriate, inform him that the test monitors his response to therapy.

• For histocompatibility typing, explain that this test helps determine the best match for a transplant.

• Advise the patient that he needn't restrict food or fluids.

• Tell the patient that the test requires a blood sample and who will perform the venipuncture and when.

• Reassure the patient that although he may feel transient discomfort from the needle puncture and the pressure of the tourniquet, collecting the sample takes less than 3 minutes.

• If a radioisotope scan is scheduled, be sure the serum sample for this test is drawn first.

Procedure and posttest care

• Perform a venipuncture. If the patient is an adult, collect the sample in a 7-ml *green-top* (heparinized) tube; for a child, use a 5-ml *green-top* tube.

• Because many of these patients may have a compromised immune system, take special care to keep the venipuncture site clean and dry.

• If a hematoma develops at the venipuncture site, apply warm soaks.

Precautions

• Completely fill the collection tube, and invert it gently several times to mix the sample and anticoagulant.

• Send the sample to the laboratory immediately.

Reference values

Results are dependent on the mitogens used. Reference ranges accompany test results.

Abnormal findings

In the mitogen and antigen assays, a low stimulation index or unresponsiveness indicates a depressed or defective immune system. Serial testing can be performed to monitor the effectiveness of therapy in a patient with an immunodeficiency disease.

In the MLC test, the stimulation index is a measure of compatibility. A high index indicates poor compatibility. Conversely, a low stimulation index indicates good compatibility.

A high stimulation index, in response to the relevant pathogen, can also demonstrate exposure to malaria, hepatitis, mycoplasmal pneumonia, periodontal disease, and certain viral infections in patients who no longer have detectable serum antibodies.

TERMINAL DEOXYNUCLEOTIDYL TRANSFERASE TEST

Using indirect immunofluorescence, this test measures levels of terminal deoxynucleotidyl transferase (TdT). The TdT test is useful in differentiating certain types of leukemias and lymphomas marked by primitive cells that can't be identified by histology alone.

Purpose

• To help differentiate acute lymphocytic leukemia (ALL) from acute non-lymphocytic leukemia

• To help differentiate lymphoblastic lymphomas from non-Hodgkin's lymphomas

• To monitor response to therapy, help determine the patient's prognosis, or obtain early diagnosis of a relapse

Patient preparation

Explain to the patient that this test detects an enzyme that can help classify tissue origin.

If the patient is scheduled for a blood test, prepare him in the following manner:
• Tell him to fast for 12 to 14 hours before the test.
• Tell him the test requires a blood sample and who will perform the venipuncture and when.
• Reassure the patient that although he may experience transient discomfort from the needle puncture and the pressure of the tourniquet, collecting the sample takes less than 3 minutes.

If the patient is scheduled for a bone marrow aspiration, prepare him in the following manner:
• Describe the procedure to him and answer any questions.
• Inform the patient that he needn't restrict food or fluids before the test.
• Tell him who will perform the biopsy and where and that it usually takes only 5 to 10 minutes to perform.
• Make sure the patient or a responsible family member has signed a consent form.
• Check the patient's history for hypersensitivity to the local anesthetic.
• After checking with the doctor, tell the patient which bone will be the biopsy site.
• Inform him that he will receive a local anesthetic but will feel pressure on insertion of the biopsy needle and a brief, pulling pain when the marrow is withdrawn.
• Administer a mild sedative 1 hour before the test.

Procedure and posttest care
• If a blood test is scheduled, perform a venipuncture and collect the sample in one 10-ml heparinized blood tube and one *lavender-top* EDTA tube; send the sample to the laboratory immediately.

• If assisting with a bone marrow aspiration, inject 1 ml of bone marrow into a 7-ml *green-top* tube and dilute it with 5 ml of sterile saline or submit four air-dried marrow smears; send the sample to the laboratory immediately.
• Because patients with leukemia may bleed excessively, apply pressure to the venipuncture site until bleeding stops completely.
• If a hematoma develops at the venipuncture site, apply warm soaks.
• Check the bone marrow aspiration site for bleeding and inflammation, and observe the patient for signs of hemorrhage and infection.

Precautions
• Contact the laboratory before performing the venipuncture to ensure that it is able to process the sample and to find out how much blood to draw.
• Because patients with leukemia are more susceptible to infection, clean the skin thoroughly before performing the venipuncture.
• Send the sample to the laboratory immediately.

Reference values
TdT is present in less than 2% of marrow cells and is undetectable in normal peripheral blood.

Abnormal findings
Positive cells are present in more than 90% of the cases of ALL, in 33% of patients with chronic myelogenous leukemia in blast crisis, and in 5% of patients with nonlymphocytic leukemias. TdT-positive cells are absent in patients with ALL who are in remission.

GENERAL HUMORAL FUNCTION

IMMUNOGLOBULINS G, A, AND M

Immunoglobulins, proteins that can function as specific antibodies in response to antigen stimulation, are responsible for the humoral aspects of immunity. Deviations from normal immunoglobulin percentages are characteristic in many immune disorders, including cancer, hepatic disorders, rheumatoid arthritis, and systemic lupus erythematosus.

Immunoelectrophoresis identifies immunoglobulin G (IgG), immunoglobulin A (IgA), and immunoglobulin M (IgM) in a serum sample; the level of each is measured by radial immunodiffusion or nephelometry. Some laboratories detect immunoglobulin by indirect immunofluorescence and radioimmunoassay.

Purpose

• To diagnose paraproteinemias, such as multiple myeloma and Waldenström's macroglobulinemia
• To detect hypogammaglobulinemia and hypergammaglobulinemia, as well as nonimmunologic diseases, such as cirrhosis and hepatitis, that are associated with abnormally high immunoglobulin levels
• To assess the effectiveness of chemotherapy or radiation therapy

Patient preparation

• Explain to the patient that this test measures antibody levels.

• If appropriate, tell the patient that the test evaluates the effectiveness of treatment.
• Instruct him to restrict food and fluids, except for water, for 12 to 14 hours before the test.
• Tell him the test requires a blood sample and who will perform the venipuncture and when.
• Reassure him that although he may experience transient discomfort from the needle puncture and the pressure of the tourniquet, collecting the sample takes less than 3 minutes.
• Check the patient's medication history for drugs that may affect test results. These include phenytoin and other anticonvulsants, asparaginase, hydralazine, hydantoin derivatives, oral contraceptives, phenylbutazone, dextran, methotrexate, methylprednisolone, prednisolone, and methadone. If medications must be continued, note this on the laboratory slip. Be aware that alcohol or narcotic abuse may affect results. Also note that patients with severe hypersensitivity to BCG (bacille Calmette-Guérin) vaccine may have altered test results.

Procedure and posttest care

• Perform a venipuncture, and collect the sample in a 7-ml *red-top* tube.
• Advise the patient with abnormally low immunoglobulin levels (especially of IgG or IgM) to protect himself against bacterial infection. When caring for such a patient, watch for signs of infection, such as fever, chills, rash, or skin ulcers.
• Instruct the patient with abnormally high immunoglobulin levels and symptoms of monoclonal gammopathies to report bone pain and tenderness. Such a patient has numerous antibody-producing malignant plasma cells in bone marrow, which hamper production of other blood components. Watch for signs of

SERUM IMMUNOGLOBULIN LEVELS IN VARIOUS DISORDERS

DISORDER	IgG	IgA	IgM
Immunoglobulin disorders			
Lymphoid aplasia	D	D	D
Agammaglobulinemia	D	D	D
Type I dysgammaglobulinemia (selective IgG and IgA deficiency)	D	D	N or I
Type II dysgammaglobulinemia (absent IgA and IgM)	N	D	D
IgA globulinemia	N	D	N
Ataxia-telangiectasia	N	D	N
Multiple myeloma, macroglobulinemia, lymphomas			
Heavy chain disease (Franklin's disease)	D	D	D
IgG myeloma	I	D	D
IgA myeloma	D	I	D
Macroglobulinemia	D	D	I
Acute lymphocytic leukemia	N	D	N
Chronic lymphocytic leukemia	D	D	D
Acute myelocytic leukemia	N	N	N
Chronic myelocytic leukemia	N	D	N
Hodgkin's disease	N	N	N
Hepatic disorders			
Hepatitis	I	I	I
Laënnec's cirrhosis	I	I	N
Biliary cirrhosis	N	N	I
Hepatoma	N	N	D
Other disorders			
Rheumatoid arthritis	I	I	I
Systemic lupus erythematosus	I	I	I
Nephrotic syndrome	D	D	N
Trypanosomiasis	N	N	I
Pulmonary tuberculosis	I	N	N

KEY: N = normal; I = increased; D = decreased.

hypercalcemia, renal failure, and spontaneous pathologic fractures.
• If a hematoma develops at the venipuncture site, apply warm soaks.
• Inform the patient that he may resume his normal diet.
• Resume administration of medications withheld before the test.

Precautions
• Send the sample to the laboratory immediately to prevent deterioration of immunoglobulins.

Reference values
When using nephelometry, serum immunoglobulin levels for adults range as follows:
• IgG: 700 to 1,800 mg/dl
• IgA: 70 to 440 mg/dl
• IgM: 60 to 290 mg/dl.

Abnormal findings
The accompanying chart (*Serum immunoglobulin levels in various disorders,* page 245) shows IgG, IgA, and IgM levels in various disorders. In congenital and acquired hypogammaglobulinemias, myelomas, and macroglobulinemia, the findings confirm diagnosis. In hepatic and autoimmune diseases, leukemias, and lymphomas, such findings are less important but can support diagnosis based on other tests, such as biopsies and white blood cell differential, and on physical examination.

IMMUNE COMPLEX ASSAYS

When immune complexes are produced faster than they can be cleared by the lymphoreticular system, immune complex disease may occur; for example, postinfectious syndromes, serum sickness, drug sensitivity, rheumatoid arthritis, and systemic lupus erythematosus (SLE).

Histologic examination of tissue obtained by biopsy and the use of fluorescence or peroxidase staining with antibodies specific for immunologic types generally detect immune complexes. However, since tissue biopsies cannot provide information about titers of complexes still in circulation, serum assays, which detect circulating immune complexes indirectly, may be required. Because of the inherent variability of these complexes, several serum test methods may be appropriate.

Because most immune complex assays haven't been standardized, more than one test may be required to achieve accurate results.

Purpose
• To demonstrate circulating immune complexes in serum
• To monitor response to therapy
• To estimate severity of disease

Patient preparation
• Explain to the patient that these tests help evaluate his immune system.
• If appropriate, inform him that the test will be repeated to monitor his response to therapy.
• Advise him he needn't restrict food or fluids before the test.
• Tell him the test requires a blood sample and who will perform the venipuncture and when.
• Reassure him that although he may experience transient discomfort from the needle puncture and the pressure of the tourniquet, collecting the sample takes less than 3 minutes.
• If the patient is scheduled for C1q assays, check his history for recent heparin therapy and report your findings to the laboratory.

Procedure and posttest care
• Perform a venipuncture, and collect the sample in a 7-ml *red-top* tube.
• Because many patients with immune complexes have compromised immune systems, take special care to keep the venipuncture site clean and dry.
• If a hematoma develops at the site, apply warm soaks.

Precautions
• Send the sample to the laboratory immediately to prevent deterioration of immune complexes.

Normal findings
Normally, immune complexes are not detectable in serum.

Abnormal findings
The presence of detectable immune complexes in serum has etiologic importance in many autoimmune diseases, such as SLE and rheumatoid arthritis. However, for definitive diagnosis, the presence of these complexes must be considered with the results of other studies. For example, in SLE, immune complexes are associated with high titers of antinuclear antibodies and circulating antinative deoxyribonucleic acid antibodies.

Because of their filtering function, renal glomeruli seem most vulnerable to immune complex deposition, although blood vessel walls and choroid plexuses (vascular folds in the ventricles of the brain) can be affected. Renal biopsy to detect immune complexes can provide conclusive evidence for immune complex (Type III) glomerulonephritis, differentiating it from other types of glomerulonephritis.

RAJI CELL ASSAY

This assay, which is performed to detect the presence of circulating immune complexes, studies the Raji lymphoblastoid cell line. Identifying these cells, which have receptors for immunoglobulin G complement, is helpful in evaluating autoimmune disease.

Purpose
• To detect circulating immune complexes
• To aid the study of autoimmune disease

Patient preparation
• As appropriate, explain to the patient the purpose of the test.
• Tell him that the test requires a blood sample and who will perform the venipuncture and when.
• Reassure him that although he may experience discomfort from the puncture and the tourniquet, collecting the sample takes less than 3 minutes.

Procedure and posttest care
• Perform a venipuncture. Collect a sample in a *red-top* or *red-marble-top* tube. Promptly send it to the laboratory for assay.
• If a hematoma develops at the venipuncture site, apply warm soaks.

Precautions
• Handle the specimen gently to avoid hemolysis.

Normal findings
Normally, no Raji cells are present.

Abnormal findings
A positive Raji cell assay can detect immune complexes including those found in viral, microbial, and parasitic infec-

tions, metastasis, autoimmune disorders, and drug reactions. This test may also detect immune complexes associated with celiac disease, cirrhosis, Crohn's disease, cryoglobulinemia, dermatitis herpetiformis, sickle cell anemia, and ulcerative colitis.

COMPLEMENT ASSAYS

Complement is a collective term for a system of at least 20 serum proteins designed to destroy foreign cells and to help remove foreign materials. Complement deficiency can increase susceptibility to infection and can predispose to other diseases. Complement assays are thus indicated in patients with known or suspected immunomediated disease or repeatedly abnormal response to infection. Various laboratory methods are used to evaluate and measure total complement and its components; hemolytic assay, laser nephelometry, and radial immunodiffusion are the most common.

Although complement assays provide valuable information about the patient's immune system, the results must be considered in light of serum immunoglobulin and autoantibody tests for definitive diagnosis of immunomediated disease or abnormal response to infection.

Purpose
• To help detect immunomediated disease and genetic complement deficiency
• To monitor effectiveness of therapy

Patient preparation
• Explain to the patient that this test measures a group of proteins that fight infection.
• Advise him he needn't restrict food or fluids.

• Tell him the test requires a blood sample and who will perform the venipuncture and when.
• Reassure him that although he may experience transient discomfort from the needle puncture and the pressure of the tourniquet, collecting the sample usually takes less than 3 minutes.
• If the patient is scheduled for C1q assay, check his history for recent heparin therapy. Report such therapy to the laboratory.

Procedure and posttest care
• Perform a venipuncture, and collect the sample in a 7-ml *red-top* tube.
• Because many patients with complement defects have a compromised immune system, keep the venipuncture site clean and dry.
• If a hematoma develops at the venipuncture site, apply warm soaks.

Precautions
• Handle the sample gently to prevent hemolysis.
• Send it to the laboratory immediately because complement is heat labile and deteriorates rapidly.

Reference values
Normal values for complement range as follows:
• Total complement: 330 to 730/CH$_{50}$ units
• C1 esterase inhibitor: 7.8 to 23.4 mg/dl
• C3: 57 to 125 mg/dl
• C4: 10 to 54 mg/dl.

Abnormal findings
Complement abnormalities may be genetic or acquired; acquired abnormalities are most common. Depressed total complement levels (which are clinically more significant than elevations) may result from excessive formation of antigen-antibody complexes, insufficient synthesis of complement, inhibitor formation, or increased complement

catabolism, and are characteristic in conditions such as systemic lupus erythematosus (SLE), acute poststreptococcal glomerulonephritis, and acute serum sickness. Low levels may also occur in some patients with advanced cirrhosis of the liver, multiple myeloma, hypogammaglobulinemia, and rapidly rejecting allografts.

Elevated total complement may occur in obstructive jaundice, thyroiditis, acute rheumatic fever, rheumatoid arthritis, acute myocardial infarction, ulcerative colitis, and diabetes.

C1 esterase inhibitor deficiency is characteristic in hereditary angioedema, the most common genetic abnormality associated with complement; C3 deficiency is characteristic in recurrent pyogenic infection; C4 deficiency is characteristic in SLE.

RADIOALLERGOSORBENT TEST

The radioallergosorbent test (RAST) measures immunoglobulin E (IgE) antibodies in serum by radioimmunoassay and identifies specific allergens that cause rashes, asthma, hay fever, drug reactions, or other atopic complaints. RAST is easier to perform and more specific than skin testing; it is also less painful for and less dangerous to the patient. However, careful selection of specific allergens, based on the patient's clinical history, is crucial for effective testing.

Although skin testing is still the preferred means of diagnosing IgE-mediated hypersensitivities, RAST may be more useful when a skin disorder makes accurate reading of skin tests difficult, when a patient requires continual antihistamine therapy, or when

skin tests are negative but the patient's clinical history supports IgE-mediated hypersensitivity.

Purpose
• To identify allergens to which the patient has an immediate (IgE-mediated) hypersensitivity
• To monitor response to therapy

Patient preparation
• Explain to the patient that this test may detect the cause of allergy or monitor the effectiveness of allergy treatment.
• Inform him he needn't restrict food or fluids.
• Tell him that the test requires a blood sample and who will perform the venipuncture and when.
• Reassure him that although he may experience transient discomfort from the needle puncture and the pressure of the tourniquet, collecting the sample takes less than 3 minutes.
• If the patient is scheduled for a radioactive scan, be sure the sample is collected before the scan.

Procedure and posttest care
• Perform a venipuncture, and collect the sample in a 7-ml *red-top* tube. Generally, 1 ml of serum is sufficient for five allergen assays.
• Be sure to note on the laboratory slip the specific allergens to be tested.
• If a hematoma develops at the venipuncture site, apply warm soaks.

Normal findings
RAST results are interpreted in relationship to a control or reference serum that differs among laboratories.

Abnormal findings
Elevated serum IgE levels suggest hypersensitivity to the specific allergen or allergens used.

HAM TEST

The Ham test or acidified serum lysis test is performed to determine the cause of undiagnosed hemolytic anemia, hemoglobinuria, and bone marrow aplasia. It helps establish a diagnosis of paroxysmal nocturnal hemoglobinuria (PNH), a rare hematologic disease.

Purpose
• To help establish a diagnosis of PNH

Patient preparation
• Explain to the patient that this test helps determine the cause of his anemia or other signs.
• Advise him he needn't restrict food or fluids.
• Tell him that the test requires a blood sample and who will perform the venipuncture and when.
• Reassure him that although he may experience transient discomfort from the needle puncture and the pressure of the tourniquet, collecting the sample takes less than 3 minutes.

Procedure and posttest care
• Because the blood sample must be defibrinated immediately, laboratory personnel will perform the venipuncture and collect the sample.
• If a hematoma develops at the venipuncture site, apply warm soaks.

Normal findings
Normally, red blood cells (RBCs) do not undergo hemolysis.

Abnormal findings
Hemolysis of RBCs indicates PNH.

HUMAN LEUKOCYTE ANTIGEN TEST

The human leukocyte antigen (HLA) test identifies a group of antigens present on the surfaces of all nucleated cells but most easily detected on lymphocytes. There are four types of HLA: HLA-A, HLA-B, HLA-C, and HLA-D. These antigens are essential to immunity and determine the degree of histocompatibility between transplant recipients and donors. Numerous antigenic determinants (over 60, for instance, at the HLA-B locus) are present for each site; one set of each antigen is inherited from each parent.

High incidence of specific HLA types has been linked to specific diseases, such as rheumatoid arthritis and multiple sclerosis, but these findings have little diagnostic significance.

Purpose
• To provide histocompatibility typing of tissue recipients and donors
• To aid genetic counseling
• To aid paternity testing

Patient preparation
• Explain to the patient that this test detects antigens on white blood cells.
• Advise him he needn't restrict food or fluids before the test.
• Tell the patient that this test requires a blood sample and who will perform the venipuncture and when.
• Reassure him that although he may experience transient discomfort from the needle puncture and the pressure of the tourniquet, collecting the blood sample usually takes less than 3 minutes.
• Check the patient's history for recent blood transfusions. HLA testing may

need to be postponed if he has recently undergone a transfusion.

Procedure and posttest care
• Perform a venipuncture, and collect the sample in a collection tube containing anticoagulant acid citrate dextrose solution.
• If a hematoma develops at the venipuncture site, apply warm soaks.

Precautions
• Handle the sample gently to avoid hemolysis.

Normal findings
In HLA-A, HLA-B, and HLA-C testing, lymphocytes that react with the test antiserum undergo lysis; they're detected by phase microscopy. In HLA-D testing, leukocyte incompatibility is marked by blast formation, deoxyribonucleic acid synthesis, and proliferation.

Abnormal findings
Incompatible HLA-A, HLA-B, HLA-C, or HLA-D groups may cause unsuccessful tissue transplantation.

Many diseases have a strong association with certain types of HLAs. For example, HLA-DR5 is associated with Hashimoto's thyroiditis. B8 and Dw3 are associated with Graves' disease, whereas B8 alone is associated with chronic autoimmune hepatitis, celiac disease, and myasthenia gravis. Dw3 alone is associated with Addison's disease, Sjögren's syndrome, dermatitis herpetiformis, and systemic lupus erythematosus.

In paternity testing, a putative father who presents a phenotype (two haplotypes: one from the father and one from the mother) with no haplotype or antigen pair identical to one of the child's is excluded as the father. A putative father with one haplotype identical to one of the child's may be the father; the prob-

ability varies with the incidence of the haplotype in the population.

AUTOANTIBODIES

ANTINUCLEAR ANTIBODIES

In conditions such as systemic lupus erythematosus (SLE), scleroderma, and certain infections, the body's immune system may perceive portions of its own cell nuclei as foreign and may produce antinuclear antibodies (ANA). Specific ANA include antibodies to deoxyribonucleic acid (DNA), nucleoprotein, histones, nuclear ribonucleoprotein, and other nuclear constituents. Because they don't penetrate living cells, ANA are harmless in themselves, but they sometimes form antigen-antibody complexes that cause tissue damage (as in SLE). Because of multiorgan involvement, test results are not diagnostic and can only partially confirm clinical evidence. (See *Comparative incidence of antinuclear antibodies,* page 252.)

Purpose
• To screen for SLE (failure to detect ANA essentially rules out active SLE)
• To monitor the effectiveness of immunosuppressive therapy for SLE

Patient preparation
• Explain to the patient that this test evaluates the immune system and that further testing is usually required for diagnosis.

COMPARATIVE INCIDENCE OF ANTINUCLEAR ANTIBODIES

CONDITION	INCIDENCE OF POSITIVE A.N.A.
Healthy patient	~ 5%
Patient age 65 or older	~ 40%
Systemic lupus erythematosus (SLE)	95% to 100%
Healthy family member of SLE patient	~ 25%
Lupoid hepatitis	95% to 100%
Felty's syndrome	95% to 100%
Progressive systemic sclerosis (scleroderma)	75% to 80%
Drug-associated SLE-like syndrome: use of hydralazine, procainamide, or isoniazid	~ 50%
Sjögren's syndrome	40% to 75%
Rheumatoid arthritis	25% to 60%
Chronic discoid lupus erythematosus	15% to 50%
Juvenile arthritis	15% to 30%
Polyarteritis nodosa	15% to 25%
Dermatomyositis, polymyositis	10% to 30%
Rheumatic fever	~ 5%
Miscellaneous diseases	10% to 50%

• If appropriate, inform the patient that the test will be repeated to monitor his response to therapy.
• Advise him he needn't restrict food or fluids.
• Tell him the test requires a blood sample and who will perform the venipuncture and when.
• Reassure him that although he may experience discomfort from the puncture and the tourniquet, collecting the sample takes less than 3 minutes.
• Check the patient's history for drugs that may affect test results, such as isoniazid, hydralazine, and procainamide. Note findings on the laboratory slip.

Procedure and posttest care
• Perform a venipuncture, and collect the sample in a 7-ml *red-top* tube.
• Because a patient with an autoimmune disease has a compromised immune system, observe the venipuncture site for signs of infection, and report any changes to the doctor immediately.
• Keep a clean, dry bandage over the site for at least 24 hours.
• If a hematoma develops at the venipuncture site, apply warm soaks.

Reference values
Using Hep-2 cells, the test for ANA is negative at a titer of 1:40 or below. If

mouse kidney substrate is used, the test is negative at a titer less than 1:20.

Abnormal findings

Although the test is a sensitive indicator of ANA, it is not specific for SLE. Low titers may occur in patients with viral diseases, chronic hepatic disease, collagen vascular disease, and autoimmune diseases, and in some healthy adults; incidence increases with age. The higher the titer, the more specific the test is for SLE (titer often exceeds 1:256).

The pattern of nuclear fluorescence helps identify the type of immune disease present. A peripheral pattern is almost exclusively associated with SLE because it indicates the presence of anti-DNA antibodies; anti-DNA antibodies are sometimes measured by radioimmunoassay if ANA titers are high or a peripheral pattern is observed. A homogeneous, or diffuse, pattern is also associated with SLE, as well as with related connective tissue disorders; a nucleolar pattern, with scleroderma; and a speckled, irregular pattern, with infectious mononucleosis and mixed connective tissue disorders (for example, SLE and scleroderma).

A single serum sample, especially one collected from a patient with collagen vascular disease, may contain antibodies to several parts of the cell's nucleus. In addition, as serum dilution increases, the fluorescent pattern may change because different antibodies are reactive at different titers.

EXTRACTABLE NUCLEAR ANTIGEN ANTIBODIES

Extractable nuclear antigen (ENA) is a complex of at least two and possibly three antigens. One of these — ribonucleoprotein (RNP) — is susceptible to degradation by ribonuclease. The second — Smith (Sm) antigen — is an acidic nuclear protein that resists ribonuclease degradation. The third antigen that's sometimes included in this group — Sjögren's (SS-B) antigen — forms a precipitate when antibody is present. Antibodies to these antigens are associated with certain autoimmune disorders. Tests to detect ENA antibodies help differentiate autoimmune disorders with similar signs and symptoms.

Purpose

• To aid differential diagnosis of autoimmune disease

• To distinguish between anti-RNP and anti-Sm antibodies

• To screen for anti-RNP antibodies (common in systemic lupus erythematosus [SLE], progressive systemic sclerosis, and other rheumatic disorders)

• To screen for anti-Sm antibodies (a specific marker for SLE)

• To detect the SS-B autoantibodies produced in Sjögren's syndrome

• To monitor response to therapy in patients with autoimmune disease

Patient preparation

• Explain to the patient that this test detects certain antibodies and that test results help determine diagnosis and treatment.

• When appropriate, explain that the test assesses the effectiveness of treatment.

• Advise the patient he needn't restrict food or fluids.

• Tell him the test requires a blood sample and who will perform the venipuncture and when.

• Reassure him that although he may experience transient discomfort from the needle puncture and the pressure of the tourniquet, collecting the sample takes less than 3 minutes.

Procedure and posttest care

• Perform a venipuncture, and collect the sample in a 7-ml *red-top* tube.

• Because a patient with an autoimmune disease has a compromised immune system, check the venipuncture site for infection, and report any change promptly.

• Keep a clean, dry bandage over the site for at least 24 hours.

• If a hematoma develops at the venipuncture site, apply warm soaks.

Precautions

• Send the sample to the laboratory immediately.

Normal findings

Normally, serum is negative for anti-RNP, anti-Sm, and SS-B antibodies.

Abnormal findings

The presence of anti-Sm antibodies is highly diagnostic of SLE. A high level of anti-RNP antibodies with a low titer of anti-Sm antibodies suggests mixed connective tissue disease. Although SS-B antibodies are associated with primary Sjögren's syndrome, their presence is not considered diagnostic of this disorder; however, a positive test for SS-B antibodies mandates further testing.

ANTIMITOCHONDRIAL ANTIBODIES

Usually performed with the test for anti–smooth-muscle antibodies, this test detects antimitochondrial antibodies in serum by indirect immunofluorescence. These autoantibodies are present in several hepatic diseases, although their etiologic role is unknown, and there's no evidence they cause hepatic damage. Most commonly, they are associated with primary biliary cirrhosis and, sometimes, chronic active hepatitis and drug-induced jaundice. Antimitochondrial antibodies are also associated with autoimmune diseases, such as systemic lupus erythematosus, rheumatoid arthritis, pernicious anemia, and idiopathic Addison's disease. (See *Incidence of serum antibodies in various conditions*.)

Purpose

• To aid diagnosis of primary biliary cirrhosis

• To distinguish between extrahepatic jaundice and biliary cirrhosis

Patient preparation

• Explain to the patient that this test evaluates liver function.

• Advise the patient not to restrict food or fluids.

• Tell him the test requires a blood sample and who will perform the venipuncture and when.

• Reassure him that although he may feel some discomfort from the needle puncture and the pressure of the tourniquet, collecting the sample takes less than 3 minutes.

• Check the patient's medication history for oxyphenisatin use, and report it to

INCIDENCE OF SERUM ANTIBODIES IN VARIOUS CONDITIONS

DISEASE OR CONDITION	PERCENTAGE OF PATIENTS SHOWING ANTIBODIES TO:	
	Mitochondria	Smooth muscle
Primary biliary cirrhosis	75% to 95%	0% to 50%
Chronic active hepatitis	0% to 30%	50% to 80%
Extrahepatic biliary obstruction	0% to 5%	0%
Cryptogenic cirrhosis	0% to 25%	0% to 1%
Viral (infectious) hepatitis	0%	1% to 2%
Drug-induced jaundice	50% to 80%	
Intrinsic asthma		20%
Rheumatoid arthritis and other collagen diseases	1% to 2%	
Systemic lupus erythematosus	3% to 5%	0%
Normal	0% to 1%	

the laboratory because it may produce antimitochondrial antibodies.

Procedure and posttest care
• Perform a venipuncture, and collect the sample in a 7-ml *red-top* tube.
• Because patients with hepatic disease may bleed excessively, apply pressure to the venipuncture site until bleeding stops.
• If a hematoma develops at the venipuncture site, apply warm soaks.

Normal findings
Serum is negative for antimitochondrial antibodies at a titer below 20.

Abnormal findings
Although antimitochondrial antibodies appear in 79% to 94% of patients with primary biliary cirrhosis, this test alone doesn't confirm diagnosis. Further tests, such as serum alkaline phosphatase; serum bilirubin; aspartate aminotransferase; alanine aminotransferase; or possibly, liver biopsy or cholangiography, may also be necessary. The autoantibodies also appear in some patients with chronic active hepatitis, drug-induced jaundice, and cryptogenic cirrhosis. However, antimitochondrial antibodies rarely appear in patients with extrahepatic biliary obstruction, and a positive test helps rule out this condition.

ANTI–SMOOTH-MUSCLE ANTIBODIES

Using indirect immunofluorescence, this test measures the relative concentration of anti–smooth-muscle antibodies in serum; it is usually performed with the test for antimitochondrial antibodies.

Anti–smooth-muscle antibodies appear in several hepatic diseases, especially chronic active hepatitis and, less often, primary biliary cirrhosis. Although anti–smooth-muscle antibodies are most commonly associated with hepatic diseases, their etiologic role is unknown, and there's no evidence that they cause hepatic damage.

Purpose
• To aid diagnosis of chronic active hepatitis and primary biliary cirrhosis

Patient preparation
• Explain to the patient that this test helps evaluate liver function.
• Inform him that he needn't restrict food or fluids.
• Tell him that this test requires a blood sample and who will perform the venipuncture and when.
• Reassure him that although he may experience transient discomfort from the needle puncture and the pressure of the tourniquet, collecting the blood sample usually takes less than 3 minutes.

Procedure and posttest care
• Perform a venipuncture, and collect the sample in a 7-ml *red-top* tube.
• Because patients with hepatic disease may bleed excessively, apply pressure to the venipuncture site until bleeding stops.

• If a hematoma develops at the venipuncture site, apply warm soaks.

Reference findings
Normal titer of anti–smooth-muscle antibodies is less than 1:20.

Abnormal values
The test for anti–smooth-muscle antibodies is not very specific; these antibodies appear in about 66% of patients with chronic active hepatitis and 30% to 40% of patients with primary biliary cirrhosis.

Anti–smooth-muscle antibodies may also be present in patients with infectious mononucleosis, acute viral hepatitis, malignant tumor of the liver, and intrinsic asthma.

ANTITHYROID ANTIBODIES

In autoimmune disorders such as Hashimoto's thyroiditis and Graves' disease (hyperthyroidism), thyroglobulin, the major colloidal storage compound, is released into the blood. Antithyroglobulin antibodies come into existence to attack this foreign substance; the ensuing autoimmune response damages the thyroid gland.

Purpose
• To detect circulating antithyroglobulin antibodies when clinical evidence indicates Hashimoto's thyroiditis, Graves' disease, or other thyroid diseases

Patient preparation
• Explain to the patient that this test evaluates thyroid function.
• Advise him that he needn't restrict food or fluids.

INCIDENCE OF THYROID AUTOANTIBODIES IN VARIOUS DISEASES

DISORDER	PRESENCE OF ANTITHYROGLOBULIN	PRESENCE OF ANTIMICROSOMAL ANTIBODIES
Hashimoto's disease	60% to 95%	70% to 90%
Idiopathic myxedema	75%	65%
Graves' disease	30% to 40%	50% to 85%
Adenomatous goiter	20% to 30%	20%
Thyroid carcinoma	40%	15%
Pernicious anemia	25%	10%

• Tell him that the test requires a blood sample and who will perform the venipuncture and when.

• Reassure him that although he may experience transient discomfort from the needle puncture and the pressure of the tourniquet, collecting the sample takes less than 3 minutes.

Procedure and posttest care

• Perform a venipuncture, and collect the sample in a 7-ml *red-top* tube.

• If a hematoma develops at the venipuncture site, apply warm soaks.

Reference values

The normal titer is less than 1:100 for both antithyroglobulin and antimicrosomal antibodies. Low levels of these antibodies are normal in 10% of the general population and in 20% or more of people age 70 or older.

Abnormal findings

The presence of antithyroglobulin or antimicrosomal antibodies in serum can indicate subclinical autoimmune thyroid disease, Graves' disease, or idiopathic myxedema. High titers, which may be in the millions, strongly suggest Hashimoto's thyroiditis. The accompanying chart (*Incidence of thyroid autoantibodies in various diseases*) shows the approximate incidence of antithyroglobulin antibodies in selected diseases. Such antibodies may also occur in some patients with other autoimmune disorders, such as systemic lupus erythematosus, rheumatoid arthritis, and autoimmune hemolytic anemia.

THYROID-STIMULATING IMMUNOGLOBULIN

Thyroid-stimulating immunoglobulin (TSI), formerly called long-acting thyroid stimulator, appears in the blood of most patients with Graves' disease. It stimulates the thyroid gland to produce and excrete excessive amounts of thyroid hormones.

Reportedly, 50% to 90% of people with thyrotoxicosis have elevated TSI levels. Positive results of this test strongly suggest Graves' disease but don't always correlate with overt signs of hyperthyroidism.

Purpose
• To aid evaluation of suspected thyroid disease
• To aid diagnosis of suspected thyrotoxicosis, especially in patients with exophthalmos
• To monitor treatment of thyrotoxicosis

Patient preparation
• As appropriate, explain to the patient that this test evaluates thyroid function.
• Tell him that the test requires a blood sample and who will perform the venipuncture and when.
• Reassure him that although he may experience transient discomfort from the needle puncture and the pressure of the tourniquet, collecting the sample takes less than 3 minutes.

Procedure and posttest care
• Perform a venipuncture, and collect a 5-ml sample in a *red-top* tube.
• If a hematoma develops at the venipuncture site, apply warm soaks.

Precautions
• Handle the sample gently to prevent hemolysis.
• Send it to the laboratory promptly.
• Note on the laboratory slip if the patient had a radioactive iodine scan within 48 hours of the test.

Reference values
TSI doesn't normally appear in serum. However, it may be present in 5% of people without hyperthyroidism or exophthalmos.

Abnormal findings
Increased TSI levels are associated with exophthalmos, Graves' disease (thyrotoxicosis), and recurrence of hyperthyroidism.

LUPUS ERYTHEMATOSUS CELL PREPARATION

Lupus erythematosus (LE) cell preparation is an in vitro procedure used in the diagnosis of systemic lupus erythematosus (SLE). Although this test is less sensitive and reliable than either the antinuclear antibody (ANA) or the anti–deoxyribonucleic acid (DNA) antibody test, it's often used because it requires minimal equipment and reagents.

In this test, a blood sample is mixed with laboratory-treated nucleoprotein (the antigen). If the sample contains ANA, the ANA reacts with the nucleoprotein, causing swelling and rupture. Phagocytes from the serum then engulf the extruded nuclei, forming LE cells, which are then detected by microscopic examination of the sample.

Purpose
• To aid diagnosis of SLE
• To monitor treatment of SLE: about 60% of successfully treated patients fail to show LE cells after 4 to 6 weeks of therapy

Patient preparation
• Explain to the patient that this test helps detect antibodies to his own tissue.
• If appropriate, inform him that the test will be repeated to monitor his response to therapy.
• Advise him that he needn't restrict food or fluids.
• Tell him the test requires a blood sample and who will perform the venipuncture and when.

• Reassure him that although he may experience transient discomfort from the needle puncture and the pressure of the tourniquet, collecting the sample takes less than 3 minutes.

• Check the patient's medication history for drugs, such as isoniazid, hydralazine, and procainamide, that may affect test results. If such drugs must be continued, be sure to note this on the laboratory slip.

Procedure and posttest care

• Perform a venipuncture, and collect the sample in a 7-ml *red-top* tube.

• Because many patients with SLE have compromised immune systems, keep a clean, dry bandage over the venipuncture site for at least 24 hours.

• Check for infection.

• If a hematoma develops at the venipuncture site, apply warm soaks.

• If test results indicate SLE, tell the patient further diagnostic tests may be required to monitor treatment.

Precautions

• Handle the sample gently to prevent hemolysis.

Normal findings

Normally, no LE cells are present.

Abnormal findings

The presence of at least two LE cells may indicate SLE. Although these cells occur primarily in SLE, they may also form in chronic active hepatitis, rheumatoid arthritis, scleroderma, and drug reactions. Also, up to 25% of patients with SLE demonstrate no LE cells. Apart from supportive clinical signs, definitive diagnosis of SLE may necessitate a confirming ANA or anti-DNA test. The ANA test detects autoantibodies in the sera of many SLE patients with negative LE cell tests. Anti-DNA antibodies appear in two-thirds of all SLE patients but are rare in other conditions; the presence of such antibodies is strong evidence of SLE.

CARDIOLIPIN ANTIBODIES

This test measures serum concentrations of immunoglobulin G or immunoglobulin M antibodies in relation to the phospholipid cardiolipin. These antibodies appear in some lupus erythematosus (LE) patients whose serum also contains a coagulation inhibitor (lupus anticoagulant). They also appear in some patients who do not fulfill all the diagnostic criteria for LE but who experience recurrent episodes of spontaneous thrombosis, fetal loss, or thrombocytopenia. Serum concentrations of cardiolipin antibodies are measured by enzyme-linked immunosorbent assay.

Purpose

• To aid diagnosis of cardiolipin antibody syndrome in patients with or without LE who experience recurrent episodes of spontaneous thrombosis, thrombocytopenia, or fetal loss

Patient preparation

• Explain to the patient the purpose of the test.

• Tell him that food or fluids needn't be restricted before the test.

• Tell him that the test requires a blood sample and who will perform the venipuncture and when.

• Reassure him that although he may experience transient discomfort from the needle puncture and the pressure of the tourniquet, collecting the sample takes less than 3 minutes.

Procedure and posttest care

• Perform a venipuncture, and collect the sample in a 5-ml *red-top* tube.
• If a hematoma develops, apply warm soaks.

Precautions

• Handle the sample gently to prevent hemolysis, and send it to the laboratory immediately.

Reference values

Cardiolipin antibody results are reported as dilution titers obtained by making 1:2 serial dilutions of serum. The highest dilution is reported. A 1:4 titer is a borderline result. A lower titer (1:2) is negative; a higher titer (1:8, 1:16), positive.

Abnormal findings

A positive result along with a history of recurrent spontaneous thrombosis, thrombocytopenia, or repeated fetal loss suggests cardiolipin antibody syndrome. Treatment may involve anticoagulant or platelet-inhibitor therapy.

RHEUMATOID FACTOR

The rheumatoid factor (RF) test is the most useful immunologic test for confirming rheumatoid arthritis (RA). In this disease, "renegade" immunoglobulin G (IgG) antibodies, produced by lymphocytes in the synovial joints, react with other IgG or immunoglobulin M (IgM) to produce immune complexes, complement activation, and tissue destruction. How IgG molecules become antigenic is still unknown, but they may be altered by aggregating with viruses or other antigens. Techniques for detecting RF include the sheep cell agglutination test and the latex fixation test.

Purpose

• To confirm RA, especially when clinical diagnosis is doubtful

Patient preparation

• Explain to the patient that this test helps confirm RA.
• Advise him he needn't restrict food or fluids before the test.
• Tell him that the test requires a blood sample and who will perform the venipuncture and when.
• Reassure him that although he may experience transient discomfort from the needle puncture and the pressure of the tourniquet, collecting the blood sample usually takes less than 3 minutes.

Procedure and posttest care

• Perform a venipuncture, and collect the sample in a 7-ml *red-top* tube.
• Because a patient with RA may be immunologically compromised from the disease or from corticosteroid therapy, keep the venipuncture site covered with a clean, dry bandage for 24 hours.
• Check regularly for signs of infection.
• If a hematoma develops at the venipuncture site, apply warm soaks.

Reference values

Normal RF titer is less than 1:20; normal rheumatoid screening test is nonreactive.

Abnormal findings

Positive RF titers are found in 80% of patients with RA. Titers above 1:80 are usually considered diagnostic for RA; titers between 1:20 and 1:80 are difficult to interpret since they occur in many other diseases, such as systemic lupus erythematosus, scleroderma, polymyositis, tuberculosis, infectious mononucleosis, leprosy, syphilis, sarcoidosis, chronic hepatic disease, subacute bacterial endocarditis, and chronic pulmonary interstitial fibrosis. In addition, 5% of the general population, including as many as 25% of elderly people, have positive RF titers.

Conversely, a negative RF titer doesn't rule out RA; 20% to 25% of patients with RA lack reactive RF titers, and RF itself isn't reactive until 6 months after onset of active disease. Repeating the test is sometimes useful. However, correlation between RF and RA is inconclusive, and positive diagnosis always requires correlation with clinical status.

COLD AGGLUTININS

Cold agglutinins are antibodies, usually of the immunoglobulin M (IgM) type, that cause red blood cells (RBCs) to aggregate at low temperatures and may occur in small amounts in healthy people. Transient elevations of these antibodies develop during certain infectious diseases, notably primary atypical pneumonia. This test reliably detects such pneumonia within 1 to 2 weeks after onset.

Patients with high cold agglutinin titers, such as those with primary atypical pneumonia, may develop acute transient hemolytic anemia after repeated exposure to cold; patients with persistently high titers may develop chronic hemolytic anemia.

Purpose
• To help confirm primary atypical pneumonia
• To provide additional diagnostic evidence for cold agglutinin disease associated with many viral infections or lymphoreticular malignancy

Patient preparation
• Explain to the patient that this test detects antibodies in the blood that attack RBCs after exposure to low temperatures.
• If appropriate, inform him that the test will be repeated to monitor his response to therapy.
• Advise him that it isn't necessary to restrict food or fluids.
• Tell him that the test requires a blood sample and who will perform the venipuncture and when.
• Reassure him that although he may experience transient discomfort from the needle puncture and the pressure of the tourniquet, collecting the sample takes less than 3 minutes.
• If the patient is receiving antimicrobial drugs, note this on the laboratory slip, because use of such drugs may interfere with the development of cold agglutinins.

Procedure and posttest care
• Perform a venipuncture, and collect the sample in a 7-ml *red-top* tube that has been prewarmed to 98.6° F (37° C).
• If cold agglutinin disease is suspected, keep the patient warm. If the patient is exposed to low temperatures, agglutination may occur within peripheral vessels, possibly leading to frostbite, anemia, Raynaud's phenomenon, or, rarely, focal gangrene.
• Watch for signs of vascular abnormalities, such as mottled skin, purpura, jaundice, or pallor; pain or swelling of extremities; and cramping of fingers and toes. Hemoglobinuria may result from severe intravascular hemolysis on exposure to severe cold.
• If a hematoma develops at the venipuncture site, apply warm soaks.

Precautions
• Handle the sample gently to prevent hemolysis, and send it to the laboratory immediately.

• Don't refrigerate the sample; cold agglutinins will coat the RBCs, leaving none in the serum for testing.

Reference values
Normal titers are less than 1:32 but may be higher in elderly people.

Abnormal findings
High titers may occur as primary phenomena, or secondary to infections or lymphoreticular malignancy. They may be present in infectious mononucleosis, cytomegalovirus infection, hemolytic anemia, multiple myeloma, scleroderma, malaria, cirrhosis, congenital syphilis, peripheral vascular disease, pulmonary embolism, trypanosomiasis, tonsillitis, staphylococcemia, scarlatina, influenza, and, occasionally, in pregnancy. Chronically elevated titers are most commonly associated with pneumonia and lymphoreticular malignancy; an acute transient elevation commonly accompanies many viral infections.

In primary atypical pneumonia, cold agglutinins appear in serum in one-half to two-thirds of all patients during the first week of acute infection, even before antimycoplasmal antibodies can be detected by complement fixation or metabolic inhibition tests. Thus, titers usually become positive at 7 days, peak above 1:32 in 4 weeks, and commonly disappear rapidly after 6 weeks. When sequential titers verify this pattern and clinical evidence of pneumonia exists, diagnosis is confirmed.

Extremely high titers (1:1,000 to 1:1,000,000) can occur with idiopathic cold agglutinin disease that precedes development of lymphoma. Patients with titers this high are susceptible to intravascular agglutination, which causes significant clinical problems.

CRYOGLOBULINS

Cryoglobulins are abnormal serum proteins that precipitate at low laboratory temperatures (39.2° F [4° C]) and redissolve after being warmed. Their presence in the blood (cryoglobulinemia) is usually associated with immunologic disease but can also occur without known immunopathology. If patients with cryoglobulinemia are subjected to cold, they may experience Raynaud-like symptoms (pain, cyanosis, and coldness of fingers and toes), which generally result from precipitation of cryoglobulins in cooler parts of the body. In some patients, for example, cryoglobulins may precipitate at temperatures as high as 86° F (30° C); such temperatures are possible in some peripheral blood vessels.

The cryoglobulin test involves refrigerating a serum sample at 39.2° F (4° C) for at least 72 hours and observing for formation of a heat-reversible precipitate. Such a precipitate requires further study by immunoelectrophoresis or double diffusion to identify cryoglobulin components.

Purpose
• To detect cryoglobulinemia in patients with Raynaud-like vascular symptoms

Patient preparation
• Explain to the patient that this test detects antibodies in blood that may cause sensitivity to low temperatures.
• Instruct him to fast for 4 to 6 hours before the test.
• Tell him that the test requires a blood sample and who will perform the venipuncture and when.
• Reassure him that although he may experience transient discomfort from

CRYOGLOBULIN LEVELS IN ASSOCIATED DISEASES

TYPE OF CRYOGLOBULIN	SERUM LEVEL	ASSOCIATED DISEASES
Type I Monoclonal cryoglobulin	> 5 mg/ml	• Myeloma • Waldenström's macroglobulinemia • Chronic lymphocytic leukemia
Type II Mixed cryoglobulin	> 1 mg/ml	• Rheumatoid arthritis • Sjögren's syndrome • Mixed essential cryoglobulinemia
Type III Mixed polyclonal cryoglobulin	< 1 mg/ml (50% below 80 mcg/ml)	• Systemic lupus erythematosus • Rheumatoid arthritis, Sjögren's syndrome • Infectious mononucleosis • Cytomegalovirus infections • Acute viral hepatitis • Chronic active hepatitis • Primary biliary cirrhosis • Poststreptococcal glomerulonephritis • Infective endocarditis • Leprosy • Kala-azar • Tropical splenomegaly syndrome

the needle puncture and the pressure of the tourniquet, collecting the blood sample usually takes less than 3 minutes.

Procedure and posttest care
• Perform a venipuncture, and collect the sample in a prewarmed 10-ml *red-top* tube.
• Tell the patient that he may resume usual diet.
• If the test is positive for cryoglobulins, tell the patient to avoid cold temperatures or contact with cold objects.
• If a hematoma develops at the venipuncture site, apply warm soaks.
• Observe for signs of intravascular coagulation, such as decreased color and temperature in distal extremities, and increased pain.

Precautions
• Warm the syringe and collection tube to 98.6° F (37° C) before venipuncture and keep it at that temperature to prevent loss of cryoglobulins.
• Send the sample to the laboratory immediately.

Normal findings
Normally, serum is negative for cryoglobulins.

Abnormal findings
The presence of cryoglobulins in the blood confirms cryoglobulinemia (see *Cryoglobulin levels in associated diseases*); however, this finding doesn't always mean the presence of clinical disease.

ACETYLCHOLINE RECEPTOR ANTIBODIES

The acetylcholine receptor (AChR) antibodies test is the most useful immunologic test for confirming acquired (autoimmune) myasthenia gravis (MG), a disorder of neuromuscular transmission. In MG, antibodies block and destroy AChR sites, causing muscle weakness that can be either generalized or localized to the ocular muscles.

Two test methods — a binding assay and a blocking assay — are now available to determine the relative concentration of AChR antibodies in serum. The blocking assay is relatively new, and its clinical significance is not yet fully known. However, it is specific for the autoimmune form of MG and is useful for research. Determination of AChR antibodies by either method also helps monitor immunosuppressive therapy for MG, although antibody levels do not usually parallel the severity of disease.

Purpose
• To confirm diagnosis of MG
• To monitor the effectiveness of immunosuppressive therapy for MG

Patient preparation
• Explain to the patient that this test helps confirm MG.
• If appropriate, tell him the test assesses the effectiveness of treatment.
• Advise him he needn't restrict food or fluids.
• Tell him that the test requires a blood sample and who will perform the test and when.

• Reassure him that although he may experience transient discomfort from the needle puncture and the pressure of the tourniquet, collecting the sample takes less than 3 minutes.
• Check patient history for immunosuppressive drugs that may affect test results, and note use on laboratory slip.

Procedure and posttest care
• Perform a venipuncture, and collect the sample in a 7-ml *red-top* tube.
• Because a patient with an autoimmune disease has a compromised immune system, check the venipuncture site for infection, and promptly report any change.
• Keep a clean, dry bandage over the site for at least 24 hours.
• If a hematoma develops at the venipuncture site, apply warm soaks.

Precautions
• Keep the sample at room temperature, and send it to the laboratory immediately.

Reference values
Normal serum is negative or less than 0.03 nmol/ liter for AChR-binding antibodies and is negative for AChR-blocking antibodies.

Abnormal findings
Positive AChR antibodies in symptomatic adults confirm diagnosis of MG. Patients who have only ocular symptoms of MG tend to have lower antibody titers than those who have generalized symptoms.

VIRUSES

RUBELLA ANTIBODIES

Although rubella (German measles) is generally a mild viral infection in children and young adults, it can produce severe infection in the fetus, resulting in spontaneous abortion, stillbirth, or congenital rubella syndrome. Because rubella infection normally induces immunoglobulin G (IgG) and immunoglobulin M (IgM) antibody production, measuring rubella antibodies can determine present infection and immunity resulting from past infection. The hemagglutination inhibition (HI) test is the most commonly used serologic test for rubella antibodies.

Purpose
• To diagnose rubella infection, especially congenital infection
• To determine susceptibility to rubella in children and in women of childbearing age

Patient preparation
• Explain to the patient that this test diagnoses or evaluates susceptibility to rubella.
• Inform her that she needn't restrict food or fluids before the test.
• Tell her that this test requires a blood sample and that if a current infection is suspected, a second blood sample will be needed in 2 to 3 weeks to identify a rise in the titer.
• Inform her who will perform the venipuncture and when.
• Reassure her that although she may experience transient discomfort from the needle puncture and the pressure of the tourniquet, collecting the sample takes less than 3 minutes.

Procedure and posttest care
• Perform a venipuncture, and collect the sample in a 7-ml *red-top* tube.
• If a hematoma develops at the venipuncture site, apply warm soaks.
• When appropriate, instruct the patient to return for an additional blood test.
• If a woman of childbearing age is found susceptible to rubella (titer of 1:8 or less), explain that vaccination can prevent rubella, and that she must wait at least 3 months after the vaccination before becoming pregnant, or risk permanent damage or death to the fetus.
• If the pregnant patient is found susceptible to rubella, instruct her to return for follow-up rubella antibody tests to detect possible subsequent infection.
• If the test confirms rubella in a pregnant patient, provide emotional support. As needed, refer her for appropriate counseling.

Precautions
• Handle the specimen gently to prevent hemolysis.

Reference values
Titer less than 1:8 or 1:10 (depending on the test) indicates susceptibility to rubella; titer greater than 1:10 indicates adequate protection against rubella.

Abnormal findings
The HI antibodies normally appear 2 to 4 days after the onset of the rash, peak in 2 to 3 weeks, then slowly decline but remain detectable for life. In rubella infection, acute serum titers range from 1:8 to 1:16; convalescent serum titers, from 1:64 to 1:1,024 or more. A fourfold rise or greater from the acute to the convalescent titer indicates a recent rubella infection.

Because maternal antibodies cross the placenta and persist in the infant's serum for up to 6 months, congenital rubella can be detected only after this period. An antibody titer greater than

SERODIAGNOSIS OF ACUTE VIRAL HEPATITIS

TEST RESULTS			INTERPRETATION
HB$_s$Ag	Anti-HBc IgM	Anti-HAV IgM	
−	−	+	Recent acute hepatitis A infection
+	+	−	Acute hepatitis B infection
+	−	−	Early acute hepatitis B infection or chronic hepatitis B
−	+	−	Confirms acute or recent infection with hepatitis B virus
−	−	−	Possible non-A, non-B hepatitis infection, other viral infection, or liver toxin
+	+	+	Recent probable hepatitis A infection and superimposed acute hepatitis B infection; uncommon profile

KEY: + positive − negative

1:8 in an infant age 6 months or older who hasn't been exposed to rubella postnatally confirms congenital rubella.

HEPATITIS B SURFACE ANTIGEN

Hepatitis B surface antigen (HB$_s$Ag), also called hepatitis associated antigen or australia antigen, appears in the sera of patients with hepatitis B virus. It can be detected by radioimmunoassay or, less commonly, by reverse passive hemagglutination during the extended incubation period and usually during the first 3 weeks of acute infection or if the patient is a carrier.

Because transmission of hepatitis is one of the gravest complications asso-ciated with blood transfusion, all donors must be screened for hepatitis B before their blood is stored. This screening, required by the Food and Drug Administration's Bureau of Biologics, has helped reduce the incidence of hepatitis. However, this test does not screen for hepatitis A virus (infectious hepatitis). (See *Serodiagnosis of acute viral hepatitis*.)

Purpose
• To screen blood donors for hepatitis B

• To screen people at high risk for contacting hepatitis B, such as hemodialysis nurses

• To aid differential diagnosis of viral hepatitis

VIRAL HEPATITIS TEST PANEL

Different types of viral hepatitis produce similar symptoms but differ in terms of transmission, course of treatment, prognosis, and carrier status. When clinical history is insufficient for differentiation, serologic tests can aid diagnosis. Hepatitis A and hepatitis B antigens induce type-specific antibodies detectable by radioimmunoassay. Other types of viral hepatitis — for example, non-A, non-B — must be distinguished from types A and B to be identified.

Typical sequence of hepatitis A markers after exposure

Testing for Hepatitis A: Present in blood and feces only briefly before symptoms appear, hepatitis A virus may elude detection. However, anti-HAV, the antibody to hepatitis A virus, appears early in the acute phase of the disease, persists for many years after recovery, and ultimately gives the patient immunity. A single positive anti-HAV test may indicate previous exposure to the virus, but because this antibody persists so long in the bloodstream, only evidence of *rising* anti-HAV titers confirms hepatitis A as the cause of current or very recent infection. Determining recent infection relies on identifying the antibody as immunoglobulin M (associated with recent infection). A negative anti-HAV test rules out hepatitis A.

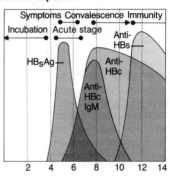

Typical sequence of hepatitis B markers after exposure

Testing for Hepatitis B: Hepatitis B viral cells are composed of a core protein and a surface protein. The surface antigen (HB_sAg) appears in serum during the long incubation period (up to 26 weeks) or during the early acute phase of infection (2 to 3 weeks) and normally peaks after symptoms begin. High levels of HB_sAg, continuing 3 or more months after onset of acute infection, suggest the development of chronic hepatitis or carrier status. Potential blood donors are screened for this antigen to

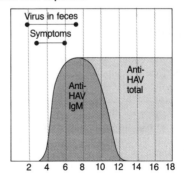

(continued)

VIRAL HEPATITIS TEST PANEL *(continued)*

prevent transmission of hepatitis B to recipients.

Another antibody to develop after exposure to hepatitis B is anti-HBc, induced by the core component of the B antigen. An early indicator of acute infection, antibody (IgM) to core antigen (anti-HBc IgM) is rarely detected in chronic infection. Thus, it's also useful in distinguishing acute from chronic infection and hepatitis B from non-A, non-B.

Anti-HBs, antibody to the surface component of the B virus, appears long after symptoms have subsided and after the antigen itself (HB$_s$Ag) has disappeared from blood. Detection of the antibody signals late convalescence or recovery from infection. Anti-HBs remains in the blood to provide immunity to reinfection.

Patient preparation
• Explain to the patient that this test helps identify a type of viral hepatitis.
• Inform him that he needn't restrict food or fluids before the test.
• Tell him that the test requires a blood sample and who will perform the venipuncture and when.
• Reassure him that although he may feel discomfort from the needle puncture and the pressure of the tourniquet, collecting the sample takes less than 3 minutes.
• Check the patient's history for hepatitis B vaccine.
• If the patient is giving blood, explain the donation procedure to him.

Procedure and posttest care
• Perform a venipuncture, and collect the sample in a 10-ml *red-top* tube.
• Notify the blood donor if test results are positive for the antigen.
• Report confirmed viral hepatitis to public health authorities. This is a reportable disease in most states.

Precautions
• Wash your hands carefully after the procedure.

• Remember to wear gloves when drawing blood.
• Be sure to dispose of the needle properly.

Normal findings
Normal serum is negative for HB$_s$Ag.

Abnormal findings
Presence of HB$_s$Ag in a patient with hepatitis confirms hepatitis B. In chronic carriers and people with chronic active hepatitis, HB$_s$Ag may be present in serum several months after onset of acute infection. HB$_s$Ag may also occur in more than 5% of patients with certain diseases other than hepatitis, such as hemophilia, Hodgkin's disease, and leukemia. If the antigen is found in donor blood, this blood must be discarded, because it carries a 40% to 70% risk of transmitting hepatitis. Blood samples that test positive should be retested because inaccurate results do occur. For related tests to diagnose viral hepatitis, see the *Viral hepatitis test panel.*

SPOT TEST FOR INFECTIOUS MONONUCLEOSIS

Several screening tests can detect the heterophil infectious mononucleosis (IM) antibody. One of these tests — the monospot — converts the Paul-Bunnell and the Davidsohn's differential absorption tests into one rapid slide test without titration. Monospot relies on agglutination of horse red blood cells (RBCs) by heterophil antibodies.

Distinguishing antibodies

Because horse RBCs contain both Forssman and IM antigens, differential absorption of the patient's serum is necessary to distinguish between them. This is done by mixing the serum sample with guinea pig kidney antigen (containing only Forssman antigen) on one end of a slide, and with beef RBC stroma (containing only IM antigen) on the other. Each absorbs only the heterophil antibody specific to it. After addition of horse RBCs to each spot, agglutination on the beef cell end of the slide indicates the presence of the IM heterophil antibody and confirms IM. Monospot rivals the classic heterophil agglutination test for sensitivity. False-positives may occur in the presence of lymphoma, hepatitis A and hepatitis B, leukemia, and pancreatic cancer.

HETEROPHIL AGGLUTINATION TESTS

Heterophil agglutination tests detect and identify two immunoglobulin M (IgM) antibodies in human serum, Epstein-Barr virus (EBV) antibodies and Forssman antibodies, that react against foreign red blood cells (RBCs).

In the Paul-Bunnell test — also called the "presumptive" test — EBV antibodies, found in the sera of patients with infectious mononucleosis, agglutinate with sheep RBCs in a test tube. However, Forssman antibodies, present in some normal serum as well as in conditions such as serum sickness, also agglutinate with sheep RBCs, thus rendering test results inconclusive for infectious mononucleosis.

If the Paul-Bunnell test establishes a presumptive titer, Davidsohn's differential absorption test can then distinguish between EBV antibodies and Forssman antibodies. (See *Spot test for infectious mononucleosis*.)

Purpose

• To aid differential diagnosis of infectious mononucleosis

Patient preparation

• Explain to the patient that this test helps detect infectious mononucleosis.

• Tell him the test requires a blood sample and who will perform the venipuncture and when.

• Reassure him that although he may experience transient discomfort from the needle puncture and the pressure of the tourniquet, collecting the sample takes less than 3 minutes.

Procedure and posttest care

• Perform a venipuncture, and collect the sample in a 7-ml *red-top* tube.

• If a hematoma develops at the venipuncture site, apply warm soaks.

• If the titer is positive and infectious mononucleosis is confirmed, instruct the patient in the treatment plan.

• If the titer is positive but infectious mononucleosis isn't confirmed, or if the titer is negative but symptoms persist, explain that additional testing will be necessary in a few days or weeks to confirm diagnosis and plan effective treatment.

Reference values

Normally, the titer is less than 1:56 but may be higher in elderly people. Some laboratories refer to a normal titer as "negative" or as having "no reaction."

Abnormal findings

Although heterophil antibodies are present in the sera of approximately 80% of patients with infectious mononucleosis 1 month after onset, a positive finding — a titer higher than 1:56 — does not confirm this disorder; for example, a high titer can result from systemic lupus erythematosus, syphilis, cryoglobulinemia, or the presence of antibodies to nonsyphilitic treponemata (yaws, pinta, bejel). A gradual increase in titer to about 1:224 during week 3 or 4, followed by a gradual decrease during weeks 4 to 8, proves most conclusive for infectious mononucleosis. However, a negative titer doesn't always rule out this disorder; occasionally, the titer becomes reactive 2 weeks later. Therefore, if symptoms persist, the test should be repeated in 2 weeks.

Confirmation of infectious mononucleosis depends on heterophil agglutination tests and hematologic tests that show absolute lymphocytosis, with 10% to 30% or more atypical lymphocytes.

EPSTEIN-BARR VIRUS ANTIBODIES

Epstein-Barr virus (EBV), a member of the herpesvirus group, is the causative agent of heterophile-positive infectious mononucleosis, Burkitt's lymphoma, and nasopharyngeal carcinoma. Although the virus does not replicate in standard cell cultures, most EBV infections can be recognized by testing the patient's serum for heterophile antibodies (monospot test), which usually appear within the first 3 weeks of illness and then decline rapidly within a few weeks.

In about 10% of adults, and a larger percentage of children, the monospot test is negative despite primary infection with EBV. Further, EBV has been associated with lymphoproliferative processes in immunosuppressed patients. These disorders occur with reactivated, rather than primary, EBV infections and, therefore, are also monospot-negative.

Alternatively, EBV-specific antibodies, which develop to several antigens of the virus during active infection, can be measured with a high level of sensitivity and specificity by indirect immunofluorescence tests.

Purpose

• To provide a laboratory diagnosis of heterophile- (or monospot-) negative cases of infectious mononucleosis

• To determine the antibody status to EBV of immunosuppressed patients with lymphoproliferative processes

Patient preparation

• Explain to the patient the purpose of the test.

CLINICAL IMPLICATIONS OF ANTIBODY RESPONSE

ANTIGEN	ACUTE INFECTIOUS MONONUCLEOSIS	REMOTE EPSTEIN-BARR VIRUS INFECTION	BURKITT'S LYMPHOMA	NASO-PHARYNGEAL CARCINOMA
Viral capsid antigen *Antibody class*				
IgM	+++	−	−	−
IgG	+++	++	++++	+++
IgA				++
Epstein-Barr nuclear antigen	−	++	++	++
Heterophil antibody (monospot)	++++	−	−	−

KEY: + antibody titer − negative for antibody titer

• Inform him that the test requires a blood specimen, and who will perform the venipuncture and when.

• Reassure him that although he may experience transient discomfort from the needle puncture and the pressure of the tourniquet, collecting the sample takes less than 3 minutes.

Procedure and posttest care
• Perform a venipuncture to collect 5 ml of sterile blood in a *red-top* tube.

• Allow the blood to clot for at least 1 hour at room temperature.

• If a hematoma develops at the venipuncture site, apply warm soaks.

Precautions
• Handle the sample gently because excessive agitation will cause hemolysis of the sample.

• Transfer the serum to a sterile tube or vial and send it to the laboratory.

• If transfer is unavoidably delayed, be careful to store the serum at 39.2° F (4° C) for 1 or 2 days, or at −4° F (−20° C) for longer periods to prevent bacterial contamination.

Reference values
Sera from patients who have never been infected with EBV will have no detectable antibodies to the virus measured by either the monospot or indirect immunofluorescence test. The monospot test is positive only during the acute phase of infection with EBV; the indirect immunofluorescence test will detect and discriminate between acute and past infection with the virus. For the profile of test results and their clinical implications, see *Clinical implications of antibody response.*

Abnormal findings
EBV infection can be ruled out if no antibodies to EBV antigens are detected in the indirect immunofluorescence test. A positive monospot test or an indirect immunofluorescence test that is either immunoglobulin M (IgM)-positive or Epstein-Barr nuclear antigen (EBNA)-

negative indicates acute EBV infection. However, a monospot-negative result does not necessarily rule out acute or past infection with EBV. Conversely, immunoglobulin G (IgG) class antibody to viral capsid antigen (VCA) and EBNA antigens (IgM-negative) indicates remote (more than 2 months) infection with EBV. Recognize that most cases of monospot-negative infectious mononucleosis are caused by cytomegalovirus infections.

RESPIRATORY SYNCYTIAL VIRUS ANTIBODIES

Respiratory syncytial virus (RSV), a member of the paramyxovirus group, is the major viral cause of severe lower respiratory tract disease in infants, but may cause infections in people of any age. RSV infections are most common and produce the most severe disease during the first 6 months of life. Initial infection involves viral replication in epithelial cells of the upper respiratory tract, but in younger children especially, the infection spreads to the bronchi, bronchioli, and even to the parenchyma of the lungs. In this test, immunoglobulin G (IgG) and immunoglobulin M (IgM) class antibodies are quantified using indirect immunofluorescence.

Purpose
• To diagnose infections caused by RSV

Patient preparation
• Explain to the patient the purpose of the test.
• Tell the patient (or parents of the patient) that the test requires a blood sample and who will perform the venipuncture and when.
• Reassure the patient that although he may experience transient discomfort from the needle puncture and the pressure of the tourniquet, collecting the sample takes less than 3 minutes.

Procedure and posttest care
• Perform a venipuncture to collect 5 ml of sterile blood in a *red-top* tube.
• Allow the blood to clot for at least 1 hour at room temperature.
• If a hematoma develops at the venipuncture site, apply warm soaks.

Precautions
• Handle the sample gently to prevent hemolysis.
• Transfer the serum to a sterile tube or vial and send it to the laboratory.
• If transfer must be delayed, store the serum at 39.2° F (4° C) for 1 to 2 days or for longer periods at −4° F (−20° C) to avoid microbial contamination.

Reference values
Sera from patients who have never been infected with RSV will have no detectable antibodies to the virus (less than 1:5).

Abnormal findings
The qualitative presence of IgM or a fourfold or greater increase in IgG antibodies indicates active RSV infection. Note that in infants, serologic diagnosis of RSV infections is difficult because of the presence of maternal IgG antibodies. Therefore, the presence of IgM antibodies is most significant.

HERPES SIMPLEX ANTIBODIES

Herpes simplex virus (HSV), a member of the herpesvirus group, causes various clinically severe manifestations, including genital lesions, keratitis or conjunctivitis, generalized dermal lesions, and pneumonia. Severe involvement is associated with intrauterine or neonatal infections and encephalitis; such infections are most severe in immunosuppressed patients. Of the two closely related antigenic types, type 1 usually causes infections above the waistline; type 2 infections predominantly involve the external genitalia. Primary contact with this virus occurs in early childhood as acute stomatitis or, more commonly, as an inapparent infection. Generally, the prevalence of antibodies to HSV in adults exceeds 50%.

Sensitive assays, such as indirect immunofluorescence or enzyme immunoassay are used to demonstrate immunoglobulin M (IgM) class antibodies to HSV or to detect a fourfold or greater increase in immunoglobulin G (IgG) class antibodies between acute- and convalescent-phase sera.

Purpose
• To confirm systemic infections caused by HSV

Patient preparation
• Explain to the patient the purpose of the test.
• Tell him that the test will require a blood sample and who will perform the venipuncture and when.
• Reassure him that although he may experience transient discomfort from the needle puncture and the pressure of the tourniquet, collecting the sample takes less than 3 minutes.

Procedure and posttest care
• Perform a venipuncture to collect 5 ml of sterile blood in a *red-top* tube.
• Allow the blood to clot for at least 1 hour at room temperature.
• If a hematoma develops at the venipuncture site, apply warm soaks.

Precautions
• Handle the sample gently to prevent hemolysis.
• Transfer the serum to a sterile tube or vial and send it to the laboratory promptly.
• If transfer must be delayed for 1 or 2 days, store the serum at 39.2° F (4° C) or, if longer, store at −4° F (−20° C) to avoid contamination.

Reference values
Sera from patients who have never been infected with HSV will have no detectable antibodies (less than 1:5).

Abnormal findings
The presence of IgM or a fourfold or greater increase in IgG antibodies indicates active HSV infection. Reportedly, more than 50% of adults have IgG class antibodies to HSV because of prior infection. Reactivated infections caused by HSV can be recognized serologically only by an increase in IgG class antibodies between acute- and convalescent-phase sera.

CYTOMEGALOVIRUS ANTIBODY SCREEN

After primary infection, cytomegalovirus (CMV) remains latent in white blood cells. The presence of CMV antibodies indicates past infection with this virus. In an immunocompromised patient, CMV can be reactivated to cause active infection. Administration of blood or tissue from a seropositive donor may cause active CMV infection in CMV-sero negative organ transplant recipients or neonates, especially those born prematurely.

Antibodies to CMV can be detected by several methods that include passive hemagglutination, latex agglutination, enzyme immunoassay, and indirect immunofluorescence. The complement fixation test is only 60% sensitive compared with these other assays and should not be used to screen for CMV antibodies. Screening tests for CMV antibodies is qualitative; it detects the presence of antibody at a single low dilution. In quantitative methods, several dilutions of the serum specimen are tested to indicate acute infection with CMV.

Purpose
• To detect past CMV infection in organ transplant or blood donors and recipients
• To screen for CMV infection in infants who require blood administration or tissue transplants
• To detect past CMV infection in immunocompromised patients

Patient preparation
• As appropriate, explain the purpose of the test to the patient or to the parents of an infant.
• Tell the patient that the test requires a blood sample and who will perform the venipuncture and when.
• Reassure him that although he may experience transient discomfort from the needle puncture and the pressure of the tourniquet, collecting the sample takes less than 3 minutes.

Procedure and posttest care
• Perform a venipuncture to collect 5 ml of blood in a *red-top* tube.
• Allow the blood to clot for at least 1 hour at room temperature.

Precautions
• Handle the sample gently to prevent hemolysis.
• Transfer the serum to a sterile tube or vial and send it to the laboratory.
• If transport must be delayed, store the serum at 39.2° F (4° C) for 1 or 2 days or at $-4°$ F ($-20°$ C) for longer periods to avoid microbial contamination.

Reference values
Patients who have never been infected with CMV have no detectable antibodies to the virus (less than 1:5).

Abnormal findings
A serum specimen positive for antibody at this single dilution indicates that the patient has been infected with CMV and that the patient's white blood cells contain latent virus capable of being reactivated in an immunocompromised host. Immunosuppressed patients who lack antibodies to CMV should receive blood products or organ transplants from donors who are also seronegative. Patients with CMV antibodies do not require seronegative blood products.

HUMAN IMMUNODEFICIENCY VIRUS ANTIBODY

This test detects antibodies to human immunodeficiency virus (HIV) in serum. HIV is the virus that causes acquired immunodeficiency syndrome (AIDS). Transmission occurs by direct exposure of a person's blood to body fluids containing the virus. The virus may be transmitted when contaminated blood and blood products are exchanged from one person to another; during sexual intercourse with an infected partner; when intravenous drugs are shared; and during pregnancy or breast-feeding, from an infected mother to her child.

Initial identification of HIV virus is usually achieved through the enzyme-linked immunosorbent assay (ELISA). Positive findings are confirmed by Western Blot and immunofluorescence assay.

Purpose
• To screen for HIV in high-risk patients.
• To screen donated blood for HIV

Patient preparation
• Inform the patient that this test detects HIV infection.
• Provide adequate counseling about the reasons for performing the test, usually requested by the patient's doctor.
• If your patient has questions about his condition, be sure to provide full and accurate information.
• Tell the patient who will perform the venipuncture and when.
• Reassure him that although he may experience transient discomfort from the needle puncture and the pressure of the tourniquet, collecting the sample takes less than 3 minutes.

Procedure and posttest care
• Perform a venipuncture, and collect a blood sample in a 10-ml *red-top* barrier tube. Barrier tubes help prevent contamination when pouring the serum in the laboratory.
• If a hematoma develops at the venipuncture site, apply warm soaks.
• Keep test results confidential.

• When the results are received, give the patient another opportunity to ask questions.
• Encourage the patient with positive screening tests to seek medical follow-up care, even if he's asymptomatic.
• Tell him to report early signs of AIDS, such as fever, weight loss, axillary or inguinal lymphadenopathy, rash, and persistent cough or diarrhea. Women should also report gynecological symptoms.
• Tell the patient to assume that he can transmit AIDS to others until conclusively proven otherwise. To prevent possible contagion, advise him about safe sex precautions.
• Instruct him not to share razors, toothbrushes, or utensils (which may be contaminated with blood) and to clean such items with household bleach diluted 1:10 in water.
• Advise against donating blood, tissues, or an organ.
• Warn the patient to inform his doctor and dentist about his condition, so they can take proper precautions.

Precautions
• When drawing a blood sample, employ universal precautions.
• Use gloves, properly dispose of needles, and use blood-fluid precaution labels on tubes, as necessary.

Reference values
Test results should normally be nonreactive.

Abnormal findings
The test detects previous exposure to the virus. However, it doesn't identify patients who have been exposed to the virus but who haven't yet made antibodies. Most patients with AIDS have antibodies to HIV. A positive test for the HIV antibody can't determine whether a patient harbors actively replicating vi-

rus or when the patient will present signs and symptoms of AIDS.

Many apparently healthy people have been exposed to HIV and have circulating antibodies. These are not false-positives. Furthermore, patients in the later stages of AIDS may exhibit no detectable antibody in their sera because they can no longer mount an antibody response.

BACTERIA AND FUNGI

ANTISTREPTOLYSIN-O TEST

This test measures the relative serum concentrations of the antibody to streptolysin O. A serum sample is diluted with a commercial preparation of streptolysin O and incubated. After the addition of rabbit or human red blood cells, the tube is reincubated and examined visually. If hemolysis fails to develop, it indicates recent beta-hemolytic streptococcal infection.

Purpose
• To confirm recent or ongoing infection with beta-hemolytic streptococci
• To help diagnose rheumatic fever and poststreptococcal glomerulonephritis in the presence of clinical symptoms
• To distinguish between rheumatic fever and rheumatoid arthritis when joint pains are present

Patient preparation
• Explain to the patient that this test detects an immunologic response to certain bacteria (streptococci).
• Inform him he needn't restrict food or fluids.
• Tell him that the test requires a blood sample and who will perform the venipuncture and when.
• Reassure him that although he may experience transient discomfort from the needle puncture and the pressure of the tourniquet, collecting the sample takes less than 3 minutes.
• If the test is to be repeated at regular intervals to identify active and inactive states of rheumatic fever or to confirm acute glomerulonephritis, tell the patient that measuring changes in antibody levels helps determine the effectiveness of therapy.
• Check the patient's medication history for drugs, such as antibiotics or corticosteroids, that may suppress the streptococcal antibody response. If such drugs must be continued, note this on the laboratory slip.

Procedure and posttest care
• Perform a venipuncture, and collect the sample in a 7-ml *red-top* tube.
• If a hematoma develops at the venipuncture site, apply warm soaks.

Precautions
• Handle the sample gently to prevent hemolysis.

Reference values
Even healthy people have some detectable antistreptolysin-O (ASO) titer from previous minor streptococcal infections. Normal ASO titer is:
• Adults: 120 Todd units/ml
• School-age children: 170 Todd units/ml
• Preschoolers: 120 Todd units/ml.

Abnormal findings

High ASO titers usually occur only after prolonged or recurrent infections. Roughly 15% to 20% of patients with poststreptococcal disease don't have elevated ASO titers. Titers ranging to 250 Todd units may indicate inactive rheumatic fever. Higher titers of 500 to 5,000 Todd units suggest acute rheumatic fever or acute poststreptococcal glomerulonephritis.

Serial titers, determined at 10- to 14-day intervals, provide more reliable information than a single titer. A rise in titer 2 to 5 weeks after the acute infection, which peaks 4 to 6 weeks after the initial rise, confirms poststreptococcal disease.

FEBRILE AGGLUTINATION TESTS

Bacterial infections (such as tularemia, brucellosis, and the disorders caused by *Salmonella*) and rickettsial infections (such as Rocky Mountain spotted fever and typhus) sometimes cause puzzling fevers, called fevers of undetermined origin (FUO). In these infections and others in which microorganisms are difficult to isolate from blood or excreta, febrile agglutination tests can provide important diagnostic information.

The Weil-Felix reaction for rickettsial disease, Widal's test for *Salmonella*, and tests for brucellosis and tularemia are essentially the same. In these tests, a serum sample is mixed with a few drops of prepared antigens in normal saline solution on a slide and the reaction is observed.

The Weil-Felix reaction establishes rickettsial antibody titers. This test uses three forms of *Proteus* antigens (OX-19, OX-2, and OX-K) that cross-react

with the various strains of rickettsiae. Antibodies to certain rickettsial strains react with more than one *Proteus* antigen, while antibodies to other strains fail to react with any *Proteus* antigens.

Widal's test establishes their titers for flagellar (H) and somatic (O) antigens, which may indicate *Salmonella* gastroenteritis and extraintestinal focal infections caused by *Salmonella enteritidis* or enteric (typhoid) fever, caused by *Salmonella typhosa*. A third antigen, the Vi, or envelope, antigen may indicate typhoid carrier status, which often tests negative for H and O antigens. Widal's test isn't recommended for diagnosing *Salmonella* gastroenteritis.

Slide-agglutination and tube dilution tests, using killed suspensions of the disease organisms as antigens, establish titers for the gram-negative coccobacilli *Brucella* and *Francisella tularensis*, which cause brucellosis and tularemia, respectively.

Purpose

• To support clinical findings in diagnosis of disorders caused by *Salmonella, Rickettsia, F. tularensis,* or *Brucella* organisms
• To identify the cause of FUO

Patient preparation

• Explain to the patient that this test detects and quantifies microorganisms that may cause fever and other symptoms.
• Inform him that he needn't restrict food or fluids.
• Tell him the test requires a blood sample and who will perform the venipuncture and when.
• Reassure him that although he may experience transient discomfort from the needle puncture and the pressure of the tourniquet, collecting the blood sample takes less than 3 minutes.
• If appropriate, explain to the patient that this test requires a series of blood

samples to detect a pattern of titers that is characteristic of the suspected disorder. Reassure him that a positive titer only suggests a disorder.

• Note on the laboratory slip when antimicrobial therapy, if any, began.

Procedure and posttest care
• Perform a venipuncture, and collect the sample in a 7-ml *red-top* tube.
• If a hematoma develops at the venipuncture site, apply warm soaks.
• In FUO and suspected infection, contact the hospital infection control department. Isolation may be necessary.

Precautions
• Use standard hospital isolation procedures when collecting and handling samples.
• Send samples to the laboratory immediately.

Reference values
Normal dilutions are as follows:
• *Salmonella* antibody: < 1:80
• Brucellosis antibody: < 1:80
• Tularemia antibody: < 1:40
• Rickettsial antibody: < 1:40.

Abnormal findings
Observed rise and fall of titers are crucial for detecting active infection. If this is not possible, certain titer levels can suggest the disorder. For all febrile agglutinins, a fourfold increase in titers is strong evidence of infection.

The Weil-Felix reaction is positive for rickettsiae with antibodies to *Proteus* 6 to 12 days after infection; titers peak in 1 month and usually drop to negative in 5 or 6 months. However, this test cannot be used for diagnosing rickettsialpox or Q fever, because the antibodies of these diseases don't cross-react with *Proteus* antigens; the test shows positive titers in *Proteus* infections and, in such cases, is nonspecific for rickettsiae.

In *Salmonella* infection, H and O agglutinins usually appear in serum after 1 week, and titers rise for 3 to 6 weeks. O agglutinins usually fall to insignificant levels in 6 to 12 months. H agglutinin titers may remain elevated for years.

In brucellosis, titers usually rise after 2 or 3 weeks and reach their highest levels between 4 and 8 weeks. Absence of *Brucella* agglutinins doesn't rule out brucellosis. In tularemia, titers usually become positive in the second week of infection, exceed 1:320 by the third week, peak in 4 to 7 weeks, and usually decline gradually 1 year after recovery.

FUNGAL SEROLOGY

Most fungal organisms enter the body as spores inhaled into the lungs or infiltrated through wounds in the skin or mucosa. If the body's defenses can't destroy the organisms initially, the fungi multiply to form lesions; blood and lymph vessels may then spread the mycoses throughout the body. Most healthy people easily overcome initial mycotic infection, but elderly people and others with deficient immune systems are more susceptible to acute or chronic mycotic infection and to disorders secondary to such infection. Fungal serology may find evidence of blastomycosis, coccidioidomycosis, histoplasmosis, aspergillosis, and sporotrichosis antibodies or cryptococcosis antigen.

Mycosis may be deep-seated or superficial: deep-seated mycosis occurs primarily in the lungs; superficial mycosis, in the skin or the mucosal linings. Although cultures are usually performed to diagnose mycoses by identifying the causative organism, occasionally serologic tests provide the sole evi-

SERUM TEST METHODS FOR FUNGAL INFECTIONS

DISEASE AND NORMAL VALUES	CLINICAL SIGNIFICANCE OF ABNORMAL RESULTS
Blastomycosis Complement fixation: titers < 1:8	Titers ranging from 1:8 to 1:16 suggest infection; titers > 1:32 denote active disease. A rising titer in serial samples taken every 3 to 4 weeks indicates disease progression; a falling titer indicates regression. This test has limited diagnostic value due to high percentage of false-negatives.
Immunodiffusion: negative	A more sensitive test for blastomycosis; detects 80% of infected persons.
Coccidioidomycosis Complement fixation: titers < 1:2	Most sensitive test for this fungus. Titers ranging from 1:2 to 1:4 suggest active infection; titers > 1:16 usually denote active disease. Test may remain negative in mild infections.
Immunodiffusion: negative	Most useful for screening, followed by complement fixation test for confirmation
Precipitin: titers < 1:16	Good screening test; titers > 1:16 usually indicate infection. 80% of infected persons show positive titers by 2 weeks: most revert to negative by 6 months. Early primary disease is shown by positive precipitin and negative complement fixation test. A positive complement fixation and negative precipitin test indicate chronic disease.
Histoplasmosis Complement fixation (histoplasmin): titers < 1:8	Titers ranging from 1:8 to 1:16 suggest infection; titers >1:32 indicate active disease. Antibodies generally appear 10 to 21 days after initial infection. Test is positive in 10% to 15% of cases.
Complement fixation (yeast): titers < 1:18	More sensitive than histoplasmin complement fixation test; gives positive results in 75% to 80% of cases. (Both histoplasmin and yeast antigens are positive in 10% of cases.) A rising titer in serial samples taken every 2 to 3 weeks indicates progressive infection; a decreasing titer indicates regression. Titers ranging from 1:8 to 1:16 suggest infection; titers > 1:32 indicate active disease.
Immunodiffusion (histoplasmin): negative	Appearance of both H and M bands indicates active infection. If the M band appears first and lasts longer than the H band, the infection may be regressing. The M band alone may indicate early infection, chronic disease, or a recent skin test.

(continued)

dence for mycosis. Such serologic tests employ immunodiffusion, complement fixation, precipitin, latex agglutination, or agglutination methods to demonstrate the presence of specific mycotic antibodies.

Purpose
• To rapidly detect the presence of antifungal antibodies, aiding in the diagnosis of mycoses
• To monitor effectiveness of therapy for mycoses

SERUM TEST METHODS FOR FUNGAL INFECTIONS *(continued)*

DISEASE AND NORMAL VALUES	CLINICAL SIGNIFICANCE OF ABNORMAL RESULTS
Aspergillosis Complement fixation: titer < 1:8	Titers of > 1:8 suggest infection; 70% to 90% of patients with known pulmonary aspergillosis or aspergillus allergy present antibodies, as does about 5% of the general population. This test cannot detect invasive aspergillosis because patients with this disease do not present antibodies; biopsy is required.
Immunodiffusion: negative	One or more precipitin bands suggests infection; precipitins appear in 95% of patients with pulmonary fungus balls and in 50% of those with allergic bronchopulmonary disorders. The number of bands is related to complement fixation titers; the more precipitin bands, the higher the titer.
Sporotrichosis Agglutination: titers < 1:40	Titers of > 1:80 usually indicate active disease. The test usually is negative in cutaneous infections, positive in extracutaneous infections.
Cryptococcosis Latex agglutination for cryptococcal antigen: negative	About 90% of patients with cryptococcal meningoencephalitis present capsular antigen in cerebrospinal fluid (CSF) serum. (Serum is less frequently positive than CSF.) Culturing is definitive because false-positives do occur. (Presence of rheumatoid factor may cause a positive reaction.) Serum antigen tests are positive in 33% of patients with pulmonary cryptococcosis; biopsy is usually required.

Patient preparation

• Explain to the patient that this test aids diagnosis of certain fungal infections. If appropriate, tell him this test monitors his response to mycoses therapy and that it may be necessary to repeat the test.

• Instruct him to restrict food and fluids for 12 to 24 hours before the test.

• Tell him that the test requires a blood sample, and who will perform the venipuncture and when.

• Reassure him that although he may experience brief discomfort from the needle puncture and the pressure of the tourniquet, collecting the sample takes less than 3 minutes.

Procedure and posttest care

• Perform a venipuncture, and collect the sample in a 10-ml sterile *red-top* tube.

• If a hematoma develops at the venipuncture site, apply warm soaks.

Precautions

• Send the blood sample to the laboratory immediately.

• If transport to the laboratory is delayed, store the blood sample at 39.2° F (4° C).

Findings

Depending on the test method, a negative finding, or normal titer, usually indicates the absence of mycosis. The chart entitled *Serum test methods for fungal infections* explains the significance of findings for specific organisms.

CANDIDA ANTIBODY

Commonly present in the body, *Candida albicans* is a saprophytic yeast that can become pathogenic when the environment favors proliferation or the host's defenses have been significantly weakened.

Candidiasis is usually limited to the skin and mucous membranes but may cause life-threatening systemic infection. Susceptibility to candidiasis is associated with antibacterial, antimetabolic, or corticosteroid therapy and with immunologic defects, pregnancy, obesity, diabetes, and debilitating diseases. Oral candidiasis is common and benign in children; in adults, it may be an early indication of acquired immunodeficiency syndrome (AIDS).

Diagnosis of candidiasis is usually made by culture or histologic study. However, when such diagnosis cannot be made, identifying the *Candida* antibody may be helpful in diagnosing systemic candidiasis. Be cautioned that serologic testing for detecting antibodies in candidiasis is not reliable, and investigators continue to disagree about its usefulness.

Purpose
• To aid diagnosis of candidiasis when culture or histologic study can't confirm diagnosis

Patient preparation
• As appropriate, explain the purpose of the test to the patient.
• Tell him that the test doesn't require restriction of food or fluids.

• Tell him that the test requires a blood sample and who will perform the venipuncture and when.
• Reassure him that although he may experience transient discomfort from the needle puncture and the pressure of the tourniquet, collecting the sample takes less than 3 minutes.

Procedure and posttest care
• Perform a venipuncture, and collect 5 ml of sterile blood in a *red-top* tube.
• If a hematoma develops at the venipuncture site, apply warm soaks.

Precautions
• Handle the sample gently because excessive agitation or rough handling may cause hemolysis.
• Send the sample to the laboratory promptly.
• Be certain to note any recent antimicrobial therapy on the laboratory request form.

Reference values
A normal test result is negative for the *Candida* antigen.

Abnormal findings
A positive test for *C. albicans* antigen is common in patients with disseminated candidiasis. However, this test yields a significant percentage of false-positive results.

BACTERIAL MENINGITIS ANTIGEN

This test, performed by counterimmunoelectrophoresis, can detect specific antigens of *Streptococcus pneumoniae*, *Neisseria meningitidis*, and *Haemophilus influenzae* type B, the principal etiologic agents in meningitis. This test can be performed on samples of serum, cerebrospinal fluid (CSF), urine, pleural fluid, or joint fluid; however, the preferred specimen is either CSF or urine.

Purpose
• To identify the etiologic agent in meningitis
• To aid diagnosis of bacterial meningitis
• To aid diagnosis of meningitis when the Gram-stained smear and culture are negative

Patient preparation
• As appropriate, explain the purpose of the test to the patient.
• Inform the patient that this test requires a urine sample or a sample of CSF.
• If a CSF sample is required, describe how it will be obtained.
• Tell him who will perform the procedure and when and that he may experience transient discomfort from the needle puncture.
• Advise the patient that a headache is the most common adverse effect of lumbar puncture but that his cooperation during the test minimizes such an effect.
• Make sure the patient or a family member has signed a consent form.

Procedure and posttest care
• Collect a 10-ml sample of urine or a 1-ml sample of CSF in a sterile container.

Precautions
• It's important to maintain specimen sterility during collection.
• Wear gloves when obtaining or handling all specimens.
• Make sure all caps are tightly fastened on specimen containers.
• Promptly send the specimen to the laboratory on a refrigerated coolant.

Normal findings
Normally, results are negative for bacterial antigens.

Abnormal findings
Positive results identify the specific bacterial antigen: *S. pneumoniae, N. meningitidis, Haemophilus influenzae* type B, or *Streptococci* group B.

LYME DISEASE SEROLOGY

Lyme disease is a multisystem disorder characterized by dermatologic, neurologic, cardiac, and rheumatic manifestations in various stages. Epidemiologic and serologic studies implicate a commonly tickborne spirochete, *Borrelia burgdorferi*, as the causative agent. Serologic tests are able to identify 50% of patients with early-stage Lyme disease and all patients with later complications of carditis, neuritis, and arthritis or who are in remission.

Purpose
• To confirm diagnosis of Lyme disease

Patient preparation
• Explain to the patient that this test helps determine whether his symptoms are caused by Lyme disease.
• Instruct the patient to fast for 12 hours before the blood sample is drawn but to drink fluids as usual.
• Tell the patient that the test requires a blood sample and who will perform the venipuncture and when.
• Reassure him that although he may experience transient discomfort from the needle puncture and the pressure of the tourniquet, collecting the sample takes less than 3 minutes.

Procedure and posttest care

• Perform a venipuncture, and collect the sample in a 7-ml *red-top* tube.
• If a hematoma develops at the venipuncture site, apply warm soaks.

Precautions

• Handle the specimen carefully to prevent hemolysis.
• Send the specimen to the laboratory immediately.

Reference values

Normal serum values are nonreactive. Serum titer should be less than 1:256. A serum titer of 1:128 is considered borderline and calls for repeat testing in 4 to 6 weeks.

Abnormal findings

A positive Lyme serology can help confirm diagnosis but is not definitive. Other treponemal diseases and high rheumatoid factor titers can cause false-positive results. More than 15% of patients with Lyme disease fail to develop antibodies.

MISCELLANEOUS TESTS

VDRL

The Venereal Disease Research Laboratory (VDRL) test is widely used to screen for primary and secondary syphilis. Usually, a serum sample is used in the VDRL test, but this test may also be performed on a specimen of cerebrospinal fluid (CSF), obtained by lumbar puncture, to test for tertiary syphilis. However, the VDRL test of CSF is less sensitive than the fluorescent treponemal antibody absorption test.

Purpose

• To screen for primary and secondary syphilis
• To confirm primary or secondary syphilis in the presence of syphilitic lesions
• To monitor response to treatment

Patient preparation

• Explain to the patient that this test detects syphilis.
• Inform him that the disease often goes undetected in the general population because infected people remain untreated.
• Tell the patient he needn't restrict food, fluids, or medications, but should abstain from alcohol for 24 hours before the test.
• Tell him that the test requires a blood sample and who will perform the venipuncture and when.
• Reassure him that although he may experience transient discomfort from the needle puncture and the tourniquet pressure, collecting the sample takes less than 3 minutes.

Procedure and posttest care

• Perform a venipuncture, and collect the sample in a 7-ml *red-top* tube.
• If a hematoma develops at the venipuncture site, apply warm soaks.
• If the test is nonreactive or borderline but syphilis hasn't been ruled out, instruct the patient to return for follow-up testing. Explain that borderline test results don't necessarily mean he is free of the disease.
• If the test is reactive, explain the importance of proper treatment. Provide the patient with further information about venereal disease and how it is spread, and stress the need for antibiotic therapy. Prepare him for mandatory inquiries from public health authorities.

• If the test is reactive but the patient shows no clinical signs of syphilis, explain that many uninfected people show false-positive reactions. However, stress the need for further specific tests to rule out syphilis.

Precautions
• Handle the specimen carefully to prevent hemolysis.

Normal findings
Normal serum shows no flocculation and is reported as a nonreactive test.

Abnormal findings
Definite flocculation is reported as a reactive test; slight flocculation is reported as a weakly reactive test. A reactive VDRL test occurs in about 50% of patients with primary syphilis and in nearly all patients with secondary syphilis. If syphilitic lesions exist, a reactive VDRL test is diagnostic. If no lesions are evident, a reactive VDRL test necessitates repeated testing. However, biological false-positive reactions can be caused by conditions unrelated to syphilis, for example, infectious mononucleosis, malaria, leprosy, hepatitis, systemic lupus erythematosus, rheumatoid arthritis, and nonsyphilitic treponemal diseases, such as pinta or yaws.

A nonreactive test doesn't rule out syphilis, because *T. pallidum* causes no detectable immunologic changes in the serum for 14 to 21 days after infection. However, dark-field microscopic examination of exudate from suspicious lesions can provide early diagnosis by identifying the causative spirochetes.

A reactive VDRL test using a CSF specimen indicates neurosyphilis, which can follow the primary and secondary stages in patients who remain untreated.

FLUORESCENT TREPONEMAL ANTIBODY ABSORPTION TEST

The fluorescent treponemal antibody absorption (FTA-ABS or simply FTA) test uses indirect immunofluorescence to detect antibodies to the spirochete *Treponema pallidum* in the serum. This spirochete causes syphilis.

Although the FTA-ABS test is generally performed on a serum sample to detect primary or secondary syphilis, a cerebrospinal fluid (CSF) specimen is required to detect tertiary syphilis. Because antibody levels remain constant for long periods, the FTA-ABS test is not recommended for monitoring response to therapy. (See *Two new tests for* Treponema pallidum.)

Purpose
• To confirm primary or secondary syphilis
• To screen for suspected false-positive results of VDRL tests

Patient preparation
• Explain to the patient that this test can confirm or rule out syphilis.
• Inform him that he needn't restrict food or fluids.
• Tell him the test requires a blood sample and who will perform the venipuncture and when.
• Reassure him that although he may experience transient discomfort from the needle puncture and the pressure of the tourniquet, collecting the blood sample usually takes less than 3 minutes.

Procedure and posttest care
• Perform a venipuncture, and collect the sample in a 7-ml *red-top* tube.
• If a hematoma develops at the venipuncture site, apply warm soaks.
• If the test is reactive, explain the nature of syphilis, and stress the importance of proper treatment and the need to find and treat the patient's sexual contacts.
• If appropriate, provide the patient with additional information about syphilis and how it is spread; emphasize the need for antibiotic therapy. Also, prepare him for inquiries from the public health authorities.
• If the test is nonreactive, or findings are borderline but syphilis has not been ruled out, instruct the patient to return for follow-up testing; explain that inconclusive results don't necessarily indicate he is free of the disease.

Precautions
• Handle the sample gently to prevent hemolysis.

Normal findings
Normally, reaction to the FTA-ABS test is negative (no fluorescence).

Abnormal findings
The presence of treponemal antibodies in the serum — a reactive test result — does not indicate the stage or the severity of infection. (However, the presence of these antibodies in CSF is strong evidence of tertiary neurosyphilis.) Elevated antibody levels appear in 80% to 90% of patients with primary syphilis and in 100% of patients with secondary syphilis. Higher antibody levels persist for several years, with treatment or without treatment.

The absence of treponemal antibodies — a nonreactive test — doesn't necessarily rule out syphilis. *T. pallidum* causes no detectable immunologic changes in the blood for 14 to 21 days

---

TWO NEW TESTS FOR TREPONEMA PALLIDUM

The recently developed microhemagglutination assay for *Treponema pallidum* antibody increases the specificity of syphilis testing by eliminating methodologic interference. In this assay, tanned sheep red blood cells are coated with *T. pallidum* antigen and are combined with absorbed test serum. Hemagglutination occurs in the presence of specific anti–*T. pallidum* antibodies in the serum.

In the enzyme-linked immunosorbent assay, tubes coated with *T. pallidum* are washed and then treated with enzyme-labeled antihuman globulin. After the substrate for the enzymes is added to the tubes, the enzymatic activity is measured by quantitating the reaction product formed.

---

after initial infection. Organisms may be detected earlier by examining suspicious lesions with a dark-field microscope. Low antibody levels or other nonspecific factors produce borderline findings. In such cases, repeated testing and a thorough review of patient history may be productive.

Although the FTA-ABS test is specific, some patients with nonsyphilitic conditions — such as systemic lupus erythematosus, genital herpes, or increased or abnormal globulins — or those who are pregnant may show minimally reactive levels. In addition, the FTA-ABS test doesn't always distinguish between *T. pallidum* and certain other treponemas, such as those that cause pinta, yaws, and bejel.

CARCINOEMBRYONIC ANTIGEN

Carcinoembryonic antigen (CEA), a glycoprotein secreted onto the glycocalyx surface of cells lining the gastrointestinal tract, appears during the first or second trimester of fetal life. Normally, production of CEA is halted before birth but may begin again later, if a neoplasm develops. Because CEA levels are also raised by biliary obstruction, alcoholic hepatitis, chronic heavy smoking, and other conditions, this test can't be used as a general indicator of cancer. However, measurement of enzyme CEA levels by immunoassay is useful for staging and monitoring treatment of certain cancers.

Purpose
• To monitor the effectiveness of cancer therapy
• To assist in preoperative staging of colorectal cancers, assess adequacy of surgical resection, and to test for recurrence of colorectal cancers

Patient preparation
• Explain to the patient that this test detects and measures a special protein that's not normally present in adults.
• If appropriate, inform him that the test will be repeated to monitor the effectiveness of therapy.
• Advise him that he needn't restrict food, fluids, or medications before the test.
• Tell him the test requires a blood sample and who will perform the venipuncture and when.
• Reassure him that although he may experience discomfort from the puncture and the tourniquet, collecting the sample takes less than 3 minutes.

Procedure and posttest care
• Perform a venipuncture, and collect the sample in a 7-ml *red-top* tube.
• If a hematoma develops at the venipuncture site, apply warm soaks.

Precautions
• Handle the sample gently to prevent hemolysis, and send it to the laboratory immediately to ensure integrity of test results.

Reference values
Normal serum CEA values are less than 5 ng/ml in healthy nonsmokers. However, about 5% of the population has above-normal CEA concentrations.

Abnormal findings
Persistent elevation of CEA levels suggests residual or recurrent tumor. If levels exceed normal before surgical resection, chemotherapy, or radiation therapy, their return to normal within 6 weeks suggests successful treatment.

High CEA levels are characteristic in various malignant conditions, particularly endodermally derived neoplasms of the gastrointestinal organs and the lungs, and in certain nonmalignant conditions, such as benign hepatic disease, hepatic cirrhosis, alcoholic pancreatitis, and inflammatory bowel disease.

Elevated CEA concentrations may occur in nonendodermal carcinomas, such as breast cancer or ovarian cancer.

ALPHA-FETOPROTEIN

Alpha-fetoprotein (AFP) is a glycoprotein produced by fetal tissue and tumors that differentiate from midline embryonic structures. During fetal development, AFP levels in serum and amniotic fluid rise. AFP crosses the placenta and appears in maternal serum.

High maternal serum AFP levels at 14 to 22 weeks' gestation may suggest fetal neural tube defects, such as spina bifida or anencephaly, but positive confirmation requires amniocentesis and ultrasonography. Other congenital anomalies may also be associated with high maternal serum AFP concentrations: evaluation for Down's syndrome can be performed on serum samples drawn at 15 to 20 weeks' gestation.

Elevated AFP levels in patients who aren't pregnant may occur in malignancy, such as hepatocellular carcinoma, or in certain nonmalignant conditions, such as ataxia-telangiectasia. In these conditions, AFP assays are more useful for monitoring response to therapy than for diagnosis. AFP levels are best determined by enzyme-immunoassay on amniotic fluid or serum.

Purpose
• To monitor the effectiveness of therapy in malignant conditions, such as hepatomas and germ cell tumors, and in certain nonmalignant conditions, such as ataxia-telangiectasia
• To screen for the need for amniocentesis or high-resolution ultrasound in a pregnant woman

Patient preparation
• Explain to the patient that this test monitors response to therapy by measuring a specific blood protein. Advise her that she may need further testing.
• Tell her she needn't restrict food, fluids, or medications before the test.
• Tell her that this test requires a blood sample and who will perform the venipuncture and when. Reassure her that although she may experience discomfort, collecting the sample takes less than 3 minutes.

Procedure and posttest care
• Perform a venipuncture, and collect the sample in a 7-ml *red-top* tube.

• Record the patient's age, race, weight, and gestational period on the laboratory slip.
• If a hematoma develops at the venipuncture site, apply warm soaks.

Precautions
• Handle the sample gently.

Reference values
When testing by immunoassay, AFP values are 0 to 6.4 IU/ml in men and nonpregnant women. Values in maternal serum are shown in *Alpha-fetoprotein values for maternal serum,* page 288.

Abnormal findings
Elevated maternal serum AFP levels may suggest neural tube defect or other tube anomalies after 14 weeks' gestation. AFP levels rise sharply in approximately 90% of fetuses with anencephaly and in 50% of those with spina bifida. Definitive diagnosis requires ultrasonography and amniocentesis. High AFP levels may indicate intrauterine death. Sometimes, high levels indicate other anomalies such as duodenal atresia, omphalocele, tetralogy of Fallot, and Turner's syndrome.

Elevated serum AFP levels in nonpregnant patients may indicate hepatocellular carcinoma or germ cell tumor of gonadal, retroperitoneal, or mediastinal origin. Serum AFP rises in ataxia-telangiectasia and, sometimes, in cancer of the pancreas, the stomach, or the biliary system. Transient modest elevations can occur in nonneoplastic hepatocellular disease, such as alcoholic cirrhosis and acute or chronic hepatitis.

In hepatocellular carcinoma, a gradual decrease in serum AFP levels indicates a favorable response to therapy. In germ cell tumors, serum AFP levels and serum human chorionic gonadotropin levels should be measured concurrently.

ALPHA-FETOPROTEIN VALUES FOR MATERNAL SERUM

GESTATIONAL AGE (weeks)	MEDIAN VALUE (IU/ml)	MEDIAN VALUE (IU/ml)
	White women	Black women
14	19.9	23.2
15	23.2	26.9
16	27.0	31.1
17	31.5	35.9
18	36.7	41.6
19	42.7	48.0
20	49.8	55.6
21	58.1	64.2
22	67.8	74.2

TORCH TEST

This test helps detect exposure to pathogens involved in congenital and neonatal infections. TORCH is an acronym for toxoplasmosis, rubella, cytomegalovirus, syphilis, and herpes simplex. These pathogens are commonly associated with congenital or neonatal infections that are not clinically apparent and may cause severe central nervous system impairment. This test detects specific immunoglobulin M–associated antibodies in infant blood.

Purpose
• To aid diagnosis of acute, congenital, and intrapartum infections

Patient preparation
• Explain to the infant's parents the purpose of the test and mention that the test requires a blood sample.

• Tell them who will perform the venipuncture and when. Reassure them that although their child may experience transient discomfort, collecting the sample takes less than 3 minutes.

Procedure and posttest care
• Obtain a 3-ml sample of venous or cord blood.
• Send it to the laboratory promptly for serologic testing.
• If a hematoma develops at the venipuncture site, apply warm soaks.

Precautions
• Send the blood sample to the laboratory immediately.
• Don't freeze the sample.
• Handle the sample gently to prevent hemolysis.

Reference values
Normal test result is negative for TORCH agents.

Abnormal findings

Toxoplasmosis is diagnosed by sequential examination that shows rising antibody titers, changing titers, and serologic conversion from negative to positive; a titer of 1:256 suggests recent *Toxoplasma* infection.

In infants less than 6 months old, rubella infection is associated with a marked and persistent rise in complement-fixing antibody titer over time. Persistence of rubella antibody in an infant after age 6 months strongly suggests congenital infection. Congenital rubella is associated with cardiac anomalies, neurosensory deafness, growth retardation, and encephalitic symptoms. Detection of herpes antibodies in cerebrospinal fluid with signs of herpetic encephalitis and persistent herpesvirus type 2 antibody levels confirm herpes simplex infection in a neonate without obvious herpetic lesions.

TUBERCULIN SKIN TESTS

These skin tests are used to screen for previous infection by the tubercle bacillus. They are routinely performed in children, young adults, and patients with radiographic findings that suggest this infection. In both the old tuberculin (OT) and purified protein derivative (PPD) tests, intradermal injection of the tuberculin antigen causes a delayed hypersensitivity reaction in patients with active or dormant tuberculosis.

The Mantoux test employs a single-needle intradermal injection of PPD, permitting precise measurement of dosage. Multipuncture tests such as the tine test, Mono-Vacc tests, and Aplitest employ intradermal injections using tines impregnated with OT or PPD. Because they require less skill and are more rapidly administered, multipuncture tests are generally used for screening. However, a positive multipuncture test usually requires a Mantoux test for confirmation.

Purpose

• To distinguish tuberculosis from blastomycosis, coccidioidomycosis, and histoplasmosis
• To identify persons who need diagnostic investigation for tuberculosis

Patient preparation

• Explain to the patient that this test helps detect tuberculosis.
• Tell him the test requires an intradermal injection, which may cause him transient discomfort.
• Check the patient's history for active tuberculosis, the results of previous skin tests, or hypersensitivities.
• If the patient has had tuberculosis, don't perform a skin test.
• If he's had a positive reaction to previous skin tests, consult the doctor or follow hospital policy.
• If he's had an allergic reaction to acacia, don't perform an OT test, because this product contains acacia.
• If you're performing a tuberculin test on an outpatient, instruct him to return at the specified time so that test results can be read.
• Inform the patient that a positive reaction to a skin test appears as a red, hard, raised area at the injection site. Although the area may itch, instruct him not to scratch it.
• Stress that a positive reaction doesn't always indicate active tuberculosis.

Procedure and posttest care

• Ask the patient to sit and to support his extended arm on a flat surface.
• Clean the volar surface of the upper forearm with alcohol, and allow the area to dry completely.

• For a Mantoux test, perform an intradermal injection.

• For a multipuncture test, remove the protective cap on the injection device to expose the four tines.

• Hold the patient's forearm in one hand, stretching the skin of the forearm tightly. Then, with your other hand, firmly depress the device into the patient's skin, without twisting it.

• Hold the device in place for at least 1 second before removing it.

• If you've applied sufficient pressure, you'll see four puncture sites and a circular depression made by the device on the patient's skin.

• For both tests, record where the test was given, the date and time, and when it's to be read. Tuberculin skin tests are generally read 48 to 72 hours after injection; however, the Mono-Vacc test can be read 48 to 96 hours after the test.

• If ulceration or necrosis develops at the injection site, apply cold soaks or a topical steroid.

Precautions

• Tuberculin skin tests are contraindicated in patients with current reactions to smallpox vaccinations, any rash, skin disorder, or active tuberculosis.

• Don't perform a skin test in areas with excess hair, acne, or insufficient subcutaneous tissue, such as over a tendon or bone.

• If the patient is known to be hypersensitive to skin tests, use a first-strength dose in the Mantoux test to avoid necrosis at the puncture site.

• Have epinephrine available to treat a possible anaphylactoid or acute hypersensitivity reaction.

Normal findings

In tuberculin skin tests, normal findings show negative or minimal reactions. In the Mantoux test, no induration may appear, or the patient may develop induration of less than 5 mm in diameter.

In the tine and Aplitest tests, no vesiculation or induration may appear, or the patient may develop an induration of less than 2 mm in diameter. In the Mono-Vacc tests, there is no induration.

Abnormal findings

A positive tuberculin reaction indicates previous infection by tubercle bacilli. It does not distinguish between an active and dormant infection, nor does it provide a definitive diagnosis. If a positive reaction occurs, sputum smear and culture and chest radiography are necessary for further information.

In the Mantoux test, induration of 5 to 9 mm in diameter indicates a borderline reaction; larger induration, a positive reaction. Because patients infected with atypical mycobacteria other than tubercle bacilli may have borderline reactions, repeat testing is necessary.

In the tine or Aplitest tests, vesiculation indicates a positive reaction; induration of 2 mm in diameter without vesiculation requires confirmation by the Mantoux test. Any induration in the Mono-Vacc test indicates a positive reaction; however, it requires confirmation by the Mantoux test.

DELAYED HYPERSENSITIVITY SKIN TESTS

Skin testing is used to evaluate the cellular immune response of patients with severe recurrent infection, infection caused by unusual organisms, or suspected disorders associated with delayed hypersensitivity. Because diminished delayed hypersensitivity may be associated with a poor prognosis in patients with certain malignancies, this test may also be useful in determining prognosis in some cancer patients.

In skin tests, a small amount of antigen, or group of antigens, is injected intradermally or applied topically, and the test site is later examined for a visible reaction. Skin tests have only limited value in infants.

Purpose

• To evaluate primary and secondary immune responses

• To assess effectiveness of immunotherapy, when the patient's immune response is augmented by adjuvants

• To diagnose fungal diseases (coccidioidomycosis, histoplasmosis), bacterial diseases (tuberculosis, brucellosis, leprosy), and viral diseases (infectious mononucleosis)

• To monitor the course of certain diseases, such as Hodgkin's disease and coccidioidomycosis

Patient preparation

• Explain to the patient that this test evaluates the immune system after application or injection of small doses of antigens.

• Inform him he needn't restrict food or fluids before the test.

• Tell him who will perform the test and where.

• Explain that it takes about 10 minutes for each antigen to be administered and that reactions should appear in 48 to 72 hours.

• Explain that some antigens are readministered after 2 weeks or, if the test is negative, that a stronger dose of antigen may be given.

• Check the patient's history for hypersensitivity to any of the test antigens.

• If not listed in his history, ask the patient if he's had a skin test previously and, if so, what his reactions were.

• Check for previous bacille Calmette-Guérin vaccination or tuberculosis.

• If the patient's history reveals no sensitivity or hypersensitivity, it's appropriate to test with intermediate-strength antigens.

• If skin tests are to be performed, check the standardized hospital procedure.

• Because many antigens are approved by the Food and Drug Administration (FDA) for use as vaccines but not for skin testing, check with the pharmacy about FDA approval for this purpose.

• If the tests require the patient's informed consent, such as for use of dinitrochlorobenzene (DNCB) in research studies, check with the appropriate hospital committee for guidelines.

Procedure and posttest care

For the DNCB test:

• Wear gloves and a mask to avoid sensitizing yourself to DNCB.

• Dissolve DNCB in acetone.

• Position the patient's forearm comfortably, ventral side up, with his elbow slightly flexed.

• Clean a small, hairless area midway between the wrist and elbow with an alcohol swab, allow it to dry, and apply the prescribed amount of DNCB with a cotton swab.

• Allow this to dry, then cover the area with a sterile gauze pad for 24 to 48 hours.

• Instruct the patient to watch for a spontaneous flare reaction 10 to 14 days after application of DNCB. (If a reaction occurs, a lower dose of the test solution can be used for the challenge dose of DNCB.)

• After 14 days, apply a challenge dose of DNCB to the same spot and in the same manner.

• Inspect the site 48 to 96 hours after application of DNCB for reactivity.

• The challenge dose can be repeated 2 weeks later (1 month after the sensitizing dose) when test results are negative.

For the recall antigen test:
• Inject each antigen intradermally, using a separate tuberculin syringe, on the patient's forearm.
• Circle each injection site with a pen and label each according to the antigen given.
• Tell the patient to avoid washing off the circles until the test is completed.
• Inject the control allergy diluent on the other forearm.
• Inspect injection sites for reactivity after 48 and 72 hours.
• Record induration and erythema in millimeters.
• A negative test at the first concentration of antigen should be confirmed using a higher concentration.
• Watch the patient closely for severe local reactions at the test site, such as pain, blistering, swelling, induration, itching, and ulceration. Scarring or hyperpigmentation may result.
• Look for swelling and tenderness in the lymph nodes at the elbow or axillary region. Check for tachycardia and fever (rare). Symptoms generally appear in 15 to 30 minutes.
• Tell the patient experiencing hypersensitivity that steroids will control the reaction, but skin lesions may persist for 10 to 14 days. Instruct him to avoid scratching the affected area.

Precautions
• Store antigens in lyophilized (freeze-dried) form at 39.2° F (4° C), protected from light.
• Reconstitute them shortly before use, and check their expiration dates.
• If the patient is suspected of hypersensitivity to the antigens, apply them first in low concentrations.
• Because excess DNCB can burn the patient's skin, apply only the prescribed amount.
• If the forearms are not free from disease (for example, in a patient with atopic dermatitis), use other sites, such as the back.
• Observe the patient carefully for signs of anaphylactic shock, urticaria, respiratory distress, and hypotension. If such signs develop, administer epinephrine and notify the doctor immediately.

Normal findings
In the DNCB test, a positive reaction (erythema, edema, induration) appears 48 to 96 hours after the second (challenge) dose; 95% of the population reacts positively to DNCB. In the recall antigen test, a positive response (5 mm or more of induration at the test site) appears 48 hours after injection.

Abnormal findings
In the DNCB test, failure to react to the challenge dose indicates diminished delayed hypersensitivity. In the recall antigen test, a positive response to less than two of the six test antigens, a persistent unresponsiveness to intradermal injection of higher-strength antigens, or a generalized diminished reaction (causing less than 10 mm combined induration) indicates diminished delayed hypersensitivity.

Diminished delayed hypersensitivity can result from conditions such as Hodgkin's disease (common); sarcoidosis; liver disease; congenital immunodeficiency disease, such as DiGeorge's syndrome, ataxia-telangiectasia, and Wiskott-Aldrich syndrome; uremia; acute leukemia; viral diseases, such as influenza, infectious mononucleosis, measles, mumps, and rubella; fungal diseases, such as coccidioidomycosis and cryptococcosis; bacterial diseases, such as leprosy and tuberculosis; and terminal cancer. Diminished delayed hypersensitivity can also result from immunosuppressive or steroid therapy or viral vaccination.

CHAPTER 6

Urine Tests

VITAMINS

MINERALS

URINALYSIS

ROUTINE URINALYSIS

Routine urinalysis tests screen for urinary and systemic disorders. These tests evaluate physical characteristics (color, odor, and opacity) of urine; determine specific gravity and pH; detect and measure protein, glucose, and ketone bodies; and examine sediment for blood cells, casts, and crystals.

Diagnostic laboratory methods include visual examination, reagent strip screening, refractometry for specific gravity, and microscopic inspection of centrifuged sediment.

Purpose
• To screen patient's urine for renal or urinary tract disease
• To help detect metabolic or systemic disease unrelated to renal disorders

Patient preparation
• Explain to the patient that this test aids diagnosis of renal or urinary tract disease and helps evaluate overall body function.
• Inform him that food or fluids need not be restricted before the test.
• Check his medication history; many drugs may affect test results.

Procedure and posttest care
• Collect a random urine specimen of at least 15 ml.
• Obtain a first-voided morning specimen if possible.

Precautions
• Strain the specimen to catch stones or stone fragments if the patient is being evaluated for renal colic.

• Carefully pour the urine through an unfolded 4″ x 4″ gauze pad or a fine-mesh sieve placed over the specimen container.
• Send the specimen to the laboratory immediately.
• Refrigerate the specimen if analysis will be delayed longer than 1 hour.

Normal findings
See *Normal findings in routine urinalysis,* page 296.

Abnormal findings
Nonpathologic variations in normal values may result from diet, nonpathologic conditions, specimen collection time, and other factors.

Urine pH, which is greatly affected by diet and medications, influences the appearance of urine and the composition of crystals. An alkaline pH (above 7.0)—characteristic of a vegetarian diet—causes turbidity and the formation of phosphate, carbonate, and amorphous crystals. An acid pH (below 7.0)—typical of a high-protein diet—produces turbidity and the formation of oxalate, cystine, leucine, tyrosine, amorphous urate, and uric acid crystals.

Protein, normally absent from the urine, may be present in a benign condition known as orthostatic (postural) proteinuria. Most common in patients ages 10 to 20, this condition is intermittent, appears after prolonged standing, and disappears after recumbency. Transient benign proteinuria can also occur with fever, exposure to cold, emotional stress, or strenuous exercise.

Sugars, usually absent from the urine, may appear under normal conditions. The most common sugar in urine is glucose. Transient nonpathologic glycosuria may result from emotional stress or pregnancy and may follow ingestion of a high-carbohydrate meal.

Centrifuged urine sediment contains cells, casts, crystals, bacteria, yeast, and

NORMAL FINDINGS IN ROUTINE URINALYSIS

ELEMENT	FINDINGS
Macroscopic	
Color	Straw to dark yellow
Odor	Slightly aromatic
Appearance	Clear
Specific gravity	1.005 to 1.035
pH	4.5 to 8.0
Protein	None
Glucose	None
Ketone bodies	None
Bilirubin	None
Urobilinogen	Normal
Hemoglobin	None
Erythrocytes (RBCs)	None
Nitrite (Bacteria)	None
Leukocytes (WBCs)	None
Microscopic	
RBCs	0 to 2/high-power field
WBCs	0 to 5/high-power field
Epithelial cells	0 to 5/high-power field
Casts	None, except 1 to 2 hyaline casts/low-power field
Crystals	Present
Bacteria	None
Yeast cells	None
Parasites	None

parasites. Red blood cells (RBCs) don't often appear in urine without pathologic significance, but hard exercise can cause hematuria.

The following abnormal findings generally suggest pathologic conditions:

• *Color:* Color change can result from diet, drugs, and many diseases.

• *Odor:* In diabetes mellitus, starvation, and dehydration, a fruity odor accompanies formation of ketone bodies. In urinary tract infections, a fetid odor commonly is associated with *Escherichia coli.* Maple syrup urine disease and phenylketonuria also cause distinctive odors.

• *Turbidity:* Turbid urine may contain red or white cells, bacteria, fat, or chyle and may reflect renal infection.

• *Specific gravity:* Low specific gravity (< 1.005) is characteristic of diabetes insipidus, nephrogenic diabetes insipidus, acute tubular necrosis, and pyelonephritis. Fixed specific gravity, in which values remain 1.010 regardless of fluid intake, occurs in chronic glomerulonephritis with severe renal damage. High specific gravity (> 1.035) occurs in nephrotic syndrome, dehydration, acute glomerulonephritis, congestive heart failure, liver failure, and shock.

• *pH:* Alkaline urine pH may result from Fanconi's syndrome, urinary tract infection, and metabolic or respiratory alkalosis. Acid urine pH is associated with renal tuberculosis, pyrexia, phenylketonuria, alkaptonuria, and acidosis.

• *Protein:* Proteinuria suggests renal failure or disease (including nephrosis, glomerulosclerosis, glomerulonephritis, nephrolithiasis, and polycystic kidney disease), or possibly multiple myeloma.

• *Sugars:* Glycosuria usually indicates diabetes mellitus but may result from pheochromocytoma, Cushing's syndrome, impaired tubular reabsorption, advanced renal disease, and increased intracranial pressure. Fructosuria, galactosuria, and pentosuria generally suggest rare hereditary metabolic disorders (except for lactosuria during pregnancy and lactation). However, an alimentary form of pentosuria and fructosuria may follow excessive ingestion of pentose or fructose. When the liver fails

to metabolize these sugars, they spill into the urine because the renal tubules don't reabsorb them.

• *Ketone bodies:* Ketonuria occurs in diabetes mellitus when cellular energy needs exceed available cellular glucose. In the absence of glucose, cells metabolize fat for energy. Ketone bodies—the end products of incomplete fat metabolism—accumulate in plasma and are excreted in the urine. Ketonuria may also occur in starvation states and following diarrhea or vomiting.

• *Bilirubin:* Bilirubin in urine may occur in liver disease resulting from obstructive jaundice or hepatotoxic drugs or toxins, or from fibrosis of the biliary canaliculi (which may occur in cirrhosis).

• *Urobilinogen:* Bilirubin is changed into urobilinogen in the duodenum by intestinal bacteria. The liver reprocesses the remainder into bile. Increased urobilinogen in the urine may indicate liver damage, hemolytic disease, or severe infection. Decreased levels may occur with biliary obstruction, inflammatory disease, antimicrobial therapy, severe diarrhea, or renal insufficiency.

• *Cells:* Hematuria indicates bleeding within the genitourinary tract and may result from infection, obstruction, inflammation, trauma, tumors, glomerulonephritis, renal hypertension, lupus nephritis, renal tuberculosis, renal vein thrombosis, renal calculi, hydronephrosis, pyelonephritis, scurvy, malaria, parasitic infection of the bladder, subacute bacterial endocarditis, polyarteritis nodosa, and hemorrhagic disorders. Strenuous exercise or exposure to toxic chemicals may also cause hematuria. An excess of white cells in urine usually implies urinary tract inflammation, especially cystitis or pyelonephritis. White cells and white cell casts in urine suggest renal infection. Numerous epithelial cells suggest renal tubular degeneration.

• *Casts* (plugs of gelled proteinaceous material [high-molecular-weight mucoprotein]): Casts form in the renal tubules and collecting ducts by agglutination of protein cells or cellular debris and are flushed loose by urine flow. Excessive numbers of casts indicate renal disease. Hyaline casts are associated with renal parenchymal disease, inflammation, and trauma to the glomerular capillary membrane; epithelial casts, with renal tubular damage, nephrosis, eclampsia, amyloidosis, and heavy metal poisoning; coarse and fine granular casts, with acute or chronic renal failure, pyelonephritis, and chronic lead intoxication; fatty and waxy casts, with nephrotic syndrome, chronic renal disease, and diabetes mellitus; RBC casts, with renal parenchymal disease (especially glomerulonephritis), renal infarction, subacute bacterial endocarditis, vascular disorders, sickle cell anemia, scurvy, blood dyscrasias, malignant hypertension, collagen disease, and acute inflammation; and white blood cell casts, with acute pyelonephritis and glomerulonephritis, nephrotic syndrome, pyogenic infection, and lupus nephritis.

• *Crystals:* Some crystals normally appear in urine, but numerous calcium oxalate crystals suggest hypercalcemia. Cystine crystals (cystinuria) reflect an inborn error of metabolism.

• *Other components:* Bacteria, yeast cells, and parasites in urinary sediment reflect genitourinary tract infection or contamination of external genitalia. Yeast cells, which may be mistaken for red cells, are identifiable by their ovoid shape, lack of color, variable size, and frequently, signs of budding. The most common parasite in sediment is *Trichomonas vaginalis,* which causes vaginitis, urethritis, and prostatovesiculitis.

URINARY CALCULI

Urinary calculi (urinary stones) are insoluble substances most commonly formed of the mineral salts calcium oxalate, calcium phosphate, magnesium ammonium phosphate, urate, or cystine. They may appear anywhere in the urinary tract and range in size from microscopic to several centimeters.

Formation of calculi can result from reduced urinary volume, increased excretion of mineral salts, urinary stasis, pH changes, and decreased protective substances. Calculi commonly form in the kidney, pass into the ureter, and are excreted in the urine. Because not all calculi pass spontaneously, they may require surgical extraction. Calculi don't always cause symptoms, but when they do, hematuria is most common. If calculi obstruct the ureter, they may cause severe flank pain, dysuria, and urinary retention, frequency, and urgency.

Purpose
• To detect and identify calculi in the urine

Patient preparation
• Explain to the patient that this test detects urinary stones and that laboratory analysis will reveal their composition.
• Tell him that his urine will be collected and strained.
• Advise him that no prior restriction of food or fluids is required.
• Reassure him that symptoms will subside immediately after excretion of any stones.
• Inform him that medication to control pain will be administered.

Equipment

Strainer (an unfolded 4″ × 4″ dressing or a fine-mesh sieve), specimen container.

Procedure and posttest care

• Have the patient void into the strainer.
• Inspect the strainer carefully because calculi may be minute, looking like gravel or sand.
• Document the appearance of the calculi and the number if possible.
• Place the calculi in a properly labeled container.
• Send the container to the laboratory immediately for prompt analysis.
• Observe for severe flank pain, dysuria, and urinary retention, frequency, or urgency. Hematuria should subside.

Precautions

• Keep the strainer and urinal or bedpan within the patient's reach if he has received analgesics because he may be drowsy and unable to get out of bed to void.

Normal findings

Normally, calculi are not present in urine.

Abnormal findings

More than half of all calculi in urine are of mixed composition, containing two or more mineral salts; calcium oxalate is the most common component. Determination of the composition of calculi helps identify various metabolic disorders.

INULIN CLEARANCE

Inulin, a polysaccharide of fructose obtained from dahlias and artichokes, is metabolically inert within the body. When injected I.V., inulin is almost entirely filtered by the glomeruli but is reabsorbed by the tubules. Inulin clearance is, therefore, a precise measure of the glomerular filtration rate (GFR).

Despite its sensitivity and low incidence of adverse effects, the inulin clearance test is time-consuming, complex, and uncomfortable for the patient and thus is infrequently performed. Less accurate tests, such as urea and creatinine clearance, are used instead. Iothalamate ^{125}I can be substituted for inulin and usually follows the same procedure as inulin clearance. Because the iodine content is negligible, ^{125}I can be given to patients with iodine hypersensitivity but is contraindicated during pregnancy, lactation, and periods of growth.

Purpose

• To measure GFR
• To evaluate renal function

Patient preparation

• Explain to the patient that this test evaluates kidney function.
• Instruct him to fast for 4 hours before the test, to abstain from exercise the morning of the test, and to drink 1 liter of water 1 hour before the test.
• Encourage liquids during the test to maintain adequate urine flow.
• Tell him who will perform the test, that five blood samples and five urine specimens are required, and that he will receive an I.V. infusion of inulin, with a doctor in attendance.
• Reassure him that although he may experience transient discomfort from the venipunctures, collecting each sample takes less than 3 minutes.
• Advise him that he may feel bloated or have the urge to void during urine collection because a catheter will be in place for 2 hours.

Equipment
25 ml of 10% inulin and 500 ml of 1.5% inulin, five 10 ml *green-top* (heparinized) tubes, equipment for venipuncture, equipment for indwelling urinary catheterization, clamp, five urine specimen containers, I.V. pump, I.V. solution (250 ml of dextrose 5% in water, I.V. tubing with a Y-port).

Procedure and posttest care
• Perform a venipuncture, and collect 10 ml of blood in a *green-top* (heparinized) tube, to be used as a control sample.
• Catheterize the patient, make sure the bladder is empty, and save the urine for a baseline specimen.
• Infuse the recommended priming dose of 25 ml of 10% inulin by I.V. bolus over 4 minutes. Allow 30 minutes for distribution.
• Using an I.V. pump, infuse the maintenance solution of 500 ml of 1.5% inulin at a constant rate of 4 ml/minute.
• Tell the patient not to exert pressure on the arm with the I.V. site or to touch the control, and to notify you if he feels a burning sensation.
• Collect a urine specimen 30 minutes after starting the I.V., and three additional specimens at 20-minute intervals thereafter.
• Clamp the catheter between collections.
• Draw a blood sample at the midpoint of each 20-minute period and at the end of the test.
• Record the inulin dosage on the laboratory slip.
• Properly label each specimen, and include the collection time.
• Apply warm soaks if a hematoma develops at the venipuncture site.
• Elevate the arm, and apply warm soaks if phlebitis develops at the I.V. site.
• Be sure the patient voids within 8 to 10 hours after the catheter is removed.

• Tell him he can resume normal diet and activities.

Precautions
• Inulin clearance testing should be performed cautiously in patients with cardiac disease because increased fluid intake may cause congestive heart failure.
• Use the solution for I.V. bolus within 1 hour of preparation. Shake the ampul and heat it in boiling water to dissolve all crystals before administration. Then, cool to body temperature.
• Don't use the urine in the drainage bag if the patient already has a catheter in place. Empty the bag, and clamp the catheter for 1 hour before obtaining a baseline specimen.
• Handle blood samples gently to prevent hemolysis, and send specimens to the laboratory immediately after each collection.
• Refrigerate the urine specimen if more than 10 minutes will elapse before transportation.

Reference values
Inulin clearance is normally 90 to 130 ml/minute for age 21 and older, 86 to 126 ml/minute for ages 11 to 20, and 82 to 122 ml/minute from birth to age 10. Clearance may decrease as much as 45% after age 70.

Abnormal findings
Depressed clearance is characteristic in congestive heart failure, decreased renal blood flow, acute tubular necrosis, acute and chronic glomerulonephritis, advanced chronic bilateral pyelonephritis, nephrosclerosis, advanced bilateral renal lesions, bilateral ureteral obstruction, and dehydration.

PHENOLSULFON-PHTHALEIN EXCRETION

This test for evaluating kidney function is indicated in patients with abnormal results in the urine concentration test, one of the earliest signs of renal dysfunction.

Purpose
• To determine renal plasma flow
• To evaluate tubular function

Patient preparation
• Explain to the patient that this test evaluates kidney function.
• Inform him he needn't restrict food and encourage him to take fluids before and during the test to maintain adequate urine flow.
• Tell him the test requires an I.V. injection and collection of urine specimens 15 minutes, 30 minutes, 1 hour and, if ordered, 2 hours after the I.V. injection.
• Inform him who will administer the I.V. injection and when.
• Advise him that he may feel transient discomfort from the needle puncture and the pressure of the tourniquet and that the dye temporarily turns the urine red.
• If the patient is unable to void and requires catheterization, tell him that he may have the urge to void when the catheter is in place.
• Withhold drugs that may affect test results, such as chlorothiazide, aspirin, phenylbutazone, sulfonamides, penicillin, and probenecid. If they must be continued, note this on the laboratory slip.

Equipment
6 mg of phenolsulfonphthalein (PSP) dye in 1 ml solution, equipment for indwelling urinary catheterization, four urine specimen containers.

Procedure and posttest care
• Instruct the patient to empty his bladder, and discard the urine.
• The doctor will administer 1 ml of PSP, which equals 6 mg of dye, I.V.
• Collect a urine specimen at 15 minutes, 30 minutes, 1 hour and, if ordered, 2 hours after the injection.
• Because 40 ml of urine is required for each specimen, encourage fluid intake.
• If the patient is catheterized, make sure to clamp the catheter between collections.
• Record the PSP dosage on the laboratory slip.
• Properly label each specimen, and include the collection time.
• Elevate the arm and apply warm soaks if phlebitis develops at the I.V. site.
• If the patient is catheterized, make sure he voids within 8 to 10 hours after the catheter is removed.
• Resume administration of medications withheld during the test.

Precautions
• Use this test cautiously in a patient with cardiac dysfunction or renal insufficiency because the increased fluid intake necessary for proper hydration may precipitate congestive heart failure.
• Keep epinephrine available because allergic reactions to PSP occasionally occur.
• Don't use the urine in the drainage bag if the patient already has a catheter in place.
• Empty the bag, and clamp the catheter for 1 hour before the test.
• Send specimens to the laboratory immediately after each collection.
• Refrigerate the specimen if more than 10 minutes will elapse before transport.

Reference values

Normally, 25% of the PSP dose is excreted in 15 minutes, 50% to 60% in 30 minutes, 60% to 70% in 1 hour, and 70% to 80% in 2 hours. Normal excretion for children (excluding infants) is 5% to 10% higher than for adults.

Abnormal findings

The 15-minute value is the most sensitive indicator of both tubular function and renal plasma flow because depressed excretion at this interval but normal excretion at later ones suggests relatively mild or early-stage bilateral renal disease. However, a depressed 2-hour value may reveal moderate-to-severe renal impairment. Depressed PSP excretion is also characteristic in renal vascular disease, urinary tract obstruction, congestive heart failure, and gout.

Elevated PSP excretion is characteristic in hypoalbuminemia, hepatic disease, and multiple myeloma.

CONCENTRATION AND DILUTION TESTS

The kidneys normally concentrate or dilute urine according to fluid intake. When such intake is excessive, the kidneys excrete more water in the urine; when intake is limited, they excrete less. This test evaluates renal capacity to concentrate urine in response to fluid deprivation, or to dilute it in response to fluid overload.

Purpose

• To evaluate renal tubular function
• To detect renal impairment

Patient preparation

• Explain to the patient that this test evaluates kidney function.

• Tell him the test requires multiple urine specimens. Explain how many specimens will be collected and at what intervals.
• Instruct him to discard any urine voided during the night.
• Withhold diuretics as needed.
  For the concentration test:
• Provide a high-protein meal and only 200 ml of fluid the night before the test.
• Instruct the patient to restrict food and fluids for at least 14 hours. (Some concentration tests require that water be withheld for 24 hours but permit relatively normal food intake.)
• Limit salt intake at the evening meal to prevent excessive thirst.
• Emphasize to the patient that his cooperation is necessary to obtain accurate results.
  For the dilution test:
• Generally, this test directly follows the concentration test and necessitates no additional patient preparation. If it's performed alone, simply withhold breakfast.

Procedure and posttest care

Concentration test:
• Collect urine specimens at 6 a.m., 8 a.m., and 10 a.m.
  Dilution test:
• Instruct the patient to void and discard the urine.
• Give him 1,500 ml of water to drink within 30 minutes.
• Collect urine specimens every half hour or every hour for 4 hours thereafter.
  Both tests:
• Provide a balanced meal or a snack after collecting the final specimen.
• Make sure the patient voids within 8 to 10 hours after the catheter is removed.

Precautions

• Perform tests cautiously in patients with advanced renal disease or cardiac dysfunction because fluid overload can precipitate water intoxication, sodium diuresis, or congestive heart failure.

• Send each specimen to the laboratory immediately after collection.

• Provide the patient with a clean bedpan, urinal, or toilet specimen pan if he is unable to urinate into the specimen containers.

• Rinse the collection device after each use.

• If the patient is catheterized, empty the drainage bag before the test. Obtain the specimens from the catheter, and clamp the catheter between collections.

Reference values

Concentration test: Specific gravity ranges from 1.025 to 1.032 and osmolality rises above 800 mOsm/kg of water in patients with normal renal function.

Dilution test: Normally, specific gravity falls below 1.003 and osmolality below 100 mOsm/kg for at least one specimen; 80% or more of the ingested water is eliminated in 4 hours. In elderly persons, depressed values can be associated with normal renal function.

Abnormal findings

Decreased renal capacity to concentrate urine in response to fluid deprivation, or to dilute urine in response to fluid overload, may indicate tubular epithelial damage, decreased renal blood flow, loss of functional nephrons, or pituitary or cardiac dysfunction.

TUBULAR REABSORPTION OF PHOSPHATE

This test is an indirect measure of parathyroid hormone (PTH) levels. PTH helps maintain optimum blood levels of ionized calcium and controls renal excretion of calcium and phosphate. In this test urine and serum phosphate and creatinine are measured and these values are used to calculate the tubular reabsorption of phosphate.

Purpose

• To evaluate parathyroid function

• To aid diagnosis of primary hyperparathyroidism

• To distinguish between hypercalcemia due to hyperparathyroidism and hypercalcemia due to other causes

Patient preparation

• Explain to the patient that this test evaluates the function of the parathyroid glands.

• Advise him that the test requires a blood sample and urine collection over a 24-hour period.

• Tell the patient who will perform the venipuncture and when.

• Advise the patient that he may experience transient discomfort from the needle puncture and the pressure of the tourniquet.

• Reassure him that collecting the blood sample generally takes less than 3 minutes.

• Instruct the patient to maintain a normal phosphate diet for 3 days before the test because low phosphate intake (less than 500 mg/day) may elevate tubular reabsorption values and a high-phosphate diet (3,000 mg/day) may lower them. Common nutritional sources of phosphorus include legumes, nuts, milk, egg yolks, meat, poultry, fish, cereals, and cheese. These foods should be eaten in moderate amounts.

• Instruct the patient to fast after midnight the night before the test.

• As necessary, withhold drugs, such as amphotericin B, chlorothiazide diuretics, furosemide, and gentamicin, that may influence test results. If these medications must be continued throughout the test period, note this on the laboratory slip.

Procedure and posttest care
• Perform a venipuncture, and collect the sample in a 10-ml *red-top* tube.
• Instruct the patient to empty his bladder, and discard the urine; record this as time zero.
• Collect the patient's urine over a 24-hour period; occasionally, a 4-hour collection is ordered instead.
• Allow the patient to eat, and encourage fluid intake to maintain adequate urine flow after the venipuncture.
• Apply warm soaks if a hematoma develops at the venipuncture site.
• Resume administration of medications withheld during the test.
• Tell the patient that he may resume his usual diet.

Precautions
• Handle the collection tube gently to prevent hemolysis, and send it to the laboratory immediately.
• Keep the urine specimen container refrigerated or on ice during the collection period.
• Tell the patient to avoid contaminating the specimen with toilet paper or stool.
• Label the specimen and send it to the laboratory immediately at the end of the collection period.

Normal findings
Renal tubules normally reabsorb 80% or more of phosphate.

Abnormal findings
Reabsorption of less than 74% of phosphate strongly suggests primary hyperparathyroidism. Hypercalcemia is the most common manifestation of primary hyperparathyroidism. However, a patient with hypercalcemia may still re-

quire additional testing to confirm primary hyperparathyroidism as the cause.

Depressed reabsorption occurs in a small number of patients with renal calculi who do not have parathyroid tumor. Also, about one-fifth of patients with parathyroid tumor exhibit normal reabsorption.

Increased reabsorption of phosphate may result from uremia, renal tubular disease, osteomalacia, sarcoidosis, and myeloma.

ENZYMES

AMYLASE

Amylase is a starch-splitting enzyme produced primarily in the pancreas and salivary glands, which is usually secreted into the alimentary tract and absorbed into the blood; small amounts of amylase are also absorbed into the blood directly from these organs. Following glomerular filtration, amylase is excreted in the urine.

In the presence of adequate renal function, serum and urine levels usually rise in tandem. However, within 2 or 3 days of onset of acute pancreatitis, serum amylase levels fall to normal, but elevated urine amylase persists for 7 to 10 days. One method for determining urine amylase levels is the dye-coupled starch method.

Purpose
• To diagnose acute pancreatitis when serum amylase levels are normal or borderline
• To aid diagnosis of chronic pancreatitis and salivary gland disorders

SERUM AND URINE AMYLASE VALUES IN ACUTE PANCREATITIS

SERUM	URINE
Normal	
• 138 to 404 amylase units/liter (Mayo Clinic)	• 10 to 80 amylase units/hour (Mayo Clinic)
Elevation	
• Rises rapidly within 3 to 6 hours after onset of attack • May rise to 40 times normal value • Increase not proportional to severity of attack	• Reflects rise in serum level, but lags 6 to 10 hours
Duration	
• Peaks 20 to 30 hours after onset • Returns to normal level within 2 or 3 days, although active inflammation of pancreas may persist • Persistent elevation suggests pseudocyst, necrosis, or renal disease that inhibits amylase excretion.	• Elevation persists for 7 to 10 days. • Allows retrospective diagnosis of acute or relapsing pancreatitis when serum level registers in normal range • Persistent elevation in the absence of renal disease suggests pseudocyst formation.

Patient preparation
• Explain to the patient that this test evaluates the function of the pancreas and the salivary glands.
• Inform him that he needn't restrict food or fluids.
• Tell him the test requires urine collection for 2, 6, 8, or 24 hours, and teach him how to collect a timed specimen.
• Advise him that the laboratory requires 2 days to complete the analysis.
• Withhold morphine, meperidine, codeine, pentazocine, bethanechol, thiazide diuretics, indomethacin, and alcohol for 24 hours before the test. If these medications must be continued, note this on the laboratory slip.

Procedure and posttest care
• Collect the patient's urine over a 2-, 6-, 8-, or 24-hour period.

Precautions
• If a woman is menstruating, the test may have to be rescheduled.
• Cover and refrigerate the specimen during the collection period.
• If the patient is catheterized, keep the collection bag on ice.
• Instruct the patient not to contaminate the specimen with toilet tissue or stool.
• Send the specimens to the laboratory immediately when the test is completed.

Reference values
Because urine amylase is reported in various units of measure, values differ from laboratory to laboratory. The Mayo Clinic reports urinary excretion of 10 to 80 amylase units/hour as normal.

Abnormal findings
Elevated amylase levels occur in acute pancreatitis; obstruction of the pancre-

atic duct, intestines, or salivary duct; carcinoma of the head of the pancreas; mumps; acute injury of the spleen; renal disease, with impaired absorption; perforated peptic or duodenal ulcers; and gallbladder disease. (See *Serum and urine amylase values in acute pancreatitis*, page 305.)

Depressed levels occur in pancreatitis, cachexia, alcoholism, cancer of the liver, cirrhosis, hepatitis, hepatic abscess.

ARYLSULFATASE A

Arylsulfatase A (ARSA), a lysosomal enzyme found in every cell except the mature erythrocyte, is principally active in the liver, the pancreas, and the kidneys, where exogenous substances are detoxified into ester sulfates.

Urine ARSA levels rise in transitional bladder cancer, colorectal cancer, and leukemia. However, research hasn't resolved whether elevated ARSA levels provoke malignant growths or are simply an enzymatic response to their presence. This test measures urine ARSA levels by colorimetric or kinetic techniques.

Purpose
• To aid diagnosis of cancer of the bladder, the colon, or the rectum; of myeloid (granulocytic) leukemia; and of metachromatic leukodystrophy (an inherited lipid storage disease)

Patient preparation
• Tell the patient that this test measures an enzyme that's present throughout the body.
• Advise him that he needn't restrict food or fluids before the test.
• Tell him the test requires urine collection over a 24-hour period, and teach him how to collect a timed specimen.

• Advise him that test results are generally available in 2 or 3 days.

Procedure and posttest care
• Collect the patient's urine over a 24-hour period.

Precautions
• If a woman is menstruating, the test may have to be rescheduled.
• Tell the patient not to contaminate the urine specimen with toilet tissue or stool.
• Keep the collection container refrigerated or on ice during the collection period.
• Send the specimens to the laboratory immediately at the end of the collection period.
• If the patient has an indwelling urinary catheter in place, keep the collection bag on ice for the duration of the test.
• Change the continuous urinary drainage apparatus before beginning the test.

Reference values
Normal ARSA values are as follows:
• Men: 1.4 to 19.3 U/liter
• Women: 1.4 to 11 U/liter
• Children: over 1 U/liter.

Abnormal findings
Elevated ARSA levels may result from cancer of the bladder, the colon, or the rectum or from myeloid leukemia.

Depressed ARSA levels can result from metachromatic leukodystrophy. In patients with this condition, urine studies show metachromatic granules in the urinary sediment.

LYSOZYME

Lysozyme (or muramidase), a low-molecular-weight enzyme, is present in mucus, saliva, tears, skin secretions, and various internal body cells and fluids. This enzyme splits, or lyses, the cell walls of gram-positive bacteria and, with complement and other blood factors, acts to destroy them. Lysozyme seems to be synthesized in granulocytes and monocytes, and it first appears in serum after destruction of such cells. When serum lysozyme levels exceed three times normal, the enzyme appears in the urine. However, since renal tissue also contains lysozyme, renal injury alone can cause measurable excretion of this enzyme.

This test measures urine lysozyme levels turbidimetrically. Serum lysozyme determinations, using the same method, confirm the results of urine testing.

Purpose
• To aid diagnosis of acute monocytic or granulocytic leukemia and to monitor the progression of these diseases
• To evaluate proximal tubular function and to diagnose renal impairment
• To detect rejection or infarction of kidney transplantation

Patient preparation
• Explain to the patient that this test evaluates renal function and the immune system.
• Advise him that he needn't restrict food or fluids before the test.
• Tell him the test requires collection of urine over a 24-hour period and teach him how to collect the specimen correctly.
• Tell him that test results should be available in 1 day.

Procedure and posttest care
• Collect the patient's urine over a 24-hour period.

Precautions
• If a woman is menstruating, the test may have to be rescheduled for a later date.
• Tell the patient to avoid contaminating the urine specimen with toilet tissue or stool.
• Cover and refrigerate the specimen throughout the collection period.
• Keep the collection bag on ice if the patient has an indwelling urinary catheter in place.
• Send the specimens to the laboratory immediately when the test is completed.

Reference values
Normally, urine lysozyme values are less than 3 mg/24 hours.

Abnormal findings
Elevated urine lysozyme levels are characteristic of impaired renal proximal tubular reabsorption, acute pyelonephritis, nephrotic syndrome, tuberculosis of the kidney, severe extrarenal infection, rejection or infarction of kidney transplantation (levels normally increase during first few days after transplantation), and polycythemia vera.

Urine levels rise markedly after acute onset or relapse of monocytic or myelomonocytic leukemia and rise moderately after acute onset or relapse of granulocytic (myeloid) leukemia.

Urine lysozyme levels remain normal or decrease in lymphocytic leukemia and remain normal in myeloblastic and myelocytic leukemias.

CYCLIC ADENOSINE MONOPHOSPHATE

Formed from adenosine triphosphate by the action of the enzyme adenylate cyclase, the nucleotide cyclic adenosine monophosphate (cAMP) influences the protein synthesis rate within cells. Measurement of urinary excretion of cAMP after I.V. infusion of a standard dose of parathyroid hormone can show renal tubular resistance in a patient with hypoparathyroid symptoms and high levels of parathyroid hormone. Such findings suggest Type I pseudohypoparathyroidism, a rare inherited disorder. (Urinary cAMP levels respond normally with Type II pseudohypoparathyroidism because the defect is beyond the level of cAMP generation.)

Purpose
• To aid differential diagnosis of pseudohypoparathyroidism

Patient preparation
• Explain to the patient that this test evaluates parathyroid function.
• Tell him the test requires a 15-minute I.V. infusion of parathyroid hormone and a 3- to 4-hour urine specimen collection.
• Perform a skin test to detect a possible allergy to parathyroid hormone; keep epinephrine readily available in case of an adverse reaction.
• Just before the procedure is performed, instruct the patient not to touch the I.V. or exert pressure on the arm receiving the infusion.
• Tell him he may experience transient discomfort from the needle puncture. Ask him to notify you if he feels severe burning or if the site becomes inflamed or swollen.

Equipment
Parathyroid hormone (300 units, in refrigerated ampules), vial of sterile water (saline solution causes precipitate to form), urine collection container with hydrochloric acid added as a preservative.

Procedure and posttest care
• Instruct the patient to empty his bladder.
• If the patient has an indwelling urinary catheter in place, change the collection bag.
• Send this specimen to the laboratory if ordered; otherwise, discard it.
• Prepare the parathyroid hormone for infusion as directed, using sterile water for dilution.
• Start the I.V. with dextrose 5% in water, and infuse the parathyroid hormone over 15 minutes. Record the start of the I.V. as time zero.
• Collect a urine specimen 3 to 4 hours after infusion.
• Discontinue the I.V.
• Observe the patient for symptoms of hypercalcemia, including lethargy, anorexia, nausea, vomiting, vertigo, and abdominal cramps.
• Apply warm soaks if a hematoma or irritation develops at the venipuncture site.

Precautions
• This test is contraindicated in patients with high calcium levels (because parathyroid hormone further raises calcium levels).
• Measurement of cAMP should be performed cautiously in patients receiving a digitalis glycoside and in those with sarcoidosis or renal or cardiac disease.
• Tell the patient to avoid contaminating the urine specimen with toilet tissue or stool.
• Send the specimen to the laboratory immediately; if transport is delayed, refrigerate the specimen.
• Keep the collection bag on ice if the patient has a catheter in place.

Reference values
A ten- to twentyfold increase (3.6 to 4 micromoles) in cAMP demonstrates a normal response or hypoparathyroidism.

Abnormal findings

Failure to respond to parathyroid hormone, indicated by normal urinary excretion of cAMP, suggests Type I pseudohypoparathyroidism.

HORMONES

ALDOSTERONE

This test measures urine levels of aldosterone, the principal mineralocorticoid secreted by the adrenal cortex. Aldosterone promotes retention of sodium and excretion of potassium by the renal tubules, thereby helping to regulate blood pressure and fluid and electrolyte balance. In turn, aldosterone secretion is controlled by the renin-angiotensin system. This feedback mechanism is vital to maintaining fluid and electrolyte balance.

Urine aldosterone levels, measured through radioimmunoassay, are usually evaluated after measurement of serum electrolyte and renin levels.

Purpose

• To aid diagnosis of primary and secondary aldosteronism

Patient preparation

• Explain to the patient that this test evaluates hormonal balance.
• Instruct him to maintain a normal sodium diet (3 g/day) before the test and to avoid sodium-rich foods, such as bacon, barbecue sauce, corned beef, bouillon cubes or powder, and olives.
• Advise him to avoid strenuous physical exercise and stressful situations during the collection period.

• Tell him the test requires collection of urine during a 24-hour period, and teach him the proper collection technique.
• Check the patient's medication history for drugs that may affect aldosterone levels, including antihypertensives, diuretics, and corticosteroids. Review your findings with the laboratory, and then notify the doctor; he may want to restrict these medications before the test.

Procedure and posttest care

• Collect the patient's urine over a 24-hour period. Use a bottle containing a preservative to keep the specimen at a pH of 4.0 to 4.5.
• Resume administration of medications withheld during the test.
• Tell the patient he may resume normal physical activity that was restricted before the test.

Precautions

• Refrigerate the specimen or place it on ice during the collection period.
• Send the specimen to the laboratory immediately after the collection is completed.

Reference values

Normally, urine aldosterone levels range from 2 to 16 mcg/24 hours.

Abnormal findings

Elevated urine aldosterone levels suggest primary or secondary aldosteronism. The primary form usually arises from an aldosterone-secreting adenoma of the adrenal cortex but may also result from adrenocortical hyperplasia. Secondary aldosteronism, the more common form, results from external stimulation of the adrenal cortex, such as that produced when the renin-angiotensin system is activated by hypertensive and edematous disorders.

Disorders that may result in secondary aldosteronism are malignant hypertension, congestive heart failure, cirrhosis of the liver, nephrotic syndrome, and idiopathic cyclic edema.

Low urine aldosterone levels may result from Addison's disease, salt-losing syndrome, and toxemia of pregnancy. These levels normally rise during pregnancy but rapidly decline following parturition.

FREE CORTISOL

Used as a screen for adrenocortical hyperfunction, this test measures urine levels of the portion of cortisol not bound to the corticosteroid-binding globulin transcortin. It is one of the best diagnostic tools for detecting Cushing's syndrome.

Radioimmunoassay determinations of free cortisol levels in a 24-hour urine specimen, unlike a single measurement of plasma cortisol, reflect overall secretion levels instead of diurnal variations. Concurrent measurements of plasma cortisol and corticotropin, with urine 17-hydroxycorticosteroids and the dexamethasone suppression test, may be used to confirm diagnosis.

Purpose
• To aid diagnosis of Cushing's syndrome

Patient preparation
• Explain to the patient that this test helps evaluate adrenal gland function.
• Advise him that he should maintain food and fluid intake before the test but should avoid stressful situations and excessive physical exercise during the collection period.
• Tell him the test requires collection of urine over a 24-hour period.

• Teach him the proper collection technique for a 24-hour urine specimen.
• Check the patient's recent drug history for medications that may interfere with test results, including steroids, reserpine, phenothiazines, and amphetamines. Review your findings with the laboratory; then notify the doctor.

Procedure and posttest care
• Collect the patient's urine over a 24-hour period. Use a bottle containing a preservative to keep the specimen at a pH of 4.0 to 4.5.
• Tell the patient he may resume normal activity restricted during the test.
• Resume administration of medications withheld during the test.

Precautions
• Refrigerate the specimen or place it on ice during the collection period.

Reference values
Normally, free cortisol values range from 24 to 108 mcg/24 hours.

Abnormal findings
Elevated free cortisol levels may indicate Cushing's syndrome resulting from adrenal hyperplasia, adrenal or pituitary tumor, or ectopic corticotropin production. Hepatic disease and obesity, which can raise plasma cortisol levels, generally don't appreciably raise urine levels of free cortisol. Low levels have little diagnostic significance and don't necessarily indicate adrenocortical hypofunction.

CATECHOLAMINES

This test uses spectrophotofluorometry to measure urine levels of the major catecholamines—epinephrine, norepinephrine, and dopamine. Epinephrine is secreted by the adrenal medulla; dopamine, by the central nervous system; and norepinephrine, by both. Catecholamines help regulate metabolism and prepare the body for the fight-or-flight response to stress. Certain tumors can also secrete catecholamines.

The specimen of choice for this test is a 24-hour urine specimen because catecholamine secretion fluctuates diurnally and in response to pain, heat, cold, emotional stress, physical exercise, hypoglycemia, injury, hemorrhage, asphyxia, and drugs. However, a random specimen may be useful for evaluating catecholamine levels after a hypertensive episode.

For a complete diagnostic workup of catecholamine secretion, urine levels of catecholamine metabolites are measured concurrently. These metabolites — metanephrine, normetanephrine, homovanillic acid (HVA), and vanillylmandelic acid (VMA) — normally appear in the urine in greater quantities than the catecholamines.

Purpose
• To aid diagnosis of pheochromocytoma in a patient with unexplained hypertension
• To aid diagnosis of neuroblastoma, ganglioneuroma, and dysautonomia

Patient preparation
• Explain to the patient that this test evaluates adrenal function.
• Inform him that he needn't restrict food or fluids before the test but should avoid stressful situations and excessive physical activity during the collection period.
• Tell him that either a specimen collected over 24 hours or a random specimen is required, and explain the collection procedure.
• Check the patient's drug history for medications that may affect catecholamine levels, including caffeine, insulin, nitroglycerin, aminophylline, ethanol,

sympathomimetics, methyldopa, tricyclic antidepressants, chloral hydrate, quinidine, quinine, tetracycline, B-complex vitamins, isoproterenol, levodopa, and monoamine oxidase inhibitors. Review your findings with a laboratory technician, and then notify the doctor; he may want to restrict such medications before the test.

Procedure and posttest care
• Collect the patient's urine over a 24-hour period. Use a bottle containing a preservative to keep the specimen acidified to a pH of 3.0 or less. (If a random specimen is ordered, collect it immediately after a hypertensive episode.)
• Tell the patient that he may resume activity restricted during the test.
• Resume administration of medications withheld before the test.

Precautions
• Refrigerate a 24-hour specimen or place it on ice during the collection period.
• Send the specimen to the laboratory immediately at the end of the collection period.

Reference values
Normally, urine catecholamine values range from undetectable to 135 mcg/24 hours or from undetectable to 18 mcg/dl in a random specimen.

Abnormal findings
In a patient with undiagnosed hypertension, elevated urine catecholamine levels following a hypertensive episode usually indicate a pheochromocytoma. If tests indicate a pheochromocytoma, the patient may also be tested for multiple endocrine neoplasia. With the exception of HVA — a metabolite of dopamine — catecholamine metabolites may also be elevated. Abnormally high HVA levels rule out a pheochromocytoma, because this tumor mainly

secretes epinephrine, whose primary metabolite is VMA, not HVA.

Elevated catecholamine levels, without marked hypertension, may be due to a neuroblastoma or a ganglioneuroma, although HVA levels reflect these conditions more accurately. Myasthenia gravis and progressive muscular dystrophy commonly cause urine catecholamine levels to rise above normal, but this test is rarely performed to diagnose these disorders. Consistently low-normal catecholamine levels may indicate dysautonomia, marked by orthostatic hypotension.

TOTAL URINE ESTROGENS

This test is a quantitative analysis of total urine levels of estradiol, estrone, and estriol — the major estrogens present in significant amounts in urine. A common method for measuring total urine estrogen levels involves purification by gel filtration, followed by spectrophotofluorometry. Supplementary tests that may provide further information about ovarian function include cytologic examination of vaginal smears, measurement of urine levels of pregnanediol and follicle-stimulating hormone, and evaluation of response to an injection of progesterone.

Purpose
• To evaluate ovarian activity and help determine the cause of amenorrhea and female hyperestrogenism
• To aid diagnosis of tumors of ovarian, adrenocortical, or testicular origin
• To assess fetoplacental status

Patient preparation
• Explain to the female patient that this test helps evaluate ovarian function; to the pregnant patient that this test helps evaluate fetal development and placental function; and to the male patient that this test helps evaluate testicular function.
• Inform the patient that the test requires collection of urine over a 24-hour period.
• Advise her that no pretest restrictions of food or fluids are necessary.
• If the 24-hour specimen is to be collected at home, teach the patient the proper collection technique.
• Check the patient's medication history for use of drugs that may influence estrogen levels, including steroid hormones, methenamine mandelate, phenazopyridine hydrochloride, phenothiazines, tetracyclines, phenolphthalein, ampicillin, meprobamate, senna, cascara sagrada, and hydrochlorothiazide.

Procedure and posttest care
• Collect the patient's urine over a 24-hour period. Use a bottle containing a preservative to keep the specimen at a pH of 3.0 to 5.0.
• If the patient is pregnant, note the approximate week of gestation on the laboratory slip.
• If the patient is a nonpregnant female, note the stage of her menstrual cycle.
• Resume administration of medications withheld before the test.

Precautions
• Refrigerate the specimen or keep it on ice during the collection period.

Reference values
In nonpregnant females, total urine estrogen levels rise and fall during the menstrual cycle, peaking shortly before midcycle, decreasing immediately following ovulation, increasing through the life of the corpus luteum, and de-

creasing greatly as the corpus luteum degenerates and menstruation begins.

Normal values for nonpregnant females are as follows: preovulatory phase, 5 to 25 mcg/24 hours; ovulatory phase, 24 to 100 mcg/24 hours; luteal phase, 12 to 80 mcg/24 hours.

In postmenopausal females, values are less than 10 mcg/24 hours; in males, from 4 to 25 mcg/24 hours.

Abnormal findings

Decreased total urine estrogen levels may reflect ovarian agenesis, primary ovarian insufficiency (due to Stein-Leventhal syndrome, for example), or secondary ovarian insufficiency (due to pituitary or adrenal hypofunction or metabolic disturbances).

Elevated total estrogen levels in nonpregnant females may indicate tumors of ovarian or adrenocortical origin, adrenocortical hyperplasia, or a metabolic or hepatic disorder. In males, elevated total estrogen levels are associated with testicular tumors.

Elevated total urine estrogen levels are normal during pregnancy; serial determinations should show a rising titer.

PLACENTAL ESTRIOL

This test monitors fetal viability by measuring urine levels of placental estriol, the predominant estrogen excreted in urine during pregnancy. A steady rise in estriol reflects a properly functioning placenta and, in most cases, a healthy, growing fetus. Normally, estriol is secreted in much smaller amounts by the ovaries in nonpregnant females, by the testes in males, and by the adrenal cortex in both sexes.

The usual clinical indication for this test is high-risk pregnancy. Serial testing is necessary to plot the expected rise in estriol levels, or to show the absence of such a rise. The specimen of choice for this test is a 24-hour urine specimen because estriol levels fluctuate diurnally. Radioimmunoassay is the usual test method. Generally, serum estriol levels are considered more reliable than urine levels.

Purpose

• To assess fetoplacental status, especially in high-risk pregnancy, such as one complicated by maternal hypertension, diabetes mellitus, preeclampsia, toxemia, or a history of stillbirth

Patient preparation

• Explain to the patient that this test helps determine if the placenta is functioning properly, which is essential to the health of the fetus.

• Tell her she needn't restrict food or fluids.

• Advise her that this test requires urine collection over a 24-hour period, and instruct her how to collect the specimen. Emphasize that proper collection technique is necessary for results to be valid.

• Check the patient's medication history for use of drugs that may affect urine estriol levels, including steroid hormones, methenamine mandelate, phenothiazines, phenazopyridine hydrochloride, tetracyclines, phenolphthalein, ampicillin, meprobamate, senna, cascara sagrada, and hydrochlorothiazide.

Procedure and posttest care

• Collect the patient's urine over a 24-hour period. Use a bottle containing a preservative to keep the specimen at a pH of 3.0 to 5.0.

• Send the specimen to the laboratory. If the patient is pregnant, note the week of gestation on the laboratory slip.

• Resume administration of medications withheld during the test.

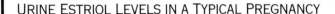

URINE ESTRIOL LEVELS IN A TYPICAL PREGNANCY

Urine estriol rises as normal gestation proceeds. Significant changes in serial urine determinations suggest abnormal conditions that may require prompt medical intervention.

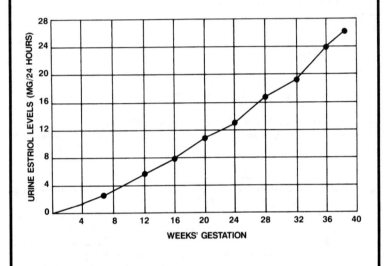

Precautions
• Refrigerate the specimen or keep it on ice during the collection period.

Reference values
Normal values vary considerably, but serial measurements of urine estriol levels, when plotted on a graph, should describe a steadily rising curve. (See *Urine estriol levels in a typical pregnancy.*)

Abnormal findings
A 40% drop from baseline values that occurs on 2 consecutive days strongly suggests placental insufficiency and impending fetal distress. A 20% drop over 2 weeks or failure of consecutive estriol levels to rise in a normal curve similarly indicates inadequate placental function and undesirable fetal status. These developments may necessitate cesarean section, depending on the patient's condition and other apparent signs of fetal distress.

A chronically low urine estriol curve may result from fetal adrenal insufficiency, congenital anomalies (such as anencephaly), Rh isoimmunization, or placental sulfatase deficiency.

A high-risk pregnancy in which maternal glomerular filtration rate decreases may cause a low-normal estriol curve. Such a pregnancy may occur in a patient with hypertension or diabetes mellitus, for example. The pregnancy may continue, as long as no complications develop and estriol levels continue to rise. However, falling estriol levels or a sudden drop from baseline values indicates severe fetal distress.

High urine estriol levels may occur in multiple pregnancy.

HUMAN CHORIONIC GONADOTROPIN

Qualitative analysis of urine levels of human chorionic gonadotropin (hCG) allows for detection of pregnancy as early as 10 days after a missed menstrual period. Production of hCG, a glycoprotein, which prevents degeneration of the corpus luteum at the end of the normal menstrual cycle, begins after conception. During the first trimester, hCG levels rise steadily and rapidly, peaking around the 10th week of gestation, subsequently tapering off to less than 10% of peak levels.

The most common method of evaluating hCG in urine is hemagglutination inhibition. This laboratory procedure can provide both qualitative and quantitative information. The qualitative urine test is easier and less expensive than the serum hCG test (beta-subunit assay); therefore it's used more frequently to detect pregnancy.

Purpose
• To detect and confirm pregnancy
• To aid diagnosis of hydatidiform mole or hCG-secreting tumors

Patient preparation
• If appropriate, explain to the patient that this test determines whether she is pregnant or the status of her pregnancy. Alternatively, explain how the test functions as a screen for some types of cancer.
• Tell her she needn't restrict food or fluids before the test.

• Inform her that the test requires a first-voided morning specimen or urine collection over a 24-hour period, depending on whether the test is qualitative or quantitative.
• Check the patient's recent medication history for use of drugs that may affect hCG levels, including phenothiazines.

Procedure and posttest care
• For verification of pregnancy (qualitative analysis), collect a first-voided morning specimen. If this is not possible, collect a random specimen.
• For quantitative analysis of hCG, collect the patient's urine over a 24-hour period.
• Specify the date of the patient's last menstrual period on the laboratory slip.
• Resume administration of medications withheld during the test.

Precautions
• Refrigerate the 24-hour specimen or keep it on ice during the collection period.

Reference values
In qualitative analysis, if agglutination fails to occur, test results are positive, indicating pregnancy. In quantitative analysis, urine hCG levels in the first trimester of a normal pregnancy may be as high as 500,000 IU/24 hours; in the second trimester, they range from 10,000 to 25,000 IU/24 hours; and in the third trimester, from 5,000 to 15,000 IU/24 hours. After delivery, hCG levels decline rapidly and within a few days are undetectable.

Measurable hCG levels don't normally appear in the urine of men or nonpregnant women.

Abnormal findings
During pregnancy, elevated urine hCG levels may indicate multiple pregnancy or erythroblastosis fetalis; depressed

urine hCG levels may indicate threatened abortion or ectopic pregnancy.

Measurable levels of hCG in males and nonpregnant females may indicate choriocarcinoma, ovarian or testicular tumors, melanoma, multiple myeloma, or gastric, hepatic, pancreatic, or breast cancer.

METABOLITES

PREGNANETRIOL

Using spectrophotometry, this test determines urine levels of pregnanetriol, the metabolite of the cortisol precursor 17-hydroxyprogesterone. Pregnanetriol is normally excreted in the urine in minute amounts. However, when cortisol biosynthesis is impaired at the point of 17-hydroxyprogesterone conversion, urinary excretion of pregnanetriol rises significantly.

Elevated urine pregnanetriol levels suggest adrenogenital syndrome. Urine 17-ketosteroids and urine 17-ketogenic steroids may be measured concurrently to assess androgen levels. Elevated androgen levels are characteristic of adrenogenital syndrome (congenital adrenal hyperplasia).

Purpose
• To aid diagnosis of adrenogenital syndrome
• To monitor cortisol replacement

Patient preparation
• Explain to the patient (or to his parents if the patient is a child) that this test evaluates hormonal secretion.
• Inform him that he need not restrict food or fluids before the test.

• Tell him the test requires collection of urine over a 24-hour period, and teach him the proper collection technique.

Procedure and posttest care
• Collect the patient's urine over a 24-hour period. Use a bottle containing a preservative to keep the specimen at a pH of 4.0 to 4.5.

Precautions
• Refrigerate the specimen or keep it on ice during the collection period.
• Send the specimen to the laboratory immediately after the collection is completed.

Reference values
The normal rate of pregnanetriol excretion is as follows:
• Adults: less than 3.5 mg/24 hours
• Children ages 7 to 16: 0.3 to 1.1 mg/24 hours
• Children younger than age 6 (including infants): up to 0.2 mg/24 hours.

Abnormal findings
Elevated urine pregnanetriol levels suggest adrenogenital syndrome, marked by excessive adrenal androgen secretion and resulting virilization. Females with this condition fail to develop normal secondary sex characteristics and show marked masculinization of external genitalia at birth. Males usually appear normal at birth but later develop signs of somatic and sexual precocity.

In monitoring treatment with cortisol replacement, elevated urine pregnanetriol levels indicate insufficient dosage of cortisol. When cortisol replacement adequately inhibits hypersecretion of corticotropin and subsequent overproduction of 17-hydroxyprogesterone, pregnanetriol levels fall within the normal range.

17-HYDROXY-CORTICOSTEROIDS

This test measures urine levels of 17-hydroxycorticosteroids (17-OHCS) — metabolites of the hormones that regulate glyconeogenesis. More than 80% of all urinary 17-OHCS are metabolites of cortisol, the primary adrenocortical steroid. Test findings thus reflect cortisol secretion and, indirectly, adrenocortical function.

Because cortisol secretion varies diurnally and in response to stress and many other factors, urine 17-OHCS levels are most accurately determined from a 24-hour specimen. Column chromatography and spectrophotofluorometry with the Porter-Silber reagent are used to measure 17-OHCS levels. Levels of plasma cortisol, urine free cortisol, and urine 17-ketosteroids may be measured and corticotropin stimulation and suppression testing performed to confirm results of this test.

Purpose
• To assess adrenocortical function

Patient preparation
• Explain to the patient that this test evaluates how his adrenal glands are functioning.
• Inform him he needn't restrict food or fluids but should avoid excessive physical exercise and stressful situations during the testing period.
• Tell him the test requires collection of urine over a 24-hour period, and instruct him in the proper collection technique.
• Check the patient's medication history for drugs that may affect 17-OHCS levels, including meprobamate, phenothiazines, spironolactone, ascorbic acid, chloral hydrate, glutethimide, chlordiazepoxide, penicillin G, hydroxyzine, quinidine, quinine, iodides, and methenamine. Review your findings with the laboratory, and then notify the doctor; he may restrict medications before the test.

Procedure and posttest care
• Collect the patient's urine over a 24-hour period. Use a bottle containing a preservative to prevent deterioration of the specimen.
• Tell the patient that he may resume activity restricted during the test.
• Resume administration of any medications restricted before the test.

Precautions
• Refrigerate the specimen or place it on ice during the collection period.

Reference values
Normally, urine 17-OHCS values range from 4.5 to 12 mg/24 hours in males, and from 2.5 to 10 mg/24 hours in females. Children ages 8 to 12 years normally excrete less than 4.5 mg/24 hours; younger children excrete less than 1.5 mg/24 hours. Levels normally increase slightly during the first trimester of pregnancy. Patients who are obese or very muscular may excrete slightly higher amounts of 17-OHCS, due to increased cortisol catabolism.

Abnormal findings
Elevated urine 17-OHCS levels may indicate Cushing's syndrome, adrenal carcinoma or adenoma, or pituitary tumor. Increased levels may also occur in patients with virilism, hyperthyroidism, and severe hypertension. Extreme stress induced by conditions such as acute pancreatitis and eclampsia also cause urine 17-OHCS levels to rise above normal.

Low urine 17-OHCS levels may indicate Addison's disease, hypopituitarism, or myxedema.

17-KETOSTEROIDS

This test uses the spectrophotofluorometric technique to measure urine levels of 17-ketosteroids (17-KS). Steroids and steroid metabolites characterized by a ketone group on carbon 17 in the steroid nucleus, 17-KS originate primarily in the adrenal glands but also in the testes and in the ovaries.

Although not all 17-KS are androgens, they cause androgenic effects. For example, excessive secretion of 17-KS may result in hirsutism and may increase clitoral or phallic size; in utero, elevated 17-KS levels may cause a female fetus to develop a male urogenital tract. Because 17-KS do not include all the androgens (testosterone, for example, the most potent androgen, is not a 17-KS), these levels provide only a rough estimate of androgenic activity. To provide additional information about androgen secretion, plasma testosterone levels may be measured concurrently.

Purpose
• To aid diagnosis of adrenal and gonadal dysfunction
• To aid diagnosis of adrenogenital syndrome (congenital adrenal hyperplasia)
• To monitor cortisol therapy in the treatment of adrenogenital syndrome

Patient preparation
• Explain to the patient that this test evaluates hormonal balance
• Inform him that he needn't restrict food or fluids before the test but should avoid excessive physical exercise and stressful situations during the collection period.

• Tell him the test requires urine collection over a 24-hour period, and instruct him in the proper collection technique.
• Check the patient's medication history for drugs that may affect test results, including meprobamate, phenothiazines, spironolactone, oleandomycin, estrogens, ethacrynic acid, phenytoin, nalidixic acid, and quinine. Review your findings with the laboratory, and then notify the doctor; he may want to restrict such drugs before the test.

Procedure and posttest care
• Collect the patient's urine over a 24-hour period. Use a bottle containing a preservative to keep the specimen at a pH of 4.0 to 4.5.
• Tell the patient that he may resume activity restricted during the test.
• Resume administration of medications withheld before the test.

Precautions
• If a woman is menstruating, urine collection may have to be postponed because presence of blood in the specimen interferes with test findings.
• Refrigerate the specimen or place it on ice during the collection period.
• When the collection is completed, send the specimen to the laboratory immediately.

Reference values
Normally, urine 17-KS values range from 6 to 21 mg/24 hours in men and from 4 to 17 mg/24 hours in women. Children between ages 11 and 14 excrete 2 to 7 mg/24 hours; younger children and infants excrete 0.1 to 3 mg/24 hours.

For more information about specific steroids in the 17-KS group, the 17-KS fractionation test may be performed. (See *Normal values for the 17-ketosteroid fractionation test.*)

NORMAL VALUES FOR THE 17-KETOSTEROID FRACTIONATION TEST

Through gas-liquid chromatography, this fractionation test shows which specific steroids in the 17-ketosteroid (KS) group are elevated or suppressed and thus aids differential diagnosis of conditions suggested by abnormal 17-KS levels. Note that 17-KS levels are measured in milligrams per 24 hours.

STEROID	ADULT MALE	ADULT FEMALE	MALE AGES 10 TO 15	FEMALE AGES 10 TO 15	BOTH SEXES (BIRTH TO AGE 9)
Androsterone	2.2 to 5	0.5 to 2.4	0.2 to 2	0.2 to 2.5	≤ 1
Dehydroepian-drosterone	0 to 2.3	0 to 1.2	< 0.4	< 0.4	< 0.2
Etiocholanolon	1.9 to 4.7	1.1 to 3	0.1 to 1.6	0.7 to 3	≤ 1
11-Hydroxy-androsterone	0.5 to 1.3	0.2 to 0.6	0.1 to 1.1	0.2 to 1	< 1
11-Hydroxy-etiocholanolone	0.3 to 0.7	0.2 to 0.6	< 0.3	0.1 to 0.5	≤ 0.5
11-Ketoandros-terone	0 to 0.1	0 to 0.2	< 0.1	< 0.1	< 0.1
11-Ketoetioch-olanolone	0.2 to 0.7	0.2 to 0.6	0.2 to 0.6	0.1 to 0.6	≤ 0.7
Pregnanediol	0.6 to 1.6	0.2 to 2.4	0.1 to 0.7	0.1 to 1.2	< 0.5
Pregnanetriol	0.6 to 1.3	0.1 to 1	0.2 to 0.6	0.1 to 0.6	< 0.3
5-Pregnanetriol	0 to 0.3	0 to 0.3	< 0.3	< 0.3	< 0.2
11-Ketopreg-nanetriol	0 to 0.2	0 to 0.4	< 0.3	< 0.2	< 0.2

Abnormal findings

Elevated urine 17-KS levels may result from adrenal hyperplasia, carcinoma or adenoma, or adrenogenital syndrome. In women, elevated levels may also indicate ovarian dysfunction — such as polycystic ovarian disease (Stein-Leventhal syndrome) — or lutein cell tumor of the ovary or androgenic arrhenoblastoma. In men, elevated 17-KS may indicate interstitial cell tumor of the testis. Characteristically, 17-KS levels also rise during pregnancy, severe stress, chronic illness, or debilitating disease.

Depressed urine 17-KS levels may result from Addison's disease, panhypopituitarism, eunuchoidism, or castration and may occur in cretinism, myxedema, and nephrosis. When this test is used to monitor cortisol therapy for adrenogenital syndrome, 17-KS levels typically return to normal with adequate cortisol administration.

17-KETOGENIC STEROIDS

Using spectrophotofluorometry, this test determines urine levels of 17-ketogenic steroids (17-KGS), which consist of the 17-hydroxycorticosteroids — cortisol and its metabolites, for example — and other adrenocortical steroids, such as pregnanetriol, that can be oxidized in the laboratory to 17-ketosteroids. Because 17-KGS represent such a large group of steroids, this test provides an excellent overall assessment of adrenocortical function. For accurate diagnosis of specific disease, 17-KGS must be compared with results of other tests, including plasma corticotropin, plasma cortisol, corticotropin stimulation, single-dose metyrapone, and dexamethasone suppression.

Purpose
• To evaluate adrenocortical function
• To aid diagnosis of Cushing's syndrome and Addison's disease

Patient preparation
• Explain to the patient that this test evaluates adrenal function.
• Inform him that he needn't restrict food or fluids before the test but should avoid excessive physical exercise and stressful situations during the collection period.
• Tell him the test requires urine collection over a 24-hour period, and teach him how to collect such a specimen correctly.
• Check the patient's medication history for drugs that may affect 17-KGS levels, including meprobamate, phenothiazines, spironolactone, penicillin, oleandomycin, hydralazine, estrogens, quinine, reserpine, thiazides, or corticosteroids (long-term therapy). Review your findings with the laboratory, and then notify the doctor; he may want to withhold medications before the test.

Procedure and posttest care
• Collect the patient's urine over a 24-hour period. Use a bottle containing a preservative to keep the specimen at a pH of 4.0 to 4.5.
• Tell the patient he may resume activity restricted during the test.
• Resume administration of drugs withheld before the test.

Precautions
• Refrigerate the specimen or keep it on ice during the collection period.
• Send the specimen to the laboratory immediately after the collection is completed.

Reference values
Normally, urine 17-KGS levels range from 4 to 14 mg/24 hours in men and from 2 to 12 mg/24 hours in women. Children ages 11 to 14 excrete 2 to 9 mg/24 hours; younger children and infants excrete 0.1 to 4 mg/24 hours.

Abnormal findings
Elevated urine 17-KGS levels indicate hyperadrenalism, which may occur in Cushing's syndrome, adrenogenital syndrome (congenital adrenal hyperplasia), and adrenal carcinoma or adenoma. Levels also rise with severe physical stress (burns, infections, or surgery, for example) or emotional stress.

Low levels may reflect hypoadrenalism, which may occur in Addison's disease and may also be associated with panhypopituitarism, cretinism, and general wasting.

VANILLYLMANDELIC ACID

Using spectrophotofluorometry, this test determines urine levels of vanillylmandelic acid (VMA), a phenolic acid. VMA is the catecholamine metabolite that is normally most prevalent in the urine and is the product of hepatic conversion of epinephrine and norepinephrine; urine VMA levels reflect endogenous production of these major catecholamines. Like the test for urine total catecholamines, this test helps to detect catecholamine-secreting tumors — especially pheochromocytoma — and helps evaluate the function of the adrenal medulla, the primary site of catecholamine production. This test is performed preferably on a 24-hour urine specimen (not a random specimen) to overcome the effects of diurnal variations in catecholamine secretion. Other catecholamine metabolites — metanephrine, normetanephrine, and homovanillic acid (HVA) — may be measured at the same time.

Purpose
• To help detect pheochromocytoma, neuroblastoma, and ganglioneuroma
• To evaluate the function of the adrenal medulla

Patient preparation
• Explain to the patient that this test evaluates hormonal secretion.
• Instruct him to restrict foods and beverages containing phenolic acid, such as coffee, tea, bananas, citrus fruits, chocolate, and vanilla, for 3 days before the test.
• Advise him to avoid stressful situations and excessive physical activity during the urine collection period.

• Tell him the test requires collection of urine over a 24-hour period, and teach him the proper collection technique.
• Check the patient's medication history for drugs that may affect test results, including epinephrine, norepinephrine, lithium carbonate, methocarbamol, chlorpromazine, guanethidine, reserpine, monoamine oxidase inhibitors, levodopa, or salicylates. Review your findings with the laboratory, and then notify the doctor; he may want to withhold these drugs before the test.

Procedure and posttest care
• Collect the patient's urine over a 24-hour period. Use a bottle containing a preservative to keep the specimen at a pH of 3.0.
• Resume administration of medications withheld before the test.
• Tell the patient he may resume normal diet and activity.

Precautions
• Refrigerate the specimen or keep it on ice during the collection period.
• Send the specimen to the laboratory immediately after the collection period.

Reference values
Normally, urine VMA values range from 0.7 to 6.8 mg/24 hours.

Abnormal findings
Elevated urine VMA levels may result from a catecholamine-secreting tumor. Further testing, such as measurement of urine HVA levels to rule out pheochromocytoma, is necessary for precise diagnosis. If pheochromocytoma is confirmed, the patient may be tested for multiple endocrine neoplasia, an inherited condition commonly associated with pheochromocytoma. (Family members of a patient with confirmed pheochromocytoma should also be carefully evaluated for multiple endocrine neoplasia.)

HOMOVANILLIC ACID

This test is a quantitative analysis of urine levels of homovanillic acid (HVA), which is a metabolite of dopamine, one of the three major catecholamines. Synthesized primarily in the brain, dopamine is a precursor to epinephrine and norepinephrine, the other principal catecholamines. The liver breaks down most dopamine into HVA, for eventual excretion; a minimal amount of dopamine appears in the urine.

Using two-dimensional chromatography, urine HVA levels are usually measured simultaneously with the major catecholamines and other catecholamine metabolites — metanephrine, normetanephrine, and vanillylmandelic acid.

Purpose
• To aid diagnosis of neuroblastoma and ganglioneuroma
• To rule out pheochromocytoma

Patient preparation
• Explain to the patient that this test assesses hormone secretion.
• Inform him that he needn't restrict food or fluids before the test, but should avoid stressful situations and excessive physical exercise during the collection period.
• Tell him the test requires collection of urine over a 24-hour period, and teach him the proper collection technique.
• Check the patient's history for drugs that may affect test results, including monamine oxidase inhibitors, aspirin, methocarbamol, and levodopa. Review your findings with the laboratory, and then notify the doctor; he may want to withhold these medications before the test.

Procedure and posttest care
• Collect a the patient's urine over a 24-hour period. Use a bottle containing a preservative to keep the specimen at a pH of 2.0 to 4.0.
• Resume administration of medications withheld before the test.
• Tell the patient that he may resume activity restricted during the test.

Precautions
• Refrigerate the specimen or keep it on ice during the collection period.
• Send the specimen to the laboratory immediately after the collection is completed.

Reference values
Normally, the urine HVA value for adults is less than 8 mg/24 hours. The range of normal urine HVA values in children varies with age, as shown in the chart below.

AGE (years)	HVA (mcg/mg creatinine)
15 to 17	0.5 to 2
10 to 15	0.25 to 12
5 to 10	0.5 to 9
2 to 5	0.5 to 13.5
1 to 2	4 to 23
birth to 1	1.2 to 35

Abnormal findings
Elevated urine HVA levels suggest neuroblastoma, a malignant soft-tissue tumor that develops in infants and young children, or ganglioneuroma, a tumor of the sympathetic nervous system that develops in older children and adolescents and rarely metastasizes. HVA levels don't usually rise in patients with pheochromocytoma, because this tumor secretes mainly epinephrine, which metabolizes primarily into vanillylmandelic acid. Thus, an abnormally

high urine HVA level generally rules out pheochromocytoma.

5-HYDROXYINDOLE-ACETIC ACID

This quantitative analysis of urine levels of 5-hydroxyindoleacetic acid (5-HIAA) is used mainly to screen for carcinoid tumors (argentaffinomas). Such tumors, found generally in the intestine or appendix, secrete an excessive amount of serotonin, which is reflected by high 5-HIAA levels. This test measures 5-HIAA levels by the colorimetric technique and is most accurately performed with a 24-hour urine specimen, which can detect small or intermittently secreting carcinoid tumors.

Purpose
• To aid diagnosis of carcinoid tumors (argentaffinomas)

Patient preparation
• Explain to the patient what serotonin is and why this test is important.
• Instruct him not to eat foods containing serotonin, such as bananas, plums, pineapples, avocados, eggplants, tomatoes, or walnuts, for 4 days before the test.
• Tell him the test requires collection of urine over a 24-hour period, and teach him the proper collection technique.
• Check the patient's history for recent use of drugs that may affect test results, including melphalan, reserpine, fluorouracil, ethanol, tricyclic antidepressants, monoamine oxidase inhibitors, methyldopa, isoniazid, methenamine compounds, phenothiazines, salicylates, guaifenesin, mephenesin, methocarbamol, and acetaminophen. Review your findings with the laboratory, and then notify the doctor; he may want to withhold these drugs before the test.

Procedure and posttest care
• Collect the patient's urine over a 24-hour period. Use a bottle containing a preservative to keep the specimen at a pH of 2.0 to 4.0
• Resume administration of medications withheld before the test.
• Tell the patient that he may resume his normal diet.

Precautions
• Refrigerate the specimen or keep it on ice during the collection period.
• Send the specimen to the laboratory immediately after the collection is completed.

Reference values
Normally, urine 5-HIAA values are less than 6 mg/24 hours.

Abnormal findings
Marked elevation of urine 5-HIAA levels, possibly as high as 200 to 600 mg/24 hours, indicates a carcinoid tumor. However, because these tumors vary in their capacity to store and secrete serotonin, some patients with carcinoid syndrome (metastatic carcinoid tumors) may not show elevated levels. Repeated testing is often necessary.

PREGNANEDIOL

Using gas chromatography or radioimmunoassay, this test measures urine levels of pregnanediol, the chief metabolite of progesterone. Although biologically inert, pregnanediol has diagnostic significance because it reflects about 10% of the endogenous production of its parent hormone. Progesterone is produced in nonpregnant females by the corpus luteum during the latter half of each menstrual cycle, preparing the uterus for implantation of a fertilized ovum. If implantation doesn't occur, progesterone secretion drops sharply; if implantation does occur, the corpus luteum secretes more progesterone to further prepare the uterus for pregnancy and to begin development of the placenta. Toward the end of the first trimester, the placenta becomes the primary source of progesterone secretion, producing the progressively larger amounts needed to maintain pregnancy.

Normally, urine levels of pregnanediol reflect variations in progesterone secretion during the menstrual cycle and during pregnancy. Direct measurement of plasma progesterone levels by radioimmunoassay may also be done.

Purpose
• To evaluate placental function in pregnant females
• To evaluate ovarian function in nonpregnant females

Patient preparation
• Explain to the patient that this test evaluates placental or ovarian function.
• Inform her that she needn't restrict food or fluids.
• Tell her the test requires collection of urine over a 24-hour period, and teach her the proper collection technique.
• Advise the pregnant patient that this test may be repeated several times to obtain serial measurements.
• Check the patient's medication history for recent use of drugs that may affect pregnanediol levels, including methenamine mandelate, methenamine hippurate, progestogens, combination oral contraceptives, and drugs containing corticotropin.

Procedure and posttest care
• Collect the patient's urine over a 24-hour period.
• Resume administration of drugs withheld before the test.

Precautions
• Refrigerate the specimen or keep it on ice during the collection period.
• If the patient is pregnant, note the approximate week of gestation on the laboratory slip.
• For premenopausal women who are not pregnant, note the stage of the menstrual cycle on the laboratory slip.

Reference values
In nonpregnant females, urine pregnanediol values normally range from 0.5 to 1.5 mg/24 hours during the proliferative phase of the menstrual cycle. Within 24 hours after ovulation, pregnanediol levels begin to rise and continue to rise for 3 to 10 days, as the corpus luteum develops. During this luteal phase, normal urine pregnanediol values range from 2 to 7 mg/24 hours. In the absence of fertilization, levels drop sharply, as the corpus luteum degenerates and menstruation begins.

During pregnancy, urine pregnanediol levels rise markedly, peaking around the 36th week of gestation and returning to prepregnancy levels by day 5 to 10 postpartum. (See *Urine pregnanediol in normal pregnancy.*) Normal postmenopausal values range from 0.2 to 1 mg/24 hours. In males, urine pregnanediol levels rarely rise above 1.5 mg/24 hours.

Abnormal findings
During pregnancy, a marked decrease in urine pregnanediol levels based on a single 24-hour urine specimen or a steady decrease in pregnanediol levels in serial measurements may indicate placental insufficiency and requires immediate investigation. A precipitous

URINE PREGNANEDIOL IN NORMAL PREGNANCY

Serial determinations of the *average* levels (middle line on chart) of pregnanediol rise steadily until about 32 weeks' gestation, then level off. Excretion decreases 24 hours postpartum and drops to prepregnancy levels within 5 to 10 days. A wide range of normal values is possible — high normal, low normal, and average levels.

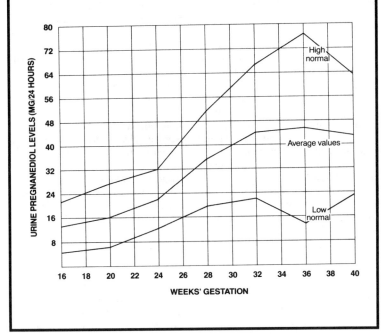

drop in pregnanediol values may suggest fetal distress — for example, threatened abortion or preeclampsia — or fetal death. However, pregnanediol measurements are not reliable indicators of fetal viability because levels can remain normal even after fetal death, as long as maternal circulation to the placenta remains adequate.

In nonpregnant females, abnormally low urine pregnanediol levels may occur with anovulation, amenorrhea, or other menstrual abnormalities. Low to normal pregnanediol levels may be associated with hydatidiform mole. Elevations may indicate luteinized granulosa or theca cell tumors, diffuse thecal luteinization, or metastatic ovarian cancer.

Adrenal hyperplasia or biliary tract obstruction may elevate urine pregnanediol values in males or females. Some forms of primary hepatic disease produce abnormally low levels in both sexes.

PROTEINS AND PROTEIN METABOLITES

PROTEINS

This is a quantitative test for proteinuria. Normally, the glomerular membrane allows only proteins of low molecular weight to enter the filtrate. The renal tubules then reabsorb most of these proteins, normally excreting a small amount that's undetectable by a screening test. A damaged glomerular capillary membrane and impaired tubular reabsorption allow excretion of proteins in the urine.

A qualitative screening often precedes this test. A positive result requires quantitative analysis of a 24-hour urine specimen by acid precipitation tests. Electrophoresis can detect Bence Jones protein, hemoglobins, myoglobins, or albumin.

Purpose
• To aid diagnosis of pathologic states characterized by proteinuria, primarily renal disease

Patient preparation
• Explain to the patient that this test detects proteins in the urine.
• Inform him that he needn't restrict food or fluids.
• Tell him that the test usually requires urine collection over a 24-hour period.
• Check the patient's history for drugs that may affect test results, including tolbutamide, para-aminosalicylic acid, acetazolamide, sodium bicarbonate, penicillin, sulfonamides, iodine contrast media, and cephalosporins. Review your findings with the laboratory, and then notify the doctor; he may want to restrict medications before the test.

Procedure and posttest care
• Collect the patient's urine over a 24-hour period. A special specimen container can be obtained from the laboratory.
• Resume administration of medications withheld before the test.

Precautions
• Tell the patient not to contaminate the urine with toilet tissue or stool.
• Refrigerate the specimen or place it on ice during the collection period.

Reference values
Normal values show up to 150 mg of protein excreted in 24 hours.

Abnormal findings
Proteinuria is a chief characteristic of renal disease. When proteinuria is present in a single specimen, 24-hour urine collection is subsequently required to identify specific renal abnormalities.

Proteinuria can result from glomerular leakage of plasma proteins (a major cause of protein excretion), from overflow of filtered proteins of low molecular weight (when these are present in excessive concentrations), from impaired tubular reabsorption of filtered proteins, and from the presence of renal proteins derived due to the breakdown of kidney tissue.

Persistent proteinuria indicates renal disease resulting from increased glomerular permeability. *Minimal proteinuria* (less than 0.5 g/24 hours), however, is most often associated with renal diseases in which glomerular involvement is not a major factor, such as chronic pyelonephritis.

Moderate proteinuria (0.5 to 4 g/ 24 hours) occurs in several types of renal disease — acute or chronic glomerulonephritis, amyloidosis, toxic nephropathies — or in diseases in which renal failure often develops as a late complication (diabetes or heart failure, for example). *Heavy proteinuria* (more than 4 g/24 hours) is commonly associated with nephrotic syndrome.

When accompanied by an elevated white blood cell count, proteinuria indicates urinary tract infection. When accompanied by hematuria, proteinuria indicates local or diffuse urinary tract disorders. Other pathologic states (infections and lesions of the central nervous system, for example) can also result in detectable amounts of proteins in the urine.

Many drugs (such as amphotericin B, gold preparations, aminoglycosides, polymyxins, and trimethadione) inflict renal damage, causing true proteinuria. This makes the routine evaluation of urine proteins essential during such treatment. In all forms of proteinuria, fractionation results obtained by electrophoresis provide more precise information than the screening test. For example, excessive hemoglobin in the urine indicates intravascular hemolysis; elevated myoglobin suggests muscle damage; albumin, increased glomerular permeability; and Bence Jones protein, multiple myeloma.

Not all forms of proteinuria have pathologic significance. *Benign proteinuria* can result from changes in body position. *Functional proteinuria* is associated with exercise, as well as emotional or physiologic stress, and is usually transient.

BENCE JONES PROTEIN

Bence Jones proteins are abnormal light-chain immunoglobulins of low molecular weight that are derived from the clone of a single plasma cell (monoclonal). This globulin appears in the urine of 50% to 80% of patients with multiple myeloma and in most patients with Waldenström's macroglobulinemia.

Screening tests, such as thermal coagulation and Bradshaw's test, can detect Bence Jones proteins, but urine immunoelectrophoresis is usually the method of choice for quantitative studies. Serum immunoelectrophoresis, which is sometimes used, is less sensitive than other tests. Nevertheless, both urine and serum studies are frequently used for patients suspected of having multiple myeloma.

Purpose
• To confirm the presence of multiple myeloma in patients with characteristic clinical signs, such as bone pain (especially in the back and thorax) and persistent anemia and fatigue.

Patient preparation
• Explain to the patient that this test can detect an abnormal protein in the urine.
• Tell him the test requires an early-morning urine specimen, and teach him how to collect a clean-catch specimen.

Procedure and posttest care
• Collect an early-morning urine specimen of at least 50 ml.

Precautions
• Instruct the patient not to contaminate the urine specimen with toilet tissue or stool.
• Send the specimen to the laboratory immediately.
• Refrigerate the specimen if transport is delayed.

Normal findings
Normal urine should contain no Bence Jones proteins.

Abnormal findings
The presence of Bence Jones proteins in urine suggests multiple myeloma or Waldenström's macroglobulinemia. Very low levels, in the absence of other symptoms, may result from benign monoclonal gammopathy. However, clinical evidence figures prominently in diagnosis of multiple myeloma.

Amino Acid Screening

This test screens for aminoaciduria — elevated urine amino acid levels — a condition that may result from inborn errors of metabolism due to the absence of specific enzymatic activities. Abnormal metabolism causes an excess of one or more amino acids to appear in plasma and, as the renal threshold is exceeded, in urine.

Aminoacidurias may be classified as either primary (overflow) aminoacidopathies or as secondary (renal) aminoacidopathies. The latter type is associated with conditions marked by defective tubular reabsorption from congenital disorders. A more specific defect, such as cystinuria, may cause one or more amino acids to appear in urine.

To screen newborns, children, and adults for congenital aminoacidurias, plasma or urine specimens may be used. The plasma test is the better indicator of overflow aminoacidurias; urine testing is used to confirm or monitor certain amino acid disorders and to screen for renal aminoacidurias.

Various laboratory techniques are available to screen for aminoacidurias, but chromatography is the preferred method. Positive findings on chromatography can be elaborated by fractionation, showing specific amino acid levels. Testing for specific amino acid levels is also necessary for infants or young children with acidosis, severe vomiting and diarrhea, and abnormal urine odor. Such testing is especially important in newborns because early diagnosis and prompt treatment of aminoacidurias may prevent mental retardation.

Purpose
• To screen for renal aminoacidurias
• To follow up on plasma test findings when results of these tests suggest overflow aminoacidurias

Patient preparation
• Explain to the patient (or to his parents if the patient is an infant or a child) that this test helps detect amino acid disorders. Advise him that additional tests may be necessary.
• Inform him he needn't restrict food or fluids before the test.
• Tell him the test requires a urine specimen.
• Check the patient's medication history for drugs that may interfere with test results. If such drugs must be continued, note this on the laboratory slip. (If the patient is a breast-fed infant, record any drugs the mother is receiving.)

Procedure and posttest care
• If the patient is an infant, clean and dry the genital area, attach the collection device, and observe for voiding. Transfer urine — at least 20 ml — to a specimen container. Remove the collection device carefully to prevent skin irritation.
• If the patient is an adult or a child, collect a fresh random specimen.

Precautions
• For an infant, apply the adhesive flanges of the collection device securely to the skin to prevent leakage.
• Send the specimen to the laboratory immediately.

Normal findings
Patterns on thin-layer chromatography are reported as normal.

Abnormal findings
If thin-layer chromatography shows gross changes or abnormal patterns, blood and 24-hour urine quantitative column chromatography are performed to identify specific amino acid abnormalities and to differentiate overflow and renal aminoacidurias. (See *Chromatographic identification of amino acid disorders*, pages 330 and 331.)

HYDROXYPROLINE

This test measures total urine levels of hydroxyproline, an amino acid found mainly in collagen (a component of skin and bone). Urine hydroxyproline levels are a good index of bone matrix turnover because levels increase when collagen breaks down during bone resorption. Bone matrix turnover and hydroxyproline levels normally rise in children during periods of rapid skeletal growth. However, they also rise in disorders that increase bone resorption, such as Paget's disease, metastatic bone tumors, and certain endocrine disorders.

Hydroxyproline levels are most often determined colorimetrically on a timed urine sample; they may also be determined by ion-exchange or gas-liquid chromatography. A collagen-restricted diet is essential for this test because hydroxyproline levels reflect collagen intake. Free hydroxyproline, a small component of total hydroxyproline and a sensitive indicator of dietary collagen intake, may be measured to validate results.

Purpose
• To monitor treatment for disorders characterized by bone resorption, including Paget's disease, metastatic bone tumors, and certain endocrine disorders
• To aid diagnosis of disorders characterized by bone resorption

Patient preparation
• Explain to the patient that this test helps monitor treatment or detect an amino acid disorder related to bone formation.
• Inform him that he must not eat meat, fish, poultry, jelly, or any foods containing gelatin for 24 hours before the test and during the test period itself.
• Tell him the test requires urine collection over a 2-hour or 24-hour period, and teach him the correct collection technique.
• Note the patient's age and sex on the laboratory slip.
• Check his history for drugs that may alter test results, including ascorbic acid, vitamin D, aspirin, glucocorticoids, calcitonin, and mithramycin. Withhold such drugs as necessary. If these medications must be continued

(Text continues on page 332.)

CHROMATOGRAPHIC IDENTIFICATION OF AMINO ACID DISORDERS

In chromatography — the preferred method for screening aminoacidurias — amino acids migrate into multicolored bands. The sequence of amino acids and their corresponding band numbers, as listed below, reflect these standard migratory patterns. When congenital enzyme deficiencies and subsequent metabolic disorders increase plasma and urine amino acid levels, these bands intensify.

		METABOLIC AMINO ACID DISORDERS						
		Phenylketon-uria		Maple syrup urine disease		Cystinuria		
Chromatographic band number	Amino acids	Plasma	Urine	Plasma	Urine	Plasma	Urine	
1	Leucine, isoleucine			+	+			
2	Phenylalanine	+	+					
3	Valine, methionine			+	+			
4	Tryptophan, beta-amino isobutyric acid							
5	Tyrosine							
6	Proline			+				
7	Alanine, ethanolamine							
8	Threonine, glutamic acid							
9	Homocitrulline, glycine, serine, hydroxyproline, aspartic acid, glutamine, citrulline			+				
10	Homocystine, asparagine							
11	Argininosuccinic acid, histidine, arginine, lysine, ornithine, cystathionine, cystine, cysteine, hydroxylysine						+	

KEY: + = Increased amino acids in the plasma or urine

Homocystinuria		Hartnup disease		Argininosuccinicaciduria		Histidinemia		Hyperprolinemia Type A		Citrullinuria	
Plasma	Urine	Plasma	Urine	Plasma	Urine	Plasma	Urine	Plasma	Urine	Plasma	Urine
			+								
			+								
+			+							+	
			+								
			+								
								+	+		
			+				+				+
							+				+
			+		+				+	+	+
	+										
			+		+	+	+				+

throughout the test period, note this on the laboratory slip.

Procedure and posttest care
• Collect the patient's urine over a 2-hour or 24-hour period. Use a container that has a preservative to prevent degradation of hydroxyproline.
• Tell the patient he may resume foods and drugs withheld before the test.

Precautions
• Refrigerate the specimen or keep it on ice during the collection period.
• Send it to the laboratory immediately.

Reference values
For adults, normal values typically range from 14 to 45 mg/24 hours or 0.4 to 5 mg/2-hour specimen (males) and 0.4 to 2.9 mg/2-hour specimen (females). Normal values for children are much higher and peak between ages 11 and 18. Values also rise during the third trimester of pregnancy, reflecting fetal skeletal growth.

Abnormal findings
Hydroxyproline levels should decrease slowly during therapy for bone resorption disorders. Elevated levels may indicate bone disease, metastatic bone tumors, or endocrine disorders that stimulate hormonal secretion.

CREATININE

This test measures urine levels of creatinine, the chief metabolite of creatine. Produced in amounts proportional to total body muscle mass, creatinine is removed from the plasma primarily by glomerular filtration and is excreted in the urine. Because the body doesn't recycle it, creatinine has a relatively high, constant clearance rate, making it an efficient indicator of renal function. However, the creatinine clearance test, which measures both urine and plasma creatinine clearance, is a more precise index than this test. A standard method for determining urine creatinine levels is based on Jaffé's reaction, in which creatinine treated with an alkaline picrate solution yields a bright orange-red complex.

Purpose
• To help assess glomerular filtration
• To check the accuracy of 24-hour urine collection, based on the relatively constant levels of creatinine excretion

Patient preparation
• Explain to the patient that this test helps evaluate kidney function.
• Inform him that he need not restrict fluids but should not eat an excessive amount of meat before the test.
• Advise him that he should avoid strenuous physical exercise during the collection period.
• Tell him the test usually requires urine collection over a 24-hour period, and teach him the proper collection technique.
• Check his medication history for drugs that may affect creatinine levels, including corticosteroids, gentamicin, tetracyclines, diuretics, and amphotericin B. Review your findings with the laboratory, and then notify the doctor; he may restrict such drugs before the test.

Procedure and posttest care
• Collect the patient's urine over a 24-hour period. Use a specimen bottle that contains a preservative to prevent the degradation of creatinine.
• Resume administration of medications withheld during the test.
• Tell the patient he may resume normal diet and activity.

Precautions
• Refrigerate the specimen or keep it on ice during the collection period.
• Once the collection is completed, send the specimen to the laboratory immediately.

Reference values
Normally, urine creatinine levels range from 1 to 1.9 g/24 hours for men and from 0.8 to 1.7 g/24 hours for women.

Abnormal findings
Decreased urine creatinine levels may result from impaired renal perfusion (associated with shock, for example) or from renal disease due to urinary tract obstruction. Chronic bilateral pyelonephritis, acute or chronic glomerulonephritis, and polycystic kidney disease may also depress creatinine levels. Increased levels generally have little diagnostic significance.

CREATININE CLEARANCE

An anhydride of creatine, creatinine is formed and excreted in constant amounts by an irreversible reaction and functions solely as the main end product of creatine. Creatinine production is proportional to total muscle mass and is relatively unaffected by urine volume or normal physical activity or diet.

An excellent diagnostic indicator of renal function, the creatinine clearance test determines how efficiently the kidneys are clearing creatinine from the blood. The rate of clearance is expressed in terms of the volume of blood (in ml) that can be cleared of creatinine in 1 minute. Creatinine levels become abnormal when more than 50% of the total nephron units have been damaged.

Purpose
• To assess renal function (primarily glomerular filtration)
• To monitor progression of renal insufficiency

Patient preparation
• Explain to the patient that this test assesses kidney function.
• Inform him that he needn't restrict fluids but should not eat an excessive amount of meat before the test.
• Advise him that he should avoid strenuous physical exercise during the collection period.
• Tell him the test requires a timed urine specimen and at least one blood sample.
• Tell him how the urine specimen will be collected. Also inform him who will perform the venipuncture and when and that he may feel some discomfort from the needle puncture. Reassure him that collecting the blood sample takes less than 3 minutes.
• Explain that more than one venipuncture may be necessary.
• Check the patient's medication history for drugs that may affect creatinine clearance, including amphotericin B, thiazide diuretics, furosemide, and aminoglycosides. Review your findings with the laboratory, and then notify the doctor; he may want to restrict these medications before the test.

Procedure and posttest care
• Collect a timed urine specimen at 2, 6, 12, or 24 hours in a bottle containing a preservative to prevent degradation of creatinine.
• Perform a venipuncture anytime during the collection period, and collect the sample in a 7-ml *red-top* tube.
• Apply warm soaks to ease discomfort if a hematoma develops at the venipuncture site.
• Resume administration of medications withheld before the test.

• Tell the patient that he may resume normal diet and activity.

Precautions
• Refrigerate the urine specimen or keep it on ice during the collection period.
• Send the specimen to the laboratory immediately after the collection is completed.

Reference values
For men, normal creatinine clearance ranges from 85 to 125 ml/minute. For women, it ranges from 75 to 115 ml/minute. For older patients, creatinine clearance normally decreases by 6 ml/minute for each decade.

Abnormal findings
Low creatinine clearance may result from reduced renal blood flow (associated with shock or renal artery obstruction), acute tubular necrosis, acute or chronic glomerulonephritis, advanced bilateral chronic pyelonephritis, advanced bilateral renal lesions (which may occur in polycystic kidney disease, renal tuberculosis, and malignancy), nephrosclerosis, congestive heart failure, or severe dehydration.

High creatinine clearance rates generally have little diagnostic significance.

UREA CLEARANCE

The urea clearance test is a quantitative analysis of urine levels of urea, the main nitrogenous component in urine and the end product of protein metabolism. This test is most useful for assessing overall renal function; the creatinine clearance test provides a more accurate evaluation of the glomerular filtration rate (GFR). In urea clearance, blood urea content and the total amount of urea excreted in the urine are proportional only when the rate of urine flow is 2 ml/minute or higher (maximal clearance). At lower flow rates, the accuracy of the test decreases.

Purpose
• To assess total renal function

Patient preparation
• Explain to the patient that this test evaluates kidney function.
• Instruct him to fast from midnight before the test and to abstain from exercise before and during the test.
• Tell him the test requires two timed urine specimens and one blood sample.
• Tell him how the urine specimens will be collected. Also inform him who will perform the venipuncture and when and that he may experience transient discomfort from the needle puncture. Reassure him that collecting the blood sample takes less than 3 minutes.
• Check the patient's medication history for drugs that may affect urea clearance, including epinephrine, corticosteroids, amphotericin B, thiazide diuretics, and streptomycin. Review your findings with the laboratory, and then notify the doctor; he may want to restrict medications before the test.

Procedure and posttest care
• Instruct the patient to empty his bladder and discard the urine.
• Give him water to drink to assure adequate urine output.
• Collect two specimens 1 hour apart, and mark the collection time on the laboratory slip.
• Perform a venipuncture anytime during the collection period, and collect the sample in a 7-ml *red-top* tube.
• Apply warm soaks if a hematoma develops at the venipuncture site.
• Resume administration of medications withheld before the test.

• Tell the patient that he may resume normal diet and activity.

Precautions

• Because this is a clearance test, make sure the patient empties his bladder and that the total amount of urine is collected from each hour's specimen.
• Send each specimen to the laboratory as soon as it is collected.
• If the patient is catheterized, empty the drainage bag before beginning the specimen collection.
• Handle the blood sample gently to prevent hemolysis, and send it to the laboratory immediately.

Reference values

Normally, the urea clearance rate ranges from 64 to 99 ml/minute with maximal clearance. If the flow rate is less than 2 ml/minute, normal clearance is 41 to 68 ml/minute. (If the urine flow rate is less than 1 ml/minute, this test should not be performed.)

Abnormal findings

Low urea clearance values may indicate decreased renal blood flow (due to shock or renal artery obstruction), acute or chronic glomerulonephritis, advanced bilateral chronic pyelonephritis, acute tubular necrosis, or nephrosclerosis. Diminished rates may also result from advanced bilateral renal lesions (which may occur in polycystic kidney disease, renal tuberculosis, or malignancy), bilateral ureteral obstruction, congestive heart failure, or dehydration.

High urea clearance usually is not diagnostically significant.

URIC ACID

A quantitative analysis of urine uric acid levels may supplement serum uric acid testing when seeking to identify disorders that alter production or excretion of uric acid (such as leukemia, gout, and renal dysfunction).

The most specific laboratory method for detecting uric acid is spectrophotometric absorption after treatment of the specimen with the enzyme uricase.

Purpose

• To detect enzyme deficiencies and metabolic disturbances that affect uric acid production
• To help measure the efficiency of renal clearance

Patient preparation

• Explain to the patient that this test measures the body's production and excretion of a waste product known as uric acid.
• Inform him that he needn't restrict food or fluids before the test.
• Tell him the test requires urine collection over a 24-hour period, and teach him the proper collection technique.
• Check the patient's medication history for recent use of drugs that may influence uric acid levels, including diuretics, pyrazinamide, salicylates, phenylbutazone, probenecid, and allopurinol. If these medications must be continued, note this on the laboratory slip.

Procedure and posttest care

• Collect the patient's urine over a 24-hour period.
• Resume administration of medications withheld before the test.

Precautions
• Send the specimen to the laboratory immediately after the collection period.

Reference values
Normal urine uric acid values vary with diet but generally range from 250 to 750 mg/24 hours.

Abnormal findings
Elevated urine uric acid levels may result from chronic myeloid leukemia, polycythemia vera, multiple myeloma, early remission in pernicious anemia, lymphosarcoma and lymphatic leukemia during radiotherapy, or tubular reabsorption defects, such as Fanconi's syndrome and hepatolenticular degeneration (Wilson's disease).

Low urine uric acid levels occur in gout (when associated with normal uric acid production but inadequate excretion) and in severe renal damage, such as that resulting from chronic glomerulonephritis, diabetic glomerulosclerosis, and collagen disorders.

PIGMENTS

HEMOGLOBIN

An abnormal finding, free hemoglobin in the urine may occur in hemolytic anemias, infection, strenuous exercise, or severe intravascular hemolysis from a transfusion reaction. Contained in red blood cells (RBCs), hemoglobin consists of an iron-protoporphyrin complex (heme) and a polypeptide (globin). Usually, RBC destruction occurs within the reticuloendothelial system. However, when RBC destruction occurs within the circulation, free hemoglobin enters the plasma and binds with haptoglobin. If the plasma level of hemoglobin exceeds that of haptoglobin, the excess of unbound hemoglobin is excreted in the urine (hemoglobinuria).

Heme proteins act like enzymes that catalyze oxidation of organic substances. This reaction produces a blue coloration; the intensity of color varies with the amount of hemoglobin present. Microscopic examination is required to identify intact RBCs in urine (hematuria), which can occur in the presence of unbound hemoglobin.

Purpose
• To aid diagnosis of hemolytic anemias, infection, or severe intravascular hemolysis from a transfusion reaction

Patient preparation
• Explain to the patient that this test detects excessive RBC destruction.
• Inform him he needn't restrict food or fluid.
• Tell him the test requires a random urine specimen, and teach him the proper collection technique.
• Check the patient's medication history for drugs that may affect free hemoglobin levels, including nephrotoxic drugs, anticoagulants, and drugs that contain vitamin C as a preservative. Review your findings with the laboratory, and then notify the doctor; he may want to restrict these medications before the test.

Procedure and posttest care
• Collect a random urine specimen. (See *Bedside testing for urine blood pigments.*)
• Resume administration of medications withheld during the test.

Precautions
• Because contamination of the specimen with menstrual blood alters results, a female patient who is menstruating should reschedule her test.

BEDSIDE TESTING FOR URINE BLOOD PIGMENTS

To test a patient's urine for blood pigments at bedside, use one of the methods that follow.

Dipstick, Multistix, or Chemstrip
- Collect a urine specimen.
- Dip the stick into the specimen and withdraw it.
- After 30 seconds, compare the stick to the color chart. Blue indicates a positive reaction; the intensity of color indicates pigment concentration.

Occult tablet
- Collect a urine specimen.
- Put one drop of urine on the filter paper. Place the tablet on the urine, and then put two drops of water on the tablet.
- After 2 minutes, inspect the filter paper around the tablet. Blue indicates

a positive reaction; the intensity of color indicates pigment concentration.

Occult solution
- Collect a urine specimen.
- After placing one drop of urine on the filter paper, close the package and turn it over. Open the opposite ends, and place two drops of solution on the filter paper.
- After 30 seconds, inspect the filter paper. Blue indicates a positive reaction; the intensity of color indicates pigment concentration.

Distinguishing hemoglobin
Because these methods detect only blood pigments, immunochemical studies are necessary to differentiate hemoglobin from other blood pigments, such as myoglobin.

- Send the specimen to the laboratory immediately.

Normal findings
Normally, hemoglobin is not present in the urine.

Abnormal findings
Hemoglobinuria may result from severe intravascular hemolysis due to a blood transfusion reaction, burns, or a crushing injury. It may result from acquired hemolytic anemias caused by chemical or drug intoxication or malaria; congenital hemolytic anemias, such as hemoglobinopathies or enzyme defects; or paroxysmal nocturnal hemoglobinuria (another type of hemolytic anemia). Less commonly, it may signal cystitis, ureteral calculi, or urethritis.

Hemoglobinuria and hematuria occur in renal epithelial damage (which

may result from acute glomerulonephritis or pyelonephritis), renal tumor, and tuberculosis.

MYOGLOBIN

This test detects the presence of myoglobin — a red pigment found in the cytoplasm of cardiac and skeletal muscle cells — in the urine. When muscle cells are extensively damaged, as by disease or severe crushing trauma, myoglobin is released into the blood, quickly cleared by renal glomerular filtration, and eliminated in the urine (myoglobinuria). For example, myoglobin appears in the urine within 24 hours after myocardial infarction.

Because of marked structural similarities, urine myoglobin must be differentiated from urine hemoglobin. The most commonly used test method is the differential precipitation test. Hemoglobin — bound to haptoglobin — precipitates when urine is mixed with ammonium sulfate. Myoglobin, however, remains soluble and can be measured.

Purpose
• To aid diagnosis of muscular disease
• To detect extensive infarction of muscle tissue
• To assess the extent of muscular damage from crushing trauma

Patient preparation
• Explain to the patient that this test detects a red pigment found in muscle cells and helps evaluate muscle injury or disease.
• Inform him that he needn't restrict food or fluids before the test.
• Tell him that this test requires a random urine specimen, and teach him the proper technique for collecting the specimen.
• Advise him that test results are generally available in 1 day.

Procedure and posttest care
• Collect a random urine specimen.

Precautions
• Send the specimen to the laboratory immediately.

Normal findings
Normally, myoglobin does not appear in urine.

Abnormal findings
Myoglobinuria occurs in acute or chronic muscular disease, alcoholic polymyopathy, familial myoglobinuria, extensive myocardial infarction, and in severe trauma to the skeletal muscles (which may result from a crushing injury, extreme hyperthermia, or severe burns). It also occurs in strenuous or prolonged exercise, but disappears after rest.

PORPHYRINS

This test is a quantitative analysis of urine porphyrins (most notably, uroporphyrins and coproporphyrins) and their precursors (porphyrinogens, such as porphobilinogen [PBG]). Porphyrins are red-orange fluorescent compounds, consisting of four pyrrole rings, that are produced during heme biosynthesis. They are present in all protoplasm, figure in energy storage and utilization, and are normally excreted in urine in small amounts. Elevated urine levels of porphyrins or porphyrinogens, therefore, reflect impaired heme biosynthesis. Such impairment may result from inherited enzyme deficiencies (congenital porphyrias) or from defects caused by disorders such as hemolytic anemias and hepatic disease (acquired porphyrias).

Determination of the specific porphyrins and porphyrinogens found in a urine specimen can help identify the impaired metabolic step in heme biosynthesis. Occasionally, a preliminary qualitative screening is performed on a random specimen; a positive finding on the screening test must be confirmed by the quantitative analysis of a 24-hour specimen. For correct diagnosis of a specific porphyria, urine porphyrin levels should be correlated with plasma and fecal porphyrin levels.

Purpose
• To aid diagnosis of congenital or acquired porphyrias

URINE PORPHYRIN LEVELS IN PORPHYRIA

In porphyria, defective heme biosynthesis increases urinary porphyrins and their corresponding precursors.

PORPHYRIA	PORPHYRIN PRECURSORS		PORPHYRINS	
	Delta-amino-levolinic acid	Porphobili-nogen	Uroporphyrins	Coproporphyrins
Erythropoietic porphyria	Normal	Normal	Highly increased	Increased
Erythropoietic protoporphyria	Normal	Normal	Normal	Normal
Acute intermittent porphyria	Highly increased	Highly increased	Variable	Variable
Variegate porphyria	Highly increased during acute attack	Normal or slightly increased; highly increased during acute attack	Normal or slightly increased; may be highly increased during acute attack	Normal or slightly increased; may be highly increased during acute attack
Coproporphyria	Increased during acute attack	Increased during acute attack	Not applicable	May be highly increased during acute attack
Porphyria cutanea tarda	Variable	Variable	Highly increased	Increased

Patient preparation
• Explain to the patient that this test detects abnormal hemoglobin formation.
• Inform him he needn't restrict food or fluids before the test.
• Tell him the test requires urine collection over a 24-hour period, and teach him the proper collection technique.
• Note whether the patient is taking any drugs that may interfere with test results, such as oral contraceptives, griseofulvin, or rifampin. Inform the laboratory and the doctor, who may reschedule the test or restrict drugs before the test.

Procedure and posttest care
• Collect the patient's urine over a 24-hour period. Use a light-resistant specimen bottle containing a preservative to prevent degradation of the light-sensitive porphyrins and their precursors.
• Resume administration of medications withheld during the test.

Precautions
• If a female patient is pregnant or menstruating, be aware that these conditions may interfere with accurate determination of test results.

- Refrigerate the specimen or keep it on ice during the collection period.
- Send it to the laboratory immediately.
- Protect the specimen from light exposure if a light-resistant container isn't available.
- Put the collection bag in a dark plastic bag if an indwelling urinary catheter is in place.

Reference values
Normal porphyrin and precursor values for urine fall in the following ranges:
- Uroporphyrins: in women, from 1 to 22 mcg/24 hours; in men, from undetectable to 42 mcg/24 hours
- Coproporphyrins: in women, from 1 to 57 mcg/24 hours; in men, from undetectable to 96 mcg/24 hours
- PBG: in both sexes, up to 1.5 mg/24 hours.

Abnormal findings
Increased urine levels of porphyrins and porphyrin precursors are characteristic of porphyria. (See *Urine porphyrin levels in porphyria,* page 339.) Infectious hepatitis, Hodgkin's disease, central nervous system disorders, cirrhosis, and heavy metal, benzene, or carbon tetrachloride toxicity may also increase porphyrin levels.

DELTA-AMINO-LEVULINIC ACID

Using the colorimetric technique, this quantitative analysis of urine delta-aminolevulinic acid (ALA) levels helps diagnose porphyrias, hepatic disease, and lead poisoning. In an emergency, a simple qualitative screening test may be performed.

ALA, the basic precursor of the porphyrins, normally converts to porphobilinogen during heme synthesis. Impaired conversion, which occurs in porphyrias and lead poisoning, causes urine ALA levels to rise before other chemical or hematologic changes occur.

Purpose
- To screen for lead poisoning
- To aid diagnosis of porphyrias and certain hepatic disorders, such as hepatitis and hepatic carcinoma

Patient preparation
- Explain to the patient that this test detects abnormal hemoglobin formation.
- If lead poisoning is suspected, tell the patient (or parents, because the patient is usually a child) that the test helps detect the presence of excessive lead in the body.
- Inform the patient or his parents that he needn't restrict food or fluids.
- Tell him that the test requires urine collection over a 24-hour period, and teach him or his parents the proper collection technique.
- Check his medication history for recent administration of drugs that may alter ALA levels, including barbiturates, griseofulvin, and vitamin E. Review your findings with the laboratory, and then notify the doctor; he may want to restrict medications before the test.

Procedure and posttest care
- Collect the patient's urine over a 24-hour period. Use a light-resistant bottle containing a preservative (usually glacial acetic acid) to prevent degradation of ALA.
- Resume administration of medications withheld during the test.

Precautions
- Refrigerate the specimen or keep it on ice during the collection period.

• Send the specimen to the laboratory immediately after the collection is completed.

• Protect the specimen from direct sunlight.

• Insert the drainage bag in a dark plastic bag if the patient has an indwelling urinary catheter in place.

Reference values

Normally, urine ALA values range from 1.5 to 7.5 mg/dl/24 hours.

Abnormal values

Elevated urine ALA levels may occur in lead poisoning, acute porphyria, hepatic carcinoma, or hepatitis.

BILIRUBIN

This screening test, based on a color reaction with a specific reagent, detects water-soluble direct (conjugated) bilirubin in the urine. Detectable amounts of bilirubin in the urine may indicate liver disease caused by infections, biliary disease, or hepatotoxicity.

When combined with urobilinogen measurements, this test helps identify disorders that can cause jaundice. The analysis can be performed at bedside, using a bilirubin reagent strip, or in the laboratory.

Purpose

• To help identify the cause of jaundice

Patient preparation

• Explain to the patient that this test helps determine the cause of jaundice.

• Inform him that he needn't restrict food or fluids before the test.

• Tell him the test requires a random urine specimen.

• Advise him that the specimen will be tested at bedside or in the laboratory.

Bedside analysis can be performed immediately; laboratory analysis is completed in 1 day.

Procedure and posttest care

• Collect a random urine specimen in the container provided.

To perform bedside analysis using the *dipstrip* procedure, take the following steps:

• Dip the reagent strip into the specimen and remove it immediately.

• Compare the strip color with the color standards after 20 seconds.

• Record the test results on the patient's chart.

To perform bedside analysis using the *ictotest* procedure:

• Place five drops of urine on the asbestos-cellulose test mat. If bilirubin is present, it will be absorbed into the mat.

• Put a reagent tablet on the wet area of the mat, and place two drops of water on the tablet. If bilirubin is present, a blue to purple coloration will develop on the mat. Pink or red indicates absence of bilirubin.

Precautions

• Use only a freshly voided specimen. Bilirubin disintegrates after 30 minutes of exposure to room temperature or light.

• If the specimen is to be analyzed in the laboratory, send it to the laboratory immediately.

• Record the time of collection on the patient's chart.

• If the specimen is tested at bedside, make sure 20 seconds elapse before interpreting the color change on the dipstrip.

• Be sure lighting is adequate to make this color determination.

Normal findings

Normally, bilirubin is not found in urine in a routine screening test.

COMPARATIVE VALUES OF BILIRUBIN AND UROBILINOGEN

CAUSES OF JAUNDICE	Indirect bilirubin	Direct bilirubin	Bilirubin	Urobil- inogen	Urobil- inogen
	SERUM		URINE		FECES
Unconjugated hyperbilirubinemia					
Hemolytic disorders: hemolytic anemia, erythroblastosis fetalis	↑	N	O	N↑	↑
Gilbert's disease: constitutional hepatic dysfunction	↑↑	N	O	N↓	N↓
Crigler-Najjar syndrome: congenital hyperbilirubinemia	↑↑↑	N	O	N↓	N↓
Conjugated hyperbilirubinemia					
Extrahepatic obstruction: calculi, tumor, scar tissue in common bile duct or hepatic excretory duct	N	↑	+	↓O	↓O
Hepatocellular disorders: viral, toxic, or alcoholic hepatitis; cirrhosis; parenchymal injury	↑	↑	+	↓N↑	N↓
• *Hepatocanalicular disorders or intrahepatic obstruction*: drug-induced cholestasis; some familial defects, such as Dubin-Johnson and Rotor's syndromes; viral hepatitis; primary biliary cirrhosis	↑	↑	+	↓N↑	N↓

KEY

↑	Increased
N↑	May be increased
↑↑	Moderately increased
↑↑↑	Markedly increased
N	Normal
O	Absent
+	Present
N↓	Normal or reduced
↓O	Decreased or absent
↓N↑	Variable

Abnormal findings

High concentrations of direct bilirubin in urine may be evident from the specimen's appearance (dark, with a yellow foam). To diagnose jaundice, however, the presence or absence of direct bilirubin in urine must be correlated with serum test results and with urine and fecal urobilinogen levels. (See *Comparative values of bilirubin and urobilinogen.*)

UROBILINOGEN

This test detects impaired liver function by measuring urine levels of urobilinogen, the colorless, water-soluble product that results from the reduction of bilirubin by intestinal bacteria. Absent or altered urobilinogen levels can indicate hepatic damage or dysfunction. Increased urine urobilinogen may indicate hemolysis of red blood cells.

Quantitative analysis of urine urobilinogen involves addition of Ehrlich's reagent to a 2-hour urine specimen. The resulting color reaction is read promptly by spectrophotometry.

Purpose

• To aid diagnosis of extrahepatic obstruction, such as blockage of the common bile duct
• To aid differential diagnosis of hepatic and hematologic disorders

Patient preparation

• Explain to the patient that this test helps assess liver and biliary tract function.
• Inform him that he needn't restrict fluids or food, except for bananas, which he should avoid for 48 hours before the test.
• Tell him that the test requires a 2-hour urine specimen, and teach him how to collect it.

• Check the patient's history for drugs that may affect urine urobilinogen levels, such as para-aminosalicylic acid, phenazopyridine, procaine, mandelate, phenothiazines, and sulfonamides. Review your findings with the laboratory and the doctor, who may restrict such drugs before the test.

Procedure and posttest care

• Most laboratories request a random urine specimen; others prefer a 2-hour specimen, usually during the afternoon (ideally, between 1 p.m. and 3 p.m.), when urobilinogen levels peak.
• Tell the patient he may resume his normal diet.
• Resume administration of drugs withheld during the test.

Precautions

• Send the specimen to the laboratory immediately. This test must be performed within 30 minutes of collection because urobilinogen quickly oxidizes to an orange compound called urobilin.

Reference values

Normally, urine urobilinogen values range from 0.1 to 1.1 Ehrlich units/ 2 hours in women and 0.3 to 2.1 Ehrlich units/2 hours in men.

Abnormal findings

Absence of urine urobilinogen may result from complete obstructive jaundice or treatment with broad-spectrum antibiotics, which destroy the intestinal bacterial flora. Low urine urobilinogen levels may result from congenital enzymatic jaundice (hyperbilirubinemia syndromes) or from treatment with drugs that acidify urine, such as ammonium chloride or ascorbic acid.

Elevated levels may indicate hemolytic jaundice, hepatitis, or cirrhosis.

SUGARS, KETONES, AND MUCOPOLY-SACCHARIDES

COPPER REDUCTION TEST

The copper reduction test measures the concentration of reducing substances in the urine through the reaction of these substances with a commercially prepared tablet called Clinitest. Clinitest, which reacts to glucose and to other reducing substances (mostly sugars), has almost replaced Benedict's test.

This test is most valuable for providing the patient with overt or latent diabetes a simple, at-home method of monitoring urine sugar level. It is sometimes used as a rapid laboratory screening tool.

Purpose
• To detect mellituria
• To monitor urine glucose levels during insulin therapy, after determination that the sugar in the urine is glucose

Patient preparation
• Explain to the patient that this test determines urine sugar level.
• If the patient has been recently diagnosed as diabetic, teach him how to perform the Clinitest tablet test.
• Check his medication history for drugs that may interfere with test results, such as aminosalicylic acid, cephalosporins, chloral hydrate, chloramphenicol, isoniazid, levodopa, metolazone, nalidixic acid, penicillin G, probenecid, salicylates, streptomycin, tetracycline, or uric acid.

• Provide written guidelines and a flow sheet to help him record Clinitest results at home, if appropriate.

Equipment
Specimen container, 10-ml test tube, medicine dropper, Clinitest tablets, Clinitest color chart.

Procedure and posttest care
• Have the patient void; then give him a drink of water.
• Collect a second-voided urine specimen after 30 to 45 minutes.
To perform the five-drop Clinitest tablet test:
• Hold the medicine dropper vertically, and instill five drops of urine from the specimen container into the test tube.
• Rinse the dropper with water, and add 10 drops of water to the test tube.
• Add one Clinitest tablet, and observe the color change, especially during effervescence (the pass-through phase).
• Wait 15 seconds after effervescence subsides, and gently agitate the test tube.
• If color develops at the 15-second interval, read the color against the Clinitest color chart, and record the results.
• Ignore any changes that develop after 15 seconds.
• Rapid color changes (bright orange to dark brown or green-brown) in the pass-through phase in a five-drop Clinitest reaction indicate glycosuria of 2% or more. Record the results as over 2% without comparison to the color chart.
To perform the two-drop Clinitest tablet test:
• Hold the medicine dropper vertically, and instill two drops of urine into the test tube.
• Flush urine residue from the dropper with water; then add 10 drops of water to the test tube.
• Add one Clinitest tablet, and observe the color change during the pass-through phase.

• Wait 15 seconds after effervescence stops; compare the color with the appropriate color reference chart, and record results.

• In a two-drop Clinitest reaction, rapid color changes (bright orange to dark brown or green-brown) in the pass-through phase indicate glycosuria of 5% or more.

Precautions

• Instruct the patient not to contaminate the specimen with toilet tissue or stool.

• Make sure hands are dry when handling Clinitest tablets and avoid contact with eyes, mucous membranes, gastrointestinal tract, and clothing because sodium hydroxide and moisture produce caustic burns.

• Store tablets in a well-marked, child-proof bottle to prevent accidental ingestion.

• Don't use discolored tablets (dark blue). The normal color of fresh tablets is light blue, with darker blue flecks.

• During effervescence, hold the test tube near the top to avoid burning your hand; it becomes boiling hot.

Normal findings

Normally, no glucose is present in urine.

Abnormal findings

Glycosuria occurs in diabetes mellitus, adrenal and thyroid disorders, hepatic and central nervous system diseases, conditions involving low renal threshold such as Fanconi's syndrome, toxic renal tubular disease, heavy metal poisoning, glomerulonephritis, nephrosis, pregnancy, and total parenteral nutrition. It also occurs with administration of large amounts of glucose and some drugs, such as asparaginase, corticosteroids, carbamazepine, ammonium chloride, thiazide diuretics, dextrothyroxine, large amounts of nicotinic acid, lithium carbonate, and long-term phenothiazines.

GLUCOSE OXIDASE TEST

The glucose oxidase test — which involves the use of commercial, plastic-coated reagent strips (Clinistix, Diastix) or Tes-Tape — is a specific, qualitative test for glycosuria. The test is used primarily to monitor urine glucose in patients with diabetes. Because of this test's simplicity and convenience, patients can perform it at home.

Purpose

• To detect glycosuria

• To monitor urine glucose levels during insulin therapy

Patient preparation

• Explain to the patient that this test determines urine glucose concentration.

• If he's a newly diagnosed patient with diabetes, teach him how to perform a reagent strip test.

• Check his drug history. If he's receiving levodopa, ascorbic acid, phenazopyridine, salicylates, peroxides, or hypochlorites, use Clinitest tablets instead.

Equipment

Specimen container, glucose test strips, reference color blocks.

Procedure and posttest care

• Have the patient void; then give him a drink of water.

• Collect a second-voided specimen after 30 to 45 minutes.

To perform the Clinistix test:

• Dip the test area of the reagent strip in the specimen for 2 seconds.

• Remove excess urine by tapping the strip against a clean surface or the side of the container, and begin timing.

• Hold the strip in the air, and "read" the color *exactly 10 seconds* after taking the strip out of the urine by comparing it with the reference color blocks on the label of the container.
• Record the results.
• Ignore color changes that develop after 10 seconds.

To perform the Diastix test:
• Dip the reagent strip in the specimen for 2 seconds.
• Remove excess urine by tapping the strip against the container, and begin timing.
• Hold the strip in the air, and compare the color to the color chart *exactly 30 seconds* after taking the strip out of the urine.
• Record the results.
• Ignore color changes that develop after 30 seconds.

To use Tes-Tape:
• Withdraw about 1½″ (3.8 cm) of the reagent tape from the dispenser; dip ¼″ (0.6 cm) in the specimen for 2 seconds.
• Remove excess urine by tapping the strip against the side of the container, and begin timing.
• Hold the tape in the air, and compare the color of the darkest part of the tape to the color chart *exactly 60 seconds* after taking the strip out of the urine.
• If the tape indicates 0.5% or higher, wait an additional 60 seconds to make the final color comparison.
• Record the results.

Precautions
• Instruct the patient not to contaminate the urine specimen with toilet tissue or stool.
• Keep the test strip container tightly closed to prevent deterioration of strips by exposure to light or moisture.
• Store it in a cool place (under 86° F [30° C]) to avoid heat degradation.
• Don't use discolored or darkened Clinistix or Diastix or dark yellow or yellow-brown Tes-Tape.

Normal findings
Normally, no glucose is present in urine.

Abnormal findings
Glycosuria occurs in diabetes mellitus, adrenal and thyroid disorders, hepatic and central nervous system diseases, conditions involving low renal threshold such as Fanconi's syndrome, toxic renal tubular disease, heavy metal poisoning, glomerulonephritis, nephrosis, pregnancy, and total parenteral nutrition. It also occurs with administration of large amounts of glucose and of certain drugs, such as asparaginase, corticosteroids, carbamazepine, ammonium chloride, thiazide diuretics, dextrothyroxine, large doses of nicotinic acid, lithium carbonate, and prolonged use of phenothiazines.

KETONE TEST

In this routine, semiquantitative screening test, a commercially prepared product is used to measure the urine level of ketone bodies. Ketone bodies are the by-products of fat metabolism; they include acetoacetic acid, acetone, and beta-hydroxybutyric acid. Excessive amounts may appear in patients with carbohydrate dehydration, which may occur in starvation or diabetic ketoacidosis.

Commercially available tests include the Acetest tablet, Chemstrip K, Ketostix, or Keto-Diastix. Each product measures a specific ketone body. For example, Acetest measures acetone and Ketostix measures acetoacetic acid.

Purpose
• To screen for ketonuria
• To identify diabetic ketoacidosis and carbohydrate deprivation

• To distinguish between a diabetic and a nondiabetic coma
• To monitor control of diabetes mellitus, ketogenic weight reduction, and treatment of diabetic ketoacidosis

Patient preparation
• Explain to the patient that this test evaluates fat metabolism.
• If he is a newly diagnosed patient with diabetes, tell him how to perform the test.
• Check his medication history. Acetest tablets must be used if the patient is taking levodopa or phenazopyridine or has recently received sulfobromophthalein.

Procedure and posttest care
• Instruct the patient to void; then give him a drink of water.
• Collect a second-voided midstream specimen about 30 minutes later.
To use Acetest:
• Lay the tablet on a piece of white paper, and place one drop of urine on the tablet.
• Compare the tablet color (white, lavender, or purple) with the color chart after 30 seconds.
To use Ketostix:
• Dip the reagent stick into the specimen and remove it immediately.
• Compare the stick color (buff or purple) with the color chart after 15 seconds.
• Record the results as negative, small, moderate, or large amounts of ketones.
To use Keto-Diastix:
• Dip the reagent strip into the specimen, and remove it immediately.
• Tap the edge of the strip against the container or a clean, dry surface to remove excess urine.
• Hold the strip horizontally to prevent mixing the chemicals from the two areas.
• Interpret each area of the strip separately. Compare the color of the ketone section (buff or purple) with the appropriate color chart after exactly 15 seconds; compare the color of the glucose section after 30 seconds.
• Ignore color changes that occur after the specified waiting periods.
• Record the results as negative or positive for small, moderate, or large amounts of ketones.

Precautions
• Test the specimen within 60 minutes after it is obtained, or you must refrigerate it.
• Allow refrigerated specimens to return to room temperature before testing.
• Don't use tablets or strips that have become discolored or darkened.

Normal findings
Normally, no ketones are present in urine.

Abnormal findings
Ketonuria may occur in uncontrolled diabetes mellitus or starvation. It also occurs as a metabolic complication of total parenteral nutrition.

ACID MUCOPOLY-SACCHARIDES

This quantitative test helps detect mucopolysaccharidoses, a rare disorder that may affect the skeleton, joints, liver, spleen, eye, ear, skin, teeth, and the cardiovascular, respiratory, and central nervous systems. This test measures the urine level of acid mucopolysaccharides (AMPs), a group of polysaccharides or carbohydrates.

Purpose
• To diagnose mucopolysaccharidoses in infants with family histories of the disease

Patient preparation
• Explain to the parents of the infant that this test helps determine the efficiency of carbohydrate metabolism.
• Inform them that they needn't restrict the child's food or fluids.
• Tell the parents that the test requires urine collection for 24 hours, and instruct them on the proper way to collect the specimen at home.
• If the infant is receiving therapy with heparin and must continue it, note this on the laboratory slip.

Equipment
Pediatric urine collectors, 24-hour collection container, 20 ml toluene (usually obtained from the laboratory).

Procedure and posttest care
• Collect the patient's urine over a 24-hour period.
• Add 20 ml toluene as a preservative at the start of the collection.
• Indicate the patient's age on the laboratory slip.
• Send the specimen to the laboratory immediately at the end of the 24-hour collection period.
• Be sure to remove all adhesive from the urine collector from the infant's perineum.
• Wash the area gently with soap and water, and watch for irritation.

Precautions
• Refrigerate the specimen or place it on ice during the collection period.

Reference values
The AMP value is expressed as milligrams of glucuronic acid divided by the amount of creatinine in the same specimen (which reflects glomerular filtration rate) to overcome irregularities in the 24-hour urine collection. Normal AMP values vary with age.

AGE	A.M.P. VALUES
2	8 to 30
4	7 to 27
6	6 to 24
8	4 to 22
10	2 to 18
12	0 to 15
14	0 to 12

Abnormal findings
Elevated AMP levels reliably indicate mucopolysaccharidoses. Supplementary quantitative analysis and detailed blood studies can identify the defective enzyme.

VITAMINS

TRYPTOPHAN CHALLENGE TEST

Measurement of urine xanthurenic acid after a challenge dose of tryptophan confirms deficiency of vitamin B_6 long before symptoms appear. This test is especially important because direct assay of vitamin B_6 isn't currently available.

Although vitamin B_6 isn't directly involved in energy metabolism, it is essential for reactions that occur in protein metabolism and for amino acid synthesis. Vitamin B_6 deficiency can cause hypochromic microcytic anemia without iron deficiency and central nervous system disturbances. When normal magnesium levels accompany a vitamin B_6 deficiency, urinary citrate and oxalate solubility may decrease, causing formation of urinary calculi.

Purpose
• To detect vitamin B_6 deficiency

Patient preparation
• Explain to the patient that this test determines the body's stores of vitamin B_6.
• Tell him he'll receive an oral dose of medication.
• Explain that this test requires urine collection over a 24-hour period.
• Check the patient's medication history for current use of drugs that may cause vitamin B_6 deficiency, including oral contraceptives, hydralazine, D-penicillamine, or isoniazid.

Procedure and posttest care
• Administer L-tryptophan by mouth (usually, 50 mg/kg for children and up to 2 g/kg for adults).
• Have the patient void and discard the urine. Immediately begin collection of a 24-hour urine specimen.
• Inform the patient with vitamin B_6 deficiency that yeast, wheat, corn, liver, and kidneys are good sources of pyridoxine.

Precautions
• Make sure the specimen bottle contains a crystal of thymol, a preservative.
• Tell the patient not to contaminate the urine specimen with toilet tissue or stool.
• Refrigerate the specimen, or place it on ice during the collection period.

Reference values
Normal excretion of xanthurenic acid after a tryptophan challenge dose is less than 50 mg/24 hours.

Abnormal findings
Urine levels of xanthurenic acid exceeding 100 mg/24 hours indicate vitamin B_6 deficiency. This rare disorder may result from malnutrition, malignancy, pregnancy, familial xanthurenic aciduria, or use of oral contraceptives, hydralazine, D-penicillamine, or isoniazid.

VITAMIN C

Through colorimetric measurement of urinary levels, this test determines body stores of vitamin C (ascorbic acid). This water-soluble vitamin, which is easily absorbed by the intestine, acts as a reversible reducing agent in metabolic processes, aids collagen formation, and helps maintain connective and osteoid tissues.

This analysis is particularly useful in diagnosing scurvy, an extreme deficiency of vitamin C characterized by the degeneration of connective and osteoid tissues, dentin, and endothelial membranes. Although now uncommon in North America, scurvy may occur in alcoholics, people on low-residue or low-citrus diets, and infants who have been weaned to cow's milk that does not contain a vitamin C supplement.

Purpose
• To aid diagnosis of scurvy, scurvy-like conditions, and metabolic disorders, such as malnutrition, that interfere with oxidative processes

Patient preparation
• Explain to the patient that this test detects vitamin C deficiency.
• Inform the patient that he should maintain a normal diet.
• Tell him the test requires urine collection over a 24-hour period.
• If the specimen is to be collected at home, instruct the patient on proper collection technique.

Procedure and posttest care
• Collect the patient's urine over a 24-hour period.
• Advise the patient with vitamin C deficiency that citrus fruits, tomatoes, potatoes, cabbage, and strawberries are good dietary sources of vitamin C.

Precautions
• Tell the patient not to contaminate the specimen with toilet tissue or stool.
• Refrigerate the specimen, or place it on ice during the collection period.

Reference values
Normal urine vitamin C excretion is 30 mg/24 hours.

Abnormal findings
Depressed urine vitamin C levels are common in patients with infection, cancer, burns, or other stress-producing conditions. Decreased vitamin C levels may also indicate malnutrition, malabsorption, renal deficiencies, or prolonged I.V. therapy without vitamin C replacement. Severe vitamin C deficiency causes scurvy.

MINERALS

SODIUM AND CHLORIDE

This test determines urine levels of sodium, the major extracellular cation, and of chloride, the major extracellular anion. Less significant than serum levels (and, consequently, performed less frequently), measurement of urine sodium and urine chloride concentrations is used to evaluate renal conservation of these two electrolytes and to confirm serum sodium and chloride values.

In the body, sodium and chloride help maintain osmotic pressure and water and acid-base balance. Normal ranges of sodium and chloride in the urine vary greatly with dietary salt intake and perspiration.

Purpose
• To help evaluate fluid and electrolyte imbalance
• To monitor the effects of a low-salt diet
• To help evaluate renal and adrenal disorders

Patient preparation
• Explain to the patient that this test helps determine the balance of salt and water in the body.
• Advise him that no special restrictions are necessary.
• Tell him the test requires urine collection over a 24-hour period.
• Advise him that the laboratory requires 1 day to complete the analysis.
• If the specimen is to be collected at home, instruct the patient on proper collection technique.
• Check the patient's history for medications that may influence test results, including ammonium chloride, potassium, sodium bicarbonate, and thiazide diuretics.

Procedure and posttest care
• Collect the patient's urine over a 24-hour period.

Precautions
• Tell the patient not to contaminate the specimen with toilet tissue or stool.

Reference values
Normal urine sodium excretion is 30 to 280 mEq/24 hours. Normal urine chloride excretion is 110 to 250 mEq/24 hours. Normal urine sodium-chloride excretion is 5 to 20 g/24 hours.

Abnormal findings

Usually, urine sodium and urine chloride levels are parallel, rising and falling in tandem. Abnormal levels of both minerals may indicate the need for more specific testing.

Elevated urine sodium levels may reflect increased salt intake, adrenal failure, salicylate toxicity, diabetic acidosis, salt-losing nephritis, and water-deficient dehydration.

Decreased urine sodium levels suggest decreased salt intake, primary aldosteronism, acute renal failure, and congestive heart failure.

Elevated urine chloride levels may result from water-deficient dehydration, salicylate toxicity, diabetic acidosis, adrenocortical insufficiency (Addison's disease), and salt-losing renal disease. Decreased levels may result from excessive diaphoresis, congestive heart failure, hypochloremic metabolic alkalosis, or from prolonged vomiting or gastric suctioning.

To evaluate fluid-electrolyte imbalance, results must be correlated with findings of serum electrolyte studies.

POTASSIUM

This quantitative test measures urine levels of potassium, a major intracellular cation that helps regulate acid-base balance and neuromuscular function. Potassium imbalance may cause such signs and symptoms as muscle weakness, nausea, diarrhea, confusion, hypotension, and electrocardiogram changes; severe imbalance may lead to cardiac arrest.

Most commonly, a serum potassium test is performed to detect hyperkalemia (abnormally high levels) or hypokalemia (abnormally low levels). A urine potassium test may be performed to evaluate hypokalemia when a history and physical examination fail to uncover the cause. If results suggest a renal disorder, additional renal function tests may be ordered.

Purpose

• To determine whether hypokalemia is caused by renal or extrarenal disorders

Patient preparation

• Explain to the patient that this test evaluates his kidney function.
• Advise him that no special dietary restrictions are necessary.
• Tell him that the test requires urine collection over a 24-hour period.
• If the specimen is to be collected at home, teach him the correct collection technique.
• Check his medication history for drugs that may alter test results, including ammonium chloride, thiazide diuretics, and acetazolamide. If they must be continued, note this on the laboratory slip.

Procedure and posttest care

• Collect the patient's urine over a 24-hour period.
• Administer potassium supplements and monitor serum levels as appropriate.
• Provide dietary supplements and nutritional counseling as necessary.
• Replace volume loss with I.V. or oral fluids as necessary.
• Resume administration of drugs withheld during the test.

Precautions

• Tell the patient not to contaminate the specimen with toilet tissue or stool.
• Refrigerate the specimen or place it on ice during the collection period.
• Send the specimen to the laboratory immediately after collection or refrigerate it.

Reference values

Normal potassium excretion is 25 to 125 mEq/24 hours, with an average potassium concentration of 25 to 100 mEq/L.

Abnormal findings

In a patient with hypokalemia, potassium concentration less than 10 mEq/L suggests normal kidney function, indicating that potassium loss is most likely the result of a gastrointestinal disorder, such as malabsorption syndrome.

In a patient with hypokalemia lasting more than 3 days, urine potassium concentration above 10 mEq/L indicates renal loss of potassium. These losses may result from such disorders as aldosteronism, renal tubular acidosis, or chronic renal failure. However, extrarenal disorders, such as dehydration, starvation, Cushing's disease, or salicylate intoxication, may also elevate urine potassium levels.

CALCIUM AND PHOSPHATES

This test measures the urine levels of calcium and phosphates, elements essential for the formation and resorption of bone. Urine calcium and phosphate levels generally parallel serum levels.

Normally absorbed in the upper intestine and excreted in feces and urine, calcium and phosphates help maintain tissue and fluid pH, electrolyte balance in cells and extracellular fluids, and permeability of cell membranes. Calcium promotes enzymatic processes, aids blood coagulation, and lowers neuromuscular irritability; phosphates aid carbohydrate metabolism.

Purpose

• To evaluate calcium and phosphate metabolism and excretion
• To monitor treatment of calcium or phosphate deficiency

Patient preparation

• Explain to the patient that this test measures the amount of calcium and phosphates in the urine.
• Encourage him to be as active as possible before the test.
• Tell him the test requires urine collection over a 24-hour period.
• If the patient is to collect the specimen, teach him the proper technique.
• Provide the Albright-Reifenstein diet (which contains about 130 mg of calcium/24 hours) for 3 days before the test or provide a copy of the diet for the patient to follow at home.
• Note recent use of thiazide diuretics, sodium phosphate, or glucocorticoids on the laboratory slip.

Procedure and posttest care

• Collect the patient's urine over a 24-hour period.
• Observe a patient with low urine calcium levels for tetany.

Precautions

• Tell the patient not to contaminate the specimen with toilet tissue or stool.

Reference values

Normal values depend on dietary intake. Males excrete less than 275 mg of calcium/24 hours. Females excrete less than 250 mg/24 hours. Normal excretion of phosphate is less than 1,000 mg/24 hours.

Abnormal findings

A variety of disorders may affect calcium and phosphorus levels. (See *Disorders that affect urine calcium and urine phosphorus levels.*)

DISORDERS THAT AFFECT URINE CALCIUM AND URINE PHOSPHORUS LEVELS

DISORDER	URINE CALCIUM LEVEL	URINE PHOSPHATE LEVEL
Hyperparathyroidism	Elevated	Elevated
Vitamin D intoxication	Elevated	Suppressed
Metastatic carcinoma	Elevated	Normal
Sarcoidosis	Elevated	Suppressed
Renal tubular acidosis	Elevated	Elevated
Multiple myeloma	Elevated or normal	Elevated or normal
Paget's disease	Normal	Normal
Milk-alkali syndrome	Suppressed or normal	Suppressed or normal
Hypoparathyroidism	Suppressed	Suppressed
Acute nephrosis	Suppressed	Suppressed or normal
Chronic nephrosis	Suppressed	Suppressed
Acute nephritis	Suppressed	Suppressed
Renal insufficiency	Suppressed	Suppressed
Osteomalacia	Suppressed	Suppressed
Steatorrhea	Suppressed	Suppressed

MAGNESIUM

Measurement of urine magnesium is especially useful because magnesium deficiency is detectable in urine before it changes serum magnesium levels. This test may be used to rule out magnesium deficiency as the cause of neurologic symptoms and to help evaluate glomerular function in suspected renal disease.

Magnesium is a cation found primarily in the bones and in intracellular fluid; a small amount is present in extracellular fluid. This element activates many enzyme systems, helps transport sodium and potassium across cell membranes, affects nucleic acid and protein metabolism, and influences intracellular calcium levels through its effect on secretion of parathyroid hormone.

Purpose
• To rule out magnesium deficiency in patients with symptoms of central nervous system irritation
• To detect excessive urinary excretion of magnesium
• To help evaluate glomerular function in renal disease

Patient preparation
• Explain to the patient that this test determines urine magnesium levels.
• Advise him that no special restrictions are necessary.
• Tell him that this test requires urine collection over a 24-hour period.
• Advise him that the laboratory requires at least 1 day to complete the analysis.
• Ask the patient if he is receiving magnesium-containing antacids, ethacrynic acid, thiazide diuretics (for example, spironolactone), or aldosterone. If so, be sure to note this on the laboratory slip.

Procedure and posttest care
• Collect the patient's urine over a 24-hour period.

Precautions
• Tell the patient to be careful not to contaminate the urine specimen with toilet tissue or stool.

Reference values
Normal urinary excretion of magnesium is less than 150 mg/24 hours (atomic absorption).

Abnormal findings
Low urine magnesium levels may result from malabsorption, acute or chronic diarrhea, diabetic acidosis, dehydration, pancreatitis, advanced renal failure, and primary aldosteronism. They may also result from decreased dietary intake of magnesium.

Elevated urine magnesium levels may result from early chronic renal disease, adrenocortical insufficiency (Addison's disease), chronic alcoholism, or chronic ingestion of magnesium-containing antacids.

COPPER

This test measures the urine level of copper, an essential trace element and a component of several metalloenzymes and proteins necessary for hemoglobin synthesis and oxidation reduction. Most copper in plasma is bound to and transported by an alpha$_2$-globulin (plasma protein) called ceruloplasmin. When copper is unbound, the ions can inhibit many enzyme reactions, resulting in copper toxicity. Urine normally contains only a small amount of free copper.

Determination of urine copper levels is frequently used to detect Wilson's disease, a rare, inborn metabolic error, most common among people of eastern European Jewish, southern Italian, or Sicilian ancestry.

Purpose
• To help detect Wilson's disease
• To screen infants with family histories of Wilson's disease

Patient preparation
• Explain to the patient that this test determines the amount of copper in urine.
• Inform him that no special restrictions are necessary.
• Tell him the test requires urine collection over a 24-hour period. If the specimen is to be collected at home, describe the proper collection technique.

Procedure and posttest care
• Collect the patient's urine over a 24-hour period.

Precautions
• Tell the patient not to contaminate the urine specimen with toilet tissue or stool.

Reference values

Normal urinary excretion of copper is 15 to 60 mcg/24 hours.

Abnormal findings

Elevated urine copper levels usually indicate Wilson's disease (a liver biopsy helps establish this diagnosis). Wilson's disease is marked by decreased ceruloplasmin, increased urinary excretion of copper, and accumulation of copper in the interstitial tissues of the liver and brain. Early detection and treatment (low-copper diet and D-penicillamine) are vital to prevent irreversible changes, such as nerve tissue degeneration and cirrhosis of the liver.

Elevated copper levels may also occur in nephrotic syndromes, chronic active hepatitis, biliary cirrhosis, and rheumatoid arthritis.

HEMOSIDERIN

This test measures the urine level of hemosiderin — a colloidal iron oxide and one of the two forms of storage iron deposited in body tissue.

When iron storage mechanisms fail to manage iron overload, excess iron may escape to cells unaccustomed to high iron concentrations and may produce toxic effects. Toxicity may affect the liver, myocardium, bone marrow, pancreas, kidneys, and skin. Subsequent tissue damage is referred to as hemochromatosis. Hemochromatosis may occur in a rare hereditary form (primary hemochromatosis) and in exogenous forms.

Purpose

• To aid diagnosis of hemochromatosis

Patient preparation

• Explain to the patient that this test helps determine if the body is accumulating excessive amounts of iron.
• Inform him that no restrictions are necessary and that the test requires a urine specimen.

Procedure and posttest care

• Collect a random urine specimen of approximately 30 ml.

Precautions

• Securely seal the container, and send the specimen to the laboratory immediately.

Normal findings

Normally, hemosiderin is not found in urine.

Abnormal findings

The presence of hemosiderin, appearing as yellow-brown granules in urinary sediment, indicates hemochromatosis; liver or bone marrow biopsy is necessary for confirmation of primary hemochromatosis. Hemosiderin may also suggest pernicious anemia, chronic hemolytic anemia, multiple blood transfusions, and paroxysmal nocturnal hemoglobinuria, the result of excessive iron injections or dietary intake of iron.

OXALATE

This test measures urine levels of oxalate, a salt of oxalic acid. Oxalate is an end product of metabolism and is excreted almost exclusively in the urine.

Most important, the test detects hyperoxaluria, a disorder in which oxalate accumulates in the soft and connective tissue, especially in the kidneys and bladder, causing chronic inflammation and fibrosis. Calcium oxalate deposits are the most common cause of renal calculi, which may produce kidney damage.

Purpose
• To detect primary hyperoxaluria in infants
• To rule out hyperoxaluria in renal insufficiency

Patient preparation
• Explain to the patient (or to the parents if the patient is a child) that this test determines if the urine contains excess oxalate.
• Instruct him to restrict intake of tomatoes, strawberries, rhubarb, and spinach for about 1 week before the test.
• Tell him the test requires urine collection over a 24-hour period.
• Advise him that the laboratory requires at least 2 days to complete the analysis.

Procedure and posttest care
• Collect the patient's urine over a 24-hour period. Use a light-protected container with hydrochloric acid.

Precautions
• Tell the patient not to urinate directly into the 24-hour specimen container, but to use an appropriate container.
• Advise him not to contaminate the urine specimen with toilet tissue or stool.

Reference values
Urine oxalate levels up to 40 mg/24 hours are considered normal.

Abnormal findings
Elevated urine oxalate levels (hyperoxaluria) may result from excessive metabolic production of oxalate or increased oxalate intake. Levels as high as 100 to 400 mg/24 hours can occur.

Primary hyperoxaluria, a rare inborn metabolic disorder, causes excessive production and urinary excretion of oxalate. In this type of hyperoxaluria, urine oxalate levels become elevated before serum levels become elevated.

Secondary hyperoxaluria can result from pancreatic insufficiency, diabetes mellitus, cirrhosis, pyridoxine deficiency, Crohn's disease, ileal resection, or ingestion of antifreeze (ethylene glycol) or stain-remover or it can occur as a reaction to a methoxyflurane anesthetic.

CHAPTER 7

Additional Specimen Tests

RESPIRATORY SYSTEM

EXAMINATION OF SPUTUM FOR OVA AND PARASITES

This test evaluates a sputum specimen for parasites. Parasite infestation is rare in North America but may result from exposure to *Entamoeba histolytica, Ascaris lumbricoides, Echinococcus granulosus, Strongyloides stercoralis, Paragonimus westermani,* or *Necator americanus.* The specimen is obtained by expectoration or by tracheal suctioning.

Purpose
• To identify pulmonary parasites

Patient preparation
• Explain to the patient that this test helps identify parasitic pulmonary infection.
• Tell him the test requires a sputum specimen or, if necessary, tracheal suctioning.
• Inform him that early morning collection is preferred because secretions accumulate overnight.
• Encourage the patient to help sputum production by drinking fluids the night before collection.
• Teach the patient how to expectorate by taking three deep breaths and forcing a deep cough.
• Tell him during tracheal suctioning, he'll experience some discomfort from the catheter.

Equipment
For expectoration: Sterile, disposable, impermeable container with screw cap or tight-fitting cap, nebulizer, intermittent positive-pressure breathing ventilator, and 10% sodium chloride, acetylcysteine, or sterile or distilled water aerosols, to induce cough.
For tracheal suctioning: #16 or #18 French suction catheter, sterile gloves, sterile specimen container or sputum trap, sterile 0.9% sodium chloride solution.

Procedure and posttest care
Expectoration:
• Instruct the patient to breathe deeply a few times and then to "deep cough" and expectorate into the container.
• Use chest physiotherapy, or heated aerosol spray (nebulization), if cough is unproductive.
• Take proper precautions in sending the specimen to the laboratory.
Tracheal suctioning:
• Administer oxygen before and after the procedure if necessary.
• Attach a sputum trap to the suction catheter.
• Wear a sterile glove to lubricate the tip of the catheter, and pass the catheter through the patient's nostril without suction. (The patient will cough when the catheter passes into the larynx.)
• Advance the catheter into the trachea.
• Apply suction for no longer than 15 seconds to obtain the specimen.
• Stop suction, and gently remove the catheter.
• Discard the catheter and glove in a proper receptacle.
• Detach the sputum trap from the suction apparatus and cap the opening.
• Label all specimens carefully.
• Provide proper mouth care. After suctioning, offer water.
• Monitor vital signs every hour until the patient is stable.

Precautions

• Be sure to wear gloves when performing procedures and handling specimens.

• Do not perform tracheal suctioning in patients with esophageal varices or cardiac disease.

• If the patient has asthma or chronic bronchitis, watch for aggravated bronchospasms with use of more than 10% concentration of sodium chloride or acetylcysteine in an aerosol.

• Suction for only 5 to 10 seconds at a time during tracheal suctioning. *Never* suction for longer than 15 seconds. If the patient shows signs of hypoxia or cyanosis, remove the suctioning catheter immediately, and administer oxygen.

• Send the specimen to the laboratory immediately, or place it in preservative.

Normal findings

Normally, no parasites or ova are present.

Abnormal findings

The parasite identified indicates the type of pulmonary infection and the presence of adult-stage intestinal infection.

• *Entamoeba histolytica* trophozoites: pulmonary amebiasis

• *A. lumbricoides* larvae and adults: pneumonitis

• *Echinococcus granulosus* cysts of larval stage: hydatid disease

• *P. westermani* ova: paragonimiasis

• *S. stercoralis* larvae: strongyloidiasis

• *N. americanus* larvae: hookworm disease.

PLEURAL FLUID ANALYSIS

The pleura, a two-layer membrane that covers the lungs and lines the thoracic cavity, maintains a small amount of lubricating fluid between its layers to minimize friction during respiration. Increased fluid in this space may result from diseases such as cancer or tuberculosis, or from blood or lymphatic disorders, and can cause respiratory difficulty.

In pleural fluid aspiration (thoracentesis), the thoracic wall is punctured to obtain a specimen of pleural fluid for analysis or to relieve pulmonary compression and resultant respiratory distress.

Purpose

• To determine the cause and nature of pleural effusion

Patient preparation

• Explain to the patient that the test assesses the space around the lungs for fluid.

• Inform him that he needn't restrict food or fluids.

• Tell him who will perform the test and where it will take place.

• Explain that chest radiography or ultrasound study may precede the test to help locate the fluid.

• Check the patient's history for hypersensitivity to local anesthetics.

• Warn the patient that he may feel a stinging sensation on injection of the anesthetic and some pressure during withdrawal of the fluid.

• Advise him not to cough, breathe deeply, or move during the test to minimize the risk of injury to the lung.

Equipment

Sterile collection bottles, sterile gloves, adhesive tape, sterile thoracentesis tray (a prepackaged, disposable tray with the following: 70% alcohol or povidone-iodine solution, drapes, local anesthetic [usually 1% lidocaine], 5-ml sterile syringe for local anesthetic, 25G needle, 50-ml syringe for removing fluid, 17G aspiration needle, sterile specimen bottle or tube, three-way stopcock or sterile tubing to prevent air from entering the pleural cavity, small sterile dressing).

Procedure and posttest care

• Record baseline vital signs.

• If necessary, shave the area around the needle insertion site.

• Position the patient to widen intercostal spaces and to allow easier access to the pleural cavity. He must be well-supported and comfortable, preferably seated at the edge of the bed with a chair or stool supporting his feet and his head and arms resting on a padded overbed table. If the patient can't sit up, he may be positioned on his unaffected side, with the arm on the affected side elevated above his head.

• Remind him not to cough, breathe deeply, or move suddenly during the procedure.

• During aspiration, observe the patient for signs of respiratory distress, such as weakness, dyspnea, pallor, cyanosis, changes in heart rate, tachypnea, diaphoresis, blood-tinged frothy mucus, and hypotension.

• After the needle is withdrawn, apply slight pressure and a small adhesive bandage to the puncture site.

• Label the specimen, and record the date and time of the test and the amount, color, and character of the fluid (clear, frothy, purulent, bloody) on the request slip.

• Note any signs of distress exhibited during the procedure.

• Record the exact location from which fluid was removed to aid diagnosis.

• Reposition the patient comfortably on the affected side. Tell him to remain on this side for at least 1 hour to seal the puncture site. Elevate the head of the bed to facilitate breathing.

• Monitor vital signs every 30 minutes for 2 hours, and then every 4 hours until they are stable.

• Tell the patient to call a nurse immediately if he experiences difficulty breathing.

• Watch for signs of pneumothorax, tension pneumothorax, fluid reaccumulation and, if a large amount of fluid was withdrawn, pulmonary edema or cardiac distress due to mediastinal shift. Usually, a posttest radiograph is ordered to detect these complications before clinical symptoms appear.

• Check the puncture site for any fluid leakage. A large amount of leakage is abnormal. Also check the site and surrounding area for subcutaneous emphysema.

Precautions

• Thoracentesis is contraindicated in patients who have histories of bleeding disorders.

• Use strict aseptic technique.

• Note the patient's temperature and whether he is receiving antimicrobial therapy on the laboratory slip.

• Add a small amount (about 0.5 ml) of sterile heparin to the container to prevent coagulation of the fluid.

• Send the specimen to the laboratory immediately.

Reference values

Normally, the pleural cavity maintains negative pressure and contains less than 20 ml of serous fluid.

Abnormal findings

Pleural effusion results from the abnormal formation or reabsorption of pleural fluid. Certain characteristics classify pleural fluid as either a transudate (a low-protein fluid that has leaked from normal blood vessels) or an exudate (a protein-rich fluid that has leaked from blood vessels with increased permeability).

Pleural fluid may contain blood (hemothorax), chyle (chylothorax), or pus and necrotic tissue. Blood-tinged fluid may indicate a traumatic tap; if so, the fluid should clear as aspiration progresses.

Transudative effusion generally results from diminished colloidal pressure, increased negative pressure within the pleural cavity, ascites, systemic and pulmonary venous hypertension, congestive heart failure, hepatic cirrhosis, and nephritis. *Exudative effusion* results from disorders that increase pleural capillary permeability (possibly with changes in hydrostatic or colloid osmotic pressures), lymphatic drainage interference, infections, pulmonary infarctions, and neoplasms. Exudative effusion associated with depressed glucose levels; elevated lactate dehydrogenase isoenzymes (LD); rheumatoid arthritis cells; and negative smears, cultures, and cytologic examination may indicate pleurisy associated with rheumatoid arthritis.

The most common pathogens that appear in culture studies of pleural fluid include *Mycobacterium tuberculosis, Staphylococcus aureus, Streptococcus pneumoniae* and other streptococci, *Haemophilus influenzae* and, in the case of a ruptured pulmonary abscess, anaerobes, such as bacteroides. Generally, cultures are positive during the early stages of infection; however, antibiotic therapy may produce a negative culture despite a positive Gram stain and grossly purulent fluid. Empyema may result from complications of pneumonia, pulmonary abscess, perforation of the esophagus, or penetration from

mediastinitis. A high percentage of neutrophils suggests septic inflammation; predominating lymphocytes suggest tuberculosis, or fungal or viral effusions.

Serosanguineous fluid may indicate pleural extension of a malignant tumor. Elevated LD in a nonpurulent, nonhemolyzed, nonbloody effusion may also suggest malignancy. Pleural fluid glucose levels that are 30 to 40 mg/dl lower than blood glucose levels may indicate malignancy, bacterial infection, nonseptic inflammation, or metastases. Increased amylase levels occur with pleural effusions associated with pancreatitis.

GASTROINTESTINAL SYSTEM

BASAL GASTRIC SECRETION TEST

This test measures basal secretion during fasting by aspirating stomach contents through a nasogastric tube. It is indicated in patients with obscure epigastric pain, anorexia, and weight loss. Because external factors — such as the sight or odor of food — and psychological stress stimulate gastric secretion, accurate testing requires that the patient be relaxed and isolated from all sources of sensory stimulation. Although abnormal basal secretion can suggest various gastric and duodenal disorders, complete evaluation of secretion requires the gastric acid stimulation test.

Purpose
• To determine gastric output while the patient is fasting

Patient preparation
• Explain to the patient that this test measures the stomach's secretion of acid.
• Instruct him to restrict food for 12 hours and fluids and smoking for 8 hours before the test.
• Tell him who will perform the test and that the procedure takes approximately 1½ hours (or 2½ hours, if followed by the gastric acid stimulation test).
• Inform the patient that the test requires insertion of a tube through the nose and into the stomach and that he may initially experience discomfort and may cough or gag.
• Withhold antacids, anticholinergics, cholinergics, alcohol, cimetidine, reserpine, adrenergic blockers, and adrenocorticosteroids for 24 hours before the test. If these medications must be continued, note this on the laboratory slip.
• Check the patient's pulse rate and blood pressure just before the test. Then encourage him to relax.

Procedure and posttest care
• Insert the nasogastric tube after seating the patient comfortably.
• Attach a 20-ml syringe to it, and aspirate the stomach contents.
• To ensure complete emptying of the stomach, ask the patient to assume three positions in sequence — supine, and right and left lateral decubitus — while the stomach contents are aspirated.
• Label the specimen container "Residual Contents."
• Connect the nasogastric tube to the suction machine. Aspirate gastric contents by continuous low suction for 1½ hours. Aspiration can also be performed manually with a syringe.

• Collect a specimen every 15 minutes, but discard the first two; this eliminates the specimen that could be affected by the stress of the intubation.
• Record the color and odor of each specimen, and note the presence of food, mucus, bile, or blood.
• Label these specimens "Basal Contents," and number them 1 through 4.
• If the nasogastric tube is to be left in place, clamp it or attach it to low intermittent suction.
• Watch for complications such as nausea, vomiting, and abdominal distention or pain following removal of the nasogastric tube.
• If the patient complains of a sore throat, provide soothing lozenges.
• Tell the patient to resume his usual diet and any medications that were withheld for the test, unless the gastric acid stimulation test will also be performed.

Precautions
• The basal gastric secretion test is contraindicated in patients with conditions that prohibit nasogastric intubation.
• During insertion, make sure the nasogastric tube enters the esophagus, and not the trachea; remove it immediately if the patient develops cyanosis or paroxysms of coughing.
• Monitor vital signs during intubation, and observe carefully for arrhythmias.
• To prevent contamination of the specimens with saliva, instruct the patient to expectorate excess saliva.
• When collection is completed, send the specimens to the laboratory immediately.

Reference values
Normally, basal secretion ranges from 0.2 to 3.8 mEq/hour in women and 1 to 5 mEq/hour in men.

Abnormal findings

Abnormal basal secretion findings are nonspecific and must be considered with the results of the gastric acid stimulation test. Elevated secretion may suggest duodenal or jejunal ulcer (after partial gastrectomy) or, when markedly elevated, Zollinger-Ellison syndrome. Depressed secretion may indicate gastric carcinoma or benign gastric ulcer. Absence of secretion may indicate pernicious anemia.

GASTRIC ACID STIMULATION TEST

The gastric acid stimulation test measures the secretion of gastric acid for 1 hour after subcutaneous injection of pentagastrin or a similar drug that stimulates gastric acid output. This test is indicated when the basal secretion test suggests abnormal gastric secretion and is commonly performed immediately afterward. Although this test detects abnormal gastric secretion, radiographic studies and endoscopy are necessary to determine the cause.

Purpose

• To aid diagnosis of duodenal ulcer, Zollinger-Ellison syndrome, pernicious anemia, and gastric carcinoma

Patient preparation

• Explain to the patient that this test determines if the stomach is secreting acid properly.
• Instruct him to refrain from eating, drinking, and smoking after midnight before the test.
• Tell him who will perform the test, where it will take place, and that it takes 1 hour.

• Explain that the test requires passing a tube through the nose and into the stomach and a subcutaneous injection of pentagastrin.
• Describe the possible adverse effects of the test, such as abdominal pain, nausea, vomiting, flushing, transitory dizziness, faintness, and numbness of extremities. Instruct him to report such symptoms immediately.
• Check the patient's history for hypersensitivity to pentagastrin.
• Withhold antacids, anticholinergics, adrenergic blockers, cimetidine, and reserpine. If these drugs must be continued, note this on the laboratory slip.
• Record baseline vital signs before beginning the procedure.

Procedure and posttest care

• After basal gastric secretions have been collected, the nasogastric tube remains in place.
• Pentagastrin is injected subcutaneously. After 15 minutes, collect a specimen every 15 minutes for 1 hour.
• Record the color and odor of each specimen and note the presence of food, mucus, bile, or blood.
• Label the specimens "Stimulated Contents," and number them 1 through 4.
• If the nasogastric tube is kept in place, it should be clamped or attached to low intermittent suction.
• Watch for nausea, vomiting, and abdominal distention and pain after the nasogastric tube is removed.
• If the patient complains of a sore throat, provide soothing lozenges.
• Tell the patient he may resume his usual diet.
• Resume any medications withheld for the test.

Precautions

• The gastric acid stimulation test is contraindicated in patients with hypersensitivity to pentagastrin or with conditions that prohibit nasogastric intubation.

• Observe for adverse effects of pentagastrin.

• To prevent contamination of the specimens with saliva, instruct the patient to expectorate excess saliva.

• When collection is completed, send the specimens to the laboratory immediately.

Reference values

Following stimulation, gastric secretion ranges from 11 to 21 mEq/hour for women and 18 to 28 mEq/hour for men.

Abnormal findings

Elevated gastric secretion may indicate duodenal ulcer; markedly elevated secretion suggests Zollinger-Ellison syndrome. Depressed secretion may indicate gastric carcinoma; achlorhydria may indicate pernicious anemia.

PERITONEAL FLUID ANALYSIS

This test assesses a sample of peritoneal fluid obtained by paracentesis. This procedure requires inserting a trocar and cannula through the abdominal wall while the patient receives a local anesthetic. If the fluid sample is removed for therapeutic purposes, the trocar may be connected to a drainage system. However, if only a small amount of fluid is removed for diagnostic purposes, an 18G needle may be used in place of the trocar and cannula. In a four-quadrant tap, fluid is aspirated from each quadrant of the abdomen to verify abdominal trauma and confirm the need for surgery.

Purpose

• To determine the cause of ascites
• To detect abdominal trauma

Patient preparation

• Explain to the patient that this procedure helps determine the cause of ascites or detects abdominal trauma.

• Inform him he needn't restrict food or fluids before the test.

• Tell him that the test requires a peritoneal fluid sample, that he will receive a local anesthetic to minimize discomfort, and that the procedure takes about 45 minutes to perform.

• Provide psychological support to decrease the patient's anxiety, and assure him that complications are rare.

• If the patient has severe ascites, inform him that the procedure will relieve his discomfort and allow him to breathe more easily.

• Tell the patient to void just before the test. This helps prevent accidental bladder injury during needle insertion.

Procedure and posttest care

• Have the patient sit on a bed or in a chair with his feet flat on the floor and his back well supported. If he cannot tolerate being out of bed, place him in high Fowler's position and make him as comfortable as possible.

• Except for the puncture site, keep him covered to prevent chilling.

• Provide a plastic sheet or absorbent pad to collect spillage and to protect the patient and bed linens.

• Shave the puncture site, prepare the skin, and drape the area.

• Inject the local anesthetic.

• Insert the needle or trocar and cannula 1″ to 2″ (2.5 to 5 cm) below the umbilicus. However, insertion may also be through the flank, the iliac fossa, the border of the rectus, or at each quadrant of the abdomen.

• If a trocar and cannula are used, make a small incision to facilitate insertion.

When the needle pierces the peritoneum, it "gives" with an audible sound. Remove the trocar and aspirate a sample of fluid with a 50-ml luer-lock syringe.

• Apply a gauze dressing to the puncture site. Make sure it's thick enough to absorb all drainage. Check the dressing frequently, whenever you check vital signs; reinforce or apply a pressure dressing, if needed.

• Monitor vital signs until stable. If the patient's recovery is poor, check vital signs every 15 minutes. Weigh the patient and measure abdominal girth; compare these with baseline measurements.

• Allow the patient to rest, and if possible, withhold treatment or procedures that may cause undue stress.

• Monitor urine output for at least 24 hours, and watch for hematuria, which may indicate bladder trauma.

• If a large amount of fluid was aspirated, watch for signs of vascular collapse (color change, elevated pulse rate and respirations, decreased blood pressure and central venous pressure, mental changes, and dizziness). Administer fluids orally if the patient is alert and can accept them.

• Watch for signs of hemorrhage and shock or for increasing pain and abdominal tenderness. These may indicate a perforated intestine or, depending on the site of the tap, puncture of the inferior epigastric artery, hematoma of the anterior cecal wall, or rupture of the iliac vein or bladder.

• Observe the patient with severe hepatic disease for signs of hepatic coma, which may result from loss of sodium and potassium accompanying hypovolemia. Watch for mental changes, drowsiness, and stupor. Such a patient is also prone to uremia, infection, hemorrhage, and protein depletion.

• Administer I.V. infusions and albumin. Check the laboratory report for electrolytes (especially sodium) and serum protein levels.

Precautions

• Peritoneal fluid analysis should be performed cautiously in pregnant patients and in patients with bleeding tendencies or unstable vital signs.

• Check vital signs every 15 minutes during the procedure. Watch for deviations from baseline findings. Observe for dizziness, pallor, perspiration, and increased anxiety.

• If rapid fluid aspiration induces hypovolemia and shock, reduce the vertical distance between the trocar and the collection bag to slow the drainage rate. If necessary, stop drainage by turning the stopcock off or by clamping the tubing.

• Avoid contamination of specimens, which alters their bacterial content. Send them to the laboratory immediately.

Reference values

For normal values for peritoneal fluid, see *Peritoneal fluid analysis,* page 366.

Abnormal findings

Milk-colored peritoneal fluid may result from chyle escaping from a thoracic duct that is damaged or blocked by carcinoma, lymphoma, tuberculosis, parasitic infection, adhesion, or hepatic cirrhosis; a pseudochylous condition may result from the presence of leukocytes or tumor cells. Differential diagnosis of true chylous ascites depends on the presence of elevated triglyceride levels (≥ 400 mg/dl) and microscopic fat globules.

Cloudy or turbid fluid may indicate peritonitis due to primary bacterial infection, ruptured bowel (after trauma), pancreatitis, strangulated or infarcted intestine, or appendicitis. Bloody fluid may result from a benign or malignant tumor, hemorrhagic pancreatitis, or a

PERITONEAL FLUID ANALYSIS

ELEMENT	NORMAL VALUE OR FINDING
Gross appearance	Sterile, odorless, clear to pale yellow color; scant amount (< 50 ml)
Red blood cells	None
White blood cells	< 300/µl
Protein	0.3 to 4.1 g/dl (albumin, 50% to 70%; globulin, 30% to 45%; fibrinogen, 0.3% to 4.5%)
Glucose	70 to 100 mg/dl
Amylase	138 to 404 amylase units/liter
Ammonia	< 50 µg/dl
Alkaline phosphatase	Male: > age 18: 90 to 239 units/liter Female: < age 45: 76 to 196 units/liter Female: > age 45: 87 to 250 units/liter
Lactate dehydrogenase isoenzymes	Equal to serum level
Cytology	No malignant cells present
Bacteria	None
Fungi	None

traumatic tap; however, if the fluid fails to clear on continued aspiration, traumatic tap isn't the cause. Bile-stained green fluid may indicate a ruptured gallbladder, acute pancreatitis, or perforated intestine or duodenal ulcer.

A red blood cell count over 100/µl indicates neoplasm or tuberculosis; a count over 100,000/µl indicates intra-abdominal trauma. A white blood cell count over 300/µl, with more than 25% neutrophils, occurs in 90% of patients with spontaneous bacterial peritonitis and in 50% of those with cirrhosis. A high percentage of lymphocytes suggests tuberculous peritonitis or chylous ascites. Numerous mesothelial cells indicate tuberculous peritonitis.

Protein levels rise above 3 g/dl in malignancy and above 4 g/dl in tuberculosis. Peritoneal fluid glucose levels fall below 60 mg/dl in 30% to 50% of patients with tuberculous peritonitis and peritoneal carcinomatosis.

Amylase levels rise in about 90% of patients with pancreatic trauma, pancreatic pseudocyst, or acute pancreatitis and may also rise in intestinal necrosis or strangulation.

Peritoneal alkaline phosphatase levels rise to more than twice the normal serum levels in about 90% of patients with ruptured or strangulated small intestine. Peritoneal ammonia levels also exceed twice the normal serum levels in ruptured or strangulated large and small intestines, and in ruptured ulcer or appendix.

A protein ascitic fluid/serum ratio of 0.5 or greater, a lactate dehydrogenase isoenzyme (LD) ascitic fluid/serum ratio over 0.6, and an ascitic fluid LD level over 400 µ/ml suggest malignant, tuberculous, or pancreatic ascites. Any two of these findings indicates a nonhepatic cause; absence of all three usually suggests uncomplicated hepatic disease. An albumin gradient between ascitic fluid and serum over 1 g/dl indicates chronic hepatic disease; a lesser value suggests malignancy.

Cytologic examination of peritoneal fluid accurately detects malignant cells. Microbiological examination can reveal coliforms, anaerobes, and enterococci, which can enter the peritoneum from a ruptured organ, or from infections accompanying appendicitis, pancreatitis, tuberculosis, or ovarian disease. Gram-positive cocci often indicate primary peritonitis; gram-negative organisms, secondary peritonitis. The presence of fungi may indicate histoplasmosis, candidiasis, or coccidioidomycosis.

TEST FOR DUODENAL PARASITES

This test evaluates duodenal contents for the presence of parasites in a specimen obtained by duodenal intubation and aspiration or by the string test (Entero test). Such parasites include trophozoites of *Giardia lamblia*, the ova and larvae of *Strongyloides stercoralis,* or the ova of *Necator americanus* or *Ancylostoma duodenale* in various stages of cleavage. This test can also detect ova of the liver flukes *Clonorchis sinensis* and *Fasciola hepatica* in the biliary tract. Liver fluke infestations are rare in North America.

Examination of duodenal contents for ova and parasites is performed only in a symptomatic patient with negative stool examinations.

Purpose
• To detect parasitic infection when stool examinations are negative

Patient preparation
• Explain to the patient that this test detects parasitic infection of the gastrointestinal tract.
• Instruct him to restrict food and fluids for 12 hours before the test.
• Tell him who will perform the test and when.
• If the test will be done with a nasoenteric tube, warn him that he may gag during the tube's passage, but assure him that following the examiner's instructions about positioning, breathing, and swallowing will minimize discomfort.
• Instruct the patient to empty his bladder just before the procedure.

Equipment
Gloves, double-lumen tube with olive tip (or weighted gelatin capsule with string attached, for string test), water-soluble jelly, 30-ml sterile syringe, emesis basin, sterile specimen container, adhesive tape (½″ wide).

Procedure and posttest care
Using a nasoenteric tube:
• After inserting the tube, place the patient in a left lateral decubitus position, with his feet elevated, to allow peristalsis to move the tube into the duodenum.
• The pH of a small amount of aspirated fluid determines tube position: If the tube is in the stomach, pH is lower than 7.0; if it's in the duodenum, pH is higher than 7.0.

• Fluoroscopy can also determine correct positioning. When position is confirmed, residual duodenal contents are aspirated.

• Transfer the entire specimen to a sterile container; label it appropriately.

Using an Entero test capsule with string:

• Tape the free end of the string to the patient's cheek.

• Instruct him to swallow the capsule (on the other end of the string) with water.

• Leave the string in place for 4 hours; then pull it out gently and place it in a sterile container.

• Label the container appropriately.

• Dispose of equipment properly.

• Provide mouth care and offer water.

• Observe carefully for signs of perforation, such as dysphagia or fever.

• Tell the patient he can resume his normal diet.

Precautions

• Use gloves when performing the procedure and handling specimens.

• Duodenal intubation is contraindicated during pregnancy or for patients with acute cholecystitis; acute pancreatitis; esophageal varices, stenosis, diverticula, or malignant neoplasms; recent severe gastric hemorrhage; aortic aneurysm; or congestive heart failure.

• When possible, obtain the specimen before the start of drug therapy.

• Send the specimen to the laboratory immediately.

• Withdraw the tube slowly (6″ to 8″ [15 to 20 cm] every 10 minutes) to the esophagus; then clamp the tube and remove it quickly. *Never* force the tube.

Findings

Normally, no ova or parasites appear.

Abnormal findings

Finding *G. lamblia* indicates giardiasis, possibly causing malabsorption syndrome; *S. stercoralis* suggests strongyloidiasis; *A. duodenale* and *N. americanus* imply hookworm disease; and *C. sinensis* and *F. hepatica* signify histopathologic changes in the bile ducts.

FECAL OCCULT BLOOD TEST

Fecal occult blood is detected by microscopic analysis or by chemical tests for hemoglobin, such as the guaiac or orthotoluidine test. Normally, feces contain small amounts of blood (2 to 2.5 ml/day); therefore, tests for occult blood detect quantities larger than this. Testing is indicated when clinical symptoms and preliminary blood studies suggest GI bleeding. Additional tests are required to pinpoint the origin of the bleeding. (See *Common sites and causes of GI blood loss.*)

Purpose

• To detect GI bleeding

• To aid early diagnosis of colorectal cancer

Patient preparation

• Explain to the patient that this test helps detect abnormal GI bleeding.

• Instruct him to maintain a high-fiber diet and to refrain from eating red meats, poultry, fish, turnips, and horseradish for 48 to 72 hours before the test, as well as throughout the collection period.

• Tell him the test requires collection of three stool specimens. Occasionally, only a random specimen is collected.

• Withhold iron preparations, bromides, iodides, rauwolfia derivatives,

COMMON SITES AND CAUSES OF GI BLOOD LOSS

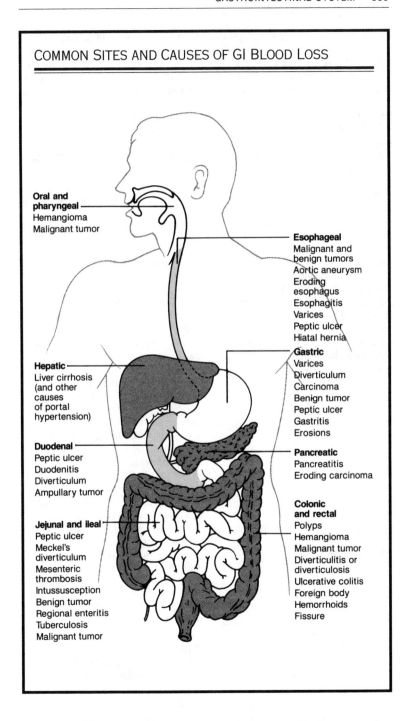

**Oral and
pharyngeal**
Hemangioma
Malignant tumor

Esophageal
Malignant and
benign tumors
Aortic aneurysm
Eroding
esophagus
Esophagitis
Varices
Peptic ulcer
Hiatal hernia

Hepatic
Liver cirrhosis
(and other
causes
of portal
hypertension)

Gastric
Varices
Diverticulum
Carcinoma
Benign tumor
Peptic ulcer
Gastritis
Erosions

Duodenal
Peptic ulcer
Duodenitis
Diverticulum
Ampullary tumor

Pancreatic
Pancreatitis
Eroding carcinoma

**Colonic
and rectal**
Polyps
Hemangioma
Malignant tumor
Diverticulitis or
diverticulosis
Ulcerative colitis
Foreign body
Hemorrhoids
Fissure

Jejunal and ileal
Peptic ulcer
Meckel's
diverticulum
Mesenteric
thrombosis
Intussusception
Benign tumor
Regional enteritis
Tuberculosis
Malignant tumor

indomethacin, colchicine, salicylates, phenylbutazone, steroids, and ascorbic acid for 48 hours before and during the test. If these medications must be continued, note this on the laboratory slip.

Procedure and posttest care
• Collect three stool specimens or a random specimen. Testing may take place in the laboratory or in a utility room on the nursing unit, depending on hospital policy.
• Place a small amount of stool on a piece of filter paper.
• Add two drops each of tap water, glacial acetic acid, 1:60 solution of gum guaiac in 95% ethyl alcohol, and 3% hydrogen peroxide *or* two drops each of 0.2% orthotoluidine and 0.3% hydrogen peroxide. Mix thoroughly with a tongue blade. Note the color immediately, and check it again after 5 minutes.
• Be sure to obtain specimens from two different areas of each stool to allow for variance in distribution of blood.
• Tell the patient to resume his usual diet and medication schedule.

Precautions
• Instruct the patient to avoid contaminating the stool specimen with toilet tissue or urine.
• Send the specimen to the laboratory or perform the test immediately.

Normal findings
Normally, less than 2.5 ml of blood is present, resulting in a green reaction.

Abnormal findings
A dark blue reaction that appears within 5 minutes indicates that the test is positive for occult blood; a strongly positive reaction within 3 to 4 minutes is always abnormal. A faint blue reaction is weakly positive and isn't necessarily abnormal. A positive test indicates GI bleeding, which may result from many disorders, such as varices, peptic ulcer, carcinoma, ulcerative colitis, dysentery, or hemorrhagic disease. This test is particularly important for early diagnosis of colorectal cancer. Further tests, such as barium swallow, analyses of gastric contents, and endoscopic procedures, are necessary to define the site and extent of bleeding.

FECAL LIPIDS

Lipids excreted in feces include monoglycerides, diglycerides, triglycerides, phospholipids, glycolipids, soaps (fatty acids and fatty acid salts), sterols, and cholesterol esters. When biliary and pancreatic secretions are adequate, emulsified dietary lipids are almost completely absorbed in the small intestine.

Excessive excretion of fecal lipids (steatorrhea) occurs in several malabsorption syndromes. Qualitative and quantitative tests are used to detect excessive excretion of lipids in patients exhibiting signs of malabsorption, such as weight loss, abdominal distention, and scaly skin. The qualitative test involves staining a specimen of stool with Sudan III dye and then examining it microscopically for evidence of malabsorption, such as undigested muscle fibers and various fats. The quantitative test involves drying and weighing a 72-hour specimen, and then using a solvent to extract the lipids, which are subsequently evaporated and weighed. Only the quantitative test confirms steatorrhea.

Purpose
• To confirm steatorrhea

Patient preparation
• Explain to the patient that this test evaluates digestion of fats.

• Instruct him to abstain from alcohol and to maintain a high-fat diet (100 g/day) for 3 days before the test and during the collection period.

• Tell him the test requires a 72-hour stool collection.

• Withhold azathioprine, bisacodyl, cholestyramine, kanamycin, neomycin, colchicine, aluminum hydroxide, calcium carbonate, alcohol, potassium chloride, and mineral oil because they may affect test results. If these medications must be continued, note this on the laboratory slip.

• Teach the patient how to collect a timed stool specimen, and provide him with the necessary equipment.

• Inform him that the laboratory requires 1 or 2 days to complete the analysis.

Procedure and posttest care

• Collect a 72-hour stool specimen.

• Tell the patient he may resume his usual diet.

• Administer medications withheld before the test.

Precautions

• Don't use a waxed collection container because the wax may become incorporated in the stool and interfere with accurate testing.

• Tell the patient to avoid contaminating the stool specimen with toilet tissue or urine.

• Refrigerate the collection container and keep it tightly covered.

Reference values

Fecal lipids normally comprise less than 20% of excreted solids, with excretion of less than 7 g/24 hours.

Abnormal findings

Both digestive and absorptive disorders cause steatorrhea. Digestive disorders may affect the production and release of pancreatic lipase or bile; absorptive disorders may affect the integrity of the intestine.

In pancreatic insufficiency, impaired lipid digestion may result from insufficient production of lipase. Pancreatic resection, cystic fibrosis, chronic pancreatitis, or ductal obstruction by stone or tumor may prevent the normal release or action of lipase.

In impaired hepatic function, faulty lipid digestion may result from inadequate production of bile salts. Biliary obstruction, which may accompany gallbladder disease, may prevent the normal release of bile salts into the duodenum.

Extensive small bowel resection or bypass may also interrupt normal enterohepatic circulation of bile salts.

Diseases of the intestinal mucosa affect normal absorption of lipids; regional ileitis and atrophy due to malnutrition cause gross structural changes in the intestinal wall, while celiac disease and tropical sprue produce mucosal abnormalities.

Scleroderma, radiation enteritis, fistulas, intestinal tuberculosis, small intestine diverticula, and altered intestinal flora may also cause steatorrhea.

Whipple's disease and lymphomas cause lymphatic obstruction that may inhibit fat absorption.

FECAL UROBILINOGEN

Urobilinogen, the end product of bilirubin metabolism, is a brown pigment formed by bacterial enzymes in the small intestine. It is excreted in feces or reabsorbed into portal blood, where it is returned to the liver and excreted in bile; a small amount is excreted in urine. Proper bilirubin metabolism depends on normal hepatobiliary system functioning and normal erythrocyte lifespan. Although measuring fecal urobilinogen is a useful indicator of hepatobiliary and hemolytic disorders, the test is rarely performed because it is easier to measure serum bilirubin and urine urobilinogen.

Purpose
• To aid diagnosis of hepatobiliary and hemolytic disorders

Patient preparation
• Explain to the patient that this test evaluates function of the liver and bile ducts or detects red blood cell disorders.
• Inform him that he needn't restrict food or fluids before the test.
• Tell him the test requires collection of a random stool specimen.
• Withhold broad-spectrum antibiotics, sulfonamides, and salicylates for 2 weeks before the test. If these medications must be continued, note this on the laboratory slip.

Procedure and posttest care
• Collect a random stool specimen.
• Tell the patient that he may resume his usual diet.
• Resume administration of medications withheld for the test.

Precautions
• Tell the patient not to contaminate the stool specimen with toilet tissue or urine.
• Use a light-resistant collection container because urobilinogen breaks down to urobilin on exposure to light.
• Send the specimen to the laboratory immediately.
• Refrigerate the specimen if transport or testing is delayed more than 30 minutes; freeze the specimen if testing is being performed by an outside laboratory.

Reference values
Normally, fecal urobilinogen values range from 50 to 300 mg/24 hours.

Abnormal findings
Low levels or absence of urobilinogen in the feces indicates obstructed bile flow, the result of intrahepatic disorders (such as hepatocellular jaundice due to cirrhosis or hepatitis), extrahepatic disorders (such as choledocholithiasis or tumor of the head of the pancreas, the ampulla of Vater, or the bile duct). Low fecal urobilinogen levels are also characteristic of depressed erythropoiesis, as in aplastic anemia.

Elevated fecal urobilinogen levels may occur in hemolytic jaundice, thalassemia, and hemolytic, sickle cell, and pernicious anemias.

EXAMINATION OF STOOL FOR OVA AND PARASITES

Examination of a stool specimen can detect several types of intestinal parasites. Some of these parasites live in nonpathogenic symbiosis; others cause intestinal disease. In North America, the most common parasites include the roundworms *Ascaris lumbricoides* and *Necator americanus* (also called hookworms); the tapeworms *Diphyllobothrium latum, Taenia saginata,* and *Taenia solium* (rare); the amoeba *Entamoeba histolytica*; and the flagellate *Giardia lamblia*.

Purpose
• To confirm or rule out intestinal parasitic infection and disease

Patient preparation

- Explain to the patient that this test detects intestinal parasitic infection.
- Instruct him to avoid treatments with castor or mineral oil, bismuth, magnesium or antidiarrheal compounds, barium enemas, and antibiotics for 7 to 10 days before the test.
- Tell him the test requires three stool specimens—one every other day or every third day. Up to six specimens may be required to confirm the presence of *E. histolytica*.
- Record recent dietary and travel history if the patient has diarrhea. Check the patient's history for antiparasitic drugs, such as carbarsone, tetracycline, paromomycin, metronidazole, and diiodohydroxyquin within 2 weeks of the test.

Equipment

Gloves, waterproof container with tight-fitting lid, bedpan (if necessary), tongue depressor.

Procedure and posttest care

- Put on gloves and collect a stool specimen directly into the container. (See *Collection procedure for pinworms*.)
- Collect the specimen into a clean, dry bedpan if the patient is bedridden; then, using a tongue depressor, transfer it into a properly labeled container.
- Note on the laboratory slip the date and time of collection and the specimen consistency.
- Remember also to record any recent or current antimicrobial therapy and any pertinent travel or dietary history.
- Resume administration of medications discontinued before the test.

Precautions

- Do not contaminate the stool specimen with urine, which can destroy trophozoites.
- Don't collect stool from a toilet bowl because water is toxic to trophozoites

COLLECTION PROCEDURE FOR PINWORMS

The ova of the pinworm *Enterobius vermicularis* seldom appear in feces because the female migrates to the anus and deposits her ova there. To collect them, place a piece of cellophane tape, sticky side out, on the end of a tongue depressor, and press it firmly on the anal area. Then transfer the tape, sticky side down, to a slide (kits with tape and a slide or a sticky paddle are available). Because the female usually deposits her ova at night, collect the specimen early in the morning before the patient bathes or defecates.

and may contain organisms that interfere with test results.

- Send the specimen to the laboratory immediately. If a liquid or soft stool specimen can't be examined within 30 minutes of passage, place some of it in a preservative; if a formed stool specimen can't be examined immediately, refrigerate it or place it in preservative.
- If the entire stool can't be sent to the laboratory, include macroscopic worms or worm segments and bloody and mucoid portions of the specimen.
- Use gloves when performing the procedure and handling the specimen, disposing of equipment, sealing the container, and transporting it. Dispose of gloves after specimen collection.

Normal findings

No parasites or ova appear in stool.

Abnormal findings

The presence of E. *histolytica* confirms amebiasis; G. *lamblia*, giardiasis. However, the extent of infection depends on the degree of tissue invasion. If amebiasis is suspected but stool examinations are negative, specimen collection after saline cathartic using buffered sodium biphosphate or during sigmoidoscopy may be necessary. If giardiasis is suspected but stool examinations are negative, examination of duodenal contents may be necessary.

Since injury to the host is difficult to detect — even when helminth ova or larvae appear — the number of worms is usually correlated with the patient's clinical symptoms to distinguish between helminth infestation and helminth diseases. Eosinophilia may also indicate parasitic infection. Helminths may migrate from the intestinal tract, producing pathologic changes in other parts of the body. For example, the roundworm *Ascaris* may perforate the bowel wall, causing peritonitis, or may migrate to the lungs, causing pneumonitis. Hookworms can cause hypochromic microcytic anemia secondary to bloodsucking and hemorrhage, especially in patients with iron-deficient diets. The tapeworm D. *latum* may cause megaloblastic anemia by removing vitamin B_{12}.

EXAMINATION OF STOOL FOR ROTAVIRUS ANTIGEN

Rotaviruses are the most frequent cause of infectious diarrhea in infants and young children. They are most prevalent in children ages 3 months to 2 years during the winter months. Clinical features include diarrhea, vomiting, fever, and abdominal pain. Symptoms of infection may range from mild in adults to severe in young children, especially hospitalized infants.

Because human rotaviruses do not replicate efficiently in laboratory cell cultures, detection typically requires sensitive, specific enzyme immunoassays that provide results within minutes or hours (depending on the assay).

Purpose

• To obtain a laboratory diagnosis of rotavirus gastroenteritis

Patient preparation

• Explain the purpose of the test to the patient or to his parents if the patient is a child.

• Inform him that the test requires a stool specimen.

• Collect the specimens during the prodromal and acute stages of clinical infection to ensure detection of the viral antigens by enzyme immunoassay.

Procedure and posttest care

• Usually, a stool specimen (1 g in a screw-capped tube or vial) is used to detect rotaviruses. If a microbiological transport swab is used, it must be heavily stained with feces to be diagnostically productive for rotavirus.

• Provide fluids to the patient to avoid dehydration caused by vomiting and diarrhea.

Precautions

• Avoid using collection containers with preservatives, metal ions, detergents, and serum, which may interfere with the assay.

• Store stool specimens for up to 24 hours at 35.6° F to 46.4° F (2° C to 8° C). If a longer period of storage or shipment is necessary, freeze specimens at − 4° F (− 20° C) or colder. Repeated freezing and thawing will

cause the specimen to deteriorate and yield misleading results.
• Don't store the specimen in a self-defrosting freezer.
• Use gloves when obtaining or handling all specimens.

Reference values

The detection of rotavirus by enzyme immunoassay is laboratory evidence of current infection with the organism. Rotavirus can infect all age groups; the severity of disease is generally greater in young children than in adults. Rotavirus infections are easily transmitted in group settings such as nursing homes, preschools, and day-care centers. Transmission is presumed to occur from person-to-person by the fecal-oral route. In a hospital setting, nosocomial spread of this viral infection can cause significant harm.

REPRODUCTIVE SYSTEM

SEX CHROMATIN TESTS

Although sex chromatin tests can screen for abnormalities in the number of sex chromosomes, the faster, simpler, and more accurate full karyotype (chromosome analysis) has all but replaced them. Sex chromatin tests are usually indicated for abnormal sexual development, ambiguous genitalia, amenorrhea, and suspected chromosomal abnormalities.

Purpose

• To quickly screen for abnormal sexual development (both X and Y chromatin tests)
• To aid assessment of an infant with ambiguous genitalia (X chromatin test only)
• To determine the number of Y chromosomes in an individual (Y chromatin test only)

Patient preparation

• Explain to the patient or to his parents, if appropriate, why the test is being performed.
• Tell him the test requires that the inside of his cheek be scraped to obtain a specimen and who will perform the test.
• Assure the patient the test takes only a few minutes, but may require a follow-up chromosome analysis.
• Inform him that the laboratory generally requires as long as 4 weeks to complete the analysis.

Equipment

Wooden or metal spatula, clean glass slide, cell fixative.

Procedure and posttest care

• Scrape the buccal mucosa firmly with a wooden or metal spatula at least twice to obtain a specimen of healthy cells (vaginal mucosa is occasionally used in young women).
• Rub the spatula over the glass slide, making sure the cells are evenly distributed.
• Spray the slide with cell fixative, and send the slide to the laboratory with a brief patient history and indications for the test.

Precautions

• Make sure the buccal mucosa is scraped firmly to ensure a sufficient number of cells.

SEX CHROMOSOME ANOMALIES

DISORDER AND CHROMOSOMAL ANEUPLOIDY	CAUSE AND INCIDENCE	PHENOTYPIC FEATURES
Klinefelter's syndrome • 47,XXY • 48,XXXY • 49,XXXXY • 48,XX,YY • 49,XXX,YY • Mosaics: XXY, XXXY, or XXXXY/XX or XY	• Nondisjunction or improper chromatid separation during anaphase I or II of oogenesis or spermatogenesis results in abnormal gamete • 1 per 500 to 600 male births	• Syndrome usually inapparent until puberty • Small penis and testes • Sparse facial and abdominal hair; feminine distribution of pubic hair • Somewhat enlarged breasts (gynecomastia) • Sexual dysfunction • Sterility • Possible mental retardation
Polysomy Y • 47,XYY	• Nondisjunction during anaphase II of spermatogenesis causes both Y chromosomes to pass to the same pole and results in a YY sperm • 1 per 1,000 male births	• Above average stature (often over 72″ [1.8 m]) • Normal fertility
Turner's syndrome • 45,XO • Mosaics: XO/XX or XO/XXX • Aberrations of X chromosomes, including deletion of short arm of one X chromosome, presence of a ring chromosome, or presence of an isochromosome on the long arm of an X chromosome	• Nondisjunction during anaphase I or II of spermatogenesis results in sperm without any sex chromosomes • 1 per 3,500 female births (most common chromosome complement in first-trimester abortions)	• Short stature (usually under 57″ [145 cm]) • Webbed neck • Low hairline • Broad chest with widely spaced nipples • Underdeveloped breasts • Juvenile external genitalia • Primary amenorrhea common • Sterility • No mental retardation but possible problems with space perception and orientation
Other X polysomes	Nondisjunction at anaphase I or II of oogenesis	
• 47,XXX	1/1,400 female births	• Often, no obvious anatomical abnormalities • Normal fertility
• 48,XXXX	Rare	• Mental retardation • Ocular hypertelorism • Reduced fertility

SEX CHROMOSOME ANOMALIES *(continued)*

DISORDER AND CHROMOSOMAL ANEUPLOIDY	CAUSE AND INCIDENCE	PHENOTYPIC FEATURES
• 49,XXXXX	Rare	• Severe mental retardation • Ocular hypertelorism, with uncoordinated eye movement • Abnormal development of sexual organs • Various skeletal anomalies

• Check that the specimen isn't saliva, which contains no cells.

Normal findings

A normal female (XX) has only one X chromatin mass (the number of X chromatin masses discernible is one less than the number of X chromosomes in the cells examined). For various reasons, an X chromatin mass is ordinarily discernible in only 20% to 50% of the buccal mucosal cells of a normal woman.

A normal male (XY) has only one Y chromatin mass (the number of Y chromatin masses equals the number of Y chromosomes in the cells examined).

Abnormal findings

In most laboratories, if less than 20% of the cells in a buccal smear contain an X chromatin mass, some cells are presumed to contain only one X chromosome, necessitating full karyotyping. Persons with female phenotypes and positive Y chromatin masses run a high risk of developing malignancies in their *intra-abdominal* gonads. In such persons, removal of these gonads is indicated and should generally be performed before age 5.

The patient or his parents require genetic counseling after the cause of chromosomal abnormal sexual development has been identified. A medical team comprising of doctors, psychologists, psychiatrists, and educators must decide the child's sex if a child is phenotypically of one sex and genotypically of the other. This careful evaluation should be made early to prevent developmental problems related to incorrect gender identification. (See *Sex chromosome anomalies*.)

CHROMOSOME ANALYSIS

Chromosome analysis studies the relationship between the microscopic appearance of chromosomes and an individual's phenotype — the expression of the genes in physical, biochemical, or physiologic traits.

Ideally, chromosomes are studied during metaphase, the middle phase of mitosis, when new cell poles appear. During metaphase, colchicine (a cell poison) is added to arrest cell division.

Cells are harvested, stained, and then examined under a microscope. These cells are then photographed to record the karyotype — the systematic arrangement of chromosomes in groupings according to size and shape.

Only rapidly dividing cells, such as bone marrow or neoplastic cells, permit direct, immediate study. In other cells, mitosis is stimulated by the addition of phytohemagglutinin. Indications for the test determine the specimen required (blood, bone marrow, amniotic fluid, skin, or placental tissue) and the specific analytic procedure.

Purpose
• To identify chromosomal abnormalities, such as hypoploidy or hyperploidy, as the underlying cause of malformation, maldevelopment, or disease

Patient preparation
• Explain to the patient or to his parents, if appropriate, the purpose of this test.
• Tell him who will perform the test and what kind of specimen will be required.
• Inform him when results will be available, according to the specimen required. For example, test results on a blood sample are generally available 72 to 96 hours after stimulation; analysis of skin biopsy specimens or amniotic fluid cells may take several weeks.

Procedure and posttest care
• Collect a blood sample (in a 5- to 10-ml *green-top* heparinized tube), a tissue specimen, 1 ml of bone marrow, or at least 20 ml of amniotic fluid.
• Provide appropriate posttest care, depending on the procedure used to collect the specimen.
• Explain the test results and their implications to the patient or to the parents of a child with a chromosomal abnormality.

• Recommend appropriate genetic or other counseling and follow-up care if necessary, such as an infant stimulation program for a patient with Down's syndrome.

Precautions
• Keep all specimens sterile, especially those requiring a tissue culture.
• To facilitate interpretation of test results, send the specimen to the laboratory immediately, with a brief patient history and indication for the test.
• Refrigerate the specimen if transport is delayed, but *never* freeze it.
• Make sure the povidone-iodine solution is thoroughly removed with alcohol before skin biopsy to prevent cell growth in tissue culture.

Normal findings
The normal cell contains 46 chromosomes: 22 pairs of nonsex chromosomes (autosomes) and 1 pair of sex chromosomes (Y for the male-determining chromosome, X for the female-determining chromosome). On a karyotype, chromosomes are arranged according to size and the location of their primary constrictions, or centromeres. The centromere may be medial (metacentric), slightly to one end of the chromosome (submetacentric), or entirely to one end (acrocentric). The largest chromosomes are displayed first; the others are arranged in order of decreasing size, with the two sex chromosomes traditionally placed last. By convention, the centromere is always placed at the top in a karyotype. Thus, if the two pairs of chromosomal arms are of unequal length, the arm above the centromere will be shorter. The letter "p" designates the short arm; the letter "q," the long arm.

Special stains identify individual chromosomes and locate and enumerate particular portions of chromosomes. Trypsin, alkali, heat denaturization, and

CHROMOSOME ANALYSIS FINDINGS

SPECIMEN AND INDICATION	RESULT	IMPLICATION
Blood		
• To evaluate abnormal appearance or development suggesting chromosomal irregularity	• Abnormal chromosome number (aneuploidy) or arrangement	• Identifies specific chromosomal abnormality
• To evaluate couples with history of miscarriages or to identify balanced translocation carriers having unbalanced offspring	• Normal chromosomes	• Miscarriage unrelated to parental chromosomal abnormality
	• Parental balanced translocation carrier	• Increased risk of repeated abortion or unbalanced offspring indicates need for amniocentesis in future pregnancies
• To detect chromosomal rearrangements in rare genetic diseases predisposing patient to malignant neoplasms	• Chromosomal rearrangements, gaps, and breaks	• Occurs in Bloom's syndrome, Fanconi's syndrome, telangiectasia; patient predisposed to malignant neoplasms
Blood or bone marrow		
• To identify Philadelphia chromosome and confirm chronic myelogenous leukemia	• Translocation of chromosome 22q (long arm) to another chromosome (often chromosome 9)	• Aids diagnosis of chronic myelogenous leukemia
	• Aneuploidy (usually due to abnormalities in chromosomes 8 and 12)	• Occurs in acute myelogenous leukemia
	• Trisomy 21	• Occasionally occurs in chronic lymphocytic leukemia cells
Skin		
• To evaluate abnormal appearance or development suggesting chromosomal irregularity	• All chromosomal abnormalities possible	• Same as chromosomal abnormality in blood; rarely, mosaic individual has normal blood but abnormal skin chromosomes

(continued)

CHROMOSOME ANALYSIS FINDINGS *(continued)*

SPECIMEN AND INDICATION	RESULT	IMPLICATION
Amniotic fluid		
• To evaluate developing fetus with possible chromosomal abnormality	• All chromosomal abnormalities possible	• Same as chromosomal abnormality in blood or fetus
Placental tissue		
• To evaluate products of conception after a miscarriage to determine if abnormality is fetal or placental in origin	• All chromosomal abnormalities possible	• Over 50% of aborted tissue is chromosomally abnormal
Tumor tissue		
• For research purposes only	• Many chromosomal abnormalities possible	• Although malignant tumors are not associated with specific chromosomal aberrations, most are aneuploid, usually hyperploid.

Giemsa's stain are used for visible light microscopy; quinacrine stain, for ultraviolet microscopy. These staining techniques produce nonuniform staining of each chromosome in a repetitive, banded pattern. The mechanism of chromosome banding is unknown, but seems related to primary deoxyribonucleic acid sequence and protein composition of the chromosome.

Abnormal findings

Chromosome abnormalities may be numerical or structural. Numerical deviation from the norm of 46 chromosomes is called aneuploidy. Less than 46 chromosomes is called hypoploidy; more than 46, hyperploidy. Special designations exist for whole multiples of the haploid number 23: diploidy for the normal somatic number of 46, triploidy for 69, tetraploidy for 92, and so forth. When the deviation occurs within a single pair of chromosomes, the suffix "-somy" is used, as in trisomy for the presence of three chromosomes instead of the usual pair or monosomy for the presence of only one chromosome.

Aneuploidy most commonly follows failure of the chromosomal pair to separate (nondisjunction) during anaphase, the mitotic stage that follows metaphase. It may also result from anaphase lag, in which one of the normally separated chromosomes fails to move to a pole and is left out of the daughter cells. If nondisjunction or anaphase lag occurs during meiosis, the cells of the zygote will all be the same. Errors in mitotic division after the formation of the zygote will produce more than one cell line (mosaicism).

Structural chromosome abnormalities result from chromosome breakage. Intrachromosomal rearrangement occurs within a single chromosome in various forms:

• *Deletion:* loss of an end (terminal) or middle (interstitial) portion of a chromosome

• *Inversion:* end-to-end reversal of a chromosome segment, which may be pericentric inversion (including the centromere) or paracentric inversion (occurring in only one arm of the chromosome)

• *Ring chromosome formation:* breakage of both ends of a chromosome and reunion of the ends

• *Isochromosome formation:* abnormal splitting of the centromere in a transverse rather than a longitudinal plane.

Interchromosomal rearrangements (of more than one chromosome, usually two) also occur. The most common rearrangement is translocation, or exchange, of genetic material between two chromosomes. Translocations may be balanced, in which the cell neither loses nor gains genetic material; unbalanced, in which a piece of genetic material is gained or lost from each cell; reciprocal (in children), in which two chromosomes exchange material; or Robertsonian, in which two chromosomes join to form one combined chromosome, with little or no loss of material.

Implications of chromosome analysis results depend on the specimen and indications for the test (see *Chromosome analysis findings*, page 379).

AMNIOTIC FLUID ANALYSIS

Amniocentesis is the transabdominal needle aspiration of 10 to 20 ml of amniotic fluid for laboratory analysis. This analysis may be used to detect certain birth defects, such as Down's syndrome or spina bifida; determine fetal maturity; detect hemolytic disease of the newborn; or, through karyotyping, detect gender and chromosomal abnormalities. This test can be performed only when the amniotic fluid level reaches 150 ml, usually after the 16th week of pregnancy.

Amniocentesis is indicated if the mother is over age 35; there is a family history of genetic, chromosomal, or neural tube defects; or a miscarriage has occurred. Although adverse effects are rare, potential complications include spontaneous abortion, trauma to the fetus or placenta, bleeding, premature labor, infection, and Rh sensitization from fetal bleeding into the maternal circulation. Due to the severity of possible complications, amniocentesis is contraindicated as a general screening test. Abnormal test results or failure of the tissue cultures to grow may necessitate repetition of the test.

Another method of detecting fetal chromosomal and biochemical disorders in early pregnancy is chorionic villi sampling. (See *Chorionic villi sampling,* pages 382 and 383.)

Purpose
• To detect fetal abnormalities, particularly chromosomal and neural tube defects
• To detect hemolytic disease of the newborn
• To diagnose metabolic disorders, amino acid disorders, and mucopolysaccharidoses
• To determine fetal age and maturity, especially pulmonary maturity
• To assess fetal health by detecting the presence of meconium or blood, or measuring amniotic levels of estriol and fetal thyroid hormone
• To identify fetal gender when one or both parents are carriers of a sex-linked disorder

CHORIONIC VILLI SAMPLING

Chorionic villi sampling (CVS), or biopsy, is a prenatal test for quick detection of fetal chromosomal and biochemical disorders that is performed during the first trimester of pregnancy. Preliminary results may be available within hours; complete results within a few days. In contrast, amniocentesis cannot be performed before the 16th week of pregnancy, and the results aren't available for at least 2 weeks. Thus, CVS can detect fetal abnormalities as much as 10 weeks sooner than amniocentesis.

The chorionic villi are finger-like projections that surround the embryonic membrane and eventually give rise to the placenta. Cells obtained from an appropriate sample are of fetal, rather than maternal, origin and thus can be analyzed for fetal abnormalities.

Collection time
Samples are best obtained between the 8th and 10th weeks of pregnancy. Before 7 weeks, the villi cover the embryo and make selective sampling difficult. After 10 weeks, maternal cells begin to grow over the villi and the amniotic sac begins to fill the uterine cavity, making the procedure difficult and potentially dangerous.

Collection method
To collect a chorionic villi sample, place the patient in the lithotomy position. The doctor checks the placement of the patient's uterus bimanually, and then inserts a Graves speculum and swabs the cervix with an antiseptic solution. If necessary, he may use a tenaculum to straighten an acutely flexed uterus, permitting cannula insertion. Guided by ultrasound and, possibly, endoscopy, he directs the catheter through the cannula to the villi. Suction is applied to the catheter to remove about 30 mg of tissue from the villi. The sample is withdrawn, placed in a Petri dish, and examined with a dissecting microscope. Part of the specimen is then cultured for further testing.

Interpretation
CVS can be used to detect about 200 diseases prenatally. For example, direct analysis of rapidly dividing fetal cells can detect chromosome disorders; deoxyribonucleic acid analysis can detect

Patient preparation
• Describe the procedure to the patient, and explain that this test detects fetal abnormalities.
• Assess her understanding of the test, and answer any questions she may have.
• Inform her that she needn't restrict food or fluids.
• Tell her the test requires a specimen of amniotic fluid and who will perform the test.
• Advise her that normal test results can't guarantee a normal fetus because some fetal disorders are undetectable.

• Make sure the patient has signed a consent form.
• Explain that she'll feel a stinging sensation when the local anesthetic is injected.
• Provide emotional support before and during the test and reassure her that adverse effects are rare.
• Ask her to void just before the test to minimize the risk of puncturing the bladder and aspirating urine instead of amniotic fluid.

hemoglobinopathies; and lysosomal enzyme assays can screen for lysosomal storage disorders, such as Tay-Sachs disease.

The test appears to provide reliable results except when the sample contains too few cells or the cells fail to grow in culture. Patient risks for this procedure appear to be similar to those for amniocentesis: a small chance of spontaneous abortion, cramps, infection, and bleeding. However, recent research reports an incidence of limb malformations in neonates when CVS has been performed.

Unlike amniocentesis, CVS can't detect complications in cases of Rh sensitization, uncover neural tube defects, or determine pulmonary maturity. However, it may prove to be the best way to detect other serious fetal abnormalities early in pregnancy.

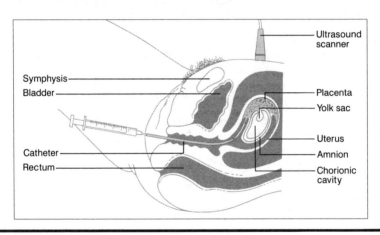

Equipment
70% alcohol or povidone-iodine solution, sponge forceps, 2″ × 2″ gauze pads, local anesthetic (1% lidocaine), 25G sterile needle, 3-ml syringe, 20G sterile spinal needle with stylet, 10-ml syringe, amber or foil-covered sterile 10-ml test tube.

Procedure and posttest care
• A pool of amniotic fluid is located after determining fetal and placental position, usually through palpation and ultrasonic visualization.

• The skin is prepared with antiseptic and alcohol; then 1 ml of 1% lidocaine is injected with a 25G needle, first intradermally and then subcutaneously
• Then a 20G spinal needle, with a stylet, is inserted into the amniotic cavity and the stylet is withdrawn.
• A 10-ml syringe is attached to the needle; then the fluid is aspirated and placed in an amber or foil-covered test tube.
• The needle is withdrawn, and an adhesive bandage is placed over the needle insertion site.

• Monitor fetal heart rate and maternal vital signs every 15 minutes for at least 30 minutes.
• Position the patient on her left side when she feels faint, nauseated, or sweats profusely to counteract uterine pressure on the vena cava.
• Instruct the patient before she is discharged to report abdominal pain or cramping, chills, fever, vaginal bleeding or leakage of serous vaginal fluid, or fetal hyperactivity or unusual fetal lethargy immediately.

Precautions
• Instruct the patient to fold her hands behind her head to prevent her from accidently touching the sterile field and causing contamination.
• Send the specimen to the laboratory immediately.

Normal findings
Normal amniotic fluid is clear but may contain white flecks of vernix caseosa when the fetus is near term. For detailed analysis of the appearance and components of amniotic fluid, see *Analysis of amniotic fluid,* page 385.

Abnormal findings
Blood in amniotic fluid is usually of maternal origin and doesn't indicate abnormality. However, it does inhibit cell growth and changes the level of other amniotic fluid constituents.

Large amounts of *bilirubin,* a breakdown product of red blood cells, may indicate hemolytic disease of the newborn. Normally, the bilirubin level increases from the 14th to the 24th week of pregnancy, then declines as the fetus matures, essentially reaching zero at term. Testing for bilirubin usually isn't performed until the 26th week because that's the earliest time successful therapy for Rh sensitization can begin. Bilirubin level is determined by spectrophotometric measurement of the optic density of the amniotic fluid. The deviation of the scan at 450 µ from a straight line drawn between 375 and 525 µ represents the bilirubin peak.

Meconium, a semisolid viscous material found in the fetal gastrointestinal tract, consists of mucopolysaccharides, desquamated cells, vernix, hair, and cholesterol. Meconium passes into the amniotic fluid when hypoxia causes fetal distress and relaxation of the anal sphincter. Meconium is a normal finding in breech presentation. Meconium in the amniotic fluid produces a peak of 410 µ on the spectrophotometric analysis. However, serial amniocentesis may show a clearing of meconium over a 2- to 3-week period. If meconium is present during labor, the newborn's nose and throat require thorough cleaning to prevent meconium aspiration.

Creatinine, a product of fetal urine, increases in the amniotic fluid as the fetal kidneys mature. Generally, the creatinine value exceeds 2 mg/dl in a mature fetus.

Alpha-fetoprotein is a fetal alpha globulin produced first in the yolk sac and, later, in the parenchymal cells of the liver and gastrointestinal tract. Fetal serum levels of alpha-fetoprotein are about 150 times more than amniotic fluid levels; maternal serum levels are far less than amniotic fluid levels. High amniotic fluid levels indicate neural tube defects, but the alpha-fetoprotein level may remain normal if the defect is small and closed. Elevated alpha-fetoprotein level may occur in multiple pregnancy; in disorders such as omphalocele, congenital nephrosis, esophageal or duodenal atresia, cystic fibrosis, exomphalos, Turner's syndrome, and fetal bladder neck obstruction with hydronephrosis; and in impending fetal death.

The amount of *uric acid* in the amniotic fluid increases as the fetus matures, but these levels fluctuate widely and

ANALYSIS OF AMNIOTIC FLUID

TEST	NORMAL FINDINGS	FETAL IMPLICATIONS OF ABNORMAL FINDINGS
Color	Clear, with white flecks of vernix caseosa in a mature fetus	Blood of maternal origin is usually harmless. "Port wine" fluid may indicate abruptio placentae. Fetal blood may indicate damage to the fetal, placental, or umbilical cord vessels.
Bilirubin	Absent at term	High levels indicate hemolytic disease of the newborn in isoimmunized pregnancy.
Meconium	Absent (except in breech presentation)	Presence indicates fetal hypotension or distress.
Creatinine	More than 2 mg/dl in a mature fetus	Less than 2 mg/dl may indicate immature fetus (less than 37 weeks).
Lecithin/sphingomye-lin ratio	More than 2 generally indicates fetal pulmonary maturity.	Less than 2 indicates pulmona-ry immaturity and subsequent respiratory distress syndrome.
Phosphatidylglycerol	Present	Absence indicates pulmonary immaturity.
Glucose	Less than 45 mg/dl	Excessive increases at term or near term indicates hypertrophy of fetal pancreas and subse-quent neonatal hypoglycemia.
Alpha-fetoprotein	Variable, depending on gestational age and laboratory technique. Highest concentration (about 18.5 mcg/ml) occurs at 13 to 14 weeks.	Inappropriate increases indi-cate neural tube defects, such as spina bifida or anencephaly, impending fetal death, congenital nephrosis, or contamination by fetal blood.
Bacteria	Absent	Presence indicates chorioamnionitis.
Chromosome	Normal karyotype	Abnormal karyotype may indicate fetal sex and chromosome disorders.
Acetycholinesterase	Absent	Presence may indicate neural tube defects, exomphalos, or other serious malformations.

can't accurately predict maturity. Laboratory studies indicate that severe erythroblastosis fetalis, familial hyperuricemia, and Lesch-Nyhan syndrome tend to increase the level of uric acid.

Estrone, estradiol, estriol, and *estriol conjugates* appear in amniotic fluid in varying amounts. Levels of estriol, the most prevalent estrogen, increase from 25.7 ng/ml during the 16th to 20th weeks to almost 1,000 ng/ml at term. Severe erythroblastosis fetalis decreases the estriol level.

Blood in the amniotic fluid occurs in about 10% of amnioceneses and results from a faulty tap. If the origin is maternal, the blood generally has no special significance; however, "port wine" fluid may be a sign of abruptio placentae, while blood of fetal origin may indicate damage to the fetal, placental, or umbilical cord vessels by the amniocentesis needle.

The Type II cells lining the fetal lung alveoli produce *lecithin* slowly in early pregnancy and then markedly increase production around the 35th week.

The *sphingomyelin* level parallels that of lecithin until the 35th week, when it gradually decreases. Measuring the ratio of lecithin to sphingomyelin (L/S ratio) confirms fetal pulmonary maturity (L/S ratio > 2) or suggests a risk of respiratory distress (L/S ratio < 2). However, fetal respiratory distress may develop in the fetus of a patient with diabetes, even though the L/S ratio is greater than 2, a level usually indicative of pulmonary maturity.

Phosphatidylglycerol levels are present with pulmonary maturity; *phosphatidylinositol* levels decrease. Measuring *glucose* levels in the fluid can aid in assessing glucose control in the patient with diabetes, but this isn't done routinely. A level greater than 45 mg/dl indicates poor maternal and fetal control. *Insulin* levels normally increase slightly from the 27th to the 40th week but increase sharply (up to 27 times normal) in a poorly controlled patient with diabetes.

Laboratory analysis can identify at least 25 different *enzymes* (usually in low concentrations) in amniotic fluid. The enzymes have few known clinical implications, although elevated acetylcholinesterase levels may occur with neural tube defects, exomphalos, and other serious malformations.

When the mother carries an *X-linked disorder,* determination of fetal sex is important. If chromosome karyotyping identifies a male fetus, there's a 50% chance he'll be affected; a female fetus won't be affected but has a 50% chance of being a carrier.

PAPANICOLAOU TEST

The Papanicolaou (Pap) test is a widely known cytologic test for early detection of cervical cancer. A doctor or specially trained nurse scrapes secretions from the patient's cervix and spreads them on a slide, which is sent to the laboratory for cytologic analysis. The test relies on the ready exfoliation of malignant cells from the cervix and shows cell maturity, metabolic activity, and morphology variations.

Although cervical scrapings are the most common test specimen, the test may involve cytologic evaluation of the vaginal pool, prostatic secretions, urine, gastric secretions, cavity fluids, bronchial aspirations, sputum, or solid tumor cells obtained by fine needle aspiration. If a Pap test is positive or suggests malignancy, cervical biopsy can confirm diagnosis.

Purpose
• To detect malignant cells
• To detect inflammatory tissue changes

- To assess response to chemotherapy and radiation therapy
- To detect viral, fungal and, occasionally, parasitic invasion

Patient preparation

- Explain to the patient that the test allows the study of cervical cells.
- Stress its importance as an aid for detection of cancer at a stage when the disease is often asymptomatic and still curable.
- The test should not be scheduled during the menstrual period; the best time is mid-cycle.
- Instruct the patient not to douche or insert vaginal medications for 24 hours before the test because doing so can wash away cellular deposits and change the vaginal pH.
- Tell her the test requires that the cervix be scraped, who will perform the procedure and when, and that she may experience slight discomfort but no pain from the speculum.
- Inform her that the procedure takes 5 to 10 minutes or slightly longer if the vagina, pelvic cavity, and rectum are examined bimanually.
- Obtain an accurate patient history, and ask the following questions: When did you last have a Pap test? Have you ever had an abnormal Pap test? When was your last menstrual period? Are your periods regular? How many days do they last? Is bleeding heavy or light? Have you taken or are you presently taking hormones or oral contraceptives? Do you use an intrauterine device? Do you have any vaginal discharge, pain, or itching? Which, if any, gynecologic disorders have occurred in your family? Have you ever had gynecologic surgery, chemotherapy, or radiation therapy? If so, describe it fully. Note any pertinent patient history data on the laboratory slip.
- Be supportive of the patient if she is anxious and tell her that test results should be available within a few days.

- Ask the patient to empty her bladder just before the test.

Equipment

Gloves; drape; vaginal speculum; collection device, such as a Pap stick (wooden spatula), cotton-tipped swab, or clean, dry glass pipette with rubber bulb; saline solution; glass microscopic slides; fixative (commercial spray or 95% ethyl alcohol solution in a jar) for slides.

Procedure and posttest care

- Instruct the patient to disrobe from the waist down and to drape herself.
- Ask her to lie on the examining table and to place her heels in the stirrups. (She may be more comfortable if she keeps her shoes on.) Tell her to slide her buttocks to the edge of the table. Adjust the drape to minimize exposure.
- Tell the patient when the examination will begin to avoid startling her.
- The examiner puts on gloves and inserts an unlubricated speculum into the vagina. To make insertion easier, the speculum may be moistened with saline solution or warm water.
- After the examiner locates the cervix, he will collect secretions from the cervix and material from the endocervical canal with a saline-moistened cotton-tipped swab or wooden spatula.
- Then the specimen is spread on the slide according to laboratory recommendations and the slide is immediately immersed in a fixative or is sprayed.
- Alternatively, posterior vaginal pool secretions and pancervical material may be collected and smeared on a single slide, which must be fixed immediately according to laboratory instructions.
- Label the specimen appropriately, including the date, the patient's name,

age, date of her last menstrual period, and the collection site and method.

• A bimanual examination may follow removal of the speculum. Help the patient up and instruct her to dress when the examination is completed.

• Supply the patient with a sanitary napkin if cervical bleeding occurs.

• Tell the patient when to return for her next Pap test.

Precautions

• Be sure the cervical specimen is aspirated and scraped from the cervix. Aspiration of the posterior fornix of the vagina can supplement a cervical specimen but should not replace it.

• Scrapings taken directly from the lesion are preferred if vaginal or vulval lesions are present.

• Use a small pipette, if necessary, in a patient whose uterus is involuting or atrophying from age, to aspirate cells from the squamocolumnar junction and the cervical canal.

• Preserve the slides *immediately*.

Normal findings

Normally, no malignant cells or other abnormalities are present.

Abnormal findings

Usually, malignant cells have relatively large nuclei and only small amounts of cytoplasm. They show abnormal nuclear chromatin patterns and marked variation in size, shape, and staining properties and may have prominent nucleoli.

A Pap smear may be graded in different ways, so check your laboratory's reporting format. The following list contains the traditional classifications:

• *Class I:* normal pattern; absence of atypical or abnormal cells

• *Class II:* benign abnormality; atypical, but nonmalignant, cells present

• *Class III:* atypical cells consistent with dysplasia

• *Class IV:* suggestive of, but inconclusive for, malignancy

• *Class V:* conclusive for malignancy.

To confirm a suggestive or positive cytology report, the test may be repeated or followed by a biopsy.

SEMEN ANALYSIS

Semen analysis is a simple, inexpensive, and reasonably definitive test that is used in a broad range of applications, including evaluation of a man's fertility. Fertility analysis usually includes measuring the volume of seminal fluid, performing sperm counts, and microscopic examination of spermatozoa. Sperm are counted in much the same way that white blood cells, red blood cells, and platelets are counted on an anticoagulated blood sample. Motility and morphology are studied microscopically after staining a drop of semen.

If analysis detects an abnormality, additional tests (for example, liver, thyroid, pituitary, or adrenal function tests) may be performed to identify the underlying cause and to screen for metabolic abnormalities (such as diabetes mellitus). Significant abnormalities — such as greatly decreased sperm count or motility, or marked increase in morphologically abnormal forms — may require testicular biopsy.

Purpose

• To evaluate male fertility in an infertile couple

• To substantiate the effectiveness of vasectomy

• To detect semen on the body or clothing of a suspected rape victim or elsewhere at the crime scene

• To identify blood group substances to exonerate or incriminate a criminal suspect

• To rule out paternity on grounds of complete sterility

Patient preparation
Evaluation of fertility:
• Provide written instructions, and inform the patient that the most desirable specimen requires masturbation, ideally in a doctor's office or a laboratory.
• Tell him to follow the instructions given to him regarding the period of sexual continence before the test because this may increase his sperm count. Some doctors specify a fixed number of days, usually between 2 and 5; others advise a period of continence equal to the usual interval between episodes of sexual intercourse.
• If the patient prefers to collect the specimen at home, emphasize the importance of delivering the specimen to the laboratory within 3 hours after collection. Warn him not to expose the specimen to extreme temperatures or to direct sunlight (which can also increase its temperature). Ideally, the specimen should remain at body temperature until liquefaction is complete (about 20 minutes). To deliver a semen specimen to the laboratory during cold weather, suggest that the patient protect the specimen from exposure to cold by keeping the specimen container in a coat pocket on the way to the laboratory.
• Alternatives to collection by masturbation include coitus interruptus or the use of a condom. For collection by coitus interruptus, instruct the patient to withdraw immediately before ejaculation during intercourse and to deposit the ejaculate in a suitable specimen container. For collection by condom, tell the patient to first wash the condom with soap and water, rinse it thoroughly, and allow it to dry completely. (Powders or lubricants applied to the condom may be spermicidal.) After collection, instruct him to tie the condom,

place it in a glass jar, and promptly deliver it to the laboratory.
• Fertility may also be determined by collecting semen from the woman after coitus to assess the ability of the spermatozoa to penetrate the cervical mucus and remain active. For the postcoital cervical mucus test, instruct the patient to report for examination during the ovulatory phase of her menstrual cycle, as determined by basal temperature records, and as soon as possible after sexual intercourse (within 8 hours). Explain to the patient scheduled for this test that the procedure takes only a few minutes. Tell her that she'll be placed in the lithotomy position and that a speculum will be inserted into the vagina to collect the specimen. She may feel some pressure but no pain during this procedure.
Semen collection from rape victim:
• Explain to the patient that the examiner will try to obtain a semen specimen from her vagina.
• Prepare her for insertion of the speculum as you would the patient scheduled for postcoital examination.
• Handle the victim's clothes as little as possible. If her clothes are moist, put them in a paper bag — not a plastic bag (which causes seminal stains and secretions to mold). Label the bag properly, and send it to the laboratory immediately.
• Provide emotional support by speaking to the patient calmly and reassuringly. Encourage her to express her fears and anxieties. Listen sympathetically.
• If she is scheduled for vaginal lavage, tell the rape victim to expect a cold sensation when saline solution is instilled to wash out the specimen.
• Help her relax during this procedure by instructing her to breathe deeply and slowly through her mouth.
• Instruct the victim to urinate just before the test, but warn her not to wipe

the vulva afterward because this may remove semen.

Equipment
For semen collection by masturbation, coitus interruptus, or condom: clean plastic specimen container (for example, disposable urine or sputum container with lid).

For semen collection from rape victim: clean plastic specimen container, vaginal speculum, rubber gloves, cotton applicator sticks, glass microscopic slides with frosted ends, physiologic (0.85%) saline solution, Pap sticks, Coplin jars containing 95% ethanol, large syringe, rubber bulb or other device suitable for vaginal lavage.

For a postcoital specimen collection: clean plastic specimen container, vaginal speculum, rubber gloves, cotton applicator sticks, glass microscopic slides with frosted ends, 1-ml tuberculin syringe without a cannula or needle.

Procedure and posttest care
• Obtain a semen specimen for a fertility study by asking the patient to collect semen in a clean plastic specimen container.

• A specimen is obtained from the vagina of a rape victim by direct aspiration, saline lavage, or a direct smear of vaginal contents, using a Pap stick or, less desirably, a cotton applicator stick. Dried smears are usually collected from the suspected rape victim's skin by gently washing the skin with a small piece of gauze moistened with physiologic saline solution.

• Prepare direct smears on glass microscopic slides after labeling the frosted end. Immediately place smeared slides in Coplin jars containing 95% ethanol.

• Before postcoital examination, the examiner wipes any excess mucus from the external cervix and collects the specimen by direct aspiration of the cervical canal, using a 1-ml tuberculin syringe without a cannula or needle.

• Inform a patient who is undergoing infertility studies that test results should be available in 24 hours.

• Refer the suspected rape victim to an appropriate specialist for counseling — a gynecologist, psychiatrist, clinical psychologist, nursing specialist, member of the clergy, or representative of a community support group, such as Women Organized Against Rape (WOAR).

Precautions
• If the patient prefers to collect the specimen during coitus interruptus, tell him he must prevent any loss of semen during ejaculation.

• Deliver all specimens, regardless of source or method of collection, to the laboratory promptly.

• Protect semen specimens for fertility studies from extremes of temperature and direct sunlight during delivery to the laboratory.

• Never lubricate the vaginal speculum. Oil or grease hinders examination of spermatozoa by interfering with smear preparation and staining and by inhibiting sperm motility through toxic ingredients. Instead, moisten the speculum with water or physiologic saline solution.

• Use extreme caution in securing, labeling, and delivering all specimens to be used for medicolegal purposes. You may be asked to testify as to when, where, and from whom the specimen was obtained; the specimen's general appearance and identifying features; steps taken to ensure the specimen's integrity; and when, where, and to whom the specimen was delivered for analysis. If your hospital or clinic uses routing slips for such specimens, fill them out carefully, and place them in the permanent medicolegal file.

Normal findings

Normal semen volume ranges from 0.7 to 6.5 ml. Paradoxically, the semen volume of men in infertile couples is frequently increased. Continence for 1 week or more results in progressively increased semen volume (sperm counts increase with abstinence up to 10 days, sperm motility progressively decreases, and sperm morphology stays the same). Liquefied semen is generally highly viscid, translucent, and gray-white, with a musty or acrid odor. After liquefaction, specimens of normal viscosity can be poured in drops. Normally, semen is slightly alkaline, with a pH of 7.3 to 7.9.

Other normal characteristics of semen: It coagulates immediately and liquefies within 20 minutes; normal spermatozoa count ranges from 20 to 150 million/ml; at least 40% of spermatozoa have normal morphology; and at least 20% of spermatozoa show progressive motility within 4 hours of collection.

The normal postcoital cervical mucus test shows at least 10 motile spermatozoa per microscopic high-power field and spinnbarkeit (a measurement of the tenacity of the mucus) of at least 4″ (10 cm). These findings indicate adequate spermatozoa and receptivity of the cervical mucus.

Abnormal findings

Abnormal semen is *not* synonymous with infertility. Only one viable spermatozoon is needed to fertilize an ovum. Although a normal sperm count is more than 20 million/ml, many men with sperm counts below 1 million/ml have fathered normal children. Only men who can't deliver *any* viable spermatozoa in their ejaculate during sexual intercourse are absolutely sterile. Nevertheless, subnormal sperm counts, decreased sperm motility, and abnormal morphology are usually associated with

decreased fertility. Other tests may be necessary to evaluate the patient's general health, metabolic status, or the function of specific endocrine glands (pituitary, thyroid, adrenal, or gonadal).

MISCELLANEOUS TESTS

CEREBROSPINAL FLUID ANALYSIS

For qualitative analysis, cerebrospinal fluid (CSF) is most commonly obtained by lumbar puncture (usually between the third and fourth lumbar vertebrae) and, rarely, by cisternal or ventricular puncture. A sample of CSF for laboratory analysis is frequently obtained during other neurologic tests, such as myelography.

Purpose

- To measure CSF pressure as an aid in detecting obstruction of CSF circulation
- To aid diagnosis of viral or bacterial meningitis, and subarachnoid or intracranial hemorrhage, tumors, and brain abscesses
- To aid diagnosis of neurosyphilis and chronic central nervous system infections

Patient preparation

- Describe the procedure to the patient, and explain that this test analyzes the fluid within the spinal cord.
- Inform him that he needn't restrict food or fluids.

• Tell him who will perform the procedure and where and that it usually takes at least 15 minutes.

• Advise the patient that a headache is the most common adverse effect of a lumbar puncture, but reassure him that his cooperation during the test helps minimize this effect.

• Be sure the patient or his legal guardian has signed the appropriate consent form.

• If the patient is unusually anxious, assess and report his vital signs.

Equipment
Lumbar puncture tray, sterile gloves, local anesthetic (usually 1% lidocaine), povidone-iodine solution, small adhesive bandage.

Procedure and posttest care
• Position the patient on his side at the edge of the bed, with his knees drawn up to his abdomen and his chin on his chest. Provide pillows to support the spine on a horizontal plane. This position allows full flexion of the spine and easy access to the lumbar subarachnoid space. Help him maintain this position by placing one arm around his knees and the other arm around his neck.

• If the sitting position is preferred, have the patient sit up and bend his chest and head toward his knees. Help him maintain this position throughout the procedure.

• After the skin is prepared for injection, the area is draped. Warn the patient that he'll probably experience a transient burning sensation when the local anesthetic is injected.

• Tell him that when the spinal needle is inserted, he may feel some transient local pain as the needle transverses the dura mater.

• Ask him to report any pain or sensations that differ from or continue after this expected discomfort because such sensations may indicate irritation or puncture of a nerve root, requiring repositioning of the needle.

• Instruct the patient to remain still and breathe normally; movement and hyperventilation can alter pressure readings or cause injury.

• The anesthetic is injected, and the spinal needle is inserted in the midline, between the spinous processes of the vertebrae (usually between the third and fourth lumbar vertebrae). At this point, initial (or opening) CSF pressure is measured and a specimen is obtained.

• After the specimen is collected, label the containers in the order in which they were filled, and determine if there are any specific instructions for the laboratory.

• Next, a final pressure reading is taken, and the needle is removed.

• Clean the puncture site with a local antiseptic, such as povidone-iodine solution, and apply a small adhesive bandage.

• Check if the patient must lie flat or if the head of his bed may be slightly elevated. In most cases, you will be instructed to keep the patient lying flat for 8 hours after lumbar puncture. Some doctors, however, allow a 30-degree elevation at the head of the bed. Remind the patient that although he must not raise his head, he can turn from side to side.

• Encourage the patient to drink fluids. Provide a flexible straw.

• Check the puncture site for redness, swelling, and drainage every hour for the first 4 hours, then every 4 hours for the first 24 hours.

• If CSF pressure is elevated, assess neurologic status every 15 minutes for 4 hours. If the patient is stable, assess him every hour for 2 hours, and then every 4 hours or according to pretest schedule.

• Watch for complications of lumbar puncture, such as reaction to the anesthetic, meningitis, bleeding into the spi-

ANALYSIS OF CEREBROSPINAL FLUID

TEST	NORMAL	ABNORMAL	IMPLICATIONS
Pressure	50 to 180 mm H_2O	Increase	Increased intracranial pressure due to hemorrhage, tumor, or edema caused by trauma
		Decrease	Spinal subarachnoid obstruction above puncture site
Appearance	Clear, colorless	Cloudy	Infection (elevated WBC count and protein levels, or many microorganisms)
		Xanthochromic or bloody	Subarachnoid, intracerebral, or intraventricular hemorrhage; spinal cord obstruction; traumatic tap (usually noted only in initial specimen)
		Brown, orange, or yellow	Elevated protein levels, RBC breakdown (blood present for at least 3 days)
Protein	15 to 45 mg/dl	Marked increase	Tumors, trauma, hemorrhage, diabetes mellitus, polyneuritis, blood in CSF
		Marked decrease	Rapid CSF production
Gamma globulin	3% to 12% of total protein	Increase	Demyelinating disease (such as multiple sclerosis), neurosyphilis, Guillain-Barré syndrome
Glucose	50 to 80 mg/dl (two-thirds of blood glucose level)	Increase	Systemic hyperglycemia
		Decrease	Systemic hypoglycemia, bacterial or fungal infection, meningitis, mumps, postsubarachnoid hemorrhage
Cell count	0 to 5 WBCs	Increase	Active disease: meningitis, acute infection, onset of chronic illness, tumor, abscess, infarction, demyelinating disease (such as multiple sclerosis)
	No RBCs	RBCs	Hemorrhage or traumatic tap
VDRL and other serologic tests	Nonreactive	Positive	Neurosyphilis
Chloride	118 to 130 mEq/liter	Decrease	Infected meninges (as in tuberculosis or meningitis)
Gram stain	No organisms	Gram-positive or gram-negative organisms	Bacterial meningitis

nal canal, and cerebellar tonsillar herniation and medullary compression. Signs of meningitis include fever, neck rigidity, and irritability; signs of herniation include decreased level of consciousness, changes in pupil size and equality, altered vital signs (including widened pulse pressure, decreased pulse rate, and irregular respirations), or respiratory failure.

Precautions
• Infection at the puncture site contraindicates removal of CSF; in a patient with increased intracranial pressure, CSF should be removed with extreme caution because the rapid reduction in pressure that follows withdrawal of fluid can cause cerebellar tonsillar herniation and medullary compression.
• During the procedure, observe closely for adverse reactions, such as elevated pulse rate, pallor, or clammy skin. Report any significant changes immediately.
• Record the collection time on the test request form. Send the form and labeled specimens to the laboratory immediately.

Findings
Normally, the CSF pressure is recorded and the appearance of the specimen is checked. Three tubes are collected routinely and are sent to the laboratory for analysis of protein, sugar, and cells as well as for serologic testing, such as the Venereal Disease Research Laboratory (VDRL) test for neurosyphilis. A separate specimen is also sent to the laboratory for culture and sensitivity testing. Electrolyte analysis and Gram stain may be ordered as supplementary tests. CSF electrolyte levels are of special interest in patients with abnormal serum electrolyte levels or CSF infection and in those receiving hyperosmolar agents. For a summary of normal and abnormal findings in CSF analysis, see *Analysis of cerebrospinal fluid,* page 393.

SYNOVIAL FLUID ANALYSIS

In synovial fluid aspiration, or arthrocentesis, a sterile needle is inserted into a joint space — most commonly the knee — to obtain a fluid specimen for analysis. This procedure is indicated for patients with undiagnosed articular disease and symptomatic joint effusion, a condition marked by the excessive accumulation of synovial fluid. Although rare, complications associated with synovial fluid aspiration include joint infection and hemorrhage leading to hemarthrosis (accumulation of blood within the joint).

Purpose
• To aid differential diagnosis of arthritis, particularly septic or crystal-induced arthritis
• To identify the cause and nature of joint effusion
• To relieve the pain and distention resulting from accumulation of fluid within the joint
• To administer a drug locally (usually corticosteroids)

Patient preparation
• Describe the procedure to the patient, and answer any questions he may have.
• Explain that this test helps determine the cause of joint inflammation and swelling and also helps relieve the associated pain.
• Instruct him to fast for 6 to 12 hours before the test if glucose testing of synovial fluid is ordered; otherwise, inform him that he needn't restrict food or fluids before the test.

NORMAL FINDINGS IN SYNOVIAL FLUID ANALYSIS

ANALYSIS	RESULTS
Gross	
Color	Colorless to pale yellow
Clarity	Clear
Quantity (in knee)	0.3 to 3.5 ml
Viscosity	High
pH	7.2 to 7.4
Mucin clot	Good
Microscopic	
WBC count	0 to 200/μl
WBC differential	
• Lymphocytes	0 to 78/μl
• Monocytes	0 to 71/μl
• Macrophages	0 to 26/μl
• Polymorphonuclears	0 to 25/μl
• Other phagocytes	0 to 21/μl
• Synovial lining cells	0 to 12/μl
Microbiological	
Formed elements	Absence of cartilage debris and crystals
Bacteria	None
Serologic	
Complement	
• For 10 mg protein/dl	3.7 to 33.7 U/ml
• For 20 mg protein/dl	7.7 to 37.7 U/ml
Rheumatoid arthritis cells	None
Lupus erythematosus cells	None
Chemical	
Total protein	10.7 to 21.3 mg/dl
Fibrinogen	None
Glucose	70 to 100 mg/dl
Uric acid	2 to 8 mg/dl (men)
	2 to 6 mg/dl (women)
Hyaluronate	0.3 to 0.4 g/dl
$PaCO_2$	40 to 60 mm Hg
PaO_2	40 to 80 mm Hg

• Tell him who will perform the test and where.
• Warn him that although he'll receive a local anesthetic, he may still feel transient pain when the needle penetrates the joint capsule.

• Make sure the patient or his legal guardian has signed a consent form.
• Check the patient's history for hypersensitivity to iodine compounds (such as povidone-iodine), procaine, lidocaine, or other local anesthetics.
• Administer a sedative.

SYNOVIAL FLUID ANALYSIS IN ARTHRITIS

DISEASE	COLOR	CLARITY	VISCOSITY	MUCIN CLOT
Group I noninflammatory				
Traumatic arthritis	Straw to bloody to yellow	Transparent to cloudy	Variable	Good to fair
Osteoarthritis	Yellow	Transparent	Variable	Good to fair
Group II inflammatory				
Systemic lupus erythematosus	Straw	Clear to slightly cloudy	Variable	Good to fair
Rheumatic fever	Yellow	Slightly cloudy	Variable	Good to fair
Pseudogout	Yellow	Slightly cloudy (if acute)	Low (if acute)	Fair to poor
Gout	Yellow to milky	Cloudy	Low	Fair to poor
Rheumatoid arthritis	Yellow to green	Cloudy	Low	Fair to poor
Group III septic				
Tuberculous arthritis	Yellow	Cloudy	Low	Poor
Septic arthritis	Gray or bloody	Turbid, purulent	Low	Poor

Equipment

Surgical detergent; skin antiseptic (usually tincture of povidone-iodine); alcohol sponges; local anesthetic (procaine or lidocaine, 1% or 2%); sterile, disposable 1½" 25G needle; sterile, disposable 1½" to 2" 20G needle; sterile 5-ml syringe for injecting anesthetic; sterile 20-ml syringe for aspiration; 3-ml syringe for administering sedative; sterile dressings; 2" × 2" sterile gauze pads; sterile drapes; elastic bandage; tubes for culture, cytologic, clot, and glucose analysis; anticoagulants (heparin, EDTA, and potassium oxalate); and venipuncture equipment.

For corticosteroid administration: corticosteroid suspension such as hydrocortisone, 2-ml and 5-ml syringes (or one 10-ml syringe if procaine and steroid are to be injected simultaneously).

Procedure and posttest care

• Position the patient.
• Explain that he will need to maintain this position throughout the procedure.
• Tell him that although he'll receive a local anesthetic to minimize pain, he will probably feel some discomfort when the needle is inserted. (A sedative may be administered to a young child.)

W.B.C. COUNT/ % NEUTROPHILS	CARTILAGE DEBRIS	CRYSTALS	R.A. CELLS	BACTERIA
1,000; 25%	None	None	None	None
700; 15%	Usually present	None	None	None
2,000; 30%	None	None	LE cells	None
14,000; 50%	None	None	LE cells may be present	None
15,000; 70%	Usually present	Calcium pyrophosphate	None	None
20,000; 70%	None	Urate	None	None
20,000; 70%	None	Occasionally cholesterol	Usually present	None
20,000; 60%	None	None	None	Usually present
90,000; 90%	None	None	None	Usually present

- Clean the skin over the puncture site with surgical detergent and alcohol.
- Paint the site with tincture of povidone-iodine, and allow it to air-dry for 2 minutes.
- After the local anesthetic is administered, the aspirating needle is quickly inserted through the skin, subcutaneous tissue, and synovial membrane into the joint space.
- As much fluid as possible is aspirated into the syringe; at least 15 ml should be obtained, although a lesser amount is usually adequate for analysis.
- The joint (except for the area around the puncture site) may be wrapped with an elastic bandage to compress the free fluid into this portion of the sac, ensuring maximal collection of fluid.
- If a corticosteroid is being injected, prepare the dose as necessary. For instillation, the syringe is detached, leaving the needle in the joint, and the syringe containing the steroid is attached to the needle instead.
- After the steroid is injected and the needle withdrawn, wipe the puncture site with an alcohol sponge.
- Apply pressure to the puncture site for about 2 minutes to prevent bleeding; then apply a sterile dressing.

• If synovial fluid glucose levels are being measured, perform a venipuncture to obtain a specimen for blood glucose analysis.

• Apply ice or cold packs to the affected joint for 24 to 36 hours after aspiration to decrease pain and swelling. Use pillows for support. If a large quantity of fluid was aspirated, apply an elastic bandage to stabilize the joint.

• If the patient's condition permits, tell him he may resume normal activity immediately after the procedure. However, warn him to avoid excessive use of the joint for a few days after the test even if pain and swelling subside.

• Watch for increased pain or fever, which may indicate joint infection.

• Carefully handle the dressings and linens of patients with drainage from the joint space, especially if septic arthritis is confirmed or suspected.

• Advise the patient that he may resume his usual diet.

Precautions

• Wear gloves when handling all specimens.

• Use strict sterile technique throughout aspiration to prevent contamination of joint space or synovial fluid specimen.

• Add an anticoagulant to the specimen, according to the laboratory tests requested. Gently invert the tube several times to mix the specimen and anticoagulant adequately.

• *For cultures,* obtain 2 to 5 ml of synovial fluid and, if possible, inoculate the medium immediately. Otherwise, add one or two drops of heparin to the specimen.

• *For cytologic analysis,* add 5 mg of EDTA or one or two drops of heparin to 2 to 5 ml of synovial fluid.

• *For glucose analysis,* add potassium oxalate, as specified by the laboratory, to 3 to 5 ml of fluid.

• *For crystal examination,* add heparin if specified by the laboratory.

• *For other studies,* such as general appearance and clot evaluation, obtain 2 to 5 ml of synovial fluid, but don't add an anticoagulant.

• Send the properly labeled specimens to the laboratory immediately — gonococci are particularly labile. If a white blood cell (WBC) count is being obtained, clearly label the specimen "Synovial Fluid" and "Caution: Don't Use Acid Diluents."

Reference values

Examination of synovial fluid in the laboratory can take many forms. Routine examination includes gross analysis for color, clarity, quantity, viscosity, pH, and the presence of a mucin clot as well as microscopic analysis for WBC count and differential. Special examination includes microbiological analysis for formed elements (including crystals) and bacteria, serologic analysis, and chemical analysis for such components as glucose, protein, and enzymes. (See *Normal findings in synovial fluid analysis,* page 395.)

Abnormal findings

Examination of synovial fluid may reveal various joint diseases, including noninflammatory disease (traumatic arthritis and osteoarthritis), inflammatory disease (systemic lupus erythematosus, rheumatic fever, pseudogout, gout, and rheumatoid arthritis), and septic disease (tuberculous and septic arthritis). (See *Synovial fluid analysis in arthritis,* pages 396 and 397.)

PERICARDIAL FLUID ANALYSIS

This test analyzes the fluid inside the pericardial sac of the heart. Testing is usually performed on patients with pericardial effusion (an accumulation of excess pericardial fluid), which may result from inflammation (as in pericarditis), rupture, or penetrating trauma.

Obtaining a specimen for analysis requires needle aspiration of pericardial fluid, a procedure called *pericardiocentesis*. This procedure must be performed cautiously because of the risk of potentially fatal complications, such as myocardial or coronary artery laceration, ventricular fibrillation or vasovagal arrest, pleural infection, or accidental puncture of the lung, liver, or stomach. If possible, echocardiography should determine the effusion site before pericardiocentesis is performed to minimize the risk of complications. (See *Aspirating pericardial fluid,* page 400.)

Purpose

• To assist in identifying the cause of pericardial effusion and to help determine appropriate therapy

Patient preparation

• Explain to the patient that this test detects excessive fluid around the heart, determines its cause, and helps determine appropriate therapy.

• Inform him that he needn't restrict food or fluids before the test.

• Tell him who will perform the test and where, and that it takes 10 to 20 minutes.

• Inform the patient that a local anesthetic will be injected before the aspiration needle is inserted.

• Warn him that although fluid aspiration isn't painful, he may experience pressure upon insertion of the needle into the pericardial sac.

• Advise him that he may be asked to briefly hold his breath to aid needle insertion and placement.

• Tell the patient that an I.V. line will be started at a slow rate in case medications need to be administered.

• Assure him that someone will remain with him during the test and that his pulse and blood pressure will be monitored after the procedure.

• Check the patient's history for current antimicrobial usage, and record such usage on the test request form.

• Make sure the patient or a responsible member of the family has signed a consent form.

• Explain the test to the family if pericardiocentesis is performed to relieve cardiac tamponade and the patient is in shock.

Equipment

70% alcohol or povidone-iodine solution; local anesthetic (1% procaine or 1% lidocaine); sterile 25G needle for the anesthetic; sterile 14G, 16G, and 18G 4″ or 5″ cardiac needles; 50-ml syringe with luer-lock tip; 7-ml sterile test tubes (one *red-top,* one *green-top* [heparin], and one *lavender-top* [EDTA]); sterile specimen container for culture; vial of heparin 1:1,000; 4″ × 4″ gauze pads; bandage; three-way stopcock. All of these items may be included in a prepackaged pericardiocentesis tray.

Also needed: electrocardiography (ECG) machine or bedside monitor, Kelly clamp, alligator clips, defibrillator, and emergency drugs.

Procedure and posttest care

• Place the patient in a supine position with the thorax elevated 60 degrees.

ASPIRATING PERICARDIAL FLUID

In pericardiocentesis, a needle and syringe assembly is inserted through the chest wall into the pericardial sac, as illustrated below. Electrocardiographic monitoring with a leadwire attached to the needle and electrodes placed on the limbs (right arm [RA], right leg [RL], left arm [LA], and left leg [LL]) helps to ensure proper needle placement and to avoid damage to the heart.

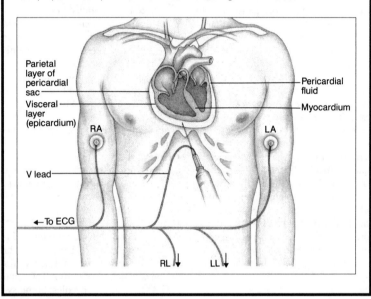

• Once he is comfortable and well-supported, instruct him to remain still during the procedure.

• A local anesthetic is administered at the insertion site after the skin is prepared with alcohol or povidone-iodine solution from the left costal margin to the xiphoid process.

• With the three-way stopcock open, a 50-ml syringe is aseptically attached to one end and the cardiac needle to the other end.

• The ECG leadwire is attached to the hub of the needle with an alligator clip. The ECG machine is set to lead V and turned on (or the patient is connected to a bedside monitor).

• The needle is inserted through the chest wall into the pericardial sac, maintaining gentle aspiration until fluid appears in the syringe.

• The needle is angled 35 to 45 degrees toward the tip of the right scapula between the left costal margin and the xiphoid process. A Kelly clamp is attached at the skin surface once the needle is properly positioned so it won't advance further.

• While the fluid is being aspirated, label and number the specimen tubes.

• When the needle is withdrawn, apply pressure to the site *immediately* with sterile gauze pads for 3 to 5 minutes. Then apply a bandage.

• Check blood pressure readings, pulse, respiration, and heart sounds every 15 minutes until stable, then every ½ hour for 2 hours, every hour for 4 hours, and every 4 hours thereafter. Reassure the patient that such monitoring is routine.

• Be alert for respiratory or cardiac distress. Watch especially for signs of cardiac tamponade: muffled and distant heart sounds, distended neck veins, paradoxical pulse, and shock. Cardiac tamponade may result from rapid reaccumulation of pericardial fluid or puncture of a coronary vessel causing bleeding into the pericardial sac.

Precautions

• Carefully observe the ECG tracing during insertion of the cardiac needle; an ST-segment elevation indicates that the needle has reached the epicardial surface and should be retracted slightly; an abnormally shaped QRS complex may indicate perforation of the myocardium. Premature ventricular contractions usually indicate that the needle has touched the ventricular wall.

• Watch for grossly bloody aspirate — a sign of inadvertent puncture of a cardiac chamber.

• Be sure to use specimen tubes with the proper additives. Although fibrin isn't a normal component of pericardial fluid, it does appear in fluid in some pericardial diseases and in carcinoma, and clotting is possible.

• If bacterial culture and sensitivity tests are scheduled, record any antimicrobial therapy on the laboratory slip.

• If anaerobic organisms are suspected, consult the laboratory concerning the proper collection technique to avoid exposing the aspirate to air. The aspirate may be placed in an anaerobic collection tube or the syringe may be filled completely, displacing all air, and the collection tube capped tightly with a sterile rubber tip.

• Send all specimens to the laboratory immediately.

• Have resuscitation equipment on hand.

Normal findings

Normally, 10 to 50 ml of sterile fluid is present in the pericardium. Pericardial fluid is clear and straw-colored, without evidence of pathogens, blood, or malignant cells. It normally contains fewer than 1,000 white blood cells/mm³. Its glucose concentration approximately equals the levels in whole blood.

Abnormal findings

Generally, pericardial effusions are classified as transudates or exudates. Transudates are protein-poor effusions that usually arise from mechanical factors altering fluid formation or resorption, such as increased hydrostatic pressure, decreased plasma oncotic pressure, or obstruction of the pericardial lymphatic drainage system by a tumor.

Most exudates result from inflammation and contain large amounts of protein. In these effusions, inflammation damages the capillary membrane, allowing protein molecules to leak into the pericardial fluid. Exudate effusions may occur in pericarditis, neoplasms, acute myocardial infarction, tuberculosis, rheumatoid disease, and systemic lupus erythematosus.

An elevated white blood cell count or neutrophil fraction may also accompany inflammatory conditions such as bacterial pericarditis; a high lymphocyte fraction may indicate fungal or tuberculous pericarditis. Turbid or milky effusions may result from the accumulation of lymph or pus in the pericardial sac, or from tuberculosis or rheumatoid disease.

Bloody pericardial fluid may indicate hemopericardium, hemorrhagic pericarditis, or a traumatic tap. Hemopericardium, the accumulation of blood in the pericardium, may result from myocardial rupture after infarction or aortic rupture secondary to dissecting aortic aneurysm or thoracic trauma. In hemopericardium, the fluid has a hematocrit level similar to that of whole blood; in hemorrhagic pericarditis, it has a relatively low hematocrit level and doesn't clot on standing.

Hemorrhagic effusions may indicate malignancies, Dressler's syndrome, closed chest trauma, or postcardiotomy syndrome. A traumatic tap is easily distinguished from hemopericardium or hemorrhagic pericarditis because the fluid becomes progressively clearer.

Glucose concentrations below whole blood levels may reflect increased local metabolism due to malignancy, inflammation, or infection. Possible causes of bacterial pericarditis include *Staphylococcus aureus, Haemophilus influenzae,* and various gram-negative organisms; possible causes of granulomatous pericarditis include *Mycobacterium tuberculosis* or various fungal agents; and causes of viral pericarditis include coxsackieviruses, echoviruses, and others.

SWEAT TEST

This test is a quantitative measurement of electrolyte concentrations (primarily sodium and chloride) in sweat, usually performed using pilocarpine iontophoresis (pilocarpine is a sweat inducer). It is used almost exclusively in children to confirm cystic fibrosis.

Purpose
• To confirm cystic fibrosis

Patient preparation
• Explain the test to the child (if he is old enough to understand) using clear, simple terms.

• Inform the child and his parents that there are no restrictions on diet, medication, or activity before the test.
• Tell the child who will perform the test and where and that it takes 20 to 45 minutes (depending on the equipment used).
• Tell him he may feel a slight tickling sensation during the procedure but won't feel any pain.
• Encourage the parents to assist with preparations and to stay with their child during the test. Their presence will minimize the child's anxiety.

Equipment
Analyzer, two skin chloride electrodes (positive and negative), distilled water, two standardizing solutions (chloride concentrations), $2'' \times 2''$ sterile gauze pads (kept in airtight container), pilocarpine pads, forceps (for handling pads), straps (for securing electrodes), gram scale, 0.9% sodium chloride solution.

Procedure and posttest care
• Wash the area that will undergo iontophoresis with distilled water and dry it. (The flexor surface of the right forearm is commonly used or, when the patient's arm is too small to secure electrodes [as with an infant], the right thigh.)
• Place a gauze pad saturated with premeasured pilocarpine solution on the positive electrode; place the pad saturated with 0.9% sodium chloride solution on the negative electrode.
• Apply both electrodes to the area to undergo iontophoresis, and secure them with straps. Leadwires to the analyzer are given a current of 4 milliamperes in 15 to 20 seconds. Iontophoresis will continue at 15- to 20-second intervals for 5 minutes.
• Try to distract the child with a book, television, a toy, or another diversion if he

becomes nervous or frightened during the test.

• Remove both electrodes after iontophoresis.

• Discard the pads, clean the skin with distilled water, and then dry it.

• Using forceps, place a dry gauze pad or filter paper (previously weighed on a gram scale) on the area that underwent iontophoresis.

• Cover the pad or filter paper with a slightly larger piece of plastic, and seal the edges of the plastic with waterproof adhesive tape.

• Leave the gauze pad or filter paper in place for about 30 to 40 minutes. (The appearance of droplets on the plastic usually indicates induction of an adequate amount of sweat.)

• Remove the pad or filter paper with the forceps, place it immediately in the weighing bottle, and insert the stopper in the bottle. (The difference between the first and second weights indicates the weight of the sweat specimen collected.)

• Wash the area that underwent iontophoresis with soap and water, and dry it thoroughly. If the area looks red, reassure the patient that this is normal and will disappear within a few hours.

• Tell the patient or his parents that he may resume his usual activities.

Precautions

• Always perform iontophoresis on the right arm (or right thigh) rather than on the left.

• Never perform iontophoresis on the chest, especially in a child, because the current can induce cardiac arrest.

• Use battery-powered equipment to prevent electric shock if possible.

• Stop the test immediately if the patient complains of a burning sensation, which usually indicates that the positive electrode is exposed or positioned improperly. Adjust the electrode and continue the test.

• Make sure at least 100 mg of sweat is collected for analysis.

• Carefully seal the gauze pad or filter paper in the weighing bottle, and send the bottle to the laboratory immediately.

Reference values

Normal sodium values in sweat range from 10 to 30 mEq/liter. Normal chloride values range from 10 to 35 mEq/liter.

Abnormal findings

Abnormal sodium values range from 50 to 130 mEq/liter; abnormal chloride values range from 50 to 110 mEq/liter. Sodium and chloride concentrations of 50 to 60 mEq/liter strongly suggest cystic fibrosis. Concentrations greater than 60 mEq/liter, with typical clinical features, confirm the diagnosis.

Only a few conditions other than cystic fibrosis cause elevated sweat electrolyte levels — most notably, untreated adrenal insufficiency, as well as type I glycogen storage disease, vasopressin-resistant diabetes insipidus, meconium ileus, and renal failure. In women, sweat electrolyte levels fluctuate cyclically: chloride concentrations usually peak 5 to 10 days before onset of menses, and most women retain fluid before menses. Men also show fluctuations (up to 70 mEq/liter). However, cystic fibrosis is the only condition that raises sweat electrolyte levels above 80 mEq/liter.

EXAMINATION OF UROGENITAL SECRETIONS FOR TRICHOMONADS

Microscopic examination of urine or vaginal, urethral, or prostatic secretions can detect urogenital infection by *Trichomonas vaginalis,* a parasitic, flagellate protozoan that's usually transmitted sexually. This test is more commonly performed on women than men because women are more likely to exhibit symptoms; men may exhibit symptoms of urethritis or prostatitis.

Purpose
• To confirm trichomoniasis

Patient preparation
• Explain that this test can identify the cause of urogenital infection.
• If the patient is a woman, tell her the test requires a specimen of vaginal secretions or urethral discharge, and ask her not to douche before the test.
• It the patient is a man, tell him the test requires a specimen of urethral or prostatic secretions.
• Inform the patient who will perform the procedure and when.

Equipment
Gloves, cotton swab, test tube containing small amount of 0.9% sodium chloride, vaginal speculum, specimen cup (if a urine specimen is being collected).

Procedure and posttest care
Vaginal secretion:
• With the patient in the lithotomy position, an unlubricated vaginal speculum is inserted, and discharge is collected with a cotton swab. The swab is then placed in the tube containing 0.9% sodium chloride solution, and the speculum is removed.
• Another method is to smear the specimen on a glass slide, allow it to air-dry, and then transport it to the laboratory.
Prostatic material:
• After prostatic massage, collect secretions with a cotton swab, and place the swab in 0.9% sodium chloride solution.

Urethral discharge:
• Collect the discharge with a cotton swab, and place the swab in 0.9% sodium chloride solution.
Urine:
• Include the first portion of a voided random specimen (not midstream).
All procedures:
• Label the specimen appropriately, including the date and time of collection.
• Provide perineal care.

Precautions
• Remember to use gloves when performing procedures and handling specimens.
• If possible, obtain the urogenital specimen before treatment with a trichomonacide begins.
• Send the specimen to the laboratory immediately because trichomonads can be identified only while still motile.

Normal findings
Trichomonads are normally absent from the urogenital tract.

Abnormal findings
Trichomonads confirm trichomoniasis. In approximately 25% of women and in most infected men, trichomonads may be present without associated pathology.

Cultures

GENERAL CULTURES

GENITAL CULTURES

GENERAL CULTURES

URINE CULTURE

Laboratory examination and culture of urine are used to evaluate urinary tract infections, especially bladder infections. Urine in the kidneys and bladder is normally sterile, but a urine specimen may contain a variety of organisms due to bacteria in the urethra and on external genitalia. Bacteriuria generally results from one prevalent bacteria type; the presence of more than two bacterial species in a specimen strongly suggests contamination during collection. A single negative culture does not always rule out infection, however; a quantitative examination of urine culture is needed.

Purpose
• To diagnose urinary tract infection
• To monitor microorganism colonization after urinary catheter insertion

Patient preparation
• Explain to the patient that this test is used to detect urinary tract infection.
• Advise him that the test requires a urine specimen and that no restriction of food or fluids is necessary.
• Provide instruction on how to collect a clean-voided midstream specimen; emphasize that external genitalia must be cleaned thoroughly.
• If appropriate, explain catheterization or suprapubic aspiration to the patient and inform him that he may experience some discomfort during specimen collection.

• For the patient with suspected tuberculosis, specimen collection may be required on three consecutive mornings.
• Check patient history for current antimicrobial therapy.

Equipment
Gloves; sterile specimen cup; towelettes or sterile water, cleansing solution (such as aqueous green soap), and cotton balls or sterile gauze sponges. Note that commercial clean-catch urine kits are available.

Procedure and posttest care
• Collect a urine specimen.
• Record the suspected diagnosis, the collection time and method, current antimicrobial therapy, and fluid- or drug-induced diuresis on the laboratory slip.

Precautions
• Use gloves when performing the procedure and handling specimens.
• Collect at least 3 ml of urine, but do not fill the specimen cup more than halfway.
• Seal the cup with a sterile lid, and send it to the laboratory immediately. If transport is delayed longer than 30 minutes, store the specimen at 39.2° F (4° C) or place it on ice, unless a urine transport tube containing preservative is used.

Normal findings
Culture results of sterile urine are normally reported as "no growth," which usually indicates the absence of urinary tract infection.

Abnormal findings
Bacterial counts of 100,000 or more organisms per milliliter of a single microbe species indicate probable urinary tract infection. Counts under 100,000/ml may be significant, depending on the patient's age, sex, history, and other individual factors. However, counts under 10,000/ml

usually suggest that the organisms are contaminants, except in symptomatic patients, those with urologic disorders, or those whose urine specimens were collected by suprapubic aspiration. A special test for acid-fast bacteria isolates *Mycobacterium tuberculosis,* thus indicating tuberculosis of the urinary tract.

Isolation of more than two species of organisms, or of vaginal or skin organisms, usually suggests contamination and requires a repeat culture. Prolonged catheterization or urinary diversion may cause polymicrobial infection.

STOOL CULTURE

Normal bacterial flora in feces include several potentially pathogenic organisms. Bacteriologic examination is valuable for identifying pathogens that cause overt GI disease — such as typhoid and dysentery — and carrier states. A sensitivity test may follow isolation of the pathogen. Stool culture may also be used to detect certain viruses, such as enterovirus, which can cause aseptic meningitis.

Purpose
• To identify pathogenic organisms — especially in a debilitated patient
• To aid treatment of disease, prevent possibly fatal complications, and confine severely infectious diseases

Patient preparation
• Explain to the patient that this test is used to determine the cause of gastrointestinal distress or to determine if the patient is a carrier of infectious organisms.
• Food or fluids need not be restricted.
• Tell the patient the test may require collection of a stool specimen on 3 consecutive days.

• Check patient history for dietary patterns, recent antimicrobial therapy, and for recent travel that might suggest endemic infections or infestations.

Equipment
Gloves; half-pint, waterproof container with tight-fitting lid or sterile swab and commercial sterile collection and transport system; tongue blade; bedpan (if needed).

Procedure and posttest care
• Collect a stool specimen directly into the container. If the patient is not ambulatory, collect the specimen in a clean, dry bedpan and, using a tongue blade, transfer the specimen to the container.
• If you must collect the specimen by rectal swab, insert the swab past the anal sphincter, rotate it gently, and withdraw it. Then, place the swab in the appropriate container.
• Check with the laboratory for the proper collection procedure before obtaining a specimen for a virus test.
• Label the specimen with the patient's name, doctor's name, hospital number, date, and time of collection.
• Indicate the suspected cause of enteritis and current antimicrobial therapy on the laboratory slip.

Precautions
• Use gloves when performing the procedure and handling the specimen.
• If the patient uses a bedpan or a diaper, avoid contaminating the stool specimen with urine.
• The specimen must represent the first, middle, and last portion of the feces passed. Be sure to include mucoid and bloody portions.
• Put the specimen container in a leakproof bag and send it to the laboratory immediately.

Normal findings

Approximately 96% to 99% of normal fecal flora consist of anaerobes, including non-spore-forming bacilli, clostridia, and anaerobic streptococci. The remaining 1% to 4% consist of aerobes, including gram-negative bacilli (predominantly *Escherichia coli* and other Enterobacteriaceae, plus small amounts of *Pseudomonas*), gram-positive cocci (mostly enterococci), and a few yeasts.

Abnormal findings

The most common pathogenic organisms of the GI tract are *Shigella, Salmonella*, and *Campylobacter jejuni*. Less common pathogenic organisms include *Vibrio cholerae, Clostridium botulinum, Clostridium difficile, Clostridium perfringens, Staphylococcus aureus*, enterotoxigenic *E. coli, Bacillus cereus, Yersinia enterocolitica, Aeromonas hydrophila*, and *Vibrio parahaemolyticus*. Isolation of some pathogens indicates bacterial infection in patients with acute diarrhea and may require antimicrobial sensitivity tests. Normal fecal flora may include *Clostridium difficile, E. coli*, and other organisms. Therefore, isolation of these may require further tests to demonstrate invasiveness or toxin production. Isolation of pathogens such as *Clostridium botulinum* indicates food poisoning; the pathogens must also be isolated from the contaminated food. In a patient undergoing long-term antimicrobial therapy, isolation of large numbers of *Staphylococcus aureus* or yeast may indicate infection. (Asymptomatic carrier states are also indicated by these enteric pathogens.) Isolation of enteroviruses may indicate aseptic meningitis.

If a stool culture shows no unusual growth, detection of viruses by immunoassay or electron microscopy may be used to diagnose nonbacterial gastroenteritis. Highly increased polymorphonuclear leukocytes in fecal material may indicate an invasive pathogen.

THROAT CULTURE

A throat culture is used primarily to isolate and identify pathogens. Culture results are considered in relation to the patient's clinical status, recent antimicrobial therapy, and amount of normal flora.

Purpose

• To isolate and identify group A beta-hemolytic streptococci *(Streptococcus pyogenes)* — allowing early treatment of pharyngitis — and to prevent sequelae, such as rheumatic heart disease or glomerulonephritis
• To screen asymptomatic carriers of pathogens, especially *Neisseria meningitidis*
• Rarely, to identify *Corynebacterium diphtheriae* or *Bordetella pertussis*
• To identify *Candida albicans*, although direct potassium hydroxide preparation usually provides the same information faster

Patient preparation

• Explain to the patient that this test is used to identify microorganisms that may be causing his symptoms or a carrier state.
• Inform him that he need not restrict food or fluids before the test.
• Tell him who will perform the procedure and when.
• Reassure him that the test takes less than 30 seconds and that test results should be available in 2 or 3 days.
• Describe the procedure, and warn him that he may gag during the swabbing.
• Check the patient's history for recent antimicrobial therapy. Determine im-

munization history if pertinent to preliminary diagnosis.

Equipment
Gloves; sterile swab and culture tube with transport medium or commercial collection and transport system.

Procedure and posttest care
• Tell the patient to tilt his head back and close his eyes.
• With the throat well illuminated, check for inflamed areas, using a tongue depressor.
• Swab the tonsillar areas from side to side; include any inflamed or purulent sites.
• *Do not* touch the tongue, cheeks, or teeth with the swab.
• Immediately place the swab in the culture tube.
• If a commercial sterile collection and transport system is used, crush the ampule and force the swab into the medium to keep the swab moist.
• Note recent antimicrobial therapy on the laboratory slip; label the specimen with the patient's name, the doctor's name, date and time of collection, and the origin of the specimen; indicate the suspected organism, especially *C. diphtheriae* (requires two swabs and special growth medium), *B. pertussis* (requires a nasopharyngeal culture and a special growth medium), and *N. meningitidis* (requires enriched selective media).
• Nonculture antigen testing methods can be used to detect group A streptococca antigen in as little as 10 minutes. Cultures are then performed on negative specimens.

Precautions
• Procure the throat specimen before beginning any antimicrobial therapy.
• Use gloves when performing the procedure and handling specimens.

• Send the specimen to the laboratory immediately. Unless a commercial sterile collection and transport system is used, keep the container upright during transport.
• To protect the specimen and prevent its exposure to pathogens, use aseptic technique during the procedure, and observe proper precautions when sending the specimen to the laboratory.

Normal findings
Normal throat flora includes non-hemolytic and alpha-hemolytic streptococci, *Neisseria* species, staphylococci, diphtheroids, some hemophilus, pneumococci, yeasts, and enteric gram-negative rods.

Abnormal findings
Possible pathogens cultured include group A beta-hemolytic streptococci (*S. pyogenes*), which can cause scarlet fever or pharyngitis; *Candida albicans,* which can cause thrush; *C. diphtheriae,* which can cause diphtheria; and *B. pertussis,* which can cause whooping cough. The laboratory report should indicate the prevalent organisms and the quantity of pathogens cultured.

NASOPHARYNGEAL CULTURE

This test is used to evaluate nasopharyngeal secretions for the presence of pathogenic organisms. It requires direct microscopic examination of a gram-stained smear of the specimen. Preliminary identification of organisms may be used to guide clinical management and determine the need for additional testing. Cultured pathogens may then require susceptibility testing to determine appropriate antimicrobial therapy.

Purpose
• To identify pathogens causing upper respiratory tract symptoms
• To identify proliferation of normal nasopharyngeal flora, which may be pathogenic in debilitated and other immunocompromised patients
• To identify *Bordetella pertussis* and *Neisseria meningitidis,* especially in very young, elderly, or debilitated patients and in asymptomatic carriers
• Infrequently, to isolate viruses, especially to identify carriers of influenza virus A and B

Patient preparation
• Explain to the patient that this test is used to isolate the cause of nasopharyngeal infection.
• Describe the procedure to the patient; tell him that secretions will be obtained from the back of the nose and the throat, using a cotton-tipped swab, and who will perform this procedure.
• Warn him that he may experience slight discomfort and may gag, but reassure him that obtaining the specimen takes less than 15 seconds.
• Inform him that initial test results are available in 48 to 72 hours or longer for viral test results.

Equipment
Gloves; penlight; sterile, flexible wire swab; small, sterile, open-ended glass Pyrex tube or sterile nasal speculum; tongue depressor; culture tube; transport medium (broth).

Procedure and posttest care
• Put on gloves.
• Ask the patient to cough before you begin collection of the specimen.
• Position the patient with his head tilted back.
• Using a penlight and a tongue depressor, inspect the nasopharyngeal area.
• Gently pass the swab through the nostril and into the nasopharynx, keeping the swab near the septum and floor of the nose. Rotate the swab quickly, and remove it.
• Alternatively, place the Pyrex tube in the patient's nostril, and carefully pass the swab through the tube into the nasopharynx. Rotate the swab for 5 seconds; then place it in the culture tube with transport medium. Remove the Pyrex tube.
• Label the specimen with the date and time of collection, the origin of the material, and the suspected organism.
• Ideally, specimens for *B. pertussis* should be inoculated to fresh culture medium at the patient's bedside due to the organism's susceptibility to environmental changes.
• If the specimen is for isolation of a virus, follow the laboratory's recommended collection technique.

Precautions
• Use gloves when performing the procedure and handling the specimen.
• Do not let the swab touch the sides of the patient's nostril or his tongue to prevent specimen contamination.
• Note recent antimicrobial therapy or chemotherapy on the laboratory slip.
• Keep the container upright.
• Tell the laboratory if *Corynebacterium diphtheriae* and *B. pertussis,* which need special growth media, are suspected.
• Refrigerate a viral specimen, according to your laboratory's procedure.

Normal findings
Flora commonly found in the nasopharynx include nonhemolytic streptococci, alpha-hemolytic streptococci, *Neisseria* species (except *N. meningitidis* and *N. gonorrhoeae*), coagulase-negative staphylococci such as *Staphylococcus epidermidis* and, occasionally, the coagulase-positive *Staphylococcus aureus.*

Abnormal findings

Pathogens include group A beta-hemolytic streptococci; occasionally groups B, C, and G beta-hemolytic streptococci; *B. pertussis; C. diphtheriae; S. aureus;* and large amounts of *Haemophilus influenzae,* pneumococci, or *Candida albicans.*

SPUTUM CULTURE

Bacteriologic examination of sputum—material raised from the lungs and bronchi — is an important aid to the management of lung disease. The usual method of specimen collection is deep coughing and expectoration, which may require ultrasonic nebulization, hydration, physiotherapy, or postural drainage; other methods include tracheal suctioning or bronchoscopy.

Purpose

• To identify the cause of pulmonary infection, thus aiding diagnosis of respiratory diseases (most frequently bronchitis, tuberculosis, lung abscess, and pneumonia)

Patient preparation

• Explain to the patient that this test is used to identify the organism causing respiratory tract infection.
• Tell him the test requires a sputum specimen and who will perform the procedure.
• If the suspected organism is *Mycobacterium tuberculosis,* tell the patient that at least three morning specimens may be required.
• Inform him that test results are usually available in 48 to 72 hours. However, because cultures for tuberculosis take up to 2 months, diagnosis of this disorder generally depends on clinical symptoms, a smear for acid-fast bacilli, a

chest X-ray, and the response to a purified protein derivative skin test.
• If the specimen is to be collected by expectoration, encourage fluid intake the night before collection to help sputum production. Teach the patient how to expectorate by taking three deep breaths and forcing a deep cough; emphasize that sputum is not the same as saliva, which is unacceptable for culturing. Tell him not to brush his teeth or use mouthwash before the specimen collection, although he may rinse his mouth with water.
• If the specimen is to be collected by tracheal suctioning, tell the patient he will experience discomfort as the catheter passes into the trachea.
• If the specimen is to be collected by bronchoscopy, instruct the patient to fast for 6 hours before the procedure. Make sure he or a responsible member of the family has signed a consent form. Tell him he'll receive a local anesthetic just before the test to minimize discomfort during passage of the tube.

Equipment

For expectoration: sterile, disposable, impermeable container with a tight-fitting cap; 10% sodium chloride, acetylcysteine, propylene glycol, or sterile or distilled water aerosols to induce cough; leakproof bag.
For tracheal suctioning: #16 or #18 French suction catheter; water-soluble lubricant; sterile gloves; sterile specimen container or in-line specimen trap; 0.9% sodium chloride solution.
For bronchoscopy: bronchoscope; local anesthetic; sterile needle and syringe; sterile specimen container; 0.9% sodium chloride solution; bronchial brush; sterile gloves.

Procedure and posttest care

Expectoration:
• Put on gloves.

• Instruct the patient to cough deeply and expectorate into the container. If the cough is nonproductive, use chest physiotherapy or heated aerosol spray (nebulization) to induce sputum. Using aseptic technique, close the container securely.

• Dispose of equipment properly; seal the container in a leakproof bag before sending it to the laboratory.

Tracheal suctioning:

• Administer oxygen to the patient before and after the procedure, if necessary.

• Attach the sputum trap to the suction catheter. Using sterile gloves, lubricate the catheter with 0.9% sodium chloride solution, and pass the catheter through the patient's nostril, without suction. (The patient will cough when the catheter passes through the larynx.) Advance the catheter into the trachea. Apply suction for no longer than 15 seconds to obtain the specimen.

• Stop suction, and gently remove the catheter. Discard the catheter and gloves in the proper receptacle. Then, detach the in-line sputum trap from the suction apparatus and cap the opening.

• After tracheal suctioning, offer the patient a drink of water.

Bronchoscopy:

• After a local anesthetic is sprayed into the patient's throat or the patient gargles with a local anesthetic, the bronchoscope is inserted through the pharynx and trachea, into the bronchus.

• Secretions are then collected with a bronchial brush or aspirated through the inner channel of the scope using an irrigating solution, such as 0.9% sodium chloride solution, if necessary.

• After the specimen is obtained, the bronchoscope is removed.

• After bronchoscopy, observe the patient carefully for signs of hypoxemia (cyanosis), laryngospasm (laryngeal stridor), bronchospasm (paroxysms of coughing or wheezing), pneumothorax (dyspnea, cyanosis, pleural pain, tachycardia), perforation of the trachea or bronchus (subcutaneous crepitus), or trauma to respiratory structures (bleeding). Also, check for difficulty in breathing or swallowing. *Do not* give liquids until the gag reflex returns.

All collection methods:

• Label the container with the patient's name. Include on the test request form the nature and origin of the specimen, the date and time of collection, the initial diagnosis, and any current antimicrobial therapy.

Precautions

• Tracheal suctioning is contraindicated in patients with esophageal varices or cardiac disease.

• In a patient with asthma or chronic bronchitis, watch for aggravated bronchospasms with use of more than 10% concentration of sodium chloride or acetylcysteine in an aerosol.

• During tracheal suctioning, suction for only 5 to 10 seconds at a time. *Never* suction longer than 15 seconds. If the patient becomes hypoxic or cyanotic, remove the catheter immediately and administer oxygen.

• Use gloves when performing the procedure and handling specimens.

• Because the patient may cough violently during suctioning, wear gloves and a mask to avoid exposure to pathogens.

• *Do not* use more than 20% propylene glycol with water as an inducer for a specimen scheduled for tuberculosis culturing because higher concentrations inhibit the growth of *M. tuberculosis.* (If propylene glycol is not available, use 10% to 20% acetylcysteine with water or sodium chloride solution.)

• Send the specimen to the laboratory immediately after collection.

Normal findings

A Gram stain of expectorated sputum must be examined to ensure that it's a representative specimen of secretions from the lower respiratory tract. Sputum is invariably contaminated with normal oropharyngeal flora, such as alpha-hemolytic streptococci, *Neisseria* species, diphtheroids, and some hemophili, pneumococci, staphylococci, and yeasts, such as *Candida*. The presence of normal flora does not rule out infection; interpretation of a culture isolate must include consideration of the patient's overall clinical condition.

Abnormal findings

Pathogenic organisms most often found in sputum include *Streptococcus pneumoniae, M. tuberculosis, Klebsiella pneumoniae* (and other Enterobacteriaceae), *Haemophilus influenzae, Staphylococcus aureus, Pseudomonas aeruginosa,* and other agents, such as *Pneumocystis carinii, Legionella,* and *Mycoplasma pneumoniae.* Isolation of *M. tuberculosis* is always a significant finding.

Respiratory viruses usually require serologic or histologic diagnosis rather than diagnosis by sputum culture.

BLOOD CULTURE

A blood culture is performed to isolate and aid identification of the pathogens in bacteremia (bacterial invasion of the bloodstream) and septicemia (systemic spread of such infection). It requires inoculating a culture medium with a blood sample and incubating it.

Purpose

• To confirm bacteremia
• To identify the causative organism in bacteremia and septicemia

Patient preparation

• Explain to the patient that this procedure is used to aid identification of the organism causing the patient's symptoms.
• Inform him he need not restrict food or fluids before the test.
• Tell him how many samples the test will require, who will perform the venipunctures and when, and that he may experience transient discomfort from the needle punctures and the pressure of the tourniquet. Reassure him that collecting each sample usually takes less than 5 minutes.

Equipment

Gloves; tourniquet; small adhesive bandages; alcohol swabs; povidone-iodine swabs; 10- to 20-ml syringe for an adult, 6-ml syringe for a child; three or four sterile needles; two blood culture bottles, one vented (aerobic) and one unvented (anaerobic), with nutritionally enriched broths and sodium polyethanol sulfonate added; or bottles with resin or a lysis-centrifugation tube.

Procedure and posttest care

• Put on gloves.
• Clean the venipuncture site with an alcohol swab and then with an iodine swab, working in a circular motion from the site outward.
• Wait at least 1 minute for the skin to dry, and remove the residual iodine with an alcohol swab. (Or remove the iodine after venipuncture.)
• Apply the tourniquet.
• Perform a venipuncture; draw 10 to 20 ml of blood for an adult, or one syringe of 2 to 6 ml for a child.
• Clean the diaphragm tops of the culture bottles with alcohol or iodine, and change the needle on the syringe.
• If broth is used, add blood to each bottle until you obtain a 1:5 or 1:10 dilution. For example, add 10 ml of blood to a 100-ml bottle. (Size of the bottle

varies, depending on hospital procedure.)

• If a special resin is used, such as Bactec resin medium or Antimicrobial Removal Device, add blood to the resin in the bottles and invert them gently to mix.

• Draw the blood directly into a special collection and processing tube if you're using the lysis-centrifugation technique (Isolator).

• Indicate the tentative diagnosis on the laboratory slip, and note any current or recent antimicrobial therapy.

• If a hematoma develops at the venipuncture site, apply warm soaks.

Precautions

• Use gloves when performing the procedure and handling specimens.

• Send each sample to the laboratory immediately after collection.

Normal findings

Normally, blood cultures are sterile.

Abnormal findings

Positive blood cultures do not necessarily confirm pathologic septicemia. Mild, transient bacteremia may occur during the course of many infectious diseases or may complicate other disorders. Persistent, continuous, or recurrent bacteremia reliably confirms the presence of serious infection. To detect most causative agents, blood cultures are ideally drawn on 2 consecutive days.

Isolation of most organisms takes about 72 hours; however, negative cultures are held for 1 week or more before being reported negative.

Common blood pathogens include *Neisseria meningitidis, Streptococcus pneumoniae, Haemophilus influenzae,* other *Streptococcus* species, *Staphylococcus aureus, Pseudomonas aeruginosa,* Bacteroidaceae, *Brucella,* and Enterobacteriaceae. Although 2% to 3% of blood samples cultured are contaminated by skin bacteria, such as *Staphylococcus epidermidis,* diphtheroids, and *Propionibacterium,* these organisms may be clinically significant when isolated from multiple cultures or from immunocompromised patients.

WOUND CULTURE

Performed to confirm infection, a wound culture is a microscopic analysis of a specimen from a lesion. Wound cultures may be aerobic (for detection of organisms that usually appear in a superficial wound) or anaerobic (for organisms that need little or no oxygen and appear in areas of poor tissue perfusion, such as postoperative wounds, ulcers, or compound fractures). Indications for wound culture include fever and inflammation and drainage in damaged tissue.

Purpose

• To identify an infectious microbe in a wound

Patient preparation

• Explain to the patient that this test is used to identify infectious microbes.

• Describe the procedure, advising him that a drainage specimen from the wound is withdrawn by a syringe or removed on cotton swabs.

• Tell him who will perform the procedure and when.

• Reassure him that collecting the drainage specimen takes less than 3 minutes.

Equipment

Sterile cotton swabs and sterile culture tube or commercial sterile collection and transport system (for aerobic culture); sterile cotton swabs or sterile 10-

ml syringe with 21G needle, and special culture tube containing carbon dioxide or nitrogen (for anaerobic culture); sterile gloves; alcohol sponges; sterile gauze and povidone-iodine solution.

Procedure and posttest care
• Using gloves, prepare a sterile field and clean the area around the wound with antiseptic solution.
• For *aerobic culture,* express the wound and swab as much exudate as possible, or insert the swab deeply into the wound and gently rotate. Immediately place the swab in the aerobic culture tube.
• For *anaerobic culture,* insert the swab deeply into the wound, gently rotate, and immediately place the swab in the anaerobic culture tube (see *Anaerobic specimen collector*). Or insert the needle into the wound, aspirate 1 to 5 ml of exudate into the syringe, and immediately inject the exudate into the anaerobic culture tube. If the needle is covered with a rubber stopper, the aspirate may be sent to the laboratory in the syringe.
• Record on the laboratory slip recent antimicrobial therapy, the source of the specimen, and the suspected organism; label the specimen container appropriately with the patient's name, the doctor's name, the hospital number, and the wound site and the time of specimen collection.
• Dress the wound.

Precautions
• Clean the area around the wound thoroughly to limit contamination of the culture by normal skin flora, such as diphtheroids, *Staphylococcus epidermidis,* and alpha-hemolytic streptococcus. However, *do not* clean the area around a perineal wound.
• Make sure no antiseptic enters the wound.

ANAEROBIC SPECIMEN COLLECTOR

Some anaerobes die when exposed to oxygen. To facilitate anaerobic collection and culturing, tubes filled with carbon dioxide (CO_2) or nitrogen are used for oxygen-free transport.

The anaerobic specimen collector shown here consists of a rubber-stoppered tube filled with CO_2, a small inner tube, and a swab attached to a plastic plunger. The drawing on the left shows the tube before specimen collection. The small inner tube containing the swab is held in place by the rubber stopper.

After specimen collection (right), the swab is quickly replaced in the inner tube and the plunger is depressed. This separates the inner tube from the stopper, forcing it into the larger tube and exposing the specimen to the CO_2-rich environment.

Keep the tube upright.

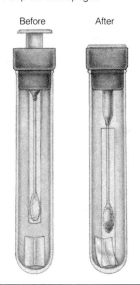

Before   After

• Obtain exudate from the entire wound, using more than one swab if necessary.

• Because some anaerobes die in the presence of even a small amount of oxygen, place the specimen in the culture tube quickly, take care that no air enters into the tube, and check that double stoppers are secure.

• Keep the specimen container upright, and send it to the laboratory within 15 minutes to prevent growth or deterioration of microbes.

• Use gloves during the procedure and when handling the specimen, and take necessary isolation precautions when sending the specimen to the laboratory.

Normal findings

Normally, no pathogenic organisms are present in a clean wound.

Abnormal findings

The most common aerobic pathogens for wound infection include *Staphylococcus aureus,* group A beta-hemolytic streptococci, *Proteus, Escherichia coli* and other Enterobacteriaceae, and some *Pseudomonas* species; the most common anaerobic pathogens include some *Clostridium* and *Bacteroides* species.

GASTRIC CULTURE

This test requires aspiration of gastric contents and cultivation of any microbes present. It is performed in conjunction with a chest X-ray and a purified protein derivative skin test and is especially useful when a sputum sample cannot be obtained by expectoration or nebulization. Gastric aspiration also provides a specimen for rapid presumptive identification of bacteria (by Gram stain) in neonatal septicemia.

Purpose

• To aid diagnosis of mycobacterial infections

• To identify the infecting bacteria in neonatal septicemia

Patient preparation

• Explain to the patient (or to the parents if the patient is a child) that gastric culture is used to diagnose tuberculosis.

• Instruct him to fast for 8 hours before the test.

• Tell him who will perform the procedure and that the same procedure may be performed on three consecutive mornings.

• Instruct him to remain in bed each morning until specimen collection has been completed to prevent premature emptying of stomach contents.

• Describe the procedure to the patient. Tell him the nasogastric tube may make him gag but passes more easily if he relaxes and follows instructions about breathing and swallowing.

• Just before the procedure, obtain baseline heart rate and rhythm, and place the patient in high Fowler's position.

• Advise the patient (or his parents) that test results may take 2 months because acid-fast bacteria generally grow slowly.

• Check medication history for recent antimicrobial therapy. Inform the doctor of your findings; he may want to discontinue medications before the test.

Equipment

Water-soluble lubricating jelly; sterile water; #16 or #18 French, disposable, plastic nasogastric tube; 50-ml sterile syringe; sterile specimen container; sterile gloves; emesis basin; stethoscope; clamp (if necessary).

Procedure and posttest care

• As soon as the patient awakens in the morning, put on gloves, perform

nasogastric intubation, and obtain gastric washings.
• Clamp the tube before quickly removing from the patient.
• Note recent antimicrobial therapy on the laboratory slip, along with the site and time of collection.
• Label the specimens with the patient's name, the doctor's name, and the hospital number.
• Resume administration of medications discontinued before the test.
• Instruct the patient not to blow his nose for at least 4 to 6 hours to prevent bleeding.
• Tell the patient that he may resume his normal diet.

Precautions
• Gastric intubation is contraindicated in conditions such as pregnancy, esophageal disorders (varices, stenosis, diverticula), malignant neoplasms, recent severe gastric hemorrhage, aortic aneurysm, heart failure, and myocardial infarction.
• If possible, obtain the specimens before the start of antimicrobial therapy.
• Watch for signs that the tube has entered the trachea, including coughing, cyanosis, or gasping.
• *Never* inject water into a nasogastric tube unless you're sure the tube is correctly placed in the patient's stomach. During lavage, use sterile, distilled water to decrease risk of contamination with saprophytic mycobacteria.
• Check the patient's pulse rate for irregularities during this procedure to detect arrhythmias.
• Use gloves when performing the procedure and when handling specimens.
• Put the specimen in a tightly capped container, wipe the outside of the container with disinfectant, place it upright in a plastic bag, and send it to the laboratory immediately.
• Handle the nasogastric tube with gloved hands, and dispose of all equipment carefully to prevent staff contamination.

Normal findings
Normally, culture specimen is negative for pathogenic mycobacteria.

Abnormal findings
Isolation and identification of the organism *Mycobacterium tuberculosis* indicates the presence of active tuberculosis; other species of *Mycobacterium*, such as *M. bovis, M. kansasii,* and *M. avium-intracellulare* complex, may cause pulmonary disease that is clinically indistinguishable from tuberculosis. Treatment of these mycobacterial diseases may be difficult and commonly requires susceptibility studies to determine effective antimicrobial therapy. Pathogenic bacteria causing neonatal septicemia may also be identified through culture.

DUODENAL CONTENTS CULTURE

This test requires duodenal intubation, aspiration of duodenal contents, and cultivation of microbes to isolate and identify pathogens that may cause duodenitis, cholecystitis, or cholangitis. Occasionally, a specimen may be obtained during surgery.

Purpose
• To detect bacterial infection of the biliary tract and duodenum
• To differentiate between infection and gallstones
• To rule out bacterial infection as the cause of persistent GI symptoms (epigastric pain, nausea, vomiting, and diarrhea)

Patient preparation
• Explain to the patient that this test is used to determine the cause of his symptoms.
• Instruct him to restrict food and fluids for 12 hours before the test.
• Tell him who will perform the procedure and where it will be done.
• Describe the intubation procedure to the patient. Assure him that although this procedure is uncomfortable, it is not dangerous; tell him that passage of the tube may cause gagging, but following the examiner's instructions about proper positioning, breathing, swallowing, and relaxing will minimize discomfort.
• Suggest that he empty his bladder before the procedure to increase his general comfort.

Equipment
Gloves; double-lumen tube with olive tip; water-soluble jelly; 30-ml sterile syringe; emesis basin; sterile specimen container; ½″ adhesive tape.

Procedure and posttest care
• After the nasoenteric tube is inserted, place the patient in a left lateral decubitus position, with his feet elevated, to allow peristalsis to move the tube into the duodenum.
• Determine the pH of a small amount of aspirated fluid to ascertain tube position: If the tube is in the stomach, pH is lower than 7.0; if the tube is in the duodenum, pH is higher than 7.0.
• Correct position of the tube can also be confirmed by fluoroscopy.
• Aspirate duodenal contents.
• Occasionally, a specimen for culture of duodenal contents is obtained during duodenoscopy (see "Esophagogastroduodenoscopy" in Chapter 10).
• Transfer specimen to a sterile container, and label it with the patient's name, doctor's name, date, and collection time.

• After duodenal intubation or duodenoscopy, observe the patient carefully for signs of perforation, such as dysphagia, epigastric or shoulder pain, dyspnea, or fever, from tube passage.
• After duodenoscopy, monitor vital signs until the patient is stable; keep the side rails up, and enforce bed rest until the patient is fully alert.
• Resume diet discontinued before the test.

Precautions
• Use gloves when performing procedures and handling specimens.
• Duodenal intubation is contraindicated in conditions such as pregnancy; acute pancreatitis or cholecystitis; esophageal varices, stenosis, and diverticular malignant neoplasms; recent severe gastric hemorrhage; aortic aneurysm; congestive heart failure; or myocardial infarction.
• Collect the specimen for culture before antimicrobial therapy begins.
• Send the specimen to the laboratory immediately.
• Withdraw the tube slowly (6″ to 8″ [15 to 20 cm] every 10 minutes) until it reaches the esophagus; then clamp the tube and remove it quickly. Report the problem if you cannot withdraw the tube easily; *never* force the tube.

Normal findings
Normally, a duodenal contents culture contains small amounts of polymorphonuclear leukocytes and epithelial cells with no pathogens. The bacterial count is usually less than 100,000 per milliliter of body fluid.

Abnormal findings
Duodenal contents (pancreatic and duodenal enzymes and bile) are subject to infection by many pathogens, such as *Escherichia coli, Staphylococcus aureus,* and *Salmonella.* Generally, bacterial counts of 100,000 or more per mil-

liliter of body fluid or the presence of pathogens in any number indicates infection. Susceptibility testing may be required. Numerous polymorphonuclear leukocytes, copious mucous debris, and bile-stained epithelial cells in the bile fluid suggest inflammation of the biliary tract; many segmented neutrophils and exfoliated epithelial cells suggest inflammation of the pancreas, the duodenum, or bile ducts. The presence of bile sand indicates cholelithiasis or calculi in the biliary tract. Differential diagnosis requires further testing.

GENITAL CULTURES

CULTURE FOR GONORRHEA

Gonorrhea nearly exclusively results from sexual transmission of *Neisseria gonorrhoeae*. A stained smear of genital exudate can confirm gonorrhea in 90% of males with characteristic symptoms, but a culture is often necessary, especially in asymptomatic females. Possible culture sites include the urethra (usual site in males), endocervix (usual site in females), anal canal, and oropharynx.

Purpose
• To confirm gonorrhea

Patient preparation
• Describe the procedure to the patient. Explain that this test is used to confirm gonorrhea.

• Inform the patient who will perform the test and when and that results are usually available within 24 to 72 hours.
• Instruct the female patient not to douche for 24 hours before the test.
• Tell the male patient that he should not void during the hour preceding the test. Warn him that males sometimes experience nausea, sweating, weakness, and fainting due to stress or discomfort when the cotton swab or wire loop is introduced into the urethra.

Equipment
Sterile gloves; sterile cotton swabs; wire bacteriologic loop or thin urogenital alginate swabs (for male); vaginal speculum; modified Thayer-Martin medium in plates (or Transgrow medium in specimen bottles if laboratory is not readily available); ring forceps; cotton balls.

Procedure and posttest care
Endocervical culture:
• Place the patient in the lithotomy position, drape her appropriately, and instruct her to take deep breaths.
• Using gloved hands, insert a vaginal speculum, lubricated only with warm water. Clean mucus from the cervix using cotton balls in ring forceps.
• Insert a dry, sterile cotton swab into the endocervical canal and rotate it from side to side. Leave the swab in place for several seconds for optimum absorption of organisms.
Urethral culture:
• Place the patient in supine position, and drape appropriately.
• Clean the urethral meatus with sterile gauze or a cotton swab; then insert a thin urogenital alginate swab or a wire bacteriologic loop $\frac{3}{8}''$ to $\frac{3}{4}''$ (1 to 2 cm) into the urethra, and rotate the swab or loop from side to side. Leave it in place for several seconds for optimum absorption of organisms. If permitted, the patient may milk the urethra, bringing

CULTURING FOR NEISSERIA GONORRHOEAE

Culturing for *Neisseria gonorrhoeae* requires use of a Modified Thayer-Martin (MTM) medium. If a laboratory isn't readily available, you may use Transgrow medium.

Modified Thayer-Martin
MTM medium is a combination of hemoglobin, gonococcal growth-enhancing chemicals, and antimicrobial agents for culturing endocervical, urethral, or rectal specimens. To inoculate a culture plate treated with MTM medium and to spread organisms out of their associated mucus, take the following steps:
- Roll the swab in a Z pattern (1).
- Using the swab or a sterile wire loop, immediately cross-streak the plate (2).
- To demonstrate *Neisseria gonorrhoeae,* incubate within 15 minutes of streaking.

Two-step method of streaking Thayer-Martin plate

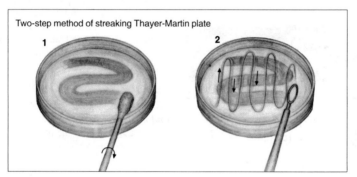

Transgrow
A modification of MTM medium, Transgrow is available in a screw-cap bottle containing air and carbon dioxide. Transgrow bottles are used to transport suspect cultures when laboratory facilities aren't available at the site of specimen collection. Use the following procedure:
- To prevent loss of carbon dioxide, inoculate the specimen bottle while it's in an upright position.
- After uncapping the bottle, immediately insert the swab and soak up all excess moisture.
- Starting at the bottom of the bottle, roll the swab from side to side across the medium.
- Recap the bottle, and send it to the laboratory immediately. Subculturing should begin within 24 to 48 hours.

One-step method of streaking Transgrow medium

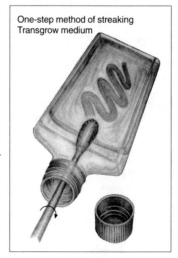

urethral secretions to the meatus for collection on a cotton swab.

Rectal culture:

• After obtaining an endocervical or urethral specimen (while the patient is still on the examining table), insert a sterile cotton swab into the anal canal about 1″ (2.5 cm), move the swab from side to side, and leave it in place for several seconds for optimum absorption.

• If the swab is contaminated with feces, discard it and repeat the procedure with a clean swab.

Throat culture:

• Position the patient with his head tilted back.

• Check his throat for inflamed areas using a tongue depressor. Rub a sterile swab from side to side over the tonsillar areas, including any inflamed or purulent sites. Be careful not to touch the teeth, cheeks, or tongue with the swab.

After collecting any of these specimens:

• Roll the swab in a Z pattern in a plate containing modified Thayer-Martin medium. Then, cross-streak the medium with a sterile wire loop or the tip of the swab, and cover the plate. (See *Culturing for* Neisseria gonorrhoeae.)

• Label the specimen with the patient's name and room number (if applicable), the doctor's name, the date, and the time of collection.

• If laboratory facilities are not readily available, do the following: Uncap the Transgrow medium specimen bottle just before inserting the swab of test material into the bottle. Keep the bottle upright to minimize loss of carbon dioxide. With the swab, absorb the excess moisture within the bottle; then roll the swab across the Transgrow medium. Discard the swab. Place the lid on the bottle, and label the bottle appropriately.

• Advise the patient to avoid intercourse and all sexual contact until test results are available.

• Explain that treatment usually begins after confirmation of positive culture, except in a patient with symptoms of gonorrhea or in a person who has had intercourse with someone known to have gonorrhea.

• Advise the patient that a repeat culture is required 1 week after completion of treatment to evaluate therapy.

• Inform the patient that positive culture findings must be reported to the local health department.

Precautions

• Use gloves when performing precautions and when handling specimens.

• Place the male patient in supine position to prevent falling if vasovagal syncope occurs during introduction of the cotton swab or wire loop into the urethra. Observe for profound hypotension, bradycardia, pallor, and sweating.

• Collect a urethral specimen at least 1 hour after the patient has voided to prevent loss of urethral secretions.

• After collecting the specimens, carefully dispose of gloves, swabs, and speculum to prevent staff exposure.

• Immediately send the specimen to the laboratory or arrange for transport of Transgrow bottle, as the specimen must be subcultured within 24 to 48 hours.

Normal findings

Normally, no *N. gonorrhoeae* appears in the culture.

Abnormal findings

A positive culture confirms gonorrhea.

CULTURE FOR HERPES SIMPLEX VIRUS

Herpes simplex virus (HSV) produces a wide spectrum of clinical manifesta-

RAPID MONOCLONAL TEST FOR CYTOMEGALOVIRUS

Cytomegalovirus (CMV), a member of the herpesvirus group, can cause systemic infection in congenitally infected infants and in immunosuppressed patients, such as transplant recipients, patients receiving chemotherapy for neoplastic disease, and patients with acquired immunodeficiency syndrome (AIDS).

Laboratory detection of CMV

In the past, CMV infections were detected in the laboratory by recognizing the distinctive cytopathic effects (CPE) produced by the virus in conventional tube cell cultures. In this slow method of detecting CMV, CPE cultures grow in 9 days on average.

The faster, shell vial assay (rapid monoclonal test) is based on centrifugal inoculation of specimens onto cell monolayers grown on round cover slips in 1 dram shell vials and the immunologic detection of early products of viral replication with specific monoclonal antibodies after 16 hours of incubation. This assay is based on the availability of a monoclonal antibody specific for the 72 kd protein of CMV synthesized during the immediate early stage of viral replication. Through indirect immunofluorescence, CMV-infected fibroblasts are recognized by their dense, homogeneous staining confined to the nucleus of these cells. Because of the smooth, regular shape of the nucleus and the surrounding nuclear membrane, infect-

ed cells are readily differentiated from nonspecific background fluorescence that may be present in some specimens.

This test is used to obtain rapid laboratory diagnosis of CMV infection, especially in immunocompromised patients who have or are at risk for developing systemic infections caused by this virus.

Specimen collection

Specimens should be collected during the prodromal and acute stages of clinical infection to ensure the best chance of detecting CMV. As required by the laboratory, collect a specimen for culture. Each type of specimen requires a specific collection device, as listed below:
- *Throat:* microbiologic transport swab
- *Urine, cerebrospinal fluid:* sterile screw-capped tube or vial
- *Bronchoalveolar lavage tissue:* sterile screw-capped jar
- *Blood:* sterile tube with anticoagulant (heparin).

CMV can be detected in urine and throat specimens from patients who are asymptomatic. However, the detection of CMV from these sites indicates active, asymptomatic infection, which may herald symptomatic involvement, especially in immunosuppressed patients. Detection of CMV in specimens of blood, tissue, and bronchoalveolar lavage generally indicates systemic infection and disease.

tions, including keratitis, gingivostomatitis, and encephalitis. In immunocompromised individuals, it may lead to disseminated illness. The herpesvirus group includes Epstein-Barr virus, cytomegalovirus (CMV), varicella-zoster virus (VZV), human herpesvirus-6, and HSV types 1 and 2. Only CMV, VZV, and HSV replicate in the standard cell cultures used in diagnostic laboratories. Approximately 50% of the strains of HSV can be detected by characteristic cytopathic effects (CPE) within 24 hours after the laboratory receives the specimen; 5 to 7 days are required to detect the remaining HSV strains. (See *Rapid monoclonal test for cytomegalovirus*.)

Purpose
• To confirm diagnosis of HSV infection by culturing the virus from specimens

Patient preparation
• Explain to the patient that this test is performed to detect infection by HSV.
• Specimens should be collected from suspected lesions during the prodromal and acute stages of clinical infection.

Procedure and posttest care
• Collect a specimen for culture into the appropriate collection device.
• For throat, skin, eye, or genital area, use a microbiologic transport swab.
• For body fluids or other respiratory specimens (washings, lavage), use a sterile screw-capped jar.
• Specimens should be stored or transported to the laboratory as soon as possible after collection. If the anticipated time between collection and inoculation of cell cultures is more than 2 hours, the specimen should be stored and transported at 39.2° F (4° C).

Precautions
• Wear gloves when obtaining and handling all specimens.
• Do not freeze specimen or allow it to dry up.

Reference values
HSV is rarely recovered from immunocompetent patients who show no overt signs of disease.

Abnormal findings
HSV detected in specimens taken from dermal lesions, the eye, cerebrospinal fluid, or tissue are highly significant. Specimens from the upper respiratory tract may be associated with intermittent shedding of the virus, particularly in an immunocompromised patient.

Like other herpesviruses, HSV can be shed from immunosuppressed patients intermittently in the absence of apparent disease. For epidemiologic purposes, HSV detected by CPE in standard tube cell cultures is confirmed and identified as type 1 or 2.

CULTURE FOR CHLAMYDIA

The most common sexually transmitted disease in North America is caused by *Chlamydia trachomatis*. Identification of this parasite requires cultivation in the laboratory by infection of susceptible cells. After incubation, *Chlamydia*-infected cells can be detected by fluorescein isothiocyanate-conjugated monoclonal antibodies or by iodine stain. Detection in cell cultures of *C. psittaci* and *C. pneumoniae* requires specific technical manipulations and reagents.

While culture is the detection method of choice, rapid noncultural (antigen detection) procedures are also available.

Purpose
• To confirm infections caused by *C. trachomatis*

Patient preparation
• Explain the purpose of the test to the patient.
• Describe the procedure for collecting a specimen for culture.
• If the specimen will be collected from the patient's genital tract, instruct the

patient not to urinate for 3 to 4 hours before the specimen is taken.

Equipment
Gloves; sterile cotton swabs; wire bacteriologic loop or thin urogenital alginate swabs (for male); vaginal speculum; sucrose phosphate (2SP) transport medium.

Procedure and posttest care
• Obtain a specimen of the epithelial cells from the infected site. In adults, these sites may include the eye, urethra (rather than from the purulent exudate that may be present), endocervix, or rectum.
• Obtain a urethral specimen by inserting a cotton-tipped applicator ¾" to 2" (2 to 5 cm) into the urethra.
• To collect a specimen from the endocervix, use a microbiologic transport swab or cytobrush.
• Extract the specimen into sucrose phosphate (2SP) transport medium.
• Specimens collected from the throat, eye, and nasopharynx and aspirates from infants should be extracted into 2SP transport medium. The specimens are sent to the laboratory at 39.2° F (4° C).
• If the anticipated time between collection of the specimen and inoculation into cell culture is more than 24 hours, freeze the 2SP transport medium and send it to the laboratory with dry ice.
• *Note:* In patients suspected of being sexually abused, be sure to process specimens by culture rather than by antigen detection methods.
• If the culture confirms infection, provide counseling for the patient regarding treatment of his sexual partners.
• Advise the patient to avoid all sexual contact until after test results are available.

Precautions
• Place the male patient in supine position to prevent falling if vasovagal syncope occurs during introduction of the cotton swab or wire loop into the urethra. Observe for profound hypotension, bradycardia, pallor, and sweating.
• Use gloves when performing procedures and when collecting and handling specimens.
• Collect a urethral specimen at least 1 hour after the patient has voided to prevent loss of urethral secretions.
• After collecting the specimens, carefully dispose of gloves, swabs, and speculum to prevent staff exposure to the organism.

Normal findings
Normally, no *C. trachomatis* appears in the culture.

Abnormal findings
A positive culture confirms *C. trachomatis* infection.

Biopsy

RESPIRATORY SYSTEM

LUNG BIOPSY

In biopsy of the lung, a specimen of pulmonary tissue is excised by closed or open technique for histologic examination. Closed technique, performed under local anesthetic, includes both needle and transbronchial biopsies; open technique, performed under general anesthetic in the operating room, includes both limited and standard thoracotomies. Needle biopsy is appropriate when the lesion is readily accessible or when it originates in the lung parenchyma, is confined to it, or is affixed to the chest wall; it provides a much smaller specimen than the open technique. Transbronchial biopsy, the removal of multiple tissue specimens through a fiber-optic bronchoscope, may be used in patients with diffuse infiltrative pulmonary disease or tumors or when severe debilitation contraindicates open biopsy. Open biopsy is appropriate for the study of a well-circumscribed lesion that may require resection.

Generally, a biopsy of the lung is recommended after chest X-ray, computed tomography scan, and bronchoscopy have failed to identify the cause of diffuse parenchymal pulmonary disease or of a pulmonary lesion. Complications of lung biopsy include bleeding, infection, and pneumothorax.

Purpose
• To confirm diagnosis of diffuse parenchymal pulmonary disease and pulmonary lesions

Patient preparation
• Explain to the patient that this test is used to assess the condition of the lungs.
• Describe the procedure to the patient, and answer any questions.
• Tell the patient that a chest X-ray and blood studies (prothrombin time, activated partial thromboplastin time, and platelet count) will be performed before the biopsy.
• Tell him who will perform the biopsy and where, that the procedure takes 30 to 60 minutes, and that test results should be available in several days.
• Instruct the patient to fast after midnight before the procedure. (Sometimes the patient is permitted to have clear liquids the morning of the test.)
• Make sure the patient or an appropriate family member has signed a consent form.
• Check patient history for hypersensitivity to the local anesthetic.
• Administer a mild sedative 30 minutes before the biopsy to help the patient relax. Tell him he'll receive a local anesthetic but may experience a sharp, transient pain when the biopsy needle touches the lung.

Procedure and posttest care
• After the biopsy site is selected, lead markers are placed on the patient's skin and X-rays are ordered to verify their correct placement.
• Place the patient in a sitting position, with arms folded on a table in front of him, and instruct him to maintain this position, remaining as still as possible, and to refrain from coughing.
• Prepare the skin over the biopsy site and drape the appropriate area.
• With a 25G needle, the local anesthetic is injected just above the lower rib to prevent damage to the intercostal nerves and vessels.
• Using a 22G needle, the examiner anesthetizes the intercostal muscles and

parietal pleura, makes a small incision (2 to 3 mm) with a scalpel, and introduces the biopsy needle through the incision, chest wall, and pleura, into the tumor or the pulmonary tissue.

• When the needle is in the tumor or pulmonary tissue, the specimen is obtained and the needle is withdrawn.

• The specimen is divided immediately: The tissue for histology is placed in a properly labeled bottle containing 10% neutral buffered formaldehyde solution; the tissue for microbiology is placed in a sterile container.

• Exert pressure on the biopsy site to stop the bleeding, and apply a small bandage.

• Check vital signs every 15 minutes for 1 hour, every hour for 4 hours, then every 4 hours. Watch for bleeding, shortness of breath, elevated pulse, diminished breath sounds on the biopsy side and, eventually, cyanosis. Make sure the chest X-ray is repeated immediately after the biopsy is completed.

• Inform the patient that he may resume his normal diet.

Precautions

• Needle biopsy is contraindicated in patients with a lesion that's separated from the chest wall or that's accompanied by emphysematous bullae, cysts, or gross emphysema and in patients with coagulopathy, hypoxia, pulmonary hypertension, or cardiac disease with cor pulmonale.

• During biopsy, observe for signs of respiratory distress — shortness of breath, elevated pulse, and cyanosis (late sign) — and if they develop, report them immediately.

• Because coughing or movement during biopsy can cause tearing of the lung by the biopsy needle, keep the patient calm and still.

Normal findings

Normal pulmonary tissue shows uniform texture of the alveolar ducts, alveolar walls, bronchioles, and small vessels.

Abnormal findings

Histologic examination of a pulmonary tissue specimen can reveal squamous cell or oat cell carcinoma and adenocarcinoma and supplements the results of microbiologic cultures, deep-cough sputum specimens, chest X-rays, and bronchoscopy and the patient's physical history in confirming cancer or parenchymal pulmonary disease.

PLEURAL BIOPSY

Pleural biopsy is the removal of pleural tissue, by needle biopsy or open biopsy, for histologic examination. Needle pleural biopsy is performed under local anesthetic. It generally follows thoracentesis (aspiration of pleural fluid), which is performed when the etiology of the effusion is unknown, but it can be performed separately.

Open pleural biopsy, performed in the absence of pleural effusion, permits direct visualization of the pleura and the underlying lung. It's performed in the operating room.

Purpose

• To differentiate between nonmalignant and malignant disease

• To diagnose viral, fungal, or parasitic disease, and collagen vascular disease of the pleura

Patient preparation

• Describe the procedure to the patient and answer his questions.

• Explain that this test permits microscopic examination of pleural tissue.

• Tell him who will perform the biopsy and where, and that it takes 30 to 45 minutes to perform, although the needle remains in the pleura for less than 1 minute.

• Explain that blood studies will precede the biopsy and that chest X-rays will be taken before and after the biopsy.

• Make sure the patient or an appropriate family member has signed a consent form.

• Check patient history for hypersensitivity to the local anesthetic.

• Tell him that he'll receive an anesthetic and should experience little pain.

• Just before the procedure, record vital signs.

Procedure and posttest care

• Seat the patient on the side of the bed, with his feet resting on a stool and his arms supported by the overbed table or upper body. Tell him to hold this position and remain still during the procedure.

• Prepare the skin and drape the area.

• The local anesthetic is then administered.

• In a *Vim-Silverman needle biopsy,* a needle is inserted through the appropriate intercostal space into the biopsy site, with the outer tip distal to the pleura and the central portion pushed in deeper and held in place. In *Cope's needle* biopsy, a trocar is introduced through the appropriate intercostal space into the biopsy site. To obtain the specimen, a hooked stylet is inserted through the trocar.

• Put the specimen immediately into 10% neutral buffered formaldehyde solution in a labeled specimen bottle and send it to the laboratory immediately.

• Clean the skin around the biopsy site and apply an adhesive bandage.

• Make sure the chest X-ray is repeated immediately after the biopsy.

• Check vital signs every 15 minutes for 1 hour, then every hour for 4 hours or until stable.

• Watch for signs of respiratory distress (shortness of breath), shoulder pain, and complications, such as pneumothorax (immediate) and pneumonia (delayed).

Precautions

• Pleural biopsy is contraindicated in patients with severe bleeding disorders.

Normal findings

The normal pleura consists primarily of mesothelial cells, flattened in a uniform layer. Layers of areolar connective tissue — containing blood vessels, nerves, and lymphatics — lie below.

Abnormal findings

Histologic examination of the tissue specimen can reveal malignant disease, tuberculosis, or viral, fungal, parasitic, or collagen vascular disease. Primary neoplasms of the pleura are generally fibrous and epithelial.

GASTROINTESTINAL SYSTEM

SMALL BOWEL BIOPSY

Small bowel biopsy is used to evaluate diseases of the intestinal mucosa, which may cause malabsorption or diarrhea. It produces larger specimens than endoscopic biopsy and allows removal of tissue from areas beyond an endoscope's reach (see *Endoscopic biopsy of the GI tract*). Several similar types of capsules are available for tissue collec-

ENDOSCOPIC BIOPSY OF THE GI TRACT

Endoscopy allows direct visualization of the GI tract and any site that requires biopsy of tissue samples for histologic analysis. This relatively painless procedure helps detect, support diagnosis of, or monitor GI tract disorders. Its complications, notably hemorrhage, perforation, and aspiration, are rare.

Patient preparation

Careful patient preparation is vital for this procedure. Describe the procedure to the patient and reassure him that he will be able to breathe with the endoscope in place. Tell him to fast for at least 8 hours before the procedure. For lower GI biopsy, clean the bowel. Make sure the patient or a responsible family member has signed a consent form.

Just before the procedure, sedate the patient. He should be relaxed but not asleep because his cooperation promotes smooth passage of the endoscope. Spray the back of his throat with a local anesthetic to suppress his gag reflex. Have suction equipment and bipolar cauterizing electrodes available to prevent aspiration and excessive bleeding.

Obtaining the sample

After the endoscope is passed into the upper or lower GI tract and a lesion, node, or other abnormal area is visualized, a biopsy forceps is pushed through a channel in the endoscope until this, too, can be seen. The forceps are then opened, positioned at the biopsy site, and closed on the tissue. The closed forceps and tissue sample are removed from the endoscope, and the tissue is taken from the forceps. The specimen is placed mucosal side up on fine mesh gauze or filter paper and then placed in a labeled biopsy bottle containing fixative. When all samples have been collected, the endoscope is removed. Samples are sent to the laboratory immediately.

Endoscopic biopsy of the GI tract can be used to diagnose cancer, lymphoma, amyloidosis, candidiasis, and gastric ulcers; to support diagnosis of Crohn's disease, chronic ulcerative colitis, gastritis, esophagitis, and melanosis coli in laxative abuse; and to monitor progression of Barrett's esophagus, multiple gastric polyps, colon cancer and polyps, and chronic ulcerative colitis.

tion. In each, a mercury-weighted bag is attached to one end of the capsule; a thin polyethylene tube about 150 cm long is attached to the other end. Once the bag, capsule, and tube are in place in the small bowel, suction on the tube draws the mucosa into the capsule and closes it, cutting off the piece of tissue within. This is an invasive procedure, but it causes little pain and complications are rare.

Biopsy verifies diagnosis of some diseases, such as Whipple's disease; it may help confirm others, such as tropical sprue.

Purpose
• To help diagnose diseases of the intestinal mucosa

Patient preparation
• Explain to the patient that this test is used to identify intestinal disorders.
• Describe the procedure to the patient, and answer any questions.

• Instruct him to restrict food and fluids for at least 8 hours before the test.

• Tell him who will perform the biopsy and where and that the procedure takes 45 to 60 minutes but causes little discomfort.

• Make sure the patient or a responsible family member has signed a consent form.

• Ensure that coagulation tests have been performed and that the results are recorded on the patient's chart.

• Withhold aspirin and anticoagulants. If these drugs must be continued, note this on the laboratory slip.

Procedure and posttest care

• Check the tubing and the mercury bag for leaks.

• Lightly lubricate the tube and the capsule with a water-soluble lubricant, and moisten the mercury bag with water.

• Spray the back of the patient's throat with a local anesthetic to decrease gagging.

• Ask the patient to sit upright.

• The capsule is placed in his pharynx, and he is asked to flex his neck and swallow as the tube is advanced.

• If a local anesthetic is used to control the gag reflex, the patient must not receive any fluids to help him swallow the capsule.

• Place the patient on his right side; the tube is then advanced another 20″ (50 cm). The tube's position is checked by fluoroscopy or by instilling air through the tube and listening with a stethoscope for air to enter the stomach.

• Next, the tube is advanced 2″ to 4″ (5 to 10 cm) at a time to pass the capsule through the pylorus. (Talk to the patient about food to stimulate the pylorus and help the capsule pass.)

• When fluoroscopy confirms that the capsule has passed the pylorus, keep the patient on his right side to allow the capsule to move into the second and third portions of the small bowel.

• Tell the patient that he may hold the tube loosely to one side of his mouth if it makes him more comfortable.

• Capsule position is checked again by fluoroscopy. When the capsule is at or beyond the ligament of Treitz, the biopsy sample can be taken. (The doctor will determine the biopsy site.)

• Place the patient supine, so the capsule's position can be verified fluoroscopically.

• The specimen is gently removed with forceps, placed mucosal side up on a piece of mesh, and then placed in a biopsy bottle with required fixative.

• Send the specimen to the laboratory immediately.

• Resume the patient's diet after confirming return of the gag reflex.

• Complications are rare. However, watch for signs of hemorrhage, bacteremia with transient fever and pain, and bowel perforation. Tell the patient to report abdominal pain or bleeding.

Precautions

• Keep suction equipment nearby to prevent aspiration if the patient vomits.

• Do not allow the patient to bite the tubing.

• Handle the tissue carefully and place it correctly on the slide.

• Biopsy is contraindicated in uncooperative patients, in those taking aspirin or anticoagulants, and in those with uncontrolled coagulation disorders.

Normal findings

A normal small-bowel biopsy sample consists of fingerlike villi, crypts, columnar epithelial cells, and round cells.

Abnormal findings

Small bowel tissue that reveals histologic changes in cell structure may indicate Whipple's disease, abetalipoproteinemia, lymphoma, lymphangiectasia, eosinophilic enteritis, and such parasitic infections as giardiasis and coccidiosis. Abnormal samples may also suggest celiac sprue, tropical sprue, infectious gastroenteritis, intraluminal bacterial over-growth, folate and B_{12} deficiency, radiation enteritis, and malnutrition, but such disorders require further studies.

PERCUTANEOUS LIVER BIOPSY

Percutaneous biopsy of the liver is the needle aspiration of a core of tissue for histologic analysis. This procedure is performed under a local or general anesthetic. Findings may help to identify hepatic disorders after ultrasonography, computerized tomography, and radionuclide studies have failed to detect them. Because many patients with hepatic disorders have clotting defects, testing for hemostasis should precede liver biopsy.

Purpose
• To diagnose hepatic parenchymal disease, malignancy, and granulomatous infections

Patient preparation
• Explain to the patient that this test is used to diagnose liver disorders.
• Describe the procedure to the patient, and answer any questions.
• Instruct the patient to restrict food and fluids for 4 to 8 hours before the test.
• Tell him who will perform the biopsy and where; that the biopsy needle remains in the liver about 1 second; that the entire procedure takes about 10 to 15 minutes; and that test results are usually available in 1 day.
• Make sure the patient or an appropriate family member has signed a consent form.

• Check patient history for hypersensitivity to the local anesthetic.
• Make sure prothrombin time and platelet count tests have been performed and that the results are recorded on the patient's chart.
• Just before the biopsy, tell the patient to void; then, record vital signs.
• Inform him that he will receive a local anesthetic but may experience pain similar to that of a punch in his right shoulder as the biopsy needle passes the phrenic nerve.

Procedure and posttest care
• For aspiration biopsy using the Menghini needle, place the patient in a supine position, with his right hand under his head. Instruct him to maintain this position and remain as still as possible during the procedure.
• The liver is palpated, the biopsy site is selected and marked, and the anesthetic is then injected.
• The needle flange is set to control the depth of penetration, and 2 ml of sterile 0.9% sodium chloride solution are drawn into the syringe.
• The syringe is attached to the biopsy needle, and the needle is introduced into the subcutaneous tissue, through the right eighth or ninth intercostal space, between the anterior and posterior axillary lines.
• Next, 1 ml of 0.9% sodium chloride solution is injected to clear the needle and the plunger; then the plunger is drawn back to the 4-ml mark to create negative pressure.
• At this point in the procedure, ask the patient to take a deep breath, exhale, and hold his breath at the end of expiration to prevent any movement of the chest wall.
• As the patient holds his breath, the biopsy needle is quickly inserted into the liver and withdrawn in 1 second.
• After the needle is withdrawn, tell the patient to resume normal respirations.

• The tissue specimen is then placed in a properly labeled specimen cup containing 10% formalin solution.

• Again, 1 ml of 0.9% sodium chloride solution is injected to clear the needle of the tissue specimen.

• Apply pressure to the biopsy site to stop bleeding.

• Position the patient on his right side for 2 hours, with a small pillow or sandbag under the costal margin to provide extra pressure. Advise bed rest for 24 hours.

• Check the patient's vital signs every 15 minutes for 1 hour, then every 30 minutes for 4 hours, and every 4 hours thereafter for 24 hours. Throughout, observe carefully for signs of shock.

• Immediately report bleeding or signs of bile peritonitis: tenderness and rigidity around the biopsy site.

• Be alert for symptoms of pneumothorax: rising respiration rate, depressed breath sounds, dyspnea, persistent shoulder pain, and pleuritic chest pain. Report such complications promptly.

• If the patient experiences pain, which may persist for several hours after the test, administer an analgesic.

• Inform the patient that he may resume his normal diet.

Precautions

• Percutaneous liver biopsy is contraindicated in a patient with a platelet count below 100,000/mm^3; prothrombin time longer than 15 seconds; empyema of the lungs, pleurae, peritoneum, biliary tract, or liver; vascular tumor; hepatic angiomas; hydatid cyst; or tense ascites. If extrahepatic obstruction is suspected, ultrasonography or subcutaneous transhepatic cholangiography should rule out this condition before the biopsy is considered.

• Send the specimen to the laboratory immediately.

Normal findings

The normal liver consists of sheets of hepatocytes supported by a reticulin framework.

Abnormal findings

Examination of the hepatic tissue may reveal diffuse hepatic disease, such as cirrhosis or hepatitis, or granulomatous infections, such as tuberculosis. Primary malignant tumors include hepatocellular carcinoma, cholangiocellular carcinoma, and angiosarcoma, but hepatic metastasis is more common.

Nonmalignant findings with a known focal lesion require further studies, such as laparotomy or laparoscopy with biopsy.

REPRODUCTIVE SYSTEM

BREAST BIOPSY

Histologic examination of breast tissue obtained by biopsy can confirm or rule out cancer after mammography, thermography, and X-rays of breast masses. Needle biopsy or fine needle biopsy provides a core of tissue or a fluid aspirate, but should be restricted to fluid-filled cysts and advanced malignant lesions. Both methods have limited diagnostic value because of the small and perhaps unrepresentative specimens they provide. Open biopsy provides a complete tissue specimen, which can be sectioned to allow more accurate evaluation. All three techniques require only a local anesthetic and can often be performed on outpatients; however, open biopsy may require a general anesthetic if the patient is fearful or uncooperative.

Breast biopsy is indicated in patients with palpable masses, suspicious areas in mammography, or persistently encrusted, inflamed, or eczematoid breast lesions or bloody discharge from the nipples. Tissue analysis often includes an estrogen and progesterone receptor assay to help select therapy if the mass proves malignant.

Purpose
• To differentiate between benign and malignant breast tumors

Patient preparation
• Obtain a complete medical history, including when the patient first noticed the lesion, the presence or absence of pain, a change in the lesion's size, association with the patient's menstrual cycle, nipple discharge, and nipple or skin changes, such as the characteristic "orange-peel" skin that may indicate an underlying inflammatory carcinoma.
• Describe the procedure to the patient, and explain that this test permits microscopic examination of a breast tissue specimen. Offer her emotional support, and assure her that breast masses do not always indicate cancer.
• If the patient is to receive a local anesthetic, tell her that it is not necessary to restrict food, fluids, or medication prior to the biopsy.
• If she's to receive a general anesthetic, advise her to fast from midnight before the test until after the biopsy.
• Tell her who will perform the biopsy and where; that it will take 15 to 30 minutes; and that pretest studies, such as blood tests, urine tests, and chest X-rays, may be required.
• Make sure the patient or an appropriate family member has signed a consent form.
• Check patient history for hypersensitivity to anesthetics.

Procedure and posttest care
• *Needle biopsy:* Instruct the patient to undress to the waist; place her in a sitting or recumbent position, with her hands at her sides; and tell her to remain still. The biopsy site is prepared, a local anesthetic is administered, and the syringe (luer-lock syringe for aspiration, Vim-Silverman needle for tissue specimen) is introduced into the lesion. Fluid aspirated from the breast is expelled into a properly labeled, heparinized tube; the tissue specimen is placed in a labeled specimen bottle containing 0.9% sodium chloride solution or formaldehyde. (With fine needle aspiration, a slide is made for cytology and viewed immediately under a microscope.) Pressure is exerted on the biopsy site and, after bleeding stops, an adhesive bandage is applied. Because breast fluid aspiration is not diagnostically accurate, some doctors aspirate fluid only from cysts. If such fluid is clear yellow and the mass disappears, the aspiration procedure is both diagnostic and therapeutic, and the aspirate is discarded. If aspiration yields no fluid, or if the lesion recurs two or three times, an open biopsy is then ordered.
• *Open biopsy:* After the patient receives a general or local anesthetic, an incision is made in the breast to expose the mass. The examiner may then *incise* a portion of tissue or *excise* the entire mass. If the mass is smaller than ¾″ (2 cm) and appears benign, it is usually excised; if it is larger or appears malignant, a specimen is usually incised before the mass is excised. The specimen is placed in a properly labeled specimen bottle containing 10% formaldehyde solution. Tissue that appears malignant is sent for frozen section and receptor assays. (Receptor assay specimens must not be placed in formaldehyde.) The wound is sutured, and an adhesive bandage is applied.

• If the patient has received a local anesthetic during needle or open biopsy, check vital signs, and provide medication for pain. Watch for and report bleeding, tenderness, or redness at the biopsy site.

• If the patient has received a general anesthetic, check vital signs every 30 minutes for the first 4 hours, every hour for the next 4 hours, and then every 4 hours. Administer an analgesic. Watch for and report bleeding, tenderness, or redness at the biopsy site.

• Provide emotional support to the patient who is awaiting diagnosis. If the biopsy confirms cancer, the patient will require follow-up tests, including radiographic tests, blood studies, bone scans, and urinalysis, to determine appropriate treatment.

Precautions

• Open breast biopsy is contraindicated in patients with conditions that preclude surgery.

• Send the specimen to the laboratory immediately.

Normal findings

Normally, breast tissue consists of cellular and noncellular connective tissue, fat lobules, and various lactiferous ducts. It's pink, more fatty than fibrous, and shows no abnormal development of cells or tissue elements.

Abnormal findings

Abnormal breast tissue may exhibit a wide range of malignant or benign pathology. Breast tumors are common in women and account for 32% of female cancers; such tumors are rare in men (0.2% of male cancers). Benign tumors include fibrocystic disease, adenofibroma, intraductal papilloma, mammary fat necrosis, and plasma cell mastitis (mammary duct ectasia). Malignant tumors include adenocarcinoma, cystosarcoma, intraductal carcinoma, infiltrating carcinoma, inflammatory carcinoma, medullary or circumscribed carcinoma, colloid carcinoma, lobular carcinoma, sarcoma, and Paget's disease.

PROSTATE GLAND BIOPSY

Prostate gland biopsy is the needle excision of a prostate tissue specimen for histologic examination. A perineal, transrectal, or transurethral approach may be used; the transrectal approach is usually used for high prostatic lesions. Indications include potentially malignant prostatic hypertrophy and prostatic nodules.

Purpose

• To confirm prostatic cancer
• To determine the cause of prostatic hyperplasia

Patient preparation

• Describe the procedure to the patient, answer his questions, and tell him the test provides a tissue specimen for microscopic study.

• Tell him who will perform the biopsy and where, that he'll receive a local anesthetic, and that the procedure takes less than 30 minutes.

• Make sure the patient or an appropriate family member has signed a consent form.

• Check patient history for hypersensitivity to the anesthetic or to other drugs.

• For a transrectal approach, administer enemas until the return is clear and administer an antibacterial agent to minimize the risk of infection.

• Just before the biopsy, check vital signs and administer a sedative.

• Tell the patient to remain still during the procedure and to follow instructions.

Procedure and posttest care

• *Perineal approach:* Place the patient in the proper position (left lateral, knee-chest, or lithotomy), and clean the perineal skin. After the local anesthetic is administered, a 2-mm incision may be made into the perineum. The examiner immobilizes the prostate by inserting a finger into the rectum, and introduces the biopsy needle into a prostate lobe. The needle is rotated gently, pulled out about 5 mm, and reinserted at another angle. The procedure is repeated at several areas. Specimens are placed immediately in a labeled specimen bottle containing 10% formaldehyde solution. Pressure is exerted on the puncture site, which is then bandaged.

• *Transrectal approach:* This approach may be performed on outpatients without an anesthetic. Place the patient in a left lateral position. A curved needle guide is attached to the finger palpating the rectum. The biopsy needle is pushed along the guide, into the prostate. As the needle enters the prostate, the patient may experience pain. The needle is rotated to cut off the tissue and then is withdrawn. The specimen is placed immediately in a labeled specimen bottle containing 10% formaldehyde solution.

• *Transurethral approach:* An endoscopic instrument is passed through the urethra, permitting direct viewing of the prostate and passage of a cutting loop. The loop is rotated to obtain tissue and is then withdrawn. The specimen is placed immediately in a labeled specimen bottle containing 10% formaldehyde solution.

• Check vital signs immediately after the procedure, every 2 hours for 4 hours, and then every 4 hours.

• Observe the biopsy site for a hematoma and for signs of infection, such as redness, swelling, and pain. Watch for urinary retention or frequency and for hematuria.

Precautions

• Complications may include transient, painless hematuria and bleeding into the prostatic urethra and bladder.

Normal findings

Normally, the prostate gland consists of a thin, fibrous capsule surrounding the stroma, which is made up of elastic and connective tissues and smooth-muscle fibers. The epithelial glands, found in these tissues and muscle fibers, drain into the chief excreting ducts.

Abnormal findings

Histologic examination can confirm cancer. Further tests—bone scans, bone marrow biopsy, tests for prostate-specific antigen, and serum acid phosphatase and prostatic acid phosphatase determinations—identify the extent of the cancer. Acid phosphatase levels usually rise in metastatic prostatic carcinoma; they tend to be low in carcinoma that is confined to the prostatic capsule. In the latter case, radical surgery and irradiation, although controversial, can provide a high cure rate. If discovery of cancer is delayed, treatment necessitates estrogen therapy, as growth of the tumor depends on secretion of testosterone.

Histologic examination can also be used to detect benign prostatic hyperplasia, prostatitis, tuberculosis, lymphomas, and rectal or bladder carcinomas.

CERVICAL PUNCH BIOPSY

Cervical punch biopsy is the excision by sharp forceps of a tissue specimen from the cervix for histologic examination. Generally, multiple biopsies are done to obtain specimens from all areas with abnormal tissue or from the squamocolumnar junction and other sites around the cervical circumference. This procedure is indicated in women with suspicious cervical lesions and should be performed when the cervix is least vascular (usually 1 week after menses). Biopsy sites are selected by direct visualization of the cervix with a colposcope — the most accurate method — or by Schiller's test, which stains normal squamous epithelium a dark mahogany but fails to color abnormal tissue.

Purpose
• To evaluate suspicious cervical lesions
• To diagnose cervical cancer

Patient preparation
• Describe the procedure to the patient, and explain that it provides a cervical tissue specimen for microscopic study.
• Tell her who will perform the biopsy and where, that the procedure takes about 15 minutes, and that she may experience mild discomfort during and after the biopsy.
• Advise the outpatient to have someone accompany her home after the biopsy.
• Make sure the patient or a responsible family member has signed a consent form.
• Just before the biopsy, ask the patient to void.

Procedure and posttest care
• Place the patient in the lithotomy position, and tell her to relax as the unlubricated speculum is inserted.
• For *direct visualization,* the colposcope is inserted through the speculum, the biopsy site is located, and the cervix is cleaned with a swab soaked in

3% acetic acid solution. The biopsy forceps are then inserted through the speculum or the colposcope, and tissue is removed from any lesion or from selected sites, starting from the posterior lip to avoid obscuring other sites with blood. Each specimen is immediately put in 10% formaldehyde solution in a labeled bottle. To control bleeding after biopsy, the cervix is swabbed with 5% silver nitrate solution (cautery or sutures may be used instead). If bleeding persists, the examiner may insert a tampon.
• For *Schiller's test,* an applicator stick saturated with iodine solution is inserted through the speculum. This stains the cervix to identify lesions for biopsy.
• Record the patient's and doctor's names and biopsy sites on the laboratory slip.
• Instruct the patient to avoid strenuous exercise for 8 to 24 hours after the biopsy. Encourage the outpatient to rest briefly before leaving the office.
• If a tampon was inserted after the biopsy, tell the patient to leave it in place for 8 to 24 hours. Inform her that some bleeding may occur, but tell her to report heavy bleeding (heavier than menstrual). Warn the patient to avoid using tampons, which can irritate the cervix and provoke bleeding.
• Tell the patient to avoid douching and intercourse for 2 weeks, or as directed.
• Inform the patient that a foul-smelling, gray-green vaginal discharge is normal for several days after biopsy and may persist for 3 weeks.

Precautions
• Send the specimens to the laboratory immediately.

Normal findings
Normal cervical tissue is composed of columnar and squamous epithelial cells, loose connective tissue, and smooth-muscle fibers, with no dysplasia or abnormal cell growth.

Abnormal findings

Histologic examination of a cervical tissue specimen is used to identify abnormal cells and to differentiate the tissue as intraepithelial neoplasia or invasive cancer. If the cause of an abnormal Papanicolaou test is not demonstrated by cervical biopsy or if the specimen shows advanced dysplasia or carcinoma in situ, a cone biopsy is performed under general anesthetic to obtain a larger tissue specimen and allow a more accurate evaluation of dysplasia.

SKELETAL SYSTEM

BONE BIOPSY

Bone biopsy is the removal of a piece or a core of bone for histologic examination. It's performed either by using a special drill needle under local anesthetic or by surgical excision under general anesthetic.

Bone biopsy is indicated in patients with bone pain and tenderness after bone scan, computed tomography scan, X-ray, or arteriography reveals a mass or deformity. Excision provides a larger specimen than drill biopsy and permits immediate surgical treatment if quick histologic analysis of the specimen reveals malignancy.

Possible complications include bone fracture, damage to surrounding tissue, and infection (osteomyelitis).

Purpose

• To distinguish between benign and malignant bone tumors

Patient preparation

• Describe the procedure to the patient, and answer any questions.
• Explain that this test permits microscopic examination of a bone specimen.
• If the patient is to have a drill biopsy, he need not restrict food or fluids; if he is to have open biopsy, he must fast overnight before the test.
• Tell him who will perform the biopsy and where and that the procedure should take no longer than 30 minutes.
• Tell the patient that he will receive a local anesthetic but will still experience discomfort and pressure when the biopsy needle enters the bone.
• Explain that a special drill forces the needle into the bone; if possible, show him a photograph of the bone drill. Stress the importance of his cooperation during the biopsy.
• Make sure the patient or a responsible family member has signed a consent form.
• Check patient history for hypersensitivity to the local anesthetic.

Procedure and posttest care

• For *drill biopsy,* the patient is properly positioned, and the biopsy site is shaved and meticulously prepared. After the local anesthetic is injected, a small incision (usually about 3 mm) is made and the biopsy needle is pushed with pointed trocar into the bone; then it's rotated about 180 degrees. When the bone core is obtained, the trocar is withdrawn, and the specimen is placed in a properly labeled bottle containing 10% formaldehyde solution. Apply pressure to the site with a sterile gauze pad. When bleeding stops, apply a topical antiseptic (povidone-iodine ointment) and an adhesive bandage or other sterile covering to close the wound and prevent infection.
• For *open biopsy,* the patient is anesthetized, and the biopsy site is prepared: The area is shaved, cleaned with surgi-

cal soap, and disinfected with an iodine wash and alcohol. An incision is made, and a piece of bone is removed and sent to the histology laboratory immediately for analysis. Further surgery can then be performed, depending on findings.

• Check vital signs and the dressing at the biopsy site. Determine how much drainage is expected and report excessive drainage.

• If the patient experiences pain, administer an analgesic.

• For several days after biopsy, watch for and report indications of bone infection: fever, headache, pain on movement, and redness or abscess near the biopsy site.

• Advise the patient that he may resume his usual diet.

Precautions
• Bone biopsy should be performed cautiously in patients with coagulopathy.

Normal findings
Normal bone tissue consists of fibers of collagen, osteocytes, and osteoblasts. It may be compact or cancellous. Compact bone has dense, concentric layers of mineral deposits, or lamellae. Cancellous bone has widely spaced lamellae, with osteocytes and red and yellow marrow between them.

Abnormal findings
Histologic examination of a bone specimen can reveal benign or malignant tumors. Benign tumors, generally well-circumscribed and nonmetastasizing, include osteoid osteoma, osteoblastoma, osteochondroma, unicameral bone cyst, benign giant-cell tumor, and fibroma. Malignant tumors, which spread irregularly and rapidly, most commonly include both multiple myeloma and osteosarcoma; the most lethal is Ewing's sarcoma. Most malignant tumors spread to bone through the blood and lymph systems from the breast, lungs, prostate, thyroid, or kidneys.

BONE MARROW ASPIRATION AND BIOPSY

The histologic and hematologic examination of bone marrow provides reliable diagnostic information about blood disorders. Marrow may be removed by aspiration or needle biopsy under local anesthetic. In aspiration biopsy, a fluid specimen in which pustulae of marrow are suspended is removed from the bone marrow. In needle biopsy, a core of marrow cells (not fluid) is removed. These methods are often used concurrently to obtain the best possible marrow specimens. Red marrow, which constitutes about 50% of an adult's marrow, actively produces red blood cells; yellow marrow contains fat cells and connective tissue and is inactive, but it can become active in response to the body's needs.

Bleeding and infection may result from bone marrow biopsy at any site, but the most serious complications occur at the sternum. Such complications are rare but include puncture of the heart and major vessels — causing severe hemorrhage — and puncture of the mediastinum — causing mediastinitis or pneumomediastinum.

Purpose
• To diagnose thrombocytopenia, leukemias, granulomas, and aplastic, hypoplastic, and pernicious anemias
• To diagnose primary and metastatic tumors
• To determine the cause of infection

• To aid staging of disease, such as Hodgkin's disease

• To evaluate the effectiveness of chemotherapy and monitor myelosuppression

Patient preparation

• Explain to the patient that the test permits microscopic examination of a bone marrow specimen.

• Describe the procedure to the patient, and answer any questions.

• Inform the patient that he need not restrict food or fluids before the test.

• Tell him who will perform the biopsy and where, that it usually takes only 5 to 10 minutes, and that test results are generally available in 1 day.

• Inform him that more than one bone marrow specimen may be required and that a blood sample will be collected before biopsy for laboratory testing.

• Make sure the patient or a responsible family member has signed a consent form.

• Check patient history for hypersensitivity to the local anesthetic.

• Tell the patient which bone — the sternum, anterior or posterior iliac crest, vertebral spinous process, rib, or tibia — will be the biopsy site.

• Inform him that he will receive a local anesthetic but will feel pressure on insertion of the biopsy needle and a brief, pulling pain on removal of the marrow. Administer a mild sedative 1 hour before the test.

Procedure and posttest care

• After positioning the patient, instruct him to remain as still as possible.

• Offer emotional support during the biopsy by talking quietly to the patient, describing what is being done and answering any questions.

• *For aspiration biopsy:* After the skin over the biopsy site is prepared and the area is draped, the local anesthetic is injected. With a twisting motion, the mar-

row aspiration needle is inserted through the skin, the subcutaneous tissue, and the cortex of the bone. The stylet is removed from the needle, and a 10- to 20-ml syringe is attached. The examiner aspirates 0.2 to 0.5 ml of marrow, then withdraws the needle. Apply pressure to the site for 5 minutes, while the marrow slides are being prepared. (If the patient has thrombocytopenia, apply pressure to the site for 10 to 15 minutes.) The biopsy site is cleaned again, and a sterile adhesive bandage is applied.

• If an adequate marrow specimen has not been obtained on the first attempt, the needle may be repositioned within the marrow cavity or may be removed and reinserted in another site within the anesthetized area. If the second attempt fails, a needle biopsy may be necessary.

• *For needle biopsy:* After preparing the biopsy site and draping the area, the examiner marks the skin at the site with an indelible pencil or marking pen. A local anesthetic is then injected intradermally, subcutaneously, and at the surface of the bone. Then the biopsy needle is inserted into the periosteum, and the needle guard is set, as indicated. The needle is advanced with a steady boring motion until the outer needle passes through the cortex of the bone. The inner needle with trephine tip is inserted into the outer needle. By alternately rotating the inner needle clockwise and counterclockwise, the examiner directs the needle into the marrow cavity and then removes a tissue plug. The needle assembly is withdrawn, and the marrow is expelled into a labeled bottle containing Zenker's acetic acid solution. After the biopsy site is cleaned, a sterile adhesive bandage or a pressure dressing is applied.

• Check the biopsy site for bleeding and inflammation.

• Observe the patient for signs of hemorrhage and infection, such as rapid pulse rate, low blood pressure, and fever.

Precautions
• Bone marrow biopsy is contraindicated in patients with severe bleeding disorders.
• Send the tissue specimen or slides to the laboratory immediately.

Normal findings
Yellow marrow contains fat cells and connective tissue; red marrow contains hematopoietic cells, fat cells, and connective tissue. An adult has a large hematopoietic capacity. An infant's marrow is mainly red, reflecting a small hematopoietic capacity.

In addition, special stains that are used to detect hematologic disorders produce these normal findings: The iron stain, which is used to measure hemosiderin (storage iron), has a +2 level; the Sudan black B (SBB) fat stain, which shows granulocytes, is negative; and the periodic acid-Schiff (PAS) stain, which is used to detect glycogen reactions, is negative.

Abnormal findings
Histologic examination of a bone marrow specimen can be used to detect myelofibrosis, granulomas, lymphoma, or cancer. Hematologic analysis, including the differential count and myeloiderythroid ratio, can implicate a wide range of disorders. (See *Bone marrow: Normal values and implications of abnormal findings.*)

In an iron stain, decreased hemosiderin levels may indicate a true iron deficiency. Increased levels may accompany other types of anemias or blood disorders. A positive SBB stain can differentiate acute granulocytic leukemia from acute lymphocytic leukemia (SBB negative) or may indicate granulation in myeloblasts. A positive PAS stain may indicate acute or chronic lymphocytic leukemia, amyloido-

sis, thalassemia, lymphomas, infectious mononucleosis, iron-deficiency anemia, or sideroblastic anemia.

SYNOVIAL MEMBRANE BIOPSY

Biopsy of the synovial membrane is needle excision of a tissue specimen for histologic examination of the thin epithelium lining the diarthrodial joint capsules. In a large joint, such as the knee, preliminary arthroscopy can aid selection of the biopsy site. Synovial membrane biopsy is performed when analysis of synovial fluid — a viscous, lubricating fluid contained within the synovial membrane — proves nondiagnostic or when the fluid is absent.

Purpose
• To diagnose gout, pseudogout, bacterial infections and lesions, and granulomatous infections
• To aid diagnosis of systemic lupus erythematosus (SLE), rheumatoid arthritis, or Reiter's disease and to monitor joint pathology

Patient preparation
• Explain to the patient that this test provides a tissue specimen from the membrane that lines the affected joint.
• Describe the procedure to the patient, and ask if he has any questions.
• Advise him he need not restrict food or fluids.
• Tell him who will perform the procedure and where, and that he'll receive a local anesthetic to minimize discomfort but will experience transient pain when the needle enters the joint.
• Advise him that the procedure takes about 30 minutes and that test results are usually available in 1 or 2 days.

BONE MARROW: NORMAL VALUES AND IMPLICATIONS OF ABNORMAL FINDINGS

CELL TYPES	NORMAL MEAN VALUES			CLINICAL IMPLICATIONS
	Adults	**Children**	**Infants**	
Normoblasts, total	25.6%	23.1%	8.0%	*Elevated values:* polycythemia vera
Pronormoblasts	0.2% to 1.3%	0.5%	0.1%	*Depressed values:* vitamin B_{12} or folic acid deficiency; hypoplastic or aplastic anemia
Basophilic	0.5% to 2.4%	1.7%	0.34%	
Polychromatic	17.9% to 29.2%	18.2%	6.9%	
Orthochromatic	0.4% to 4.6%	2.7%	0.54%	
Neutrophils, total	56.5%	57.1%	32.4%	*Elevated values:* acute myeloblastic or chronic myeloid leukemia
Myeloblasts	0.2% to 1.5%	1.2%	0.62%	*Depressed values:* lymphoblastic, lymphatic, or monocytic leukemia; aplastic anemia
Promyelocytes	2.1% to 4.1%	1.4%	0.76%	
Myelocytes	8.2% to 15.7%	18.3%	2.5%	
Metamyelocytes	9.6% to 24.6%	23.3%	11.3%	
Bands	9.5% to 15.3%	0	14.1%	
Segmented	6.0% to 12.0%	12.9%	3.6%	
Eosinophils	3.1%	3.6%	2.6%	*Elevated values:* bone marrow carcinoma, lymphadenoma, myeloid leukemia, eosinophilic leukemia, pernicious anemia (in relapse)
Plasma cells	1.3%	0.4%	0.02%	*Elevated values:* myeloma, collagen disease, infection, antigen sensitivity, malignancy

(continued)

BONE MARROW: NORMAL VALUES AND IMPLICATIONS OF ABNORMAL FINDINGS *(continued)*

CELL TYPES	NORMAL MEAN VALUES			CLINICAL IMPLICATIONS
	Adults	**Children**	**Infants**	
Basophils	0.01%	0.06%	0.07%	*Elevated values:* no relationship between basophil count and symptoms
				Depressed values: no relationship between basophil count and symptoms
Lymphocytes	16.2%	16.0%	49.0%	*Elevated values:* B- and T-cell chronic lymphocytic leukemia, other lymphatic leukemias, lymphoma, mononucleosis, aplastic anemia, macroglobulinemia
Megakaryocytes	0.1%	0.1%	0.05%	*Elevated values:* old age, chronic myeloid leukemia, polycythemia vera, megakaryocytic myelosis, infection, autoimmune thrombocytopenic purpura, thrombocytopenia
				Depressed values: pernicious anemia
Myeloid: Erythroid ratio	2.3	2.9	4.4	*Elevated values:* myeloid leukemia, infection, leukemoid reactions, depressed hematopoiesis
				Depressed values: agranulocytosis; hematopoiesis after hemorrhage or hemolysis, iron deficiency anemia, polycythemia vera

- Inform the patient that complications include infection and bleeding into the joint, but these are rare.
- Make sure the patient or an appropriate family member has signed a consent form.
- Check patient history for hypersensitivity to the local anesthetic.
- Inform the patient which site — knee (most common), elbow, wrist, ankle, or shoulder — has been chosen for this biopsy (usually, the most symptomatic joint is selected).
- Administer a sedative to help him relax.

Procedure and posttest care
- Place the patient in the proper position, clean the biopsy site, and drape the area.
- The local anesthetic is injected into the joint space; then, the trocar is forcefully thrust into the joint space.
- The biopsy needle is inserted through the trocar. The hooked notch side of the biopsy needle is positioned against the synovium, and suction is applied with a 50-ml luer-lock syringe.
- While the trocar is held stationary, the biopsy needle is twisted to cut off a tissue segment.
- The biopsy needle is withdrawn, and the specimen is placed in a properly labeled sterile container or a specimen bottle containing absolute ethyl alcohol, as indicated.
- By changing the angle of the biopsy needle, several specimens can be obtained without reinserting the trocar.
- The trocar is then removed, the biopsy site cleaned, and a pressure bandage is applied.
- Watch for signs of bleeding into the joint (swelling and tenderness) every hour for 4 hours, then every 4 hours for 12 hours.
- Administer medication if the patient experiences pain.

- Tell the patient to rest the joint for 1 day before resuming normal activity.

Precautions
- Send a specimen in a container with absolute ethyl alcohol to the histology laboratory immediately or send one in a sterile container to the microbiology laboratory.

Normal findings
The synovial membrane contains cells that are identical to those found in other connective tissue. The membrane surface is relatively smooth, except for villi, folds, and fat pads that project into the joint cavity. The membrane tissue produces synovial fluid and contains a capillary network, lymphatic vessels, and a few nerve fibers. Pathology of the synovial membrane also affects the cellular composition of the synovial fluid.

Abnormal findings
Histologic examination of synovial tissue can diagnose coccidioidomycosis, gout, pseudogout, hemochromatosis, tuberculosis, sarcoidosis, amyloidosis, pigmented villonodular synovitis, synovial tumors, or synovial malignancy (rare). Such examination can also aid diagnosis of rheumatoid arthritis, SLE, and Reiter's disease.

MISCELLANEOUS TESTS

THYROID BIOPSY

Thyroid biopsy is the excision of a thyroid tissue specimen for histologic examination. This procedure is indicated in patients with thyroid enlargement or nodules, breathing and swallowing difficulties, vocal cord paralysis, weight loss, hemoptysis, and a sensation of fullness in the neck. It's commonly performed when noninvasive tests, such as thyroid ultrasonography and scans, are abnormal or inconclusive. Coagulation studies should always precede thyroid biopsy.

Thyroid tissue may be obtained with a hollow needle under local anesthetic or during open (surgical) biopsy under general anesthetic. Open biopsy provides more information than needle biopsy; it also permits direct examination and immediate excision of suspicious tissue.

Purpose
• To differentiate between benign and malignant thyroid disease
• To help diagnose Hashimoto's thyroiditis, subacute granulomatous thyroiditis, hyperthyroidism, and nontoxic nodular goiter

Patient preparation
• Describe the procedure to the patient, and answer any questions.
• Explain that this test permits microscopic examination of a thyroid tissue specimen.
• Inform the patient that he need not restrict food or fluids (unless he'll receive a general anesthetic).
• Tell him who will perform the biopsy and where, that it takes 15 to 30 minutes, and that results should be available in 1 day.
• Make sure the patient or an appropriate family member has signed a consent form.
• Check for hypersensitivity to anesthetics or analgesics.
• Tell the patient he'll receive a local anesthetic to minimize pain during the procedure, but he may experience some pressure when the specimen is procured.
• Advise him that he may have a sore throat the day after the test.
• Administer a sedative to the patient 15 minutes before biopsy.

Procedure and posttest care
• For needle biopsy, place the patient in a supine position, with a pillow under his shoulder blades. (This position pushes the trachea and thyroid forward and allows the neck veins to fall backward.)
• Prepare the skin over the biopsy site.
• As the examiner prepares to inject the local anesthetic, warn the patient not to swallow.
• After the anesthetic is injected, the carotid artery is palpated, and the biopsy needle is inserted parallel to the thyroid cartilage to prevent damage to the deep structures and the larynx.
• When the specimen is obtained, the needle is removed and the specimen is placed immediately in formaldehyde.
• Apply pressure to the biopsy site to stop bleeding. If bleeding continues for more than a few minutes, press on the site for up to an additional 15 minutes. Apply an adhesive bandage. (Bleeding may persist in a patient with abnormal prothrombin time [PT] or abnormal activated partial thromboplastin time [APTT] or in a patient with a large vascular thyroid, with distended veins.)
• To make the patient more comfortable, place him in semi-Fowler's position; tell him to avoid straining the biopsy site by putting both hands behind his neck when he sits up.
• Watch for tenderness or redness, and report signs of bleeding at the biopsy site. Check the back of the neck and the patient's pillow for bleeding every hour for 8 hours. Observe for difficult breathing due to edema or hematoma, with resultant tracheal collapse.
• Keep the biopsy site clean and dry.

Precautions
• Thyroid biopsy should be used cautiously in patients with coagulation defects: abnormal PT or APTT.
• The specimen must be placed immediately in formaldehyde solution because cell breakdown in the tissue specimen begins immediately after excision.

Normal findings
Histologic examination of normal tissue shows fibrous networks dividing the gland into pseudolobules that comprise follicles and capillaries. Cuboidal epithelium lines the follicle walls and contains the protein thyroglobulin, which stores T_4 and T_3.

Abnormal findings
Malignant tumors appear as well-encapsulated, solitary nodules of uniform but abnormal structure. Papillary carcinoma is the most common thyroid malignancy. Follicular carcinoma, a less common form, strongly resembles normal cells.

Benign tumors — such as nontoxic nodular goiter — demonstrate hypertrophy, hyperplasia, and hypervascularity. Distinct histologic patterns characterize subacute granulomatous thyroiditis, Hashimoto's thyroiditis, and hyperthyroidism.

Because thyroid malignancies are frequently multicentric and small, a negative histologic report does not rule out malignancy.

LYMPH NODE BIOPSY

Lymph node biopsy is the surgical excision of an active lymph node or the needle aspiration of a nodal specimen for histologic examination. Both techniques usually employ a local anesthetic and sample the superficial nodes in the cervical, supraclavicular, axillary, or inguinal region. Excision is preferred as it yields a larger specimen.

Lymph nodes swell during infection, but when nodal enlargement is prolonged and is accompanied by backache, leg edema, breathing and swallowing difficulties and, later, weight loss, weakness, severe itching, fever, night sweats, cough, hemoptysis, or hoarseness, biopsy is indicated. Generalized or localized lymph node enlargement is typical of diseases such as chronic lymphatic leukemia, Hodgkin's disease, infectious mononucleosis, and rheumatoid arthritis.

Complete blood count, liver function studies, liver and spleen scans, and X-rays should precede this test.

Purpose
• To determine the cause of lymph node enlargement
• To distinguish between benign and malignant lymph node tumors
• To stage metastatic carcinoma

Patient preparation
• Explain to the patient that this test allows microscopic study of lymph node tissue.
• Describe the procedure to the patient, and ask if he has any questions.
• For excisional biopsy, instruct the patient to restrict food from midnight and to drink only clear liquids on the morning of the test (if general anesthetic is needed for deeper nodes, he must also restrict fluids).
• For needle biopsy, inform him he need not restrict food or fluids. Tell him who will perform the biopsy and where, that the procedure takes 15 to 30 minutes, and that the analysis takes 1 day to complete.
• Make sure the patient or a responsible family member has signed a consent form.

• Check patient history for hypersensitivity to the anesthetic.

• If the patient will receive a local anesthetic, explain that he may experience discomfort during injection.

• Just before the biopsy, record baseline vital signs.

Procedure and posttest care

• *Excisional biopsy:* Prepare the skin over the biopsy site, and drape the area. The anesthetic is then administered. The examiner makes an incision, removes an entire node, and places it in a properly labeled bottle containing 0.9% sodium chloride solution. The wound is sutured and dressed.

• *Needle biopsy:* After preparing the biopsy site and administering a local anesthetic, the examiner grasps the node between his thumb and forefinger, inserts the needle directly into the node, and obtains a small core specimen. The needle is removed, and the specimen is placed in a properly labeled bottle containing 0.9% sodium chloride solution. Pressure is exerted to control bleeding, and an adhesive bandage is applied.

• Check vital signs, and watch for bleeding, tenderness, and redness.

• Inform the patient that he may resume his usual diet.

Precautions

• Storing the tissue specimen in 0.9% sodium chloride solution instead of in 10% formaldehyde solution allows part of the specimen to be used for cytologic impression smears, which are studied along with the biopsy specimen.

Normal findings

The normal lymph node is encapsulated by collagenous connective tissue and is divided into smaller lobes by tissue strands called *trabeculae.* It has an outer *cortex,* comprised of lymphoid cells and nodules or follicles containing lymphocytes, and an inner *medulla,* comprised of reticular phagocytic cells that collect and drain fluid.

Abnormal findings

Histologic examination of the tissue specimen distinguishes between malignant and nonmalignant causes of lymph node enlargement. Lymphatic malignancy accounts for up to 5% of all cancers and is slightly more prevalent in males than in females. Hodgkin's disease, a lymphoma affecting the entire lymph system, is the leading cancer affecting adolescents and young adults. Lymph node malignancy may also result from metastasizing carcinoma.

When histologic results are not clear or nodular material is not involved, mediastinoscopy or laparotomy can provide another nodal specimen. Occasionally, lymphangiography can furnish additional diagnostic information.

SKIN BIOPSY

Skin biopsy is the removal of a small piece of tissue, under local anesthetic, from a lesion suspected of malignancy or other dermatoses. One of three techniques may be used: shave biopsy, punch biopsy, or excision biopsy. Shave biopsy cuts the lesion above the skin line, which allows further biopsy at the site. Punch biopsy removes an oval core from the center of a lesion. Excision biopsy removes the entire lesion and is indicated for rapidly expanding lesions; for sclerotic, bullous, or atrophic lesions; and for examination of the border of a lesion and surrounding normal skin.

Lesions suspected of malignancy usually have changed color, size, or appearance or fail to heal properly after injury. Fully developed lesions should be selected for biopsy whenever possible because they provide more diagnostic information than lesions that are resolving or in early developing stages. For example, if the skin shows blisters, biopsy should include the most mature ones.

Purpose
• To provide differential diagnosis among basal cell carcinoma, squamous cell carcinoma, malignant melanoma, and benign growths
• To diagnose chronic bacterial or fungal skin infections

Patient preparation
• Explain to the patient that the biopsy provides a sample of skin for microscopic study.
• Describe the procedure to the patient, and answer any questions.
• Inform him that he need not restrict food or fluids.
• Tell him who will perform the procedure and where, that he'll receive a local anesthetic to minimize pain, that the biopsy takes about 15 minutes, and that test results are usually available in 1 day.
• Have the patient or an appropriate family member sign a consent form.
• Check patient history for hypersensitivity to the local anesthetic.

Procedure and posttest care
• Position the patient comfortably, and clean the biopsy site before the local anesthetic is administered.
• *Shave biopsy:* The protruding growth is cut off at the skin line with a #15 scalpel. The tissue is placed immediately in a properly labeled specimen bottle containing 10% formaldehyde solution. Apply pressure to the area to stop the bleeding.
• *Punch biopsy:* The skin surrounding the lesion is pulled taut, and the punch is firmly introduced into the lesion and is rotated to obtain a tissue specimen.

The plug is lifted with forceps or a needle and is severed as deeply into the fat layer as possible. The specimen is placed in a properly labeled specimen bottle containing 10% formaldehyde solution or in a sterile container, if indicated. Closing the wound depends on the size of the punch: A 3-mm punch requires only an adhesive bandage, a 4-mm punch requires one suture, and a 6-mm punch requires two sutures.
• *Excision biopsy:* A #15 scalpel is used to totally excise the lesion; the incision is made as wide and as deep as necessary. The tissue specimen is removed and placed immediately in a properly labeled specimen bottle containing 10% formaldehyde solution. Apply pressure to the site to stop the bleeding. The wound is closed using 4-0 suture. If the incision is large, skin graft may be required.
• Check the biopsy site for bleeding.
• If the patient experiences pain, administer medication.
• Advise the patient with sutures to keep the area clean and as dry as possible. Facial sutures will be removed in 3 to 5 days; trunk sutures, in 7 to 14 days. Instruct the patient with adhesive strips to leave them in place for 14 to 21 days.

Precautions
• Send the specimen to the laboratory immediately.

Normal findings
Normal skin consists of squamous epithelium (epidermis) and fibrous connective tissue (dermis).

Abnormal findings
Histologic examination of the tissue specimen may reveal a benign or malignant lesion. Malignant tumors include basal cell carcinoma, squamous cell carcinoma, and malignant melanoma. Basal cell carcinoma occurs on hair-bearing skin; the most common loca-

tion is the face, including the nose and its folds. Squamous cell carcinoma most often appears on the lips, mouth, and genitalia. Malignant melanoma, the most deadly skin cancer, can spread throughout the body by way of the lymphatic system and the blood vessels. Benign growths include cysts, seborrheic keratoses, warts, pigmented nevi (moles), keloids, dermatofibromas, and multiple neurofibromas.

Cultures can be used to detect chronic bacterial and fungal infections in which flora are relatively sparse.

PERCUTANEOUS RENAL BIOPSY

Percutaneous renal biopsy is needle excision of a core of kidney tissue for histologic examination to obtain information about glomerular and tubular function. Biopsy may help assess histologic changes caused by acute and chronic glomerulonephritis, pyelonephritis, renal vein thrombosis, amyloid infiltration, and systemic lupus erythematosus.

Complications of percutaneous biopsy may include bleeding, hematoma, arteriovenous fistula, and infection. This procedure is safer than open biopsy, which is the preferred method for sampling a solid lesion, but noninvasive procedures, especially renal ultrasonography and computed tomography scan, have replaced percutaneous renal biopsy in many hospitals. (See *Urinary tract brush biopsy*.)

Purpose
• To aid diagnosis of renal parenchymal disease
• To monitor progression of renal disease and to assess the effectiveness of treatment

Patient preparation
• Explain to the patient that this test is used to diagnose kidney disorders.
• Describe the procedure to the patient, and ask him if he has any questions.
• Instruct the patient to restrict food and fluids for 8 hours before the test.
• Tell him who will perform the biopsy and where; that blood and urine specimens are collected and tested before the biopsy; that other tests, such as intravenous pyelography, ultrasonography, or an erect film of the abdomen, may be ordered to help determine the biopsy site; that the procedure takes only 15 minutes; and that the needle is in the kidney for only a few seconds.
• Make sure the patient or an appropriate family member has signed a consent form.
• Check patient history for hemorrhagic tendencies and hypersensitivity to the local anesthetic.
• Administer a mild sedative 30 minutes to 1 hour before the biopsy to help the patient relax.
• Inform him that he'll receive a local anesthetic but may experience a pinching pain when the needle is inserted through the back into the kidney.
• Check vital signs, and tell the patient to void just before the test.

Procedure and posttest care
• Place the patient in a prone position on a firm surface, with a sandbag beneath his abdomen.
• Tell him to take a deep breath while his kidney is being palpated.
• A 7″ 20G needle is used to inject the local anesthetic into the skin at the biopsy site. Instruct the patient to hold his breath and remain immobile as the needle is inserted through the back muscles, the deep lumbar fascia, the perinephric fat, and the kidney capsule. After the needle is inserted, tell the patient to take several deep breaths. If the needle swings smoothly during deep

URINARY TRACT BRUSH BIOPSY

Retrograde brush biopsy of the urinary tract may be used to obtain a renal tissue specimen when X-rays show a lesion in the renal pelvis or calyx. It can also be used to obtain specimens from other areas of the urinary tract. However, retrograde brush biopsy is contraindicated in patients with acute urinary tract infection or an obstruction at or below the biopsy site.

Patient preparation

To prepare the patient for brush biopsy, describe the procedure and tell him he may feel some discomfort. Inform him who will perform the biopsy and when. Reassure the patient that the procedure will take only 30 to 60 minutes.

Make sure the patient or a responsible family member has signed an appropriate consent form. Because this procedure requires use of a contrast agent and a general, local, or spinal anesthetic, check the patient's history for hypersensitivity to anesthetics, contrast media, or iodine-containing foods such as shellfish. Just before the biopsy procedure, administer a sedative to the patient.

Obtaining the biopsy

After the patient has received a sedative and an anesthetic, place him in the lithotomy position. Using a cystoscope, a guide wire is passed up the ureter and a urethral catheter is passed over the guide wire. Contrast medium is instilled through the catheter, which is positioned next to the lesion under fluoroscopic guidance. The contrast medium is washed out with 0.9% sodium chloride solution to prevent cell distortions from the dye. A nylon or steel brush is passed up the catheter and the lesion is brushed. This procedure is repeated at least six times, using a new brush each time.

As each brush is removed from the catheter, a smear is made for Papanicolaou staining and the brush tip is cut off and placed in formalin for 1 hour. The biopsy material is then removed from the brush tip for histologic examination. When the last brush is withdrawn, the catheter is irrigated with 0.9% sodium chloride solution to remove additional cells. These cells are also sent for histologic examination.

Results differentiate between malignant and benign lesions, which may appear the same on X-rays.

Posttest care

Because brush biopsy may cause complications such as perforation, hemorrhage, sepsis, or contrast medium extravasation, carefully monitor the patient's vital signs. Be sure to record the time, color, and amount of voiding, being alert for hematuria and abdominal or flank pain. Report any abnormal findings immediately, and administer analgesics and antibiotics.

breathing, it has penetrated the kidney capsule. After the penetration depth is marked on the needle shaft, instruct the patient to hold his breath and remain as still as possible while the needle is withdrawn.

• After a small incision is made in the anesthetized skin, instruct the patient to hold his breath and remain still while the Vim-Silverman needle with stylet is inserted to the measured depth.

• Tell the patient to breathe deeply. Then tell him remain still while the tissue specimen is obtained.

• After the tissue is examined immediately under a hand lens to ensure that the specimen contains tissue from both cortex and medulla, the tissue is placed on a saline-soaked gauze pad and placed in a properly labeled container.

• If an adequate tissue specimen has not been obtained, the procedure is repeated immediately.

• After an adequate specimen is secured, apply pressure to the biopsy site for 3 to 5 minutes to stop superficial bleeding. Then, apply a pressure dressing.

• Instruct the patient to lie flat on his back without moving for at least 12 hours to prevent bleeding. Check vital signs every 15 minutes for 4 hours, then every 30 minutes for 4 hours, then every hour for 4 hours, and finally every 4 hours. Report any changes.

• Examine all urine for blood; small amounts may be present after biopsy but should disappear within 8 hours. Hematocrit may be monitored after the procedure, to screen for internal bleeding.

• Encourage fluid ingestion to minimize colic and obstruction from blood clotting within the renal pelvis.

• Inform the patient that he may resume a normal diet.

Precautions

• Percutaneous renal biopsy is contraindicated in a patient with renal tumors, severe bleeding disorder, markedly reduced plasma or blood volume, severe hypertension, hydronephrosis, perinephric abscess, advanced renal failure with uremia, or only one kidney.

• Instruct the patient to hold his breath and remain still whenever the needle or prongs are advanced into or retracted from the kidney.

• Send the tissue specimen to the laboratory immediately.

Normal findings

Normally, a section of kidney tissue shows Bowman's capsule — the area between two layers of flat epithelial cells — the glomerular tuft, and the capillary lumen. The tubule sections differ depending on the area of tubule involved. The proximal tubule is one layer of epithelial cells with microvilli that form a brush border. The descending Henle's loop has flat squamous epithelial cells. The ascending, distal convoluted and collecting tubules are lined with squamous epithelial cells.

Abnormal findings

Histologic examination of renal tissue can reveal malignancy or renal disease. Malignant tumors include Wilms' tumor, which is usually present in early childhood, and renal cell carcinoma, which is most prevalent in persons over age 40. Diseases indicated by characteristic histologic changes include disseminated lupus erythematosus, amyloid infiltration, acute and chronic glomerulonephritis, renal vein thrombosis, and pyelonephritis.

CHAPTER 10

Endoscopy

RESPIRATORY SYSTEM

DIRECT LARYNGOSCOPY

This test allows visualization of the larynx by the use of a fiber-optic endoscope or laryngoscope passed through the mouth and pharynx to the larynx. It is indicated for children, for patients with strong gag reflexes due to anatomic abnormalities, for those who have had no response to short-term symptomatic therapy, or for those with symptoms of pharyngeal or laryngeal disease, such as stridor or hemoptysis. Secretions or tissue may be removed during this procedure for further study. The test is usually contraindicated in patients with epiglottitis, but may be performed on them in an operating room with resuscitative equipment available.

Purpose
• To detect lesions or strictures and to remove benign lesions or foreign bodies from the larynx
• To aid diagnosis of laryngeal cancer
• To examine the larynx when indirect laryngoscopy is inadequate

Patient preparation
• Explain to the patient that this test is used to detect laryngeal abnormalities.
• Instruct the patient to fast for 6 to 8 hours before the test.
• Tell him who will perform the laryngoscopy and that it will be performed in a dark operating room.
• Inform the patient that he'll receive a sedative to help him relax, medication to reduce secretions and, during the procedure, a general or local anesthetic. Reassure him that this procedure will not obstruct his airway.
• Make sure the patient or a responsible member of his family has signed a consent form.
• Check the patient's history for hypersensitivity to the anesthetic.
• Obtain baseline vital signs.
• Administer sedative and other medication to the patient (usually 30 minutes to 1 hour before the test).
• Just before the test, instruct the patient to remove dentures, contact lenses, and jewelry, and tell him to void.

Equipment
Laryngoscope; sedative; atropine; local anesthetic (spray or jelly) or general anesthetic; sterile container for microbiology specimen; sterile gloves; Coplin jar with 95% ethyl alcohol for cytology smears; container with 10% formaldehyde solution for histology specimen; forceps for biopsy; emesis basin; resuscitation equipment.

Procedure and posttest care
• Place the patient in a supine position.
• Encourage him to breathe through his nose and relax with his arms at his sides.
• A general anesthetic is administered or the patient's mouth and throat are sprayed with local anesthetic.
• A laryngoscope is introduced through the patient's mouth, the larynx is examined for abnormalities, and a specimen or secretions may be removed for further study; minor surgery, such as removal of polyps or nodules, may be performed at this time.
• Place specimens in their respective containers.
• Place the conscious patient in semi-Fowler's position; place the unconscious patient on his side with his head slightly elevated to prevent aspiration.

• Check vital signs every 15 minutes until stable, then every 30 minutes for 4 hours, every hour for the next 4 hours, and then every 4 hours for 24 hours. Immediately report any adverse reaction to anesthetic or sedative.

• Apply an ice collar to minimize laryngeal edema.

• Provide an emesis basin, and instruct the patient to spit out saliva rather than swallow it. Observe sputum for blood, and report excessive bleeding immediately.

• Instruct the patient to refrain from clearing his throat and coughing, to prevent hemorrhaging at the biopsy site.

• Advise the patient to avoid smoking until vital signs are stable and there is no evidence of complications.

• Immediately report any subcutaneous crepitus around the patient's face and neck, which may indicate tracheal perforation.

• Observe the patient with epiglottitis for signs of airway obstruction, and immediately report signs of respiratory difficulty. Keep emergency resuscitation equipment available; keep a tracheotomy tray nearby for 24 hours.

• Restrict food and fluids until the gag reflex returns (usually 2 hours). Then the patient may resume his usual diet, beginning with sips of water.

• Reassure the patient that voice loss, hoarseness, and sore throat are temporary. Provide throat lozenges or a soothing liquid gargle when his gag reflex returns.

Precautions
• Send the specimens to the laboratory immediately.

Normal findings
A normal larynx shows no evidence of inflammation, lesions, strictures, or foreign bodies.

Abnormal findings
The combined results of direct laryngoscopy, biopsy, and radiography may indicate laryngeal carcinoma. Direct laryngoscopy may show benign lesions, strictures, or foreign bodies and, with a biopsy, may distinguish laryngeal edema from radiation reaction or tumor.

BRONCHOSCOPY

This test allows direct visualization of the larynx, trachea, and bronchi through a flexible fiber-optic bronchoscope or a rigid metal bronchoscope. While a flexible fiber-optic bronchoscope allows a wider view and is used more often, the rigid metal bronchoscope is required to remove foreign objects, excise endobronchial lesions, and control massive hemoptysis. A brush, biopsy forceps, or a catheter may be passed through the bronchoscope to obtain specimens for cytologic examination.

Purpose
• To visually examine possible tumor, obstruction, secretion, bleeding, or foreign body in the tracheobronchial tree

• To help diagnose bronchogenic carcinoma, tuberculosis, interstitial pulmonary disease, or fungal or parasitic pulmonary infection by obtaining a specimen for bacteriologic and cytologic examination

• To remove foreign bodies, malignant or benign tumors, mucus plugs, or excessive secretions from the tracheobronchial tree

Patient preparation
• Explain to the patient that this test is used to examine the lower airways.

• Describe the procedure, and instruct the patient to fast for 6 to 12 hours before the test.
• Tell him who will perform the test and where, that the room will be darkened, and that the procedure takes 45 to 60 minutes.
• Advise him that test results are usually available in 1 day; a tuberculosis report may take up to 6 weeks, however.
• Tell the patient that chest X-ray and blood studies will be performed before the bronchoscopy.
• Advise him that he may receive a sedative I.V. to help him relax.
• If the procedure is not being performed under a general anesthetic, inform the patient that a local anesthetic will be sprayed into his nose and mouth to suppress the gag reflex. Warn him that the spray has an unpleasant taste and that he may experience some discomfort during the procedure.
• Reassure him that his airway will not be blocked during the procedure and that oxygen will be administered through the bronchoscope.
• Make sure the patient or a responsible family member has signed a consent form.
• Check the patient's history for hypersensitivity to anesthetic.
• Obtain baseline vital signs.
• Administer the preoperative sedative.
• If the patient is wearing dentures, instruct him to remove them just before the test.

Equipment
Flexible fiber-optic bronchoscope; sedative; local anesthetic (spray, jelly, or liquid); sterile gloves; sterile container for microbiology specimen; container with 10% formaldehyde solution for histology specimen; Coplin jar with 95% ethyl alcohol for cytology smears; six glass slides (frosted, if possible, or with frosted tips); emesis basin; handheld resuscitation bag with face mask;

oral and endotracheal airways; laryngoscope; oxygen delivery equipment; ventilating bronchoscope for a patient requiring controlled mechanical ventilation.

Procedure and posttest care
• Place the patient in a supine position on a table or bed or have him sit upright in a chair.
• Tell him to remain relaxed, with his arms at his sides, and to breathe through his nose.
• Provide supplemental oxygen by nasal cannula, if necessary.
• After the local anesthetic is sprayed into the patient's throat and takes effect, a bronchoscope is introduced; it's used to inspect the anatomic structure of the trachea and bronchi, observe the color of the mucosal lining, and note masses or inflamed areas.
• Biopsy forceps may be used to remove a tissue specimen from a suspect area, a bronchial brush is used to obtain cells from the surface of a lesion, or a suction apparatus is used to remove foreign bodies or mucus plugs.
• After collection, place specimens in their respective, properly labeled containers and send them to the laboratory.
• Monitor vital signs. Be certain to report adverse reactions immediately.
• Place the conscious patient in semi-Fowler's position; place the unconscious patient on his side with the head of the bed slightly elevated to prevent aspiration.
• Provide an emesis basin, and instruct the patient to spit out saliva rather than swallow it. Observe sputum for blood, and report excessive bleeding immediately.
• Tell the patient who had a biopsy to refrain from clearing his throat and coughing, which may dislodge the clot at the biopsy site and cause hemorrhaging.

• Immediately report any subcutaneous crepitus around the patient's face and neck, as this may indicate tracheal or bronchial perforation.

• Watch for and immediately report symptoms of respiratory difficulty, such as laryngeal stridor and dyspnea, resulting from laryngeal edema or laryngospasm. Observe for signs of hypoxemia, pneumothorax, bronchospasm, or bleeding.

• Restrict food and fluids until the gag reflex returns (usually in 1 hour). Then the patient may resume his usual diet, beginning with sips of clear liquid or ice chips.

• Reassure the patient that hoarseness, loss of voice, and sore throat after this procedure are only temporary. Provide lozenges or a soothing liquid gargle to ease discomfort when his gag reflex returns.

Precautions
• A patient with severe respiratory failure who cannot breathe adequately by himself should be placed on a ventilator before bronchoscopy.

• Send the specimens to the laboratory immediately.

Normal findings
The trachea normally consists of smooth muscle containing C-shaped rings of cartilage at regular intervals, and it's lined with ciliated mucosa. The bronchi appear structurally similar to the trachea; the right bronchus is slightly larger and more vertical than the left. Smaller segmental bronchi branch off from the main bronchi.

Abnormal findings
Abnormalities of the bronchial wall include inflammation, swelling, protruding cartilage, ulceration, tumors, enlargement of the mucous gland orifices, or submucosal lymph nodes.

Abnormalities of endotracheal origin include stenosis, compression, ectasia (dilation of tubular vessel), anomalous (irregular) bronchial branching, and abnormal bifurcation due to diverticulum.

Abnormal substances in the trachea or bronchi include blood, secretions, calculi, and foreign bodies.

Results of tissue and cell studies may indicate interstitial pulmonary disease, bronchogenic carcinoma, tuberculosis, or other pulmonary infections. Bronchogenic carcinomas include epidermoid or squamous cell carcinoma, small-cell (oat cell) carcinoma, adenocarcinoma, and large-cell (undifferentiated) carcinoma. Correlation of radiographic, bronchoscopic, and cytologic findings with clinical signs and symptoms is essential.

MEDIASTINOSCOPY

Using an exploring speculum with built-in fiber light and side slit, mediastinoscopy allows direct viewing of mediastinal structures. It also permits palpation and biopsy of paratracheal and carinal lymph nodes. This surgical procedure is indicated when tests such as sputum cytology, lung scans, radiography, and bronchoscopic biopsy fail to confirm diagnosis.

Scarring of the area from previous mediastinoscopy contraindicates this procedure.

Purpose
• To detect bronchogenic carcinoma, lymphoma (including Hodgkin's disease), and sarcoidosis

• To determine stages of lung cancer

Patient preparation

• Explain to the patient that this test is used to evaluate the lymph nodes and other structures in the chest.

• Describe the procedure and answer any questions.

• Instruct the patient to fast after midnight before the test.

• Tell him who will perform the procedure and where, that he'll be given general anesthesia, and that the procedure takes approximately 1 hour.

• Tell him he may have temporary chest pain, tenderness at the incision site, or a sore throat (from intubation).

• Reassure him that complications are rare with this procedure.

• Make sure the patient or a responsible family member has signed a consent form.

• Check the patient's history for hypersensitivity to the anesthetic.

• Give a sedative the night before the test and again before the procedure.

• Monitor vital signs, and check dressings for bleeding or fluid drainage.

• Observe for signs of the following complications: fever (mediastinitis); crepitus (subcutaneous emphysema); dyspnea, cyanosis, and diminished breath sounds on the affected side (pneumothorax); tachycardia and hypotension (hemorrhage).

• Administer the prescribed analgesic, as needed.

Procedure and posttest care

• After the endotracheal tube is in place, a small transverse suprasternal incision is made and the surgeon palpates the lymph nodes.

• The mediastinoscope is inserted, and tissue specimens are collected and sent to the laboratory for frozen section examination.

• If analysis confirms malignancy of a resectable tumor, thoracotomy and pneumonectomy may follow immediately.

Normal findings

Normally, lymph nodes appear as small, smooth, flat oval bodies of lymphoid tissue.

Abnormal findings

Malignant lymph nodes usually indicate lung or esophageal cancer or lymphomas. Staging of lung cancer is used to determine therapeutic regimen.

THORACOSCOPY

In this test, an endoscope is inserted directly into the chest wall to allow viewing of the pleural space. It is used for both diagnostic and therapeutic purposes and can sometimes replace traditional thoracotomy. Thoracoscopy reduces morbidity (by reducing the use of open chest surgery) and postoperative pain, decreases surgical and anesthesia time, and allows faster recovery.

Purpose

• To diagnose pleural disease

• To obtain a biopsy specimen from the mediastinum

• To treat pleural conditions, such as cysts, blebs, and effusions

• To perform wedge resections

Patient preparation

• Describe the procedure. Caution the patient that an open thoracotomy may be still be needed for diagnosis or treatment and general anesthesia may be required.

• Tell the patient that he must not eat or drink fluids for 10 to 12 hours before the procedure.

• Be sure appropriate preoperative tests (such as pulmonary function and coagulation tests, electrocardiogram, and chest X-ray) have been performed and that a consent form has been signed.

• Tell the patient that he'll have a chest tube and drainage system in place after surgery. Reassure him that analgesics will be available and that complications are rare.

Equipment

Monitors; videocassette recorder; camera; light source; insufflator; cautery; suction and irrigation equipment; trocars; endostaplers; endosutures.

Procedure and posttest care

• The patient is anesthetized and a double-lumen endobronchial tube is inserted.

• The lung on the operative side is collapsed and a small intercostal incision is made, through which a trocar is inserted.

• A lens is then inserted to view the area and assess thoracoscopy access.

• Two or three more small incisions are made and trocars are placed for insertion of suctioning and dissection instruments.

• The camera lens and instruments are moved from site to site as needed.

• After thoracoscopy, the lung is reexpanded and a chest tube is placed through one incision site and a water-sealed drainage system is attached. The other incisions are closed with adhesive strips and dressed.

• Monitor vital signs every 15 minutes for 1 hour and then every 4 hours.

• Assess respiratory status and the patency of the chest drainage system.

• Give analgesics as needed for pain.

Precautions

• Send specimens to the laboratory immediately.

• Complications, although rare, include hemorrhage, nerve injury, perforation of the diaphragm, air emboli, and tension pneumothorax.

• Thoracoscopy is not appropriate for patients who have coagulopathies or le-

sions near major blood vessels, those who have had previous thoracic surgery, or those who cannot be adequately oxygenated with one lung.

Normal findings

A normal pleural cavity contains a small amount of lubricating fluid that facilitates movement of the lung and chest wall. The parietal and visceral layers are lesion free and able to separate from each other.

Abnormal findings

Lesions adjacent to or involving the pleura or mediastinum can be seen and biopsies can be taken for diagnosis and determination of treatment. After accumulated fluid is removed, sterile talc can be blown into the pleural space to promote sclerosing and prevent future accumulations. Areas of blebs can be removed by wedge resection to reduce the risk of repeated episodes of spontaneous pneumothorax.

GASTROINTESTINAL SYSTEM

ESOPHAGOGASTRO-DUODENOSCOPY

This test permits visual examination of the lining of the esophagus, the stomach, and the upper duodenum using a flexible fiber-optic endoscope. It's indicated in patients with hematemesis, melena, or substernal or epigastric pain and in postoperative patients with recurrent or new symptoms.

Esophagogastroduodenoscopy eliminates the need for extensive exploratory surgery and can be used to detect small or surface lesions missed by radiography. Because the scope provides a channel for biopsy forceps or a cytology brush, it permits laboratory evaluation of abnormalities detected by radiography. Similarly, it allows removal of foreign bodies by suction (for small, soft objects) or by electrocautery snare or forceps (for large, hard objects).

Purpose
• To diagnose inflammatory disease, malignant and benign tumors, ulcers, Mallory-Weiss syndrome, and structural abnormalities
• To evaluate the stomach and duodenum postoperatively
• To obtain emergency diagnosis of duodenal ulcer or esophageal injury, such as that caused by ingestion of chemicals

Patient preparation
• Explain to the patient that this procedure permits visual examination of the lining of the esophagus, the stomach, and the upper duodenum.
• Instruct him to fast for 6 to 12 hours before the test.
• Tell him that a flexible instrument will be passed through his mouth; explain who will perform this procedure and where and that it takes about 30 minutes.
• If an emergency esophagogastroduodenoscopy is to be performed, tell the patient that stomach contents are aspirated through a nasogastric tube.
• Tell him that a blood sample may be drawn before the procedure.
• Inform the patient that a bitter-tasting local anesthetic will be sprayed into his mouth and throat to calm the gag reflex and that his tongue and throat may feel swollen, making swallowing seem difficult. Advise him to let the saliva drain from the side of his mouth; a suction machine may be used to remove saliva, if necessary.
• Explain that a mouth guard will be inserted to protect his teeth and the endoscope; assure him that this will not obstruct his breathing.
• Inform him that he'll receive a sedative before the endoscope is inserted to help him relax, but that he'll remain conscious. If the procedure is being done on an outpatient basis, advise the patient to arrange for transportation home.
• Tell the patient that he may experience pressure in the stomach as the endoscope is moved about and a feeling of fullness when air or carbon dioxide is insufflated (insufflation distends and flattens the stomach wall to aid visualization).
• If the patient is apprehensive, administer meperidine or another analgesic I.M. about 30 minutes before the test; also administer atropine sulfate subcutaneously to decrease GI secretions, which may interfere with test results.
• Make sure the patient or a family member has signed a consent form.
• Check the patient's history for hypersensitivity to the medications and anesthetic ordered for the test.
• Just before the procedure, instruct the patient to remove dentures, eyeglasses, necklaces, hairpins, combs, and constricting undergarments.

Procedure and posttest care
• Obtain baseline vital signs, and leave the blood pressure cuff in place for monitoring throughout the procedure.
• Ask the patient to hold his breath while his mouth and throat are sprayed with a local anesthetic.
• Instruct him to let saliva drain from the side of his mouth; provide an emesis basin to spit out saliva and tissues to wipe saliva from his mouth.

• The patient is placed in a left lateral position, his head is bent forward, and he is asked to open his mouth.

• The examiner guides the tip of the endoscope to the back of the throat and downward. As the endoscope passes through the posterior pharynx and the cricopharyngeal sphincter, the patient's head is slowly extended.

• When the endoscope is well into the esophagus (about 12″ [30 cm]), the patient's head is positioned with his chin toward the table so saliva can drain out of his mouth.

• After examination of the esophagus and the cardiac sphincter, the endoscope is advanced to examine the stomach, then the duodenum. During the examination, air or water may be introduced through the endoscope, and suction may be applied to remove insufflated air or secretions.

• A camera may be attached to the endoscope to photograph areas for later study, or a measuring tube may be passed through the endoscope to determine the size of a lesion.

• Biopsy forceps to obtain a tissue specimen or a cytology brush to obtain cells may also be passed through the scope.

• The endoscope is slowly withdrawn, and suspicious looking areas of the gastric and esophageal lining are reexamined.

• Place tissue specimens immediately in a specimen bottle containing 10% formaldehyde solution; cell specimens are smeared on glass slides and placed in a Coplin jar containing 95% ethyl alcohol.

• Observe the patient for possible perforation. Perforation in the cervical area of the esophagus produces pain on swallowing and with neck movement; thoracic perforation causes substernal or epigastric pain that increases with breathing or with movement of the trunk; diaphragmatic perforation produces shoulder pain and dyspnea; gastric perforation causes abdominal or back pain, cyanosis, fever, or pleural effusion.

• Check vital signs every 15 minutes for 4 hours, every hour for 4 hours, then every 4 hours.

• Test the gag reflex by touching the back of the throat with a tongue blade. Withhold food and fluids until the gag reflex returns — usually in 1 hour — then, allow fluids and a light meal.

• Tell the patient he may burp some insufflated air and may have a sore throat for 3 or 4 days. Provide throat lozenges and warm saline gargles to ease his discomfort.

• If the patient experiences soreness at the I.V. site, apply warm soaks.

• Make sure the outpatient has transportation home; he shouldn't drive for 12 hours because of drowsiness from sedation.

• Instruct him to immediately report persistent difficulty in swallowing, pain, fever, black stools, or bloody vomit.

Precautions

• If tissue or cell specimens are obtained during the procedure, label and send them to the appropriate laboratory immediately.

• This procedure is generally safe, but can cause perforation of the esophagus, stomach, or duodenum, especially if the patient is restless or uncooperative.

• An esophagogastroduodenoscopy is usually contraindicated in patients with Zenker's diverticulum, large aortic aneurysm, or recent ulcer perforation.

• An esophagogastroduodenoscopy shouldn't be performed within 2 days after an upper GI series.

• Observe closely for adverse effects of the medication: respiratory depression, apnea, hypotension, excessive diaphoresis, bradycardia, and laryngospasm. Have available emergency resuscitation equipment and a narcotic antagonist, such as naloxone or levallorphan tartrate. Be prepared to intervene as necessary.

Normal findings
The smooth mucosa of the esophagus is normally yellow-pink and is marked by a fine vascular network. A pulsation on the anterior wall of the esophagus between 8″ and 10″ (20 and 25 cm) from the incisor teeth represents the aortic arch. The orange-red mucosa of the stomach begins at the "Z" line, an irregular transition line slightly above the esophagogastric junction. Unlike the esophagus, the stomach has rugal folds, and its blood vessels are not visible beneath the gastric mucosa. The reddish mucosa of the duodenal bulb is marked by a few shallow longitudinal folds. However, the mucosa of the distal duodenum has prominent circular folds, is lined with villi, and appears velvety.

Abnormal findings
Esophagogastroduodenoscopy, with the results of histologic and cytologic tests, may indicate acute or chronic ulcers, benign or malignant tumors, and inflammatory disease, including esophagitis, gastritis, and duodenitis. This test may demonstrate diverticula, varices, Mallory-Weiss syndrome, esophageal rings, esophageal and pyloric stenoses, and esophageal hiatal hernia. Although esophagogastroduodenoscopy can evaluate gross abnormalities of esophageal motility, such as occurs in achalasia, manometric studies are more accurate.

COLONOSCOPY

This test employs a flexible fiber-optic endoscope to permit visual examination

of the lining of the large intestine. It is indicated for patients with histories of constipation or diarrhea, persistent rectal bleeding, or lower abdominal pain, when the results of proctosigmoidoscopy and the barium enema test are negative or inconclusive.

Purpose
• To detect or evaluate inflammatory and ulcerative bowel disease
• To locate the origin of lower gastrointestinal bleeding
• To aid diagnosis of colonic strictures and benign or malignant lesions
• To evaluate the colon postoperatively for recurrence of polyps or malignant lesions

Patient preparation
• Tell the patient that this test permits examination of the lining of the large intestine.
• Instruct him to maintain a clear liquid diet for 48 hours before the test.
• Describe the procedure, who will perform it, and where; inform the patient that the test generally takes 30 to 60 minutes.
• Explain that the large intestine must be thoroughly cleaned to be clearly visible. Give the patient a laxative, such as 10 oz (300 ml) of magnesium citrate or 3 tbsp (45 ml) of castor oil, in the evening and a warm tap-water or sodium biphosphate enema 3 to 4 hours before the test until the return is clear. Soapsuds enemas are inappropriate.
• Assure him that the colonoscope is well lubricated to ease its insertion, that it initially feels cool, and that he may feel an urge to defecate when it's inserted and advanced.
• Explain that air may be introduced through the colonoscope to distend the intestinal wall and to facilitate viewing the lining and advancing the instrument; flatus normally escapes around

the instrument due to air insufflation, and he should not attempt to control it.
• Tell him suction may be used to remove blood or liquid feces that obscure vision, but that this won't cause discomfort.
• Make sure the patient or a responsible family member has signed a consent form.
• Check the patient's vital signs 30 minutes before the test; if they are stable, administer an intramuscular or intravenous sedative to help him relax.

Procedure and posttest care
• Place the patient on his left side, with his knees flexed, and drape him.
• Instruct him to breathe deeply and slowly through his mouth as the doctor palpates the mucosa of the anus and rectum and as the colonoscope is inserted.
• The lubricated colonoscope is inserted through the patient's anus and rectum into the sigmoid colon.
• When the instrument reaches the descending sigmoid junction, assist the patient to a supine position to aid the scope's advance, if necessary, and to aid negotiation of the splenic flexure.
• The scope is next advanced through the transverse colon, through the hepatic flexure, and into the ascending colon and cecum.
• Abdominal palpation or fluoroscopy may be used to help guide the colonoscope through the large intestine.
• Suction may be used to remove blood or secretions that obscure vision.
• Biopsy forceps or a cytology brush may be passed through the colonoscope to obtain specimens for histologic and cytologic examinations; an electrocautery snare may be used to remove polyps.
• If the examiner removes a tissue specimen, immediately place it in a specimen bottle containing 10% formalin; immediately place cytology smears

in a Coplin jar containing 95% ethyl alcohol. Send specimens immediately to the laboratory.
• Observe the patient closely for signs of bowel perforation. Report such signs immediately.
• Check vital signs until stable.
• After the patient has recovered from sedation, he may resume his usual diet.
• Provide privacy while the patient rests after the test; tell him he may pass large amounts of flatus after insufflation.
• If a polyp has been removed, inform the patient that there may be some blood in his stool.

Precautions
• Colonoscopy is usually a safe procedure but can cause perforation of the large intestine, excessive bleeding, and retroperitoneal emphysema.
• This procedure is contraindicated in patients who have ischemic bowel disease, acute diverticulitis, peritonitis, fulminant granulomatous colitis, or fulminant ulcerative colitis.
• Watch closely for adverse effects of the sedative. Have available emergency resuscitation equipment and a narcotic antagonist, such as naloxone, for I.V. use, if necessary.
• If a polyp is removed but not retrieved during the examination, give enemas and strain stools to retrieve it.

Normal findings
Normally, the mucosa of the large intestine beyond the sigmoid colon appears light pink-orange and is marked by semilunar folds and deep tubular pits. Blood vessels are visible beneath the intestinal mucosa, which glistens from mucus secretions.

Abnormal findings
Visual examination of the large intestine, coupled with histologic and cytologic test results, may indicate proctitis,

granulomatous or ulcerative colitis, Crohn's disease, and malignant or benign lesions. Diverticular disease or the site of lower GI bleeding can be detected through visual examination alone.

PROCTOSIGMOIDOSCOPY

This procedure uses a proctoscope, a sigmoidoscope, and digital examination to evaluate the lining of the distal sigmoid colon, the rectum, and the anal canal. It's indicated in patients with recent changes in bowel habits, lower abdominal and perineal pain, prolapse on defecation, pruritus, or passage of mucus, blood, or pus in the stool. Specimens may be obtained from suspicious areas of the mucosa by biopsy, lavage or cytology brush, or culture swab.

Possible complications of this procedure include rectal bleeding and, rarely, bowel perforation.

Purpose
• To aid diagnosis of inflammatory, infectious, and ulcerative bowel disease
• To diagnose malignant and benign neoplasms
• To detect hemorrhoids, hypertrophic anal papilla, polyps, fissures, fistulas, and abscesses in the rectum and anal canal

Patient preparation
• Explain to the patient that this procedure allows visual examination of the lining of the distal sigmoid colon, the rectum, and the anal canal.
• Tell him the test requires passage of two special instruments through the anus, who will perform this procedure and where, and that it takes 15 to 30 minutes.
• Because dietary and bowel preparations for this procedure vary, follow the orders carefully.

• Instruct the patient to maintain a clear liquid diet for 48 hours before the test, to avoid eating fruits and vegetables before the procedure, and to fast the morning of the procedure.
• If special bowel preparation is ordered, explain to the patient that this clears the intestine to ensure a better view.
• Administer a warm tap-water or sodium biphosphate enema 3 to 4 hours before the procedure. Soapsuds enemas are inappropriate. (The procedure may be started without bowel preparation as enemas can alter intestinal markings and traumatize mucous membranes. If the examination is then hindered by excessive fecal matter, an enema may be ordered before the examination.)
• Describe the position the patient will be asked to assume and assure him that he'll be adequately draped.
• Tell him he may be secured to a tilting table that rotates into horizontal and vertical positions.
• Tell the patient that the examiner's finger and the instrument are well lubricated to ease insertion, that the instrument initially feels cool, and that he may experience the urge to defecate when it's inserted and advanced.
• Inform him that the instrument may stretch the intestinal wall and cause transient muscle spasms or colicky lower abdominal pain.
• Instruct the patient to breathe deeply and slowly through his mouth to relax the abdominal muscles; this calms the urge to defecate and eases discomfort.
• Explain to the patient that air may be introduced through the endoscope into the intestine to distend its walls. Tell him this causes flatus to escape around the endoscope and he should not attempt to control it.
• Inform him that a suction machine may remove blood, mucus, or liquid feces that obscure vision, but it will cause no discomfort.

• Make sure the patient or a responsible family member has signed a consent form.

• Check the patient's history for barium tests within the past week, as barium in the colon hinders accurate examination.

• If the patient has rectal inflammation, provide a local anesthetic about 15 to 20 minutes before the procedure to minimize discomfort.

Procedure and posttest care

• Place the patient in a knee-chest or left lateral position, with knees flexed, and drape him.

• If a left lateral position is used, a sandbag may be placed under the patient's left hip, so the buttocks project over the edge of the table. The right buttock is gently raised, and the anus and perianal region are examined.

• Instruct the patient to breathe deeply and slowly through his mouth as the anal canal, the rectum, and the rectal mucosa are digitally palpated for induration and tenderness; the examiner then withdraws his finger and checks for the presence of blood, mucus, or fecal matter.

• The sigmoidoscope is lubricated and the patient is told that the instrument is about to be inserted. The right buttock is raised, and the sigmoidoscope is inserted into the anus. As the scope is passed with steady pressure through the anal sphincters, instruct the patient to bear down as though defecating to aid its passage. The sigmoidoscope is advanced through the anal canal into the rectum.

• At the rectosigmoid junction, a small amount of air may be insufflated to open the bowel lumen. The scope is then gently advanced to its full length into the distal sigmoid colon.

• As the sigmoidoscope is slowly withdrawn, air is carefully insufflated, and the intestinal mucosa is thoroughly examined.

• If fecal matter obscures vision, the eyepiece on the scope is removed, a cotton swab is inserted through the scope, and the bowel lumen is swabbed.

• To obtain specimens from suspicious areas of the intestinal mucosa, a biopsy forceps, a cytology brush, or a culture swab is passed through the sigmoidoscope.

• Polyps may be removed for histologic examination by insertion of an electrocautery snare through the sigmoidoscope.

• Specimens are immediately placed in a specimen bottle containing 10% formalin; cytology slides are placed in a Coplin jar containing 95% ethyl alcohol; culture swabs are placed in a culture tube.

• After the sigmoidoscope is withdrawn, the proctoscope is lubricated, and the patient is told that it's about to be inserted. Assure him that he will experience less discomfort during passage of the proctoscope.

• The right buttock is raised, and the proctoscope is inserted through the anus and gently advanced to its full length.

• The obturator is removed, and the light source is inserted through the handle of the proctoscope.

• As the instrument is slowly withdrawn, the rectal and anal mucosa are carefully examined. Specimens may be obtained from suspicious areas of the intestinal mucosa.

• If a biopsy of the anal canal is required, a local anesthetic may first be administered.

• After the examination is completed, the proctoscope is withdrawn.

• If the patient has been examined in a knee-chest position, instruct him to rest in a supine position for several minutes before standing, to prevent postural hypotension.

• Observe the patient closely for signs of bowel perforation and for vasovagal attack due to emotional stress. Report such signs immediately.

• If air was introduced into the intestine, tell the patient that he may pass large amounts of flatus. Provide privacy while he rests after the test.

• If a biopsy or polypectomy was performed, inform the patient that blood may appear in his stool.

Precautions
• If a tissue specimen or culture swab has been obtained, label it and send it to the appropriate laboratory immediately.

Normal findings
The mucosa of the sigmoid colon appears light pink-orange and is marked by semilunar folds and deep tubular pits. The rectal mucosa is redder due to its rich vascular network and deepens to a purple hue at the pectinate line (the anatomic division between the rectum and anus), and has three distinct valves. The lower two-thirds of the anus (anoderm) is lined with smooth gray-tan skin and joins with the hair-fringed perianal skin.

Abnormal findings
Visual examination and palpation demonstrate abnormalities of the anal canal and rectum, including internal and external hemorrhoids, hypertrophic anal papilla, anal fissures, anal fistulas, and anorectal abscesses. However, biopsy, culture, and other laboratory tests are often necessary to detect various disorders.

REPRODUCTIVE SYSTEM

COLPOSCOPY

In this test, the cervix and vagina are visually examined by means of an instrument containing a magnifying lens and a light (colposcope). Colposcopy is used primarily to evaluate abnormal cytology or grossly suspicious lesions and to examine the cervix and vagina after a positive Papanicolaou (Pap) test. During the examination, a biopsy may be performed and photographs taken of suspicious lesions with the colposcope and its attachments. Risks of biopsy include bleeding (especially during pregnancy) and infection.

Purpose
• To help confirm cervical intraepithelial neoplasia or invasive carcinoma after a positive Pap test
• To evaluate vaginal or cervical lesions
• To monitor conservatively treated cervical intraepithelial neoplasia
• To monitor patients whose mothers received diethylstilbestrol during pregnancy

Patient preparation
• Explain to the patient that this test magnifies the image of the vagina and cervix, providing more information than routine vaginal examination.
• Inform the patient that she need not restrict food or fluids.
• Tell her who will perform the examination and where, that it's safe and painless, and it takes 10 to 15 minutes.
• Tell the patient that a biopsy may be performed at the time of examination

and that this may cause minimal but easily controlled bleeding.

Equipment

Colposcopy: gloves; colposcope; vaginal speculum; 3% acetic acid solution; swabs.

Biopsy: gloves; biopsy forceps; endocervical curette; forceps for uterine dressing; tenaculum; ring forceps; Monsel's (ferric subsulfate) solution; biopsy bottle and preservative; sterile cotton balls; Pap test equipment (glass slide, wooden spatula, swabs, and fixative).

Procedure and posttest care

• The examiner puts on gloves. With the patient in lithotomy position, the examiner inserts the speculum and, if indicated, performs a Pap test. (Help the patient relax during insertion by telling her to breathe through her mouth and to concentrate on relaxing her abdominal muscles.)

• The cervix is swabbed with acetic acid solution to remove mucus.

• After the cervix and vagina are examined, biopsy is performed on areas that appear abnormal.

• Bleeding is stopped by applying pressure or hemostatic solutions or by cautery.

• After biopsy, instruct the patient to abstain from intercourse, and tell her not to insert anything in her vagina (except a tampon) until healing of the biopsy site is confirmed.

Normal findings

Normally, cervical vessels show a network and hairpin capillary pattern, with about 100 microns between them. Surface contour is smooth and pink; columnar epithelium appears grapelike. Different tissue types are sharply demarcated.

Abnormal findings

Abnormal colposcopy findings include white epithelium or punctation and mosaic patterns, which may indicate underlying cervical intraepithelial neoplasia; keratinization in the transformation zone, which may indicate cervical intraepithelial neoplasia or invasive carcinoma; and atypical vessels, which may indicate invasive carcinoma. Other abnormalities visible on colposcopic examination include inflammatory changes (usually from infection), atrophic changes (usually from aging or, less often, the use of oral contraceptives), erosion (probably from increased pathogenicity of vaginal flora, due to changes in vaginal pH), and papilloma and condyloma (possibly from viruses).

Histologic study of the biopsy specimen confirms colposcopic findings. However, if the results of the examination and biopsy are inconsistent with the results of the Pap test and biopsy of the squamocolumnar junction, conization of the cervix for biopsy may be indicated.

LAPAROSCOPY

This test permits visualization of the peritoneal cavity by the insertion of a small fiber-optic telescope (laparoscope) through the anterior abdominal wall. This surgical technique may be used diagnostically to detect abnormalities, such as cysts, adhesions, fibroids, and infection; it can also be used therapeutically to perform procedures such as lysis of adhesions, ovarian biopsy, tubal sterilization, removal of foreign bodies, and fulguration of endometriotic implants. Although laparoscopy has largely replaced laparotomy, the latter is usually preferred when extensive surgery is indicated. Potential risks of laparoscopy include a punctured visceral organ, causing bleeding or spilling of intestinal contents into the peritoneum.

Purpose
- To identify the cause of pelvic pain
- To help detect endometriosis, ectopic pregnancy, or pelvic inflammatory disease (PID)
- To evaluate pelvic masses or the fallopian tubes of infertile patients
- To stage carcinoma

Patient preparation
- Explain the procedure to the patient and tell her the test is used to detect abnormalities of the uterus, fallopian tubes, and ovaries.
- Instruct her to fast after midnight before the test or at least 8 hours before surgery.
- Tell her who will perform the procedure and that it takes only 15 to 30 minutes.
- Tell the patient that she'll receive a local or general anesthetic and whether the procedure will require an outpatient visit or overnight hospitalization.
- Warn her that she may experience pain at the puncture site and in the shoulder.
- Make sure the patient or a responsible family member has signed a consent form.
- Check the patient's history for hypersensitivity to the anesthetic.
- Make sure all laboratory work is completed and results are reported before the test.

Equipment
Indwelling urinary or straight catheter; sterile tray with scalpel, hemostats, needle holder, suture, and suture scissors; Verees needle; gas insufflator; laparoscope; fiber-optic light source and cable; laparoscope sheath and trocar; electrosurgical generator; tenaculum and intrauterine manipulator; probes, scissors, or forceps; adhesive bandages.

Procedure and posttest care
- The patient is anesthetized and is placed in lithotomy position.
- The examiner catheterizes the bladder, and then performs a bimanual examination of the pelvic area to detect abnormalities that may contraindicate the test and to ensure that the bladder is empty.
- The tenaculum is placed on the cervix and a uterine manipulator is inserted; an incision is made at the inferior rim of the umbilicus.
- The Verees needle is inserted into the peritoneal cavity, and approximately 2 to 3 liters of carbon dioxide or nitrous oxide are insufflated to distend the abdominal wall and provide an organ-free space for insertion of the trocar; the needle is removed and a trocar and sheath are inserted into the peritoneal cavity; a second trocar may be inserted at the pubic hairline for the insertion of other instruments.
- After removal of the trocar, the laparoscope is inserted through the sheath to examine the pelvis and abdomen.
- To evaluate tubal patency, the examiner infuses a dye through the cervix and observes the fimbria of the tubes for spillage.
- Following the examination, minor surgical procedures such as ovarian biopsy may be performed.
- Monitor vital signs and urinary output. Report sudden changes immediately; they may indicate complications.
- After administration of a general anesthetic, check for allergies; monitor electrolyte balance and hemoglobin and hematocrit levels. Ambulate the patient after recovery.
- Tell the patient she may resume her usual diet.

• Instruct her to restrict activity for 2 to 7 days, as necessary.

• Reassure the patient that some abdominal and shoulder pain is normal and should disappear within 24 to 36 hours. Provide a mild pain reliever, such as acetaminophen.

Precautions

• Laparoscopy is contraindicated in patients with advanced abdominal wall malignancy, advanced respiratory or cardiovascular disease, intestinal obstruction, palpable abdominal mass, large abdominal hernia, chronic tuberculosis, or history of peritonitis.

• During the procedure, check for proper drainage of the catheter.

Normal findings

The uterus and fallopian tubes are of normal size and shape, free of adhesions, and mobile. The ovaries are of normal size and shape; cysts and endometriosis are absent. Dye injected through the cervix flows freely from the fimbria.

Abnormal findings

An ovarian cyst appears as a bubble on the surface of the ovary. The cyst may be clear, filled with follicular fluid or serous or mucous material, or red, blue, or brown if filled with blood. Adhesions appear as sheets or strands of tissue that are almost transparent or as thick and fibrous. Endometriosis resembles small, blue powder burns on the peritoneum or the serosa of any pelvic or abdominal structure. Fibroids appear as lumps on the uterus; hydrosalpinx as an enlarged fallopian tube; and ectopic pregnancy as an enlarged or ruptured fallopian tube. In PID, infection or abscess is evident.

SKELETAL SYSTEM

ARTHROSCOPY

Arthroscopy is the visual examination of the interior of a joint (most often the knee) with a specially designed fiberoptic endoscope that is inserted through a cannula in the joint cavity. It usually follows and confirms a diagnosis made through physical examination, X-rays, and arthrography. The diagnostic accuracy rate of this procedure is about 98%.

Arthroscopy permits concurrent surgery or biopsy using a technique called triangulation, in which instruments are passed through a separate cannula. Arthroscopy is commonly performed under a local anesthetic, but it may also be performed under a spinal or general anesthetic, particularly when surgery is anticipated. A camera may be attached to the arthroscope to photograph areas for later study. (See *Arthroscopy of the knee,* page 468.)

Complications associated with arthroscopy rarely occur but may include infection, hemarthrosis, swelling, synovial rupture, thrombophlebitis, infrapatellar anesthesia, and joint injury.

Purpose

• To detect and diagnose meniscal, patellar, condylar, extrasynovial, and synovial diseases

• To monitor disease progression

• To perform joint surgery

• To monitor effectiveness of therapy

Patient preparation

• Explain to the patient that this test is used to examine the interior of the joint, evaluate joint disease, or monitor his response to therapy.

ARTHROSCOPY OF THE KNEE

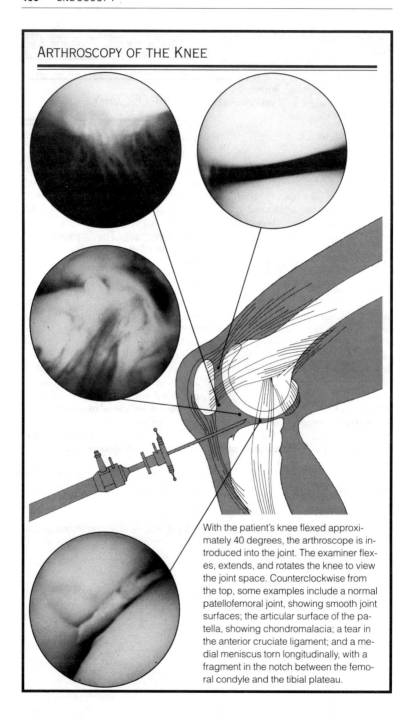

With the patient's knee flexed approximately 40 degrees, the arthroscope is introduced into the joint. The examiner flexes, extends, and rotates the knee to view the joint space. Counterclockwise from the top, some examples include a normal patellofemoral joint, showing smooth joint surfaces; the articular surface of the patella, showing chondromalacia; a tear in the anterior cruciate ligament; and a medial meniscus torn longitudinally, with a fragment in the notch between the femoral condyle and the tibial plateau.

• Describe the procedure to the patient, and answer any questions.

• If surgery or other treatment is anticipated, explain that this may be accomplished during arthroscopy.

• Instruct the patient to fast after midnight before the procedure.

• Tell him who will perform this procedure and where.

• If local anesthesia is to be used, tell the patient that he may experience transient discomfort from the injection of the local anesthetic and the pressure of the tourniquet on his leg.

• Make sure the patient or a responsible family member has signed a consent form.

• Check the patient's history for hypersensitivity to the anesthetic.

• Just before the procedure, shave the area 5″ (12.5 cm) above and below the joint; then administer a sedative.

Equipment

Skin antiseptic (povidone-iodine solution); arthroscope and accessory equipment; pointed scalpel; sterile gloves; local anesthetic; sterile needle; 12-ml and 60-ml syringes; waterproof stockinette; elastic bandages; pneumatic tourniquet; epinephrine (1:100,000 in 1% lidocaine solution); 500 ml sterile 0.9% sodium chloride solution; continuous drainage system; sponges; 2″ × 2″ sterile gauze pads; sterile drapes; small adhesive bandages.

Procedure and posttest care

Although arthroscopic techniques vary, depending on the surgeon and the type of arthroscope used, the following knee arthroscopy procedure is typical:

• After the patient is placed in a supine position on the operating table, a pneumatic tourniquet is placed around his leg but not tightened.

• The patient's leg is scrubbed according to standard surgical procedure, and a waterproof stockinette is applied.

• The patient's leg is elevated and wrapped from toes to lower thigh with an elastic bandage to drain as much blood from the leg as possible.

• The tourniquet is inflated and the elastic bandage removed; the tourniquet may be used at 300 mm Hg and may remain in place during the procedure, depending on the surgeon's preference and the patient's comfort. (For techniques that do not require a tourniquet, 50 ml of sterile 0.9% sodium chloride solution with lidocaine and epinephrine is instilled into the patient's knee immediately before insertion of the arthroscope to distend the knee and reduce bleeding.)

• The foot of the table is lowered so the patient's knee is bent at about 45 degrees, the stockinette is opened, and the local anesthetic is administered.

• A pointed scalpel is used to make a 3- to 5-mm incision in either the anteromedial or the anterolateral aspect of the knee, above the tibial plateau.

• If the procedure is being performed under a local anesthetic, warn the patient that he will feel a thumping sensation as the cannula with sharp trocar is inserted into the capsule at a point medial to the patellar tendon.

• The trocar is removed and replaced with a blunt obturator, which penetrates the synovia, causing transient pain.

• The arthroscope is then inserted through the cannula.

• A solution of 0.9% sodium chloride and epinephrine — a viewing medium — is introduced into the joint through the arthroscope and is drained into a container on the floor.

• The arthroscope is inserted in and out of various joint spaces or is held steady as the knee is bent, extended, and turned to aid visualization. The entire joint can be viewed from one puncture site, but an obstruction may necessitate additional punctures. Generally, examination of the tibial plateaus, the back recesses of the joint, the menisci, the posterior two-thirds of the femoral condyles, the cruciate structures, and the under surface of the patella takes about 10 minutes.

• After visual examination, a synovial biopsy or surgery may be performed or treatment applied, as indicated.

• When the examination is completed, the arthroscope is removed, the joint is irrigated by way of the cannula, the cannula is removed, and gentle manual pressure is applied to the knee to remove the 0.9% sodium chloride solution.

• An adhesive strip and compression dressing are applied over the incision site.

• Watch for fever, swelling, increased pain, and localized inflammation at the incision site. If the patient reports discomfort, provide a mild pain reliever, such as acetaminophen.

• Tell the patient that he may walk as soon as he's fully awake but should avoid excessive use of the joint for a few days. Tell him he may resume his usual diet.

Precautions

• Arthroscopy is contraindicated in a patient with fibrous ankylosis with flexion of less than 50 degrees and in a patient with local skin or wound infections because of the risk of subsequent joint involvement.

Normal findings

The knee is a typical diarthrodial joint surrounded by muscles, ligaments, cartilage, and tendons and lined with synovial membrane. In children, the menisci are smooth and opaque, with their thick outer edges attached to the joint capsule and their inner edges lying snugly against the condylar surfaces, unattached. Articular cartilage appears smooth and white; ligaments and tendons appear cable-like and silvery. The synovium is smooth and marked by a fine vascular network. Degenerative changes begin during adolescence.

Abnormal findings

Arthroscopic examination can reveal meniscal disease, such as torn medial or lateral meniscus or other meniscus injuries; patellar disease, such as chondromalacia, dislocation, subluxation, fracture, and parapatellar synovitis; condylar disease, such as degenerative articular cartilage, osteochondritis dissecans, and loose bodies; extrasynovial disease, such as torn anterior cruciate or tibial collateral ligaments, Baker's cyst, and ganglionic cyst; and synovial disease, such as synovitis, rheumatoid and degenerative arthritis, and foreign bodies associated with gout, pseudogout, and osteochondromatosis.

Depending on test findings, appropriate treatment or surgery can follow arthroscopy. If arthroscopic surgery cannot be performed, arthrotomy is the procedure of choice.

Ultrasonography

CARDIOVASCULAR SYSTEM

ECHOCARDIOGRAPHY

This noninvasive test shows the size, shape, and motion of cardiac structures. It is useful for evaluating patients with chest pain, enlarged cardiac silhouettes on X-ray films, electrocardiographic changes unrelated to coronary artery disease, and abnormal heart sounds on auscultation.

In echocardiography, a transducer directs ultra-high-frequency sound waves toward cardiac structures, which reflect these waves. The echoes are converted to images that are displayed on an oscilloscope screen and recorded on a strip chart or videotape. Results are correlated with clinical history, physical examination, and findings from additional tests.

The techniques most commonly used in echocardiography are M-mode (motion-mode), for recording the motion and dimensions of intracardiac structures, and two-dimensional (cross-sectional), for recording lateral motion and providing the correct spatial relationship between cardiac structures. (See *M-mode echocardiograms.*)

Purpose
• To diagnose and evaluate valvular abnormalities
• To measure the size of the heart's chambers
• To evaluate chambers and valves in congenital heart disorders
• To aid diagnosis of hypertrophic and related cardiomyopathies
• To detect atrial tumors

• To evaluate cardiac function or wall motion after myocardial infarction
• To detect pericardial effusion

Patient preparation
• Explain to the patient that this test is used to evaluate the size, shape, and motion of various cardiac structures.
• Inform him that he need not restrict food or fluids before the test.
• Tell him who will perform the test and where, that it usually takes 15 to 30 minutes, and that it is safe and painless.
• Explain that the room may be darkened slightly to aid visualization on the oscilloscope screen and that other procedures (electrocardiography and phonocardiography) may be performed simultaneously to time events in the cardiac cycle.
• Describe the procedure and instruct the patient to remain still during the test, as movement may distort results.
• Inform the patient that he may be asked to inhale a gas with a slightly sweet odor (amyl nitrite), while changes in heart function are recorded; describe the possible adverse effects of amyl nitrite (dizziness, flushing, and tachycardia), but assure the patient that such symptoms quickly subside.

Procedure and posttest care
• The patient is placed in supine position.
• Conductive jelly is applied to the third or fourth intercostal space to the left of the sternum, and the transducer is placed directly over it.
• The transducer is systematically angled to direct ultrasonic waves at specific parts of the patient's heart.
• Significant oscilloscopic findings are recorded on a strip chart recorder (M-mode echocardiography) or on a videotape recorder (two-dimensional echocardiography).
• For a different view of the heart, the transducer is placed beneath the xiph-

M-MODE ECHOCARDIOGRAMS

In this normal motion-mode echocardiogram of the mitral valve, valve movement appears as a characteristic lopsided M-shaped tracing. The anterior and posterior mitral valve leaflets separate (D) in early diastole, quickly reach maximum separation (E), then close during rapid ventricular filling (E-F). Leaflet separation varies during mid-diastole, and the valve opens widely again (A) following atrial contraction. The valve starts to close with atrial relaxation (A-B) and is completely closed during the start of ventricular systole (C). The steepness of the slope E-F indirectly shows the speed of ventricular filling, which is normally rapid.

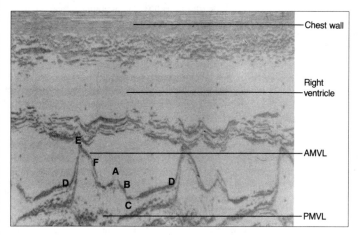

KEY:
AMVL = Anterior mitral valve leaflet
PMVL = Posterior mitral valve leaflet

Mitral stenosis is evident in this abnormal echocardiogram. The E-F slope (dashed line) is very shallow, indicating slowed left ventricular filling.

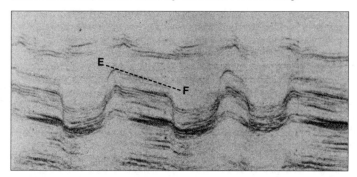

oid process or directly above the sternum.

• For a left lateral view, the patient may be positioned on his left side.

• To record heart function under various conditions, the patient is asked to inhale and exhale slowly, to hold his breath, or to inhale amyl nitrite.

• Remove conductive jelly from the skin.

Normal findings

An echocardiogram can reveal both the motion pattern and structure of the four cardiac valves. Anterior and posterior mitral valve leaflets normally separate in early diastole, with the anterior leaflet moving toward the chest wall and the posterior leaflet moving away from it. The leaflets attain maximum excursion rapidly, then move toward each other during ventricular diastole; after atrial contraction, they come together and remain so during ventricular systole. On an M-mode echocardiogram, the leaflets appear as two fine lines within the echo-free, blood-filled left ventricular cavity.

The aortic valve cusps lie between the parallel walls of the aortic root, which move anteriorly during systole and posteriorly during diastole. During ventricular systole, these cusps separate and appear as a boxlike configuration on an M-mode echocardiogram. They remain open throughout systole and normally demonstrate a characteristic fine fluttering motion. During diastole, the cusps come together and appear as a single or double line within the aortic root on an M-mode echocardiogram.

The motion of the tricuspid valve resembles that of the mitral valve. The motion of the pulmonary valve — particularly the posterior cusp — is different: During diastole, this cusp gradually moves posteriorly; during atrial systole, it is displaced posteriorly; during ventricular systole, it quickly moves poste-

riorly; and during right ventricular ejection, the cusp moves anteriorly, attaining its most anterior position during diastole.

The left ventricular cavity normally appears as an echo-free space between the interventricular septum and the posterior left ventricular wall. Echoes produced by the chordae tendineae and the mitral leaflet appear within this cavity. The right ventricular cavity normally appears as an echo-free space between the anterior chest wall and the interventricular septum.

Abnormal findings

Valvular abnormalities readily appear on the echocardiogram. In mitral stenosis, the valve narrows abnormally due to the leaflets' thickening and disordered motion. Instead of moving in opposite directions during diastole, both mitral valve leaflets move anteriorly. In mitral valve prolapse, one or both leaflets balloon into the left atrium during systole.

Aortic valve abnormalities — especially aortic insufficiency — can also affect the mitral valve because the anterior mitral leaflet is just below the aortic cusps. When blood regurgitates through the aortic valve during diastole, it strikes this leaflet, causing the flutter seen in M-mode. Although the aortic valve may appear normal, this characteristic fluttering confirms aortic insufficiency. In stenosis due to conditions such as rheumatic fever or bacterial endocarditis, the aortic valve thickens and thus generates more echoes. However, in rheumatic fever, the valve may thicken slightly and allow normal motion during systole, or it may thicken severely and curtail motion. In bacterial endocarditis, valve motion is disrupted, and shaggy or fuzzy echoes usually appear on or near the valve.

Other chamber or valve abnormalities may indicate a congenital heart disorder, such as aortic stenosis, which may require further tests. A large chamber size may indicate cardiomyopathy, valvular disorders, or congestive heart failure; a small chamber, restrictive pericarditis.

Idiopathic hypertrophic subaortic stenosis can also be identified by the echocardiogram, with systolic anterior motion of the mitral valve and asymmetric septal hypertrophy.

Left atrial tumor is usually on a pedicle, and can thus shift in and out of the mitral opening. During diastole, the tumor appears as a mass of echoes against the anterior mitral valve leaflet; during ventricular systole, these echoes shift back into the body of the atrium.

In coronary artery disease, ischemia or infarction may cause absent or paradoxical motion in ventricular walls that normally move together and thicken during systole. These affected areas may also fail to thicken or may become thinner, particularly if scar tissue is present.

The echocardiogram is especially sensitive in detecting pericardial effusion. Normally, the epicardium and pericardium are continuous membranes, and thus produce a single or near-single echo. When fluid accumulates between these membranes, it causes an abnormal echo-free space to appear. In large effusions, pressure exerted by excess fluid can restrict pericardial motion.

TRANSESOPHAGEAL ECHOCARDIOGRAPHY

In transesophageal echocardiography (TEE), ultrasound is combined with endoscopy to give a better view of the heart's structures. In this procedure, a small transducer is attached to the end of a gastroscope and inserted into the esophagus, allowing images to be taken from the posterior aspect of the heart. This causes less tissue penetration and interference from chest wall structures and produces high quality images of the thoracic aorta, except for the superior ascending aorta, which is shadowed by the trachea.

TEE is appropriate for both inpatients and outpatients, for patients under general anesthesia, and for critically ill, intubated patients.

Purpose
To visualize and evaluate:
• thoracic and aortic disorders, such as dissection and aneurysm
• valvular disease, especially in the mitral valve and in prosthetic devices
• endocarditis
• congenital heart disease
• intracardiac thrombi
• cardiac tumors
• valvular repairs

Patient preparation
• Explain to the patient that this test allows visual examination of heart function and structures.
• Tell him who will perform the test, when it's scheduled, and that he'll need to fast for 6 hours beforehand.
• Review the patient's medical history for possible contraindications to the test, such as esophageal obstruction or varices, GI bleeding, previous mediastinal radiation therapy, or severe cervical arthritis.
• Ask the patient about any allergies and note them on the chart.
• Before the test, have the patient remove any dentures or oral prostheses, and note any loose teeth.
• Explain that his throat will be sprayed with a topical anesthetic and that he may gag when the tube is inserted.
• Tell him that an I.V. line will be inserted to administer sedation before the

procedure and that he may feel some discomfort from the needle puncture and the pressure of the tourniquet. Reassure him that he'll be made as comfortable as possible during the procedure and that his blood pressure and heart rate will be monitored continuously.

• Make sure the patient or a responsible family member signs a consent form, if required.

Equipment

Cardiac monitor; sedative; topical anesthetic; bite block; gastroscope; ultrasonography equipment; suction equipment; resuscitation equipment.

Procedure and posttest care

• Connect the patient to a cardiac monitor so his blood pressure and pulse oximetry can be assessed during the procedure.

• Help him lie down on his left side, and administer the prescribed sedative.

• The back of the patient's throat is sprayed with a topical anesthetic.

• A bite block is placed in his mouth, and he's instructed to close his lips around it.

• A gastroscope is introduced and advanced 12″ to 14″ (30 to 35 cm) to the level of the right atrium. To visualize the left ventricle, the scope is advanced 16″ to 18″ (40 to 45 cm).

• Ultrasound images are recorded and then reviewed after the procedure.

• Monitor the patient's vital signs and oxygen levels for any changes.

• Keep the patient supine until the sedative wears off.

• Encourage the patient to cough after the procedure, either while lying on his side or sitting upright.

• Do not give food or water until the patient's gag response returns.

• If the procedure is done on an outpatient basis, make sure someone is available to drive the patient home.

• Treat sore throat symptomatically.

Precautions

• Keep resuscitation equipment readily available.

• Have suction equipment nearby to avoid aspiration if vomiting occurs.

• Vasovagal responses may occur with gagging, so observe the cardiac monitor closely.

• Use pulse oximetry to detect hypoxia.

• If bleeding occurs, stop the procedure immediately.

• Laryngospasm, arrhythmias, or bleeding increase the risk of complications. If any of these occurs, postpone the test.

Normal findings

TEE should reveal no cardiac problems.

Abnormal findings

TEE can reveal thoracic and aortic disorders, endocarditis, congenital heart disease, intracardiac thrombi, or tumors, or it can be used to evaluate valvular disease or repairs. Findings may include aortic dissection or aneurysm, mitral valve disease, or congenital defects such as patent ductus arteriosus.

DOPPLER ULTRASONOGRAPHY

This noninvasive test is used to evaluate blood flow in the major veins and arteries of the arms and legs and in the extracranial cerebrovascular system. An alternative to arteriography and venography, it is safer, less costly, and faster than invasive tests. Although this test can accurately detect arteriovenous disease that impairs blood flow by at least 50%, it may not reveal mild arteri-

HOW TO DETECT THROMBI WITH A DOPPLER PROBE

The Doppler probe is typically used to detect venous thrombi by first positioning the transducer and then occluding the blood vessel by compression (as illustrated with the normal leg at right). Water-soluble conductive jelly is applied to the tip of the transducer to provide coupling between the skin and the transducer.

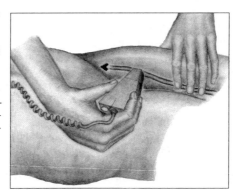

When pressure is released, allowing blood flow to resume, the transducer picks up the sudden augmentation of the flow sound and permits graphic recording of blood flow. If a thrombus is present, a compression maneuver fails to produce the augmented flow sound because the blood flow (as shown at right in the femoral vein) is significantly impaired.

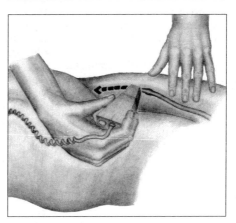

osclerotic plaques, smaller thrombi, and major calf vein thrombosis.

In Doppler ultrasonography, a handheld transducer directs high-frequency sound waves to the artery or vein being tested. The sound waves strike moving red blood cells and are reflected back to the transducer, allowing direct listening and graphic recording of blood flow. (See *How to detect thrombi with a Doppler probe.*)

Measurement of systolic pressure during this test is used to detect the presence, location, and extent of peripheral arterial occlusive disease. Changes in sound wave frequency during respiration are observed to detect venous occlusive disease. Compression maneuvers can also help detect occlusion of the veins and occlusion or stenosis of carotid arteries.

Pulse volume recorder testing may be performed with Doppler ultrasonography to record changes in blood volume or flow in an extremity or organ.

Purpose
• To aid diagnosis of chronic venous insufficiency and superficial and deep vein thromboses (popliteal, femoral, iliac)
• To aid diagnosis of peripheral artery disease and arterial occlusion
• To monitor patients who have had arterial reconstruction and bypass grafts
• To detect abnormalities of carotid artery blood flow associated with conditions such as aortic stenosis
• To evaluate possible arterial trauma

Patient preparation
• Explain to the patient that this test is used to evaluate blood flow in the arms and legs or neck.
• Tell the patient who will perform the test and that it takes about 20 minutes.
• Reassure the patient that the test does not involve risk or discomfort.
• Tell him he'll be asked to move his arms to different positions and to perform breathing exercises as measurements are taken; a small ultrasonic probe resembling a microphone is placed at various sites along veins or arteries, and blood pressure is checked at several sites.
• Check with the vascular laboratory about special equipment or instructions.

Procedure and posttest care
• Water-soluble conductive jelly is applied to the tip of the transducer.
  Peripheral arterial evaluation:
• The usual test sites in each leg are the common femoral, superficial femoral, popliteal, posterior tibial, and dorsalis pedis arteries; in each arm the test sites are usually the subclavian, brachial, radial, ulnar and, occasionally, the palmar arch and digital arteries.

• The patient is instructed to remove all clothing above or below the waist, depending on the test site, and he is placed in supine position on the examining table or bed, with his arms at his sides.
• Brachial blood pressure is measured, and the transducer is placed at various points along the test arteries.
• The signals are monitored and the waveforms recorded for later analysis.
• Segmental limb blood pressure is obtained to localize arterial occlusive disease.
• During lower extremity tests, a blood pressure cuff is wrapped around the calf, pressure readings are obtained, and waveforms recorded from the dorsalis pedis and posterior tibial arteries. Then the cuff is wrapped around the thigh, and waveforms are recorded at the popliteal artery.
• In upper extremity tests, examination is performed on one arm, with the patient first supine and then sitting; it's then repeated on the other arm. A blood pressure cuff is wrapped around the forearm, pressure readings are taken, and waveforms are recorded over both the radial and ulnar arteries. Then, the cuff is wrapped around the upper arm, pressure readings are taken, and waveforms are recorded with the transducer over the brachial artery. Blood pressure readings and waveform recordings are repeated with the arm in extreme hyperextension and hyperabduction to check for possible compression factors that may interfere with arterial blood flow.
  Peripheral venous evaluation:
• Usual test sites include the popliteal, superficial femoral, and common femoral veins in the leg and the posterior tibial vein at the ankle; the brachial, axillary, and subclavian veins in the arm; jugular veins; and, occasionally, the inferior and superior vena cava.
• The patient is instructed to remove all clothing above or below the waist, depending on the test site.

• He is placed in supine position and instructed to breathe normally.
• The transducer is placed over the appropriate vein, waveforms are recorded, and respiratory modulations noted.
• Proximal limb compression maneuvers are performed and augmentation noted after release of compression, to evaluate venous valve competency.
• Changes in respiration are monitored.
• During lower extremity tests, the patient is asked to perform Valsalva's maneuver, and venous blood flow is recorded.
• The procedure is repeated for the other arm or leg.

Extracranial cerebrovascular evaluation:
• Usual test sites include the supraorbital, common carotid, external carotid, internal carotid, and vertebral arteries.
• The patient is placed in supine position on the examining table or bed, with a pillow beneath his head for support.
• Brachial blood pressure is then recorded using the Doppler probe.
• The transducer is positioned over the test artery, and blood flow velocity is monitored and recorded.
• The influence of compression maneuvers on blood flow velocity is measured, and the procedure is repeated on the opposite side.

All procedures:
• Make sure the conductive jelly is removed from the patient's skin.

Precautions
• Do not place the Doppler probe over an open or draining lesion.

Normal findings
Arterial waveforms of the arms and legs are multiphasic, with a prominent systolic component and one or more diastolic sounds. The ankle-arm pressure index (API)—the ratio between ankle systolic pressure and brachial systolic pressure—is normally equal to or greater than 1. (The API is also known as arterial ischemia index, the ankle-brachial index, or the pedal-brachial index.) Proximal thigh pressure is normally 20 to 30 mm Hg higher than arm pressure, but pressure measurements at adjacent sites are similar. In the arms, pressure readings should remain unchanged despite postural changes.

Venous blood flow velocity is normally phasic with respiration, and is of a lower pitch than arterial flow. Distal compression or release of proximal limb compression increases blood flow velocity. In the legs, abdominal compression eliminates respiratory variations, but release increases blood flow; Valsalva's maneuver also interrupts venous flow velocity.

In cerebrovascular testing, a strong velocity signal is present. In the common carotid artery, blood flow velocity increases during diastole due to low peripheral vascular resistance of the brain. The direction of periorbital arterial flow is normally anterograde out of the orbit.

Abnormal findings
Arterial stenosis or occlusion diminishes the blood flow velocity signal, with no diastolic sound and a less prominent systolic component distal to the lesion. At the lesion, the signal is high-pitched and, occasionally, turbulent. If complete occlusion is present and collateral circulation has not taken over, the velocity signal may be absent.

A pressure gradient exceeding 20 to 30 mm Hg at adjacent sites of measurement in the leg may indicate occlusive disease. Specifically, low proximal thigh pressure signifies common femoral or aorto-iliac occlusive disease. An abnormal gradient between the proximal thigh and the above- or below-knee cuffs indicates superficial femoral or popliteal artery occlusive disease; an abnormal gradient between the below-knee and ankle cuffs indicates tibiofibular disease. Abnormal gradients of arm and forearm pressure readings may indicate brachial artery occlusion.

An abnormal API is directly proportional to the degree of circulatory impairment: mild ischemia, 1 to 0.75; claudication, 0.75 to 0.50; pain at rest, 0.50 to 0.25; and pregangrene, 0.25 to 0.

If venous blood flow velocity is unchanged by respirations, does not increase in response to compression or Valsalva's maneuvers, or is absent, venous thrombosis is indicated. In chronic venous insufficiency and varicose veins, the flow velocity signal may be reversed. Confirmation of results may require venography.

Inability to identify Doppler signals during cerebrovascular examination implies total arterial occlusion. Reversed periorbital arterial flow indicates significant arterial occlusive disease of the extracranial internal carotid artery. In addition, the audible signal may take on the acoustic characteristics of a normal peripheral artery. Stenosis of the internal carotid artery causes turbulent signals. Collateral circulation can be assessed by compression maneuvers.

Oculoplethysmography, carotid phonoangiography, or carotid imaging can further evaluate cerebrovascular disease. Retrograde blood velocity in the vertebral artery can indicate subclavian steal syndrome. Weak velocity signal on comparison of contralateral vertebral arteries can indicate diffuse vertebral artery disease.

ULTRASONOGRAPHY OF THE ABDOMINAL AORTA

In this safe, noninvasive test, a transducer directs high-frequency sound waves into the abdomen over a wide area from the xiphoid process to the umbilical region. The echoing sound waves are displayed on a monitor to indicate internal organs, the vertebral column, and the size and course of the abdominal aorta and other major vessels.

Purpose

• To detect and measure suspected abdominal aortic aneurysm (findings may be supported and refined by angiography)
• To detect and measure expansion of known abdominal aortic aneurysm and thereby assess risk of rupture

Patient preparation

• Explain to the patient that this test allows examination of the abdominal aorta.
• Instruct the patient to fast for 12 hours before the test to minimize bowel gas and motility.
• Tell him who will perform the test and where, that the lights may be lowered, that he will feel only slight pressure, and that the test takes 30 to 45 minutes.
• Describe the procedure and reassure the patient with a known aneurysm that the sound waves will not cause rupture.
• Instruct him to remain still during scanning and to hold his breath when requested.
• Give simethicone to reduce bowel gas.

Procedure and posttest care
• The patient is placed in a supine position, and acoustic coupling gel or mineral oil is applied to his abdomen.
• Longitudinal scans are made at 0.5- to 1-cm intervals left and right of the midline until the entire abdominal aorta is outlined; transverse scans are made at 1- to 2-cm intervals from the xiphoid to the bifurcation at the common iliac arteries.
• The patient may be placed in right and left lateral positions.
• Appropriate views are photographed or videotaped.
• Remove the acoustic coupling gel.
• Instruct the patient to resume his usual diet and medications.
• Aneurysms may expand and dissect rapidly, so check the patient's vital signs frequently. Remember that sudden onset of constant abdominal or back pain accompanies rapid expansion of the aneurysm; sudden, excruciating pain with weakness, sweating, tachycardia, and hypotension signals rupture.

Normal findings
In adults, the normal abdominal aorta tapers from about 2.5 to 1.5 cm in diameter along its length from the diaphragm to the bifurcation. It descends through the retroperitoneal space, anterior to the vertebral column and slightly left of the midline. Four of its major branches are usually well visualized: the celiac trunk, the renal arteries, the superior mesenteric artery, and the common iliac arteries.

Abnormal findings
Luminal diameter of the abdominal aorta greater than 1½″ (4 cm) suggests aneurysm; greater than 2¾″ (7 cm) suggests aneurysm with high risk of rupture.

GASTROINTESTINAL SYSTEM

ULTRASONOGRAPHY OF THE GALLBLADDER AND THE BILIARY SYSTEM

In ultrasonography of the gallbladder and the biliary system, a focused beam of high-frequency sound waves passes into the right upper quadrant of the abdomen, creating echoes that vary with changes in tissue density. These echoes are converted to images on a screen, indicating the size, shape, and position of the gallbladder and biliary system.

Purpose
• To confirm diagnosis of cholelithiasis (oral cholecystography may be performed if ultrasound is inconclusive)
• To diagnose acute cholecystitis
• To distinguish between obstructive and nonobstructive jaundice

Patient preparation
• Explain to the patient that this procedure allows examination of the gallbladder and the biliary system.
• Instruct him to eat a fat-free meal in the evening and then to fast for 8 to 12 hours before the procedure, if possible; this promotes accumulation of bile in the gallbladder and enhances ultrasonic visualization.
• Tell him who will perform the procedure and where. The test takes 15 to 30 minutes.
• Tell the patient that the room may be darkened slightly to aid visualization on the screen.

• Describe the procedure; assure him he'll feel only mild pressure as the transducer passes over his skin.
• Instruct him to remain as still as possible during the procedure and to hold his breath when requested to ensure that the gallbladder is in the same position for each scan.

Procedure and posttest care
• The patient is placed in supine position.
• A water-soluble lubricant is applied to the face of the transducer.
• Transverse and longitudinal oblique scans of the gallbladder are taken.
• During each scan, the patient is asked to exhale deeply and hold his breath. (If the gallbladder is positioned deeply under the right costal margin, a scan may be taken through the intercostal spaces, while the patient inhales deeply and holds his breath.)
• The patient is then placed in a left lateral decubitus position and is scanned beneath the right costal margin. (This position and scanning angle may displace and allow detection of stones lodged in the cystic duct region.)
• Scanning with the patient erect helps demonstrate mobility or fixity of suspicious echogenic areas. Oscilloscopic views may be photographed for later study.
• Remove the lubricating jelly from the patient's skin.
• Inform the patient that he may resume his usual diet.

Precautions
• Keep the patient in a fasting state to prevent the excretion of bile in the gallbladder.

Normal findings
The normal gallbladder is sonolucent; it appears circular on transverse scans and pear-shaped on longitudinal scans. Although the size of the gallbladder varies, its outer walls normally appear sharp and smooth. Intrahepatic radicles seldom appear because the flow of sonolucent bile is very fine. The cystic duct may also be indistinct—the result of folds known as Heister's valves that line the cystic duct lumen. When visualized, the cystic duct has a serpentine appearance. The common bile duct, in contrast, has a linear appearance but is sometimes obscured by overlying bowel gas.

Abnormal findings
Gallstones within the gallbladder lumen or the biliary system typically appear as mobile, echogenic areas, usually associated with an acoustic shadow. The size of gallstones generally parallels the size of their shadows; gallstones 5 mm or larger usually produce shadows. However, if the gallbladder is distended with bile, gallstones as small as 1 mm can be detected because of the acoustic contrast between liquid bile and solid gallstones. Detecting stones in the biliary ducts, which contain little bile, may be difficult. When the gallbladder is shrunken or fully impacted with gallstones, inadequate bile may likewise make gallstone detection difficult, and the gallbladder itself might not be detectable. In this case, an acoustic shadow in the gallbladder fossa indicates cholelithiasis; the presence of such a shadow in the cystic and common bile ducts can also indicate cholelithiasis.

Polyps and carcinoma within the gallbladder lumen are distinguished from gallstones by their fixity. Polyps usually appear as sharply defined, echogenic areas; carcinoma appears as a poorly defined mass, often associated with a thickened gallbladder wall.

Biliary sludge within the gallbladder lumen appears as a fine layer of echoes that slowly gravitates to the dependent portion of the gallbladder as the patient changes position. Although biliary sludge may arise without accompanying pathology, it may also result from obstruction and can predispose to gallstone formation.

Acute cholecystitis is indicated by an enlarged gallbladder with thickened, double-rimmed walls, usually with gallstones within the lumen. In chronic cholecystitis, the walls of the gallbladder appear thickened; the organ itself, however, is generally contracted. In obstructive jaundice, ultrasonography readily demonstrates a dilated biliary system and, usually, a dilated gallbladder. Dilated intrahepatic radicles appear tortuous and irregular; a dilated gallbladder usually loses its characteristic pear shape, becoming spherical.

Biliary obstruction may result from intrinsic factors, such as a gallstone or small carcinoma within the biliary system. (Ultrasonography cannot distinguish between these two echogenic masses.) Or, it may result from extrinsic factors, such as a mass in the hepatic portal that compresses the cystic duct and interferes with bile drainage from the intrahepatic radicles, or from pathology in the head of the pancreas that obstructs the common bile duct. Such pathology includes carcinoma and pancreatitis, although ultrasonography cannot distinguish between the two. When ultrasonography fails to clearly define the site of biliary obstruction, percutaneous transhepatic cholangiography or endoscopic retrograde cholangiopancreatography should be performed.

ULTRASONOGRAPHY OF THE LIVER

Ultrasonography of the liver produces images by channeling high-frequency sound waves into the right upper quadrant of the abdomen. Resultant echoes are converted to cross-sectional images on a monitor; different shades of gray depict various tissue densities. Ultrasound can show intrahepatic structures and organ size, shape, and position. This procedure is indicated in patients with jaundice of unknown etiology, with unexplained hepatomegaly and abnormal biochemical test results, with suspected metastatic tumors and elevated serum alkaline phosphatase levels, and with recent abdominal trauma.

When used with liver-spleen scanning, ultrasonography can define cold spots (focal defects that fail to pick up the radionuclide) as tumors, abscesses, or cysts; it also provides better views of the periportal and perihepatic spaces than liver-spleen scanning. If ultrasonography fails to provide definitive diagnosis, computed tomography, gallium scanning, or liver biopsy may yield more information.

Purpose
• To distinguish between obstructive and nonobstructive jaundice
• To screen for hepatocellular disease
• To detect hepatic metastases and hematoma
• To define cold spots as tumors, abscesses, or cysts

Patient preparation
• Explain to the patient that this procedure allows examination of the liver.
• Instruct him to fast for 8 to 12 hours before the test to reduce bowel gas,

which hinders transmission of ultrasound.

• Describe the procedure; tell him who will perform the test and where and that the test takes 15 to 30 minutes.

• Assure him this test is not harmful or painful, although he may feel mild pressure as the transducer is pressed against his skin.

• Instruct him to remain as still as possible during the procedure and to hold his breath when requested.

Procedure and posttest care

• The patient is placed in supine position.

• A water-soluble lubricant is applied to the face of the transducer.

• Transverse scans between the costal margins demonstrate the left lobe of the liver and part of the right lobe; sector scans through the intercostal spaces are used to view the remainder of the right lobe.

• Scans are taken longitudinally from the right border of the liver to the left.

• For better demonstration of the right lateral dome, oblique cephalad-angled scans may be taken beneath the right costal margin.

• Scans are then taken parallel to the hepatic portal, at a 45-degree angle toward the superior right lateral dome, to examine the peripheral anatomy, portal venous system, common bile duct, and biliary tree. Clear images are photographed for later study.

• During each scan, ask the patient to hold his breath briefly in deep inspiration to displace the liver caudally from the costal margin and the ribs to aid visualization.

• Remove the lubricating jelly from the patient's skin.

• Inform the patient that he may resume his usual diet.

Normal findings

The liver normally demonstrates a homogeneous, low-level echo pattern, interrupted only by the different echo patterns of its portal and hepatic veins, the aorta, and the inferior vena cava. Hepatic veins appear completely sonolucent; portal veins have margins that are highly echogenic.

Abnormal findings

In obstructive jaundice, ultrasonography shows dilated intrahepatic biliary radicles and extrahepatic ducts. Conversely, in nonobstructive jaundice, ultrasonography shows a biliary tree of normal diameter.

Ultrasonographic characteristics of hepatocellular disease are generally nonspecific, and disorders in early stages can escape detection; liver-spleen scanning is a more sensitive diagnostic tool. In cirrhosis, ultrasonography may demonstrate variable liver size; dilated, tortuous portal branches associated with portal hypertension; and an irregular echo pattern with increased echo amplitude, causing overall increased attenuation. Demonstration of splenomegaly by spleen ultrasonography or liver-spleen scanning aids diagnosis. In fatty infiltration of the liver, ultrasonography may show hepatomegaly and a regular echo pattern that, although greater in echo amplitude than that of normal parenchyma, does not alter attenuation.

Ultrasonographic characteristics of metastases in the liver vary widely; metastases may appear either hypoechoic or echogenic, poorly defined or well defined. For example, metastatic lymphomas and sarcomas are generally hypoechoic; mucin-secreting adenocarcinoma of the colon is highly echogenic. Liver biopsy is necessary to confirm tumor type. Serial ultrasonography may be used to monitor the effectiveness of therapy.

Primary hepatic tumors also present a varied appearance and may mimic metastases, requiring angiography and liver biopsy for definitive diagnosis. Hepatomas are the most common malignant tumors in adults; hepatoblastomas are most common in children. Benign tumors are far less common than malignant ones.

Abscesses usually appear as sonolucent masses with ill-defined, slightly thickened borders and accentuated posterior wall transmission; scattered internal echoes, caused by necrotic debris, may also be present. Because they produce similar echo patterns, intrahepatic abscesses are occasionally mistaken for hematomas, necrotic metastases, or hemorrhagic cysts. Gas-containing intrahepatic abscesses, which may be echogenic, are sometimes confused with solid intrahepatic lesions. Subphrenic abscesses occur between the diaphragm and the liver; subhepatic abscesses appear inferior to the liver and anterior to the upper pole of the right kidney. Ascitic fluid resembles a subhepatic abscess, but lacks internal echoes and has a more regular border.

Cysts usually appear as spherical, sonolucent areas with well-defined borders and accentuated posterior wall transmission. When a cyst cannot be distinguished from an abscess or necrotic metastases, gallium scanning, computed tomography, and angiography should be performed.

Hematomas—either intrahepatic or subcapsular—usually result from trauma. Intrahepatic hematomas appear as poorly defined, relatively sonolucent masses and may have scattered internal echoes due to clotting; serial ultrasonography can differentiate between a hematoma and a cyst or tumor as the hematoma becomes smaller. Subcapsular hematoma may appear as a focal, sonolucent mass on the periphery of the liver or as a diffuse, sonolucent area surrounding part of the liver.

ULTRASONOGRAPHY OF THE SPLEEN

In this test, a focused beam of high-frequency sound waves passes into the left upper quadrant of the abdomen, creating echoes that vary with changes in tissue density. These are displayed on a monitor as real-time images that indicate the size, shape, and position of the spleen and surrounding viscera.

Ultrasonography is indicated in patients with an upper left quadrant mass of unknown origin; with known splenomegaly, to evaluate changes in splenic size; with left upper quadrant pain and local tenderness; and with recent abdominal trauma.

Purpose
• To demonstrate splenomegaly
• To monitor progression of primary and secondary splenic disease and to evaluate effectiveness of therapy
• To evaluate the spleen after abdominal trauma
• To help detect splenic cysts and subphrenic abscess

Patient preparation
• Explain to the patient that this procedure allows examination of the spleen.
• Tell him who will perform this test and where, that the room may be darkened slightly to aid visualization on the monitor, and that this procedure takes approximately 15 to 30 minutes.
• Instruct him to fast for 8 to 12 hours before the procedure, if possible; this reduces the amount of gas in the bowel, which hinders transmission of ultrasound.

• Describe the procedure and assure him he will feel only mild pressure.

• Instruct him to remain as still as possible during the procedure and to hold his breath when requested, to aid visualization.

Procedure and posttest care

• Because the procedure for ultrasonography varies, depending on the size of the spleen or the patient's physique, the patient is usually repositioned several times; the transducer scanning angle or path is also changed.

• Generally, the patient is first placed in supine position, with his chest uncovered.

• A water-soluble lubricant is applied to the face of the transducer, and transverse scans of the spleen are taken at ⅜″ to ¾″ (1- to 2-cm) intervals.

• The patient is then placed in right lateral decubitus position, and transverse scans are taken through the intercostal spaces using a sectoring motion.

• A pillow may be placed under the patient's right side to help separate the intercostal spaces making it easier to position the transducer face between them.

• Longitudinal scans are taken from the axilla toward the iliac crest.

• To prevent rib artifacts and obtain the best view of the splenic parenchyma, oblique scans are taken by passing the transducer face along the intercostal spaces.

• During each scan, the patient may be asked to hold his breath briefly at various stages of inspiration.

• Good views are photographed for later study.

• Remove the lubricating jelly from the patient's skin.

• Inform the patient that he may resume his usual diet.

Normal findings

The splenic parenchyma normally demonstrates a homogeneous, low-level echo pattern; its individual vascular channels are not usually apparent. The superior and lateral splenic borders are clearly defined, each having a convex margin. The undersurface and medial borders, in contrast, show indentations from surrounding organs (stomach, left kidney, and pancreas). The hilar region, where the vascular pedicle enters the spleen, commonly produces an area of highly reflective echoes. The medial surface is generally concave, which helps differentiate between left upper quadrant masses and an enlarged spleen. Even when splenomegaly is present, the spleen generally remains concave medially unless a space-occupying lesion distorts this contour.

Abnormal findings

Ultrasonography can show splenomegaly, but it usually does not indicate the cause; a computed tomography (CT) scan can provide more specific information. Splenomegaly is generally characterized by increased echogenicity. Enlarged vascular channels are commonly visible, especially in the hilar region. If space-occupying lesions distort the splenic contour, liver-spleen scanning should be performed to confirm splenomegaly.

Abdominal trauma may result in splenic rupture or subcapsular hematoma. In splenic rupture, ultrasonography demonstrates splenomegaly and an irregular, sonolucent area (the presence of free intraperitoneal fluid); however, these findings must be confirmed by arteriography. In subcapsular hematoma, ultrasonography shows splenomegaly, as well as a double contour, altered splenic position, and a relatively sonolucent area on the periphery of the spleen. The double contour results from blood accumulation between the splenic parenchyma and the intact splenic capsule. As the spleen enlarges, a transverse section shows its anterior margin extending more anteriorly than the aorta. Ultrasonography may be difficult and painful after abdominal trauma because the transducer may have to pass across fractured ribs and contusions; CT scanning, which differentiates blood and fluid in the peritoneal space, should be used instead.

In subphrenic abscess, ultrasonography shows a sonolucent area beneath the diaphragm. Clinical findings may differentiate between abscess and blood or fluid accumulation.

Used with liver-spleen scanning, ultrasonography differentiates cold spots as cystic or solid lesions. It shows cysts as spherical, sonolucent areas with well-defined, regular margins with acoustic enhancement behind them. When ultrasonography fails to identify a cyst as splenic or extrasplenic—especially if the cyst is located in the upper pole of the left kidney and the adrenal gland, or in the tail of the pancreas—a CT scan and arteriography are used. Ultrasonography can readily clarify cystic cold spots, but using a CT scan with a contrast medium is superior for evaluating primary and metastatic tumors. Ultrasonography usually fails to identify tumors associated with lymphoma and chronic leukemias because these resemble tumors of the splenic parenchyma.

ULTRASONOGRAPHY OF THE PANCREAS

In this noninvasive test, cross-sectional images of the pancreas are produced by channeling high-frequency sound waves into the epigastric region, converting the resultant echoes to real time images, which are displayed on a monitor. The pattern varies with tissue density and indicates the size, shape, and position of the pancreas and surrounding viscera.

Purpose
• To help detect anatomic abnormalities and aid diagnosis of pancreatitis, pseudocysts, and pancreatic carcinoma
• To guide insertion of biopsy needles

Patient preparation
• Explain to the patient that this procedure permits examination of the pancreas.
• Instruct him to fast for 8 to 12 hours before the procedure, to reduce bowel gas.
• Tell him who will perform the procedure and where, that the room is darkened slightly to aid visualization, and that this test takes 30 minutes.
• If the patient is a smoker, ask him to abstain before the test; this eliminates the risk of swallowing air while inhaling, which interferes with test results.
• Describe the procedure and assure him this isn't harmful or painful, but he may experience mild pressure.
• Tell him he'll be asked to inhale deeply during scanning, and instruct him to remain still during the procedure.

Procedure and posttest care
• The patient is placed in supine position.
• A water-soluble lubricant or mineral oil is applied to the abdomen and, with the patient at full inspiration, transverse scans are taken at 1-cm intervals, starting from the xiphoid and moving caudally; longitudinal scans are taken to view the head, body, and tail of the pancreas in sequence; scanning the right anterior oblique view allows imaging of the head and body of the pancreas; oblique sagittal scans are used to view

the portal vein; and scanning from the sagittal view images the vena cava.

• Good oscilloscopic views are photographed for later study.

• Make sure the lubricating jelly is removed from the patient's skin.

• Inform the patient that he may resume his usual diet.

Normal findings

The pancreas normally demonstrates a coarse, uniform echo pattern and usually appears more echogenic than the adjacent liver.

Abnormal findings

Alterations in the size, contour, and parenchymal texture of the pancreas characterize pancreatic disease. An enlarged pancreas with decreased echogenicity and distinct borders suggests pancreatitis; a well-defined mass with an essentially echo-free interior indicates pseudocyst; an ill-defined mass with scattered internal echoes or a mass in the head of the pancreas (obstructing the common bile duct) and a large noncontracting gallbladder suggest pancreatic carcinoma.

Subsequent CT scan and biopsy of the pancreas may be necessary to confirm a diagnosis.

MISCELLANEOUS TESTS

THYROID ULTRASONOGRAPHY

In this safe, noninvasive procedure, ultrasonic pulses emitted from a transducer are directed at the thyroid gland and reflected back to produce structural images on an oscilloscope screen.

When a mass is located by palpation or by thyroid imaging, thyroid ultrasonography can differentiate between a cyst and a tumor larger than ⅜" (1 cm) with a high degree of accuracy. This test is also used to evaluate thyroid nodules during pregnancy because it doesn't require use of radioactive iodine.

Purpose

• To evaluate thyroid structure

• To differentiate between a cyst and a solid tumor

• To monitor the size of the thyroid gland during suppressive therapy

Patient preparation

• Describe the procedure to the patient, and explain that this test defines the size and shape of the thyroid gland.

• Inform him that he need not restrict food or fluids before the test.

• Tell him who will perform the procedure and where, that it takes approximately 30 minutes, that it is painless and safe, and that test results are usually available within 24 hours.

Equipment

Sonographic equipment; camera and film or videotape; water-soluble contact solution.

Procedure and posttest care

• The patient is placed in a supine position, with a pillow under his shoulder blades to hyperextend his neck.

• His neck is coated with water-soluble gel, and scanning proceeds.

• The image on the oscilloscope screen is photographed for subsequent examination.

• Accurate visualization of the anterior portion of the thyroid requires use of a short-focused transducer.

• Thoroughly clean the patient's neck to remove the contact solution.

Normal findings

Normally, thyroid ultrasonography exhibits a uniform echo pattern throughout the gland.

Abnormal findings

Cysts appear as smooth-bordered, echo-free areas with enhanced sound transmission; adenomas and carcinomas appear either solid and well demarcated with identical echo patterns or, less frequently, solid with cystic areas. Carcinoma infiltrating the gland may not be well demarcated.

Identification of a tumor is generally followed up by fine needle aspiration or an excisional biopsy to determine malignancy.

PELVIC ULTRASONOGRAPHY

In pelvic ultrasonography, high-frequency sound waves are reflected to a transducer to provide images of the interior pelvic area on a screen. Techniques of sound imaging include A-mode (amplitude modulation, recorded as spikes), B-mode (brightness modulation), gray scale (a representation of organ texture in shades of gray), and real-time imaging (instantaneous images of the tissues in motion, similar to fluoroscopic examination). Selected views may be photographed for later examination and a permanent record of the test.

Purpose

• To evaluate symptoms that suggest pelvic disease and to confirm tentative diagnosis

• To detect foreign bodies and distinguish between cystic and solid masses (tumors)
• To measure organ size
• To evaluate fetal viability, position, gestational age, and growth rate
• To detect multiple pregnancy
• To confirm fetal abnormalities and maternal abnormalities
• To guide amniocentesis by determining placental location and fetal position

Patient preparation

• Describe the test to the patient, and tell her the reason it is being performed.
• Assure her that this procedure is safe, noninvasive, and painless.
• Because this test requires a full bladder as a landmark to define pelvic organs, instruct the patient to drink liquids and not to void before the test.
• Tell her who will perform the procedure and where and that it can vary in length from a few minutes to several hours.
• Explain that a water enema may be necessary to produce a better outline of the large intestine.
• Reassure the patient that the test will not harm the fetus, and provide emotional support throughout.

Equipment

Mineral oil or water-soluble jelly; ultrasound machine and transducer; camera and film or videotape; oscilloscope.

Procedure and posttest care

• With the patient in supine position, the pelvic area is coated with mineral oil or water-soluble jelly to increase sound wave conduction.
• The transducer is guided over the area, images are observed on the oscilloscope screen, and a good image is photographed.
• Allow the patient to empty her bladder immediately after the test.

Normal findings

The uterus is normal in size and shape. The ovaries' size, shape, and sonographic density are normal. No other masses are visible. If the patient is pregnant, the gestational sac and fetus are of normal size in relation to gestational age.

Abnormal findings

Both cystic and solid masses have homogeneous densities, but solid masses (such as fibroids) appear more dense. Inappropriate fetal size may indicate miscalculated conception or delivery date or a dead fetus. Abnormal echo patterns may indicate foreign bodies (such as an intrauterine device), multiple pregnancy, maternal abnormalities (such as placenta previa or abruptio placentae), fetal abnormalities (such as molar pregnancy or abnormalities of the arms and legs, spine, heart, head, kidneys, and abdomen), fetal malpresentation (such as breech or shoulder presentation), and cephalopelvic disproportion.

RENAL ULTRASONOGRAPHY

In this test, high-frequency sound waves are transmitted from a transducer to the kidneys and perirenal structures. The resulting echoes are displayed on an oscilloscope screen as anatomic images.

Renal ultrasonography can be used to detect abnormalities or clarify those detected by other tests. It is especially useful in cases where excretory urography is ruled out. Unlike excretory urography, this test is not dependent on renal function and therefore may be useful in patients with renal failure.

Ultrasonography of the ureter, bladder, and gonads also may be used to evaluate urologic disorders.

Purpose

• To determine the size, shape, and position of the kidneys, their internal structures, and perirenal tissues
• To evaluate and localize urinary obstruction and abnormal fluid accumulation
• To assess and diagnose complications after kidney transplantation

Patient preparation

• Explain to the patient that this test is used to detect kidney abnormalities.
• Inform him that he need not restrict food or fluids.
• Tell him who will perform the test and where, that it takes about 30 minutes, and that it is safe and painless.

Equipment

Ultrasound transducer and jelly; cathode ray tube and amplifier; oscilloscope; Polaroid camera; dynamic or real-time imaging equipment.

Procedure and posttest care

• The patient is placed in prone position, the area to be scanned is exposed, and ultrasound jelly is applied to the area.
• The longitudinal axis of the kidneys is located by using measurements from excretory urography or by performing transverse scans through the upper and lower renal poles.
• These points are marked on the skin and connected with straight lines. Sectional images $\frac{3}{8}''$ to $\frac{3}{4}''$ (1 to 2 cm) apart can then be obtained.
• During the test, the patient may be asked to breathe deeply to assess the kidneys' movement during respiration.
• Make sure ultrasound jelly is removed from the patient's skin.

Normal findings

The kidneys are located between the superior iliac crests and the diaphragm. The renal capsule should be outlined sharply; the cortex should produce more echoes than the medulla. In the center of each kidney, the renal collecting systems appear as irregular areas of higher density than surrounding tissue. The renal veins and, depending on the scanner, some internal structures can be visualized. If the bladder is also being evaluated, its size, shape, position, and urine content can be determined.

Abnormal findings

Cysts are usually fluid-filled, circular structures that do not reflect sound waves. Tumors produce multiple echoes and appear as irregular shapes. Abscesses found within or around the kidneys usually echo sound waves poorly; their boundaries are slightly more irregular than those of cysts. A perirenal abscess may displace the kidney anteriorly.

Generally, acute pyelonephritis and glomerulonephritis are not detectable unless the renal parenchyma is significantly scarred and atrophied. In such patients, the renal capsule appears irregular and the kidney may appear smaller than normal; also, an increased number of echoes may arise from the parenchyma due to fibrosis.

In patients with hydronephrosis, renal ultrasonography may show a large, echo-free, central mass that compresses the renal cortex. Calyceal echoes are usually circularly diffused and the pelvis significantly enlarged. This test can also be used to detect congenital anomalies, such as horseshoe, ectopic, or duplicated kidneys. Ultrasonography clearly detects renal hypertrophy.

Following renal transplantation, compensatory hypertrophy of the transplanted kidney is normal but an acute increase in size indicates rejection.

This test allows identification of abnormal accumulations of fluid within or around the kidneys that sometimes arise from an obstruction. It also allows evaluation of perirenal structures and can identify abnormalities of the adrenal glands, such as tumors, cysts, and adrenal dysfunction. However, a normal adrenal gland is difficult to define ultrasonically because of its small size.

Renal ultrasonography can be used to detect changes in the shape of the bladder that result from masses and can assess urine volume. Increased urine volume or residual urine postvoiding may indicate bladder dysfunction.

TRANSCRANIAL DOPPLER STUDIES

These studies provide information about the presence, quality, and changing nature of circulation to an area of the brain by measuring the velocity of blood flow through cerebral arteries. Narrowed blood vessels produce high velocities, indicating possible stenosis or vasospasm. High velocities may also indicate an arteriovenous malformation.

Purpose

- To measure the velocity of blood flow through certain cerebral vessels
- To detect and monitor the progression of cerebral vasospasm
- To determine whether collateral blood flow exists before surgical ligation or radiologic occlusion of diseased vessels
- To help determine brain death

Patient preparation

- Explain the purpose of the study to the patient (or to his family).

• Tell him that the test will be done while he lies on a bed or stretcher or sits in a reclining chair (or it can be performed at the bedside if he's too ill to be transported to the laboratory).

• Describe the procedure and tell the patient that it usually takes less than 1 hour, depending on the number of vessels to be examined and any interfering factors (in a complete study, the middle cerebral arteries, anterior cerebral arteries, posterior cerebral arteries, ophthalmic arteries, carotid siphon, vertebral arteries, and basilar artery are studied).

• Tell the patient that fasting is not required before the test.

Equipment
Transcranial Doppler unit; probe; gel.

Procedure and posttest care
• The patient reclines in a chair or on a stretcher or bed.

• A small amount of gel is applied to the transcranial window (an area where bone is thin enough to allow the Doppler signal to enter and be detected); the most common approaches are temporal, transorbital, and through the foramen magnum.

• The technician directs the signal toward the artery being studied and records the velocities detected; waveforms may be printed for later analysis.

• The Doppler signal can be transmitted to varying depths.

• When the study is completed, wipe the gel away.

Precautions
• Be sure to remove turban head dressings or thick dressings over the test site.

Normal findings
The type of waveforms and velocities obtained indicate whether or not pathology exists.

Abnormal findings
Although this test often is not definitive, high velocities are typically abnormal and suggest that blood flow is too turbulent or the vessel is too narrow.

After the transcranial Doppler study and before surgery, the patient may undergo cerebral angiography to further define cerebral blood flow patterns and to locate the exact vascular abnormality.

Radiography

REPRODUCTIVE SYSTEM

SKELETAL SYSTEM

MISCELLANEOUS TESTS

NEUROLOGIC SYSTEM

SKULL RADIOGRAPHY

Although of limited value in assessing patients with head injuries, skull X-rays are extremely valuable for studying abnormalities of the base of the skull and the cranial vault, congenital and perinatal anomalies, and systemic diseases that produce bone defects of the skull.

Skull radiography evaluates the three groups of bones that comprise the skull: the calvaria (vault), the mandible (jaw bone), and the facial bones. The calvaria and the facial bones are closely connected by immovable joints with irregular serrated edges called sutures. The bones of the skull form an anatomic structure so complex that a complete skull examination requires several radiologic views of each area.

Purpose

• To detect fractures in patients with head trauma
• To aid diagnosis of pituitary tumors
• To detect congenital anomalies

Patient preparation

• Explain to the patient that his head will be immobilized and that several X-rays of his skull will be taken from various angles.
• Tell him that this test helps determine the presence of fractures, tumors, or other anomalies.
• Explain that a radiologic technician will perform the test. Describe where it will take place (usually the radiology department). Tell him that it takes about 15 minutes and does not cause discomfort.

• Explain that he need not restrict food or fluid before the test.
• Tell him to remove glasses, dentures, jewelry, or any metal objects that would be in the X-ray field.

Procedure and posttest care

• Have the patient recline on the X-ray table or sit in a chair.
• Tell him to remain still during the procedure.
• Use foam pads, sandbags, or a headband to immobilize the patient's head and increase comfort.
• Five views of the skull are routinely taken: left and right lateral, anteroposterior Townes, posteroanterior Caldwell, and axial (or base).
• Films are developed and checked for quality before the patient leaves the area.

Normal findings

A radiologist interprets the X-rays, evaluating the size, shape, thickness, and position of the cranial bones as well as the vascular markings, sinuses, and sutures. All should be normal for the patient's age.

Abnormal findings

Skull radiography is often used to diagnose fractures of the vault or base, although basilar fractures may not show on the film if the bone is dense. This test may confirm congenital anomalies and may show erosion, enlargement, or decalcification of the sella turcica that result from increased intracranial pressure (ICP). A marked rise in ICP may cause the brain to expand and press against the inner bony table of the skull, yielding visible marks or impressions.

In conditions such as osteomyelitis (with possible calcification of the skull itself) and chronic subdural hematomas, X-rays may show abnormal areas of calcification. The X-rays can detect neoplasms within brain substance that contains calcium (such as oligodendro-gliomas or meningiomas) or the mid-line shifting of a calcified pineal gland caused by a space-occupying lesion.

Radiography may also detect other changes in bone structure, such as those that arise from metabolic disorders like acromegaly or Paget's disease.

CEREBRAL ANGIOGRAPHY

Cerebral angiography involves inject-ing a contrast medium to allow radio-graphic examination of the cerebral vasculature. Possible injection sites in-clude the femoral, carotid, and brachial arteries. Because it allows visualization of four vessels (the carotid and the ver-tebral arteries), the femoral artery is used most often.

Usually, this test is performed on pa-tients with suspected abnormality of the cerebral vasculature; abnormalities may be suggested by intracranial com-puted tomography or lumbar puncture.

Purpose
• To detect cerebrovascular abnormali-ties such as aneurysm or arteriovenous malformation, thrombosis, narrowing, or occlusion
• To study vascular displacement caused by tumor, hematoma, edema, herniation, vasospasm, increased in-tracranial pressure (ICP), or hydro-cephalus
• To locate clips applied to blood ves-sels during surgery and to evaluate the postoperative status of affected vessels

Patient preparation
• Explain to the patient that this test shows blood circulation in the brain.

• Describe the test, including who will administer it, where it will take place, and its duration (usually 2 to 4 hours, depending on the tests ordered).
• Tell the patient to fast for 8 to 10 hours before the test.
• Explain that he will wear a hospital gown and that he must remove all jew-elry, dentures, hairpins, and other radio-paque objects before the test.
• If appropriate, administer a sedative and an anticholinergic drug 30 to 45 minutes before the test.
• Make sure the patient voids before leaving his room.
• Tell him that he'll be positioned on an X-ray table, with his head immobilized, and that he should remain still when told.
• Explain that a local anesthetic will be administered at the angiocatheter inser-tion site (some patients — especially children — receive a general anesthet-ic).
• Describe possible adverse effects as-sociated with the contrast medium, such as a transient burning sensation as the medium is injected; a warm, flushed feeling; transient headache; a salty taste in his mouth; or nausea and vomiting after the dye is injected.
• Make sure a consent form has been signed, if required.
• Check the patient's history for hyper-sensitivity to iodine, iodine-containing substances (such as shellfish), or other contrast media. Note any hypersensitiv-ities on his chart and report them as ap-propriate.

Equipment
Contrast medium, automatic contrast injector, arterial needles (18G or 19G, 2½" needle for adults; 20G, 1½" needle for children), femoral arterial catheters for femoral injection.

Procedure and posttest care

• Have the patient recline on an X-ray table and shave the injection site (femoral, carotid, or brachial artery). Instruct him to lie still with his arms at his sides.

• Clean the injection site with alcohol and povidone-iodine.

• A local anesthetic is injected. Then the artery is punctured with the appropriate needle and catheterized.

• *In the femoral artery approach,* a catheter is threaded to the aortic arch.

• *In the carotid artery approach,* the patient's neck is hyperextended, a rolled towel or sandbag is placed under his shoulders, and a restraint or tape immobilizes his head.

• *In the brachial artery approach* (least common), a blood pressure cuff is placed distal to the puncture site and inflated before injection to prevent the contrast medium from flowing into the forearm and hand.

• After X-rays or fluoroscopy verifies placement of the needle or catheter, the contrast medium is injected. Observe the patient for a reaction, such as hives, flushing, or laryngeal stridor.

• An initial series of lateral and anteroposterior radiographs is taken, developed, and reviewed. Depending on the results, more contrast medium may be injected and another series taken.

• During the test, maintain arterial catheter patency by continuous or periodic flushing. Monitor vital and neurologic signs.

• When a satisfactory series of X-rays is obtained, the needle (or catheter) is withdrawn. Apply firm pressure to the puncture site for 15 minutes.

• After the test, observe the patient for bleeding, check distal pulses, and apply a pressure bandage.

• Typically, the patient will be on bed rest for 12 to 24 hours. Administer prescribed pain medications and monitor his vital signs and neurologic status for 24 hours (hourly for the first 4 hours, and then every 4 hours).

• Observe the puncture site for signs of extravasation (redness, swelling) and apply an ice bag to ease the patient's discomfort and minimize swelling. If bleeding occurs, apply firm pressure to the puncture site.

• If the femoral approach was used, keep the affected leg straight for 12 hours or longer and routinely check pulses distal to the site (dorsalis pedis, popliteal). Monitor the leg for temperature, color, and sensation. Thrombosis or hematoma can occlude blood flow; extravasation can also impede the flow of blood by exerting pressure on the artery.

• If the carotid artery was used, monitor the patient for dysphagia or respiratory distress possibly resulting from hematoma or extravasation.

• Monitor for disorientation and weakness or numbness in the extremities (signs of thrombosis or hematoma) and for arterial spasms, which may produce symptoms of transient ischemic attacks.

• If the brachial approach was used, immobilize the affected arm for 6 hours or longer and routinely check the radial pulse.

• Place a sign near the patient's bed warning personnel not to take blood pressure readings from the affected arm.

• Observe the arm and hand for any changes in color, temperature, or sensation. If they become pale, cool, or numb, report these changes immediately.

• After the test, tell the patient he may resume his usual diet. Encourage him to drink fluids to help him pass the contrast dye.

Precautions

• Cerebral angiography is contraindicated in patients with hepatic, renal, or thyroid disease.

• This test is also contraindicated in patients with hypersensitivity to iodine or contrast media.

• If the patient has been receiving aspirin daily, take extra care when compressing the puncture site.

Normal findings

During the arterial phase of perfusion, the contrast medium fills and opacifies superficial and deep arteries and arterioles; it opacifies superficial and deep veins during the venous phase. The finding of apparently normal (symmetrical) cerebral vasculature must be correlated with the patient's history and clinical status.

Abnormal findings

Changes in the caliber of vessel lumina suggest vascular disease, possibly due to spasms, plaques, fistulas, arteriovenous malformation, or arteriosclerosis. Diminished blood flow to vessels may be related to increased ICP.

Vessel displacement may reflect the presence and size of a tumor, areas of edema, or obstruction of the cerebrospinal fluid pathway. Cerebral angiography may also show circulation within a tumor, often giving precise information on the tumor's position and nature. Meningeal blood supply originating in the external carotid artery may indicate an extracerebral tumor but usually designates a meningioma. Such a tumor may arise outside the brain substance, but it may still be within the cerebral hemisphere.

MYELOGRAPHY

Myelography uses fluoroscopy and radiography to evaluate the spinal subarachnoid space after injection of a contrast medium. Because the contrast medium is heavier than cerebrospinal fluid (CSF), it flows through the subarachnoid space to the dependent area when the patient, lying prone on a fluoroscopic table, is tilted up or down. The fluoroscope allows the doctor to see the flow of the contrast medium and the outline of the subarachnoid space. X-rays are taken to provide a permanent record.

Purpose

• To demonstrate lesions, such as tumors and herniated intervertebral disks, that partially or totally block the flow of CSF in the subarachnoid space

• To help detect arachnoiditis, spinal nerve root injury, or tumors in the posterior fossa of the skull

Patient preparation

• Explain to the patient that this test reveals obstructions in the spinal cord.

• Tell him that his food and fluid intake will be restricted for 8 hours before the test. If the test is scheduled for the afternoon, and hospital policy permits, the patient may have clear liquids before the test.

• Describe the test, including who will administer it, where it will take place, and its duration (1 hour or more).

• Describe likely adverse effects, such as a transient burning sensation as the contrast medium is injected; a warm, flushed feeling; transient headache; a salty taste; or nausea and vomiting after the dye is injected. Explain that he may feel some pain caused by his positioning, needle insertion and, in some cases, removal of the contrast medium.

• Make sure the patient or a responsible family member has signed the appropriate consent form.

• Check the patient's history for hypersensitivity to iodine and iodine-containing substances (for example, shellfish), radiographic contrast media, and associated medications. Notify the radiologist if the patient has a history of epilepsy or phenothiazine use. If metrizamide is to be used as a contrast medium, discontinue phenothiazine 48 hours before the test.

• Tell the patient to remove jewelry, metal, or other radiopaque material before the test.

• Perform pretest procedures and administer prescribed medications. For example, a cleansing enema may be prescribed, and a sedative and anticholinergic (such as atropine sulfate) may be prescribed to reduce swallowing during the procedure.

Equipment
Alcohol, 1% lidocaine solution, lumbar puncture tray, contrast medium (iophendylate or metrizamide sodium), two 10-ml syringes, spinal needle (18G for iophendylate or 11G for metrizamide), povidone-iodine solution, sterile gloves, small adhesive bandage.

Procedure and posttest care
• Position the patient on his side at the edge of the table, with his chin on his chest and knees drawn up to his abdomen. (If the patient has lumbar deformity or infection at the puncture site, cisternal puncture may be done.)

• After the lumbar puncture is performed, the fluoroscope is used to verify proper positioning of the needle in the subarachnoid space. Some CSF may be removed for routine laboratory analysis.

• Turn the patient to the prone position and secure him with straps across his upper back, under his arms, and across his ankles. Hyperextend his chin to prevent contrast medium from flowing into the cranium; place a towel or sponge under his chin for comfort.

• If the patient complains of a headache or trouble swallowing or reports that he's not breathing deeply enough, provide reassurance and explain that he'll be able to rest periodically during the procedure.

• The contrast medium is injected and the table tilted so that the dye flows through the subarachnoid space. (In rare circumstances, air is used as a negative contrast medium; however, this is typically reserved for patients with suspected congenital abnormalities, such as syringomyelia.)

• The flow of the contrast medium is observed by fluoroscope and X-rays are taken. If an obstruction in the subarachnoid space blocks the upward flow of the contrast medium, a cisternal puncture may be performed.

• The contrast medium is withdrawn, if necessary, after satisfactory X-rays are obtained, and the needle is removed. Clean the puncture site with povidone-iodine solution, and apply a small adhesive bandage.

• Based on the contrast medium used during the test, position the patient as follows: If metrizamide was used, tell him to stay in bed for the next 12 to 16 hours. Keep the head of his bed elevated for the first 6 to 8 hours. If an oil-based contrast medium was used, tell him to remain flat in bed for 6 to 24 hours.

• Monitor vital signs and neurologic status at least every 30 minutes for the first 4 hours, then every 4 hours for 24 hours.

• Encourage the patient to drink extra fluids. He should void within 8 hours after returning to his room.

• If there are no complications or adverse reactions, tell the patient that he may resume his usual diet and activities the day after the test.

• Monitor for radicular pain, fever, back pain, or signs of meningeal irritation, such as headache, irritability, or stiff neck. If these signs or symptoms occur, keep the room quiet and dark and administer an analgesic or antipyretic as needed.

Precautions

• Generally, myelography is contraindicated for patients with increased intracranial pressure, hypersensitivity to iodine or contrast media, or infection at the puncture site.

• Improper positioning after the test may affect recovery.

Normal findings

Normally, the contrast medium flows freely through the subarachnoid space, showing no obstruction or structural abnormalities.

Abnormal findings

Myelography can identify and localize lesions within or surrounding the spinal cord or subarachnoid space. Examples of common extradural lesions include herniated intervertebral disks and metastatic tumors. Neurofibromas and meningiomas are common lesions within the subarachnoid space, and ependymomas and astrocytomas are common within the spinal cord.

If the test confirms a spinal tumor, the patient may be taken directly to the operating room. Immediate surgery also may be necessary if the contrast medium causes a total block of the subarachnoid space.

Myelography may help locate or confirm a ruptured disk, spinal stenosis, or abscess and, occasionally, confirm the need for surgery. This test may also detect syringomyelia (a congenital abnormality marked by fluid-filled cavities within the spinal cord and widening of the cord itself), arachnoiditis, spinal nerve root injury, and tumors in the posterior fossa of the skull. Test results must be correlated with the patient's history and clinical status.

EYE

ORBITAL RADIOGRAPHY

The orbit is the cavity that houses the eye and the lacrimal glands, as well as blood vessels, nerves, muscles, and fat. Because portions of the orbit are composed of thin bone that fractures easily, X-rays are commonly taken following facial trauma. They are also useful in diagnosing ocular and orbital pathologies. Special radiographic techniques can reveal foreign bodies in the orbit or eye that are invisible with an ophthalmoscope. In some cases, radiography is used in conjunction with computed tomography scans and ultrasonography to better define an abnormality.

Purpose

• To aid in diagnosis of orbital fractures and pathologies

• To help locate intraorbital or intraocular foreign bodies

Patient preparation

• Explain that this test involves taking several X-rays to assess the condition of the bones around the eye.

• Describe the test, including who will perform it, where it will be performed, and the expected duration (about 15 minutes).

• Reassure the patient that the procedure is usually painless unless he has suffered facial trauma, in which case positioning may cause some discomfort. Explain that he'll be asked to turn his head from side to side and to flex or extend his neck.

• Instruct him to remove all metal objects, jewelry, and other radiopaque materials from the X-ray field.

Procedure and posttest care

• Have the patient recline on the radiographic table or sit in a chair.

• Instruct him to remain still while the X-rays are taken.

• Usually, a series of orbital X-rays includes a lateral view, posteroanterior view, submentovertical (base) view, stereo Waters' views (views from both sides), Towne's (half-axial) projection, and optic canal projections. If enlargement of the superior orbital fissure is suspected, apical views are obtained.

• The films are developed and inspected before the patient leaves the radiography department.

Normal findings

Each orbit is composed of a roof, a floor, and medial and lateral walls. The bones of the roof and floor are very thin (the floor can be less than 1 mm thick). The medial walls, which parallel each other, are slightly thicker, except for the portion formed by the ethmoid bone. The lateral walls are the thickest part of the orbit and are strongest at the orbital rim.

The superior orbital fissure, at the back of the orbit between the lateral wall and the roof, is actually a gap between the greater and lesser wings of the sphenoid bone. The optic canal, which carries the optic nerve and ophthalmic artery, is an opening in the lesser wing of the sphenoid bone located at the apex of the orbit.

Abnormal findings

Orbital fractures associated with facial trauma are most common in the thin structures of the floor and ethmoid bone. Abnormalities are detected by comparing the size and shape of orbital structures on the affected side with those on the opposite side.

Generally, orbit enlargement indicates the presence of a lesion that has caused proptosis due to increased intraorbital pressure. Any growing tumor can produce these changes. Superior orbital fissure enlargement can result from orbital meningioma, from intracranial conditions such as pituitary tumors or, more characteristically, from vascular anomalies. Optic canal enlargement may result from extraocular extension of a retinoblastoma or, in children, from an optic nerve glioma. In adults, only prolonged pathology can increase orbital size; however, in children, even a rapidly growing lesion can cause orbital enlargement because orbital bones are not fully developed. A decrease in the size of the orbit may follow childhood enucleation of the eye or conditions such as congenital microphthalmia.

Destruction of the orbital walls may indicate a malignant neoplasm or an infection. A benign tumor or cyst produces a clear-cut local indentation of the orbital wall. Lesions of adjacent structures may also produce radiographic changes due to enlargement and erosion of the orbit.

Increased bone density may be seen in conditions such as osteoblastic metastasis, sphenoid ridge meningioma, or Paget's disease. To confirm orbital pathology, however, radiographic findings must be supplemented with results from other appropriate tests and procedures.

FLUORESCEIN ANGIOGRAPHY

In this test, a special camera takes rapid-sequence photographs of the fundus following I.V. injection of sodium fluorescein (a contrast medium), thereby recording the appearance of blood vessels within the eye. This technique provides enhanced visibility of the microvascular structures of the retina and choroid, which permits evaluation of the entire retinal vascular bed, including retinal circulation.

Purpose
• To document retinal circulation when evaluating intraocular abnormalities, such as retinopathy, tumors, and circulatory or inflammatory disorders

Patient preparation
• Explain that this procedure takes about 30 minutes and evaluates the small blood vessels in the eyes.
• Make sure the patient or an appropriate family member has signed a consent form.
• Check the patient's history for glaucoma and hypersensitivity reactions, especially to contrast media and dilating eyedrops. If necessary, tell a patient with glaucoma not to use miotic eyedrops on the day of the test.
• Explain that eyedrops will be instilled to dilate his pupils and that a dye will be injected into his arm. Tell him that his eyes will be photographed with a special camera before and after the injection. Stress that these are photographs, not X-rays.
• Warn him that his skin and urine may appear yellow for 24 to 48 hours after the procedure.

Equipment
Fundus camera and film, mydriatic eyedrops, alcohol swabs, tourniquet, 21G scalp-vein needle, 5- to 10-ml syringe, 2 ml of 25% sodium fluorescein or 5 ml of 10% sodium fluorescein, small sterile dressing, emesis basin, emergency resuscitation kit.

Procedure and posttest care
• Administer mydriatic eyedrops. Usually, two instillations are necessary to achieve maximum mydriasis within 15 to 40 minutes.
• Following mydriasis, seat the patient comfortably in the examining chair, facing the camera.
• Have him loosen or remove any restrictive clothing around his neck.
• Tell the patient to place his chin in the chin rest and his forehead against the bar. Tell him to open his eyes wide and stare straight ahead, while keeping his teeth together and maintaining normal breathing and blinking.
• The antecubital vein is prepared and punctured; however, dye isn't injected yet. At this time, a few photographs may be taken. Make sure the patient keeps his arm extended; if necessary, use an arm board.
• Then the dye is injected. Warn the patient that the dye is injected rapidly. Remind him to maintain his position and to continue to stare straight ahead.
• The patient may experience nausea and a feeling of warmth. Provide reassurance and observe for hypersensitivity reactions, such as vomiting, dry mouth, metallic taste, suddenly increased salivation, sneezing, lightheadedness, fainting, or hives. In rare instances, anaphylactic shock may occur.
• As the dye is injected, 25 to 30 photographs are taken in rapid sequence. Each photograph is taken 1 second after the other.

• The needle and syringe are removed carefully; pressure and a dressing are applied to the injection site.

• If late-phase photographs are needed, tell the patient to sit and relax for 20 minutes, then reposition him for 5 to 10 photographs. If necessary, photographs may be taken up to 1 hour after the injection.

• Remind the patient that his skin and urine will be slightly discolored for 24 to 48 hours after the test.

• Explain that his near vision will be blurred for up to 12 hours and that he should avoid direct sunlight and refrain from driving during this time.

Precautions

• Don't leave the patient unattended. He may experience mild adverse reactions, such as nausea, vomiting, sneezing, paresthesia of the tongue, and dizziness.

• Have emergency resuscitation equipment at hand. Serious adverse effects (laryngeal edema, bronchospasm, and respiratory arrest) are possible. If a reaction occurs, note it on his allergy history.

• The needle must be placed in the vein correctly; extravasation of dye around the injection site is painful.

Normal findings

After rapid injection into the antecubital vein, sodium fluorescein reaches the retina in 12 to 15 seconds (filling phase). As the choroidal vessels and choriocapillaris fill, the background of the retina fluoresces, taking on an evenly mottled appearance known as the choroidal flush. Then the dye fills the arteries (arterial phase). The arteriovenous phase lasts from the complete filling of the arteries and capillaries to the earliest evidence of dye in the veins. The time the arteries begin to empty to the time the veins fill and empty is known as the venous phase. Finally, the recirculation phase occurs 30 to 60 minutes after the injection, when the fluorescein — if at all present — is barely detectable in the retinal vessels. Normally, there is no leakage from the retinal vessels.

Abnormal findings

The varying and complex findings after fluorescein angiography require interpretation by a highly skilled ophthalmologist with extensive experience in the diagnosis of retinal disorders.

Abnormalities detected in the early filling phase may include microaneurysms, arteriovenous shunts, and neovascularization. The test may identify arterial occlusion by showing delayed or absent flow of the dye through the arteries, stenosis, and prolonged venous drainage. Venous occlusion may be associated with dilation of the vessels and fluorescein leakage. Chronic obstruction may produce recanalization and collateral circulation.

In hypertensive retinopathy, abnormalities may include areas of increased vascular tortuosity, microaneurysms around zones of capillary nonperfusion, and generalized suffusion of the dye in the retina. Aneurysms and capillary hemangiomas may leak fluorescein and are often surrounded by hard yellow exudate. Tumors exhibit variable fluorescein patterns, depending on histologic type. Retinal edema or inflammation and fibrous tissue may show variable degrees of fluorescence. Papilledema produces vascular leakage in the disk area.

RESPIRATORY SYSTEM

CHEST RADIOGRAPHY

In this procedure, X-rays or electromagnetic waves penetrate the chest and cause an image to form on specially sensitized film. Normal pulmonary tissue is radiolucent, whereas abnormalities — such as infiltrates, foreign bodies, fluids, and tumors — appear as densities on the film. A chest X-ray is most useful when compared with prior films to detect changes.

Purpose
• To detect pulmonary disorders, such as pneumonia, atelectasis, pneumothorax, pulmonary bullae, and tumors
• To detect mediastinal abnormalities, such as tumors and cardiac disease
• To determine the location and size of a lesion
• To help assess pulmonary status

Patient preparation
• Explain that this test assesses respiratory status.
• Tell the patient he need not restrict food or fluid before the test.
• Describe the test, including who will perform it, where it will take place, and its expected duration.
• Provide a gown without snaps, and instruct the patient to remove jewelry that may be in the X-ray field.
• Explain that he'll be asked to take a deep breath and to hold it momentarily while the film is being taken to provide a clearer view of pulmonary structures.

Procedure and posttest care
• If a stationary X-ray machine is used, the patient stands or sits in front of the machine, so films can be taken of the posteroanterior and left lateral views.
• If a portable X-ray machine is used at the patient's bedside, the patient is moved to the top of the bed, if his tolerance permits. The head of the bed is elevated for maximum upright positioning.
• Move cardiac monitoring cables, I.V. tubing from subclavian lines, pulmonary artery catheter lines, and safety pins as far from the X-ray field as possible.

Precautions
• Chest radiography is usually contraindicated during the first trimester of pregnancy; however, when radiography is absolutely necessary, a lead apron placed over the patient's abdomen can shield the fetus.
• If the patient is intubated, check that no tubes have been dislodged during positioning.
• To avoid exposure to radiation, leave the room or the immediate area while the films are being taken. If you must stay in the area, wear a lead-lined apron or protective clothing.

Findings
For an overview of normal and abnormal chest radiography findings, see *Selected clinical implications of chest X-ray films*. For accurate diagnosis, radiography findings must be correlated with additional radiologic and pulmonary tests as well as physical assessment findings. For example, pulmonary hyperinflation with low diaphragm and generalized increased radiolucency may suggest emphysema but may also occur in a healthy person.

SELECTED CLINICAL IMPLICATIONS OF CHEST X-RAY FILMS

NORMAL ANATOMIC LOCATION AND APPEARANCE	POSSIBLE ABNORMALITY	IMPLICATIONS
Trachea		
Visible midline in the anterior mediastinal cavity; translucent tubelike appearance	• Deviation from midline	• Tension pneumothorax, atelectasis, pleural effusion, consolidation, mediastinal nodes or, in children, enlarged thymus
	• Narrowing with hour-glass appearance and deviation to one side	• Substernal thyroid
Heart		
Visible in the anterior left mediastinal cavity; solid appearance due to blood contents; edges may be clear in contrast with surrounding air density of the lung	• Large central pulmonary arteries, right ventricular enlargement	• Cor pulmonale
	• Cardiomegaly, increased pulmonary vascular markings, interstitial edema	• Congestive heart failure
Aortic knob		
Visible as water density; formed by the arch of the aorta	• Solid densities, possibly indicating calcifications	• Atherosclerosis
	• Tortuous shape	• Atherosclerosis
Mediastinum (mediastinal shadow)		
Visible as the space between the lungs; shadowy appearance that widens at the hilum of the lungs	• Deviation to nondiseased side; deviation to diseased side by traction	• Pleural effusion or tumor, fibrosis or collapsed lung
	• Gross widening	• Neoplasms of esophagus, bronchi, lungs, thyroid tissue; aortic aneurysm; mediastinitis; cor pulmonale
Ribs		
Visible as thoracic cavity encasement	• Break or misalignment	• Fractured sternum or ribs
	• Widening of intercostal spaces	• Emphysema
Spine		
Visible midline in the posterior chest; straight bony structure	• Spinal curvature	• Scoliosis, kyphosis
	• Break or misalignment	• Fractures

(continued)

SELECTED CLINICAL IMPLICATIONS OF CHEST X-RAY FILMS *(continued)*

NORMAL ANATOMIC LOCATION AND APPEARANCE	POSSIBLE ABNORMALITY	IMPLICATIONS
Clavicles		
Visible in upper thorax; intact and equidistant in properly centered X-ray films	• Break or misalignment	• Fractures
Hila (lung roots)		
Visible above the heart, where pulmonary vessels, bronchi, and lymph nodes join the lungs; appear as small, white, bilateral densities	• Shift to one side, accentuated shadows	• Atelectasis, pneumothorax, emphysema, pulmonary abscess, tumor, enlarged lymph nodes
Mainstem bronchus		
Visible; part of the hila with translucent tubelike appearance	• Spherical or oval density	• Bronchogenic cyst
Bronchi		
Usually not visible	• Visible	• Bronchial pneumonia
Lung fields		
Usually not visible throughout, except for the blood vessels	• Visible • Irregular	• Atelectasis • Resolving pneumonia, infiltrates, silicosis, fibrosis, metastatic neoplasm
Hemidiaphragm		
Rounded, visible; right side $3/8''$ to $3/4''$	• Elevation of diaphragm (difference in elevation can be measured on inspiration and expiration to detect movement) • Flattening of diaphragm • Elevation of left side only	• Active tuberculosis, pneumonia, pleurisy, acute bronchitis, active disease of the abdominal viscera, bilateral phrenic nerve involvement, atelectasis • Asthma, emphysema • Possible unilateral phrenic nerve paresis • Perforated ulcer (rare), gas distention of stomach or splenic flexure of colon, free air in abdomen

PARANASAL SINUS RADIOGRAPHY

The paranasal sinuses — air-filled cavities lined with mucous membrane — lie within the maxillary, ethmoid, sphenoid, and frontal bones. Sinus abnormalities, resulting from inflammation, trauma, cysts, mucoceles, granulomatosis, and other conditions, may include distorted bony sinus walls, altered mucous membranes, and fluid or masses within the cavities. In paranasal sinus radiography, X-rays or electromagnetic waves penetrate the paranasal sinuses and react on specially sensitized film, forming a film image that differentiates sinus structures.

When surrounding facial structures that are superimposed on the paranasal sinuses interfere with visualization of relevant areas, computed tomography scanning may be performed to provide further information.

Purpose
• To detect unilateral or bilateral abnormalities, possibly indicating trauma or disease
• To confirm diagnosis of neoplastic or inflammatory paranasal sinus disease
• To determine the location and size of a malignant neoplasm

Patient preparation
• Explain that this test helps evaluate abnormalities of the paranasal sinuses.
• Describe the test, including who will perform it, where it will take place, and its expected duration (usually 10 to 15 minutes).
• Tell the patient that his head may be immobilized in a foam vise during the test to help him maintain the correct position but that the vise doesn't hurt.

• Explain that he'll be asked to sit upright and avoid moving while the X-rays are being taken to prevent blurring of the image and to allow visualization of air-fluid levels, if present. Emphasize the importance of his cooperation.
• Instruct him to remove dentures, all jewelry, and metal objects in the X-ray field.

Procedure and posttest care
• Have the patient sit upright (his head may be placed in a foam vise) between the X-ray tube and a film cassette.
• During the test, the X-ray tube is positioned at specific angles, and the patient's head is placed in various standard positions, while his paranasal sinuses are filmed from different angles. If necessary, assist with positioning the patient.

Precautions
• Paranasal sinus radiography is usually contraindicated during pregnancy; however, when it's absolutely necessary, a lead-lined apron placed over the patient's abdomen can shield the fetus.
• To avoid exposure to radiation, leave the room or the immediate area during the test; if you must stay in the area, wear a lead-lined apron.

Normal findings
Normal paranasal sinuses are radiolucent and filled with air, which appears black on films.

Abnormal findings
See *Abnormal findings in paranasal sinus radiography,* page 508.

ABNORMAL FINDINGS IN PARANASAL SINUS RADIOGRAPHY

DISORDER	ABNORMAL FINDINGS
Paranasal sinus trauma or fracture	• Edema or hemorrhage in mucous membrane lining or sinus cavity • Clouded sinus air cells • Air-fluid level • Radiolucent, linear bone defects • Irregular, overriding bone edges • Depression or displacement of bone fragments • Foreign bodies
Acute sinusitis	• Swollen, inflamed mucous membrane • Inflammatory exudate • Hazy to opaque sinus air cells • Air-fluid level
Chronic sinusitis	• Thickened mucous membrane • Hazy to opaque sinus air cells • Air-fluid level • Thickening or sclerosis of bony wall of affected sinus
Wegener's granulomatosis	• Clouded to opaque sinus air cells • Destruction of bony sinus wall
Malignant neoplasm	• Rounded or lobulated soft-tissue mass, projecting into sinus • Destruction of bony sinus wall
Benign bone tumor	• Distortion of bony sinus wall in specific patterns
Cyst, polyp, or benign tumor	• Rounded or lobulated soft-tissue mass, projecting into sinus
Mucocele	• Clouded sinus air cells • Destruction of bony sinus wall resulting in various degrees of radiolucency

FLUOROSCOPY

In fluoroscopy, a continuous stream of X-rays passes through the patient, casting shadows of the heart, lungs, and diaphragm on a fluorescent screen. Because fluoroscopy reveals less detail than standard chest radiography, it's indicated only when diagnosis requires visualization of physiologic or pathologic motion of thoracic contents — for example, to rule out paralysis in patients with diaphragmatic elevation.

Purpose
• To assess lung expansion and contraction during quiet breathing, deep breathing, and coughing

• To assess movement and paralysis of the diaphragm
• To detect bronchial obstructions and pulmonary disease

Patient preparation
• Explain to the patient that this test assesses respiratory structures and their motion.
• Describe the test, including who will perform it, where it will take place, and its expected duration (usually 5 minutes).
• Tell the patient that he'll be asked to follow specific instructions — for example, to breathe deeply and to cough — while X-ray images depict his breathing.
• Instruct him to remove all jewelry within the X-ray field.

Procedure and posttest care
• If necessary, assist with positioning the patient.
• Move cardiac monitoring cables, I.V. tubing from subclavian lines, pulmonary artery catheter lines, and safety pins as far from the X-ray field as possible.
• During the test, the patient's cardiopulmonary motion is observed on a screen. Special equipment may be used to intensify the images, or a videotape recording of the fluoroscopy may be made, for later study.

Precautions
• Fluoroscopy is contraindicated during pregnancy.
• If the patient is intubated, check that no tubes have been dislodged during positioning.
• To avoid exposure to radiation, leave the room or the immediate area during the test; if you must stay in the area, wear a lead-lined apron.

Normal findings
Normal diaphragmatic movement is synchronous and symmetrical. Normal diaphragmatic excursion ranges from ¾″ to 1⅝″ (2 to 4 cm).

Abnormal findings
Diminished diaphragmatic movement may indicate pulmonary disease. Increased lung translucency may indicate loss of elasticity or bronchial obstruction. In elderly patients, the lowest part of the trachea may be displaced to the right by an elongated aorta.

Diminished or paradoxical diaphragmatic movement may indicate paralysis of the diaphragm; however, fluoroscopy may not detect such paralysis in patients who compensate for diminished diaphragm function by forcefully contracting their abdominal muscles to aid expiration.

CHEST TOMOGRAPHY

Also called laminagraphy, planigraphy, stratigraphy, or body section roentgenography, chest tomography provides clearly focused radiographic images of selected body sections otherwise obscured by shadows of overlying or underlying structures. In this procedure, the X-ray tube and film move around the patient in opposite directions (a motion called the linear tube sweep), producing exposures in which a selected body plane appears sharply defined and the areas above and below it are blurred. Because tomography emits high radiation levels, it's used only for evaluation of chest lesions.

Purpose
• To demonstrate pulmonary densities (for cavitation, calcification, and presence of fat), tumors (especially those obstructing the bronchial lumen), or lesions (especially those located deep

within the mediastinum, such as at lymph nodes at the hilum)

Patient preparation

• Explain to the patient that this test helps evaluate lesions inside the chest.

• Describe the test, including who will perform it, where it will take place, and its duration (30 to 60 minutes).

• Tell him that there are no food or fluid restrictions.

• Warn the patient that the equipment is noisy because of rapidly moving metal-on-metal parts and that the X-ray tube swings overhead.

• Advise him to breathe normally during the test but to remain immobile; tell him that foam wedges will be used to help him maintain a comfortable, motionless position.

• Suggest that he close his eyes to prevent involuntary movement.

• Instruct him to remove all jewelry within the X-ray field.

Procedure and posttest care

• The patient is placed in a supine position or in different degrees of lateral rotation on the X-ray table. The X-ray tube then swings over the patient, taking numerous films from different angles.

• For lung tomography, the X-ray tube is usually moved in a linear direction but may be moved in a hypocycloid, circular, elliptic, trispiral, or figure-eight pattern. Multidirectional films aid diagnosis of mediastinal lesions or tumors.

Precautions

• Tomography is contraindicated during pregnancy.

• To avoid exposure to radiation, leave the room or the immediate area during the test; if you must stay in the area, wear a lead-lined apron.

Normal findings

A normal chest tomogram shows structures equivalent to a normal chest X-ray film.

Abnormal findings

Central calcification in a nodule suggests a benign lesion; an irregularly bordered tumor suggests malignancy; a sharply defined tumor suggests granuloma or nonmalignancy. Evaluation of the hilum can help differentiate blood vessels from nodes; identify bronchial dilation, stenosis, and endobronchial lesions; and detect tumor extension into the hilar lung area. Tomography can also identify extension of a mediastinal lesion to the ribs or spine.

BRONCHOGRAPHY

Bronchography is X-ray examination of the tracheobronchial tree after instillation of a radiopaque iodine contrast agent through a catheter into the lumens of the trachea and bronchi. The contrast agent coats the bronchial tree, permitting visualization of any anatomic deviations. Bronchography of a localized lung area may be accomplished by instilling contrast dye through a fiber-optic bronchoscope placed in the area to be filmed.

Since the development of computed tomography scanning, bronchography is used less frequently. It may be performed using a local anesthetic instilled through the catheter or bronchoscope, although a general anesthetic may be necessary for children or during a concurrent bronchoscopy.

Purpose

• To help detect bronchiectasis, bronchial obstruction, pulmonary tumors,

cysts, and cavities and, indirectly, to pinpoint the cause of hemoptysis
• To provide permanent films of pathologic findings

Patient preparation
• Explain to the patient that this test helps evaluate abnormalities of the bronchial structures.
• Instruct the patient to fast for 12 hours before the test.
• Tell him to perform good oral hygiene the night before and the morning of the test.
• Explain who will perform the test, where it will take place, and its expected duration.
• Make sure the patient or a responsible family member has signed a consent form.
• Check the patient's history for hypersensitivity to anesthetics, iodine, or contrast media.
• If the patient has a productive cough, administer a prescribed expectorant and perform postural drainage 1 to 3 days before the test.
• If the procedure is to be performed under a local anesthetic, tell the patient he'll receive a sedative to help him relax and to suppress the gag reflex. Prepare him for the unpleasant taste of the anesthetic spray. Warn him that he may experience some difficulty breathing during the procedure, but reassure him that his airway won't be blocked and that he'll receive enough oxygen. Tell him the catheter or bronchoscope will pass more easily if he relaxes.
• If bronchography is to be performed under a general anesthetic, inform the patient that he'll receive a sedative before the test to help him relax.
• Just before the test, instruct the patient to remove his dentures and to void.

Equipment
Tilting table, sedative, anesthetic, catheter or bronchoscope, radiopaque oils or water-soluble contrast agent, emergency resuscitation equipment.

Procedure and posttest care
• After a local anesthetic is sprayed into the patient's mouth and throat, a bronchoscope or catheter is passed into the trachea, and the anesthetic and contrast agent are instilled.
• The patient is placed in various positions during the test to promote movement of the contrast agent into different areas of the bronchial tree. After X-rays are taken, the dye is removed through postural drainage and by having the patient cough it up.
• Watch for signs of laryngeal spasms (dyspnea) or edema (hoarseness, dyspnea, laryngeal stridor) secondary to traumatic intubation.
• Immediately report signs of allergic reaction to the contrast agent or anesthetic, such as itching, dyspnea, tachycardia, palpitations, excitation, hypotension, hypertension, or euphoria.
• Withhold food, fluids, and oral medications until the gag reflex returns (usually in 2 hours). Fluid intake before the gag reflex returns may cause aspiration.
• Encourage gentle coughing and postural drainage to facilitate clearing of the contrast agent. A postdrainage film is usually done in 24 to 48 hours.
• Watch for signs of chemical or secondary bacterial pneumonia — fever, dyspnea, crackles, or rhonchi — the result of incomplete expectoration of the contrast agent.
• If the patient has a sore throat, reassure him that it is only temporary, and provide throat lozenges or a liquid gargle when his gag reflex returns.
• Advise the outpatient not to resume his usual activities until the next day.

Precautions
• Bronchography is contraindicated during pregnancy, in persons with hypersensitivity to iodine or contrast me-

dia, and usually in persons with respiratory insufficiency.

• Observe the patient with asthma for laryngeal spasm secondary to the instillation of the contrast agent.

• Observe the patient with chronic obstructive pulmonary disease for airway occlusion secondary to the instillation of the contrast agent.

Normal findings

The right mainstem bronchus is shorter, wider, and more vertical than the left bronchus. Successive branches of the bronchi become smaller in diameter and are free of obstruction or lesions.

Abnormal findings

Bronchography may demonstrate bronchiectasis or bronchial obstruction due to tumors, cysts, cavities, or foreign objects. Findings must be correlated with physical examination, patient history, and perhaps other pulmonary studies.

PULMONARY ANGIOGRAPHY

Also called pulmonary arteriography, pulmonary angiography is the radiographic examination of the pulmonary circulation following injection of a radiopaque iodine contrast agent into the pulmonary artery or one of its branches.

Possible complications include arterial occlusion, myocardial perforation or rupture, ventricular arrhythmias from myocardial irritation, and acute renal failure from hypersensitivity to the contrast agent.

Purpose

• To detect pulmonary embolism in a patient who is symptomatic but whose lung scan is indeterminate or normal, especially before anticoagulant therapy or in patients in whom anticoagulant therapy is contraindicated

• To evaluate pulmonary circulation preoperatively in the patient with congenital heart disease

Patient preparation

• Describe the procedure to the patient. Explain that this test permits evaluation of the blood vessels to help identify the cause of his symptoms.

• Instruct him to fast for 8 hours before the test or as prescribed. Tell him who will perform the test and where and that it will take approximately 1 hour.

• Tell the patient a small incision will be made in the right arm where blood samples are usually drawn, or in the right groin, and that a local anesthetic will be used to numb the area. Inform him that a small catheter will then be inserted into the blood vessel and passed into the right side of the heart and then to the pulmonary artery.

• Tell him the contrast agent will then be injected into this artery. Warn him that he may experience an urge to cough, a flushed feeling, nausea, or a salty taste for approximately 5 minutes after the injection.

• Inform him that his heart rate will be monitored continuously during the procedure.

• Make sure the patient or a responsible family member has signed a consent form. Check the patient's history for hypersensitivity to anesthetics, iodine, seafood, or radiographic contrast agents.

Equipment

50 ml of 60% meglumine diatrizoate or of 45% diatrizoate; 60 ml thimerosal; 60 ml of 70% alcohol; 500 ml physiologic saline solution; epinephrine for emergency administration; 30 ml of 2% procaine; 3-ml, 6-ml, and 20-ml syringes; two 2½″ 18G needles; polyeth-

ylene catheter; extension tubing (Veno-tube) with stopcock; two sterile gradua-ted cups; knife blade and handle; me-chanical contrast agent injector; radio-graphic equipment.

Procedure and posttest care
• After the patient is placed in a supine position, the local anesthetic is injected and the cardiac monitor is attached to the patient.
• An incision is made, and a catheter is introduced into the antecubital or femo-ral vein. As the catheter passes through the right atrium, the right ventricle, and the pulmonary artery, pressures are measured and blood samples are drawn from various regions of the pulmonary circulatory system.
• The contrast agent is injected and cir-culates through the pulmonary artery and lung capillaries while X-rays are taken.
• Apply a pressure dressing over the catheter insertion site, and note any bleeding.
• Maintain bed rest for about 6 hours.
• Observe for signs of myocardial per-foration or rupture by monitoring vital signs.
• Be alert for signs of acute renal fail-ure, such as sudden onset of oliguria, nausea, and vomiting.
• Check the catheter insertion site for inflammation or hematoma formation and report symptoms of a delayed hy-persensitivity response to the contrast agent or to the local anesthetic (dys-pnea, itching, tachycardia, palpitations, hypotension or hypertension, excita-tion, or euphoria).
• Advise the patient about any restric-tion of activity. He may resume his usu-al diet after the test. Encourage fluid in-take.

Precautions
• Pulmonary angiography is contraindi-cated during pregnancy and in patients

who are hypersensitive to iodine, sea-food, or radiographic contrast agents.
• Monitor for ventricular arrhythmias due to myocardial irritation from pas-sage of the catheter through the heart chambers.
• Observe for signs of hypersensitivity to the contrast agent, such as dyspnea, nausea, vomiting, sweating, increased heart rate, and numbness of extremities.
• Keep emergency equipment available in case of a hypersensitivity reaction to the contrast agent.

Normal findings
Normally, the contrast agent flows symmetrically and without interruption through the pulmonary circulatory sys-tem.

Abnormal findings
Interruption of blood flow may result from emboli, vascular filling defects, or stenosis.

CARDIOVASCULAR SYSTEM

CARDIAC RADIOGRAPHY

Among the most frequently used tests for evaluating cardiac disease and its ef-fects on the pulmonary vasculature, cardiac radiography provides images of the thorax, mediastinum, heart, and lungs. In a routine evaluation, postero-anterior and left lateral views are taken. The posteroanterior view is preferable to the anteroposterior view because it places the heart slightly closer to the plane of the film, providing a sharper, less distorted image. Cardiac radiography may be performed on a bedridden patient using portable equipment, but such equipment can provide only anteroposterior views.

Purpose
• To help detect cardiac disease and abnormalities that change the size, shape, or appearance of the heart and lungs
• To ensure correct positioning of pulmonary artery and cardiac catheters and of pacemaker wires

Patient preparation
• Explain to the patient that this test reveals the size and shape of the heart. Tell him who will perform the test and where. Reassure him that the test uses little radiation and is harmless.
• Instruct the patient to remove jewelry, other metal objects, and clothing above his waist and to put on a hospital gown that has ties instead of metal snaps.

Procedure and posttest care
For a posteroanterior view:
• The patient stands erect about 6′ (1.82 m) from the X-ray machine with his back to the machine and his chin resting on top of the film cassette holder.
• The holder is adjusted to slightly hyperextend the patient's neck. The patient places his hands on his hips, with his shoulders touching the holder, and centers his chest against it.
• The patient is asked to take a deep breath and hold it during the X-ray film exposure.
For a left lateral view:
• The patient is positioned with his arms extended over his head and his left torso flush against the cassette and centered.
• The patient is asked to take a deep breath and hold it during the X-ray film exposure.

For an anteroposterior view of a bedridden patient:
• The head of the bed is elevated as much as possible.
• The patient is assisted to an upright position to reduce visceral pressure on the diaphragm and other thoracic structures.
• The film cassette is centered under the patient's back. Although the distance between the patient and the X-ray machine may vary, the path between the two should be clear.
• The patient is instructed to take a deep breath and hold it during the X-ray film exposure.

Precautions
• Cardiac radiography is usually contraindicated during the first trimester of pregnancy. If it is performed during pregnancy, a lead shield or apron should cover the abdomen and pelvic area during the X-ray exposure.
• When testing an ambulatory patient, make sure the radiographic order stipulates a posteroanterior view and not an anteroposterior view. Include on the order any pertinent findings from previous cardiac radiographs as well as the indication for this test.
• When testing a bedridden patient, make sure anyone else in the room is protected from X-rays by a lead shield, a room divider, or sufficient distance.

Normal findings
Normally, in the posteroanterior view, the thoracic cage appears at least twice as wide as the heart. However, in the anteroposterior view, relative heart size and position may look different, and the cardiac silhouette and vascular markings may increase.

If cardiac radiography is performed to evaluate the position of cardiac catheters and pacemakers, the films should confirm accurate placement.

Abnormal findings

Cardiac X-ray films must be evaluated in light of the patient's history, physical examination, electrocardiography results, and results of previous radiographic tests for cardiac abnormalities.

An abnormal cardiac silhouette usually reflects left or right ventricular or left atrial enlargement. In left ventricular enlargement, the posteroanterior view shows the border of the left side of the heart to be rounded and convex, with lateral extension of the lower left border; the lateral view shows posterior bulging of the left ventricle. In right ventricular enlargement, the posteroanterior view shows secondary prominence of the pulmonary artery segment at the border of the left side of the heart; the lateral view shows anterior bulging in the region of the right ventricular outflow tract.

In left atrial enlargement, the posteroanterior view shows double density of the enlarged left atrium, straightening of the border of the left side of the heart, elevation of the left mainstem bronchus and, rarely, lateral extension of the border of the right side of the heart superior to the right ventricle; the lateral view shows a posterior bulge at the level of the left atrium.

In the posteroanterior view, dilation of pulmonary venous shadows in the superior lateral aspect of the hilus and vascular shadows horizontally and inferiorly along the margin of the right side of the heart may be the first signs of pulmonary vascular congestion. Chronic pulmonary venous hypertension produces an antler pattern, caused by dilated superior pulmonary veins and normal or constricted inferior pulmonary veins. Acute alveolar edema may produce a butterfly appearance, with increased densities in central lung fields; interstitial pulmonary edema, a cloudy or cotton-puff appearance.

LOWER LIMB VENOGRAPHY

Venography, or ascending contrast phlebography, is the radiographic examination of a vein and is often used to assess the condition of the deep leg veins after injection of a contrast medium. It's the definitive test for deep vein thrombosis (DVT). It should not be used for routine screening because it exposes the patient to relatively high doses of radiation and can cause complications, such as phlebitis, local tissue damage and, occasionally, DVT itself.

Venography is also expensive and isn't easily repeated. A combination of three noninvasive tests — Doppler ultrasonography, impedance plethysmography, and ^{125}I fibrinogen scan — provides an acceptable though less accurate alternative to venography. Radionuclide tests, such as the ^{125}I fibrinogen scan, are used to screen for DVT or to attempt to detect the disorder in a patient who is too ill for venography or is hypersensitive to the contrast medium.

Purpose

• To confirm diagnosis of DVT
• To distinguish clot formation from venous obstruction (a large tumor of the pelvis impinging on the venous system, for example)
• To evaluate congenital venous abnormalities
• To assess deep vein valvular competence (especially helpful in identifying underlying causes of leg edema)
• To locate a suitable vein for arterial bypass grafting

Patient preparation
• Explain to the patient that this test helps detect abnormal conditions in the veins of the legs.
• Instruct him to restrict food and to drink only clear liquids for 4 hours before the test.
• Describe the test, including who will perform it, where it will take place, and its expected duration (30 to 45 minutes).
• Warn the patient that he may feel a burning sensation in his leg on injection of the contrast medium and some discomfort during the procedure.
• Make sure the patient or a responsible family member has signed a consent form.
• Check the patient's history for hypersensitivity to iodine or iodine-containing foods or to contrast media. Mark any sensitivities on the chart.
• Reassure the patient that contrast media complications are rare, but tell him to report nausea, severe burning or itching, constriction in the throat or chest, or dyspnea immediately. Restrict anticoagulant therapy, as appropriate.
• Just before the test, instruct the patient to void, to remove all clothing below the waist, and to put on a hospital gown.
• Administer a prescribed sedative to an anxious or uncooperative patient.

Procedure and posttest care
• The patient is positioned on a tilting radiographic table so that the leg being tested doesn't bear any weight. He is instructed to relax this leg and keep it still; a tourniquet may be tied around the ankle to expedite venous filling.
• A superficial vein in the dorsum of the patient's foot is injected with 0.9% sodium chloride solution.
• When needle placement is correct, the contrast medium is slowly injected.

• If a suitable superficial vein can't be found (due to edema), a surgical cutdown of the vein may be performed.
• Using a fluoroscope, the distribution of the contrast medium is monitored, and spot films are taken from the anteroposterior and oblique projections and over the thigh and femoroiliac regions. Then, overhead films are taken of the calf, knee, thigh, and femoral area.
• After filming, the patient is repositioned horizontally, the leg is quickly elevated, and 0.9% sodium chloride solution infused to flush the contrast medium from the veins.
• The fluoroscope is checked to confirm complete emptying. Then the needle is removed.
• Apply an adhesive bandage to the injection site.
• Monitor vital signs until stable; check the pulse rate on the dorsalis pedis, popliteal, and femoral arteries.
• Administer prescribed analgesics to counteract the irritating effects of the contrast medium.
• Watch for hematoma, redness, bleeding, or infection (especially if a cutdown of the vein was performed) at the puncture site, and replace the dressing when necessary.
• If the venogram indicates DVT, initiate prescribed therapy (heparin infusion, bed rest, leg elevation or support, or blood chemistry tests).
• Tell the patient he may resume his usual diet and medications.

Precautions
• Most allergic reactions to the contrast medium occur within 30 minutes of injection; carefully observe for signs of anaphylaxis (flushing, hives, urticaria, laryngeal stridor).

Normal findings

A normal venogram shows steady opacification of the superficial and deep vasculature with no filling defects.

Abnormal findings

A venogram that shows consistent filling defects on repeat views, abrupt termination of a column of contrast material, unfilled major deep veins, or diversion of flow (through collaterals, for example) is diagnostic of DVT.

GASTROINTESTINAL SYSTEM

BARIUM SWALLOW

Barium swallow (esophagography) is the cineradiographic, radiographic, or fluoroscopic examination of the pharynx and the fluoroscopic examination of the esophagus after ingestion of thick and thin mixtures of barium sulfate. This test, most commonly performed as part of the upper GI series, is indicated in patients with histories of dysphagia and regurgitation. Further testing is usually required for definitive diagnosis.

Cholangiography and the barium enema test, if necessary, should precede the barium swallow because ingested barium may obscure anatomic detail on the X-rays.

Purpose

• To diagnose hiatus hernia, diverticula, and varices
• To detect strictures, ulcers, tumors, polyps, and motility disorders

Patient preparation

• Explain to the patient that this test evaluates the function of the pharynx and esophagus.
• Instruct him to fast after midnight the night before the test. (If the patient is an infant, delay feeding to ensure complete digestion of barium).
• Describe the test, including who will perform it, where it will take place, and its expected duration (approximately 30 minutes).
• Describe the milk shake consistency and chalky taste of the barium preparation he is required to ingest. Although it's flavored, he may find it unpleasant to swallow. Tell the patient he'll first receive a thick mixture, then a thin one, and that he must drink 12 to 14 oz (355 to 415 ml) during the examination.
• Inform him that he will be placed in various positions on a tilting X-ray table and that X-ray films will be taken.
• Withhold antacids if gastric reflux is suspected.
• Just before the procedure, instruct the patient to put on a hospital gown without snap closures and to remove jewelry, dentures, hair clips, or other radiopaque objects from the X-ray field.

Procedure and posttest care

• The patient is placed in an upright position behind the fluoroscopic screen and his heart, lungs, and abdomen are examined.
• He is then instructed to take one swallow of the thick barium mixture, and the pharyngeal action is recorded using cineradiography. (This action occurs too rapidly for adequate fluoroscopic evaluation.)
• The patient is then told to take several swallows of the thin barium mixture. The passage of the barium is examined fluoroscopically and spot films of the esophageal region are taken from lateral angles and from right and left posteroanterior angles. Esophageal

strictures and obstruction of the esophageal lumen by the lower esophageal ring are best detected when the patient is upright. To accentuate small strictures or demonstrate dysphagia, the patient may be requested to swallow a special "barium marshmallow" (soft white bread that has been soaked in barium).

• The patient is then secured to the X-ray table and is rotated to the Trendelenburg position to evaluate esophageal peristalsis or demonstrate hiatus hernia and gastric reflux.

• He is instructed to take several swallows of barium while the esophagus is examined fluoroscopically, and spot films of significant findings are taken when indicated. After the table is rotated to a horizontal position, the patient is told to take several swallows of barium so that the esophagogastric junction and peristalsis may be evaluated. The passage of the barium is fluoroscopically observed, and spot films of significant findings are taken with the patient in supine and prone positions.

• During fluoroscopic examination of the esophagus, the cardia and fundus of the patient's stomach are also carefully studied because neoplasms in these areas may invade the esophagus and cause obstruction.

• Check that additional spot films and repeat fluoroscopic evaluation haven't been ordered before allowing the patient to resume his usual diet.

• Administer a cathartic, if prescribed.

• Inform the patient that stools will be chalky and light colored for 24 to 72 hours. Record description of all stools passed by the patient in the hospital.

• Barium retained in the intestine may harden, causing obstruction or fecal impaction. Notify the doctor if the patient fails to expel barium in 2 or 3 days.

Precautions

• Barium swallow is usually contraindicated in a patient with intestinal obstruction.

Normal findings

After the barium sulfate is swallowed, the bolus pours over the base of the tongue into the pharynx. A peristaltic wave propels the bolus through the entire length of the esophagus in about 2 seconds. When the peristaltic wave reaches the base of the esophagus, the cardiac sphincter opens, allowing the bolus to enter the stomach. After passage of the bolus, the cardiac sphincter closes. Normally, the bolus evenly fills and distends the lumen of the pharynx and esophagus, and the mucosa appears smooth and regular.

Abnormal findings

Barium swallow may reveal hiatus hernia, diverticula, and varices. Although strictures, tumors, polyps, ulcers, and motility disorders (pharyngeal muscular disorders, esophageal spasms, and achalasia) may be detected, definitive diagnosis commonly necessitates endoscopic biopsy or, for motility disorders, manometric studies.

UPPER GI AND SMALL-BOWEL SERIES

The upper GI and small-bowel series is the fluoroscopic examination of the esophagus, stomach, and small intestine after the patient ingests barium sulfate, a contrast agent. As the barium passes through the digestive tract, fluoroscopy outlines peristalsis and the mucosal contours of the respective organs, and spot films record significant findings. This test is indicated in patients who have upper GI symptoms (difficulty in swallowing, regurgitation, burning or gnawing epigastric pain), signs of small-bowel disease (diarrhea, weight loss), and signs of GI bleeding (hemaemesis, melena). Although this test can detect various mucosal abnormalities, subsequent biopsy is often necessary to rule out malignancy or distinguish specific inflammatory diseases. Oral cholecystography, barium enema, and routine X-rays should always precede this test because retained barium clouds anatomic detail on X-ray films.

Purpose
• To detect hiatus hernia, diverticula, and varices
• To aid diagnosis of strictures, ulcers, tumors, regional enteritis, and malabsorption syndrome
• To help detect motility disorders

Patient preparation
• Explain to the patient that this procedure uses ingested barium and X-ray films to examine the esophagus, stomach, and small intestine.
• Tell him to consume a low-residue diet for 2 or 3 days before the test and then to fast and avoid smoking after midnight the night before the test.
• Describe the test, including who will perform it, where it will take place, and its expected duration (up to 6 hours).
• Encourage the patient to bring reading material.
• Inform the patient that he'll be placed on an X-ray table that rotates into vertical, semivertical, and horizontal positions.
• Explain that he'll be adequately secured and that he will be assisted to supine, prone, and side-lying positions.
• Describe the milk shake consistency and chalky taste of the barium mixture. Although it's flavored, he may find its taste unpleasant, but tell him he must

drink 16 to 20 oz (475 to 590 ml) for a complete examination.
• Inform him that his abdomen may be compressed to ensure proper coating of the stomach or intestinal walls with barium, or to separate overlapping bowel loops.
• As prescribed, withhold most oral medications after midnight and anticholinergics and narcotics for 24 hours because these drugs affect small intestinal motility. Antacids are also sometimes withheld for several hours if gastric reflux is suspected.
• Just before the procedure, instruct the patient to put on a hospital gown without snap closures and to remove jewelry, dentures, hair clips, or other objects that might obscure anatomic detail on the X-ray films.

Procedure and posttest care
• After the patient is secured in a supine position on the radiographic table, the table is tilted until the patient is erect, and the heart, lungs, and abdomen are examined fluoroscopically.
• The patient is instructed to take several swallows of the barium suspension, and its passage through the esophagus is observed. (Occasionally, the patient is given a thick barium suspension, especially when esophageal pathology is strongly suspected.)
• During fluoroscopic examination, spot films of the esophagus are taken from lateral angles and from right and left posteroanterior angles.
• When barium enters the stomach, the patient's abdomen is palpated or compressed to ensure adequate coating of the gastric mucosa with barium.
• To perform a double-contrast examination, the patient is instructed to sip the barium through a perforated straw. As he does so, a small amount of air is also introduced into the stomach; this permits detailed examination of the gastric rugae, and spot films of signifi-

cant findings are taken. The patient is then instructed to ingest the remaining barium suspension, and the filling of the stomach and emptying into the duodenum are observed fluoroscopically.

• Two series of spot films of the stomach and duodenum are taken from posteroanterior, anteroposterior, lateral, and oblique angles, with the patient erect and then supine.

• The passage of barium into the remainder of the small intestine is then observed fluoroscopically, and spot films are taken at 30- to 60-minute intervals until the barium reaches the region of the ileocecal valve. If abnormalities in the small intestine are detected, the area is palpated and compressed to help clarify the defect, and a spot film is taken. The examination ends when the barium enters the cecum.

• Make sure additional X-rays haven't been ordered before allowing the patient food, fluids, and oral medications (if applicable).

• Administer a cathartic or enema to the patient. Tell him his stool will be lightly colored for 24 to 72 hours. Record and describe any stool passed by the patient in the hospital. Retention of barium in the intestine may cause obstruction or fecal impaction. Also, it may affect scheduling of other GI studies.

Precautions
• The upper GI and small-bowel series is contraindicated in patients with obstruction or perforation of the digestive tract. Barium may intensify the obstruction or seep into the abdominal cavity. If a perforation is suspected, gastrografin rather than barium may be used.

Normal findings
After the barium suspension is swallowed, it pours over the base of the tongue into the pharynx and is propelled by a peristaltic wave through the entire length of the esophagus in about 2 seconds. The bolus evenly fills and distends the lumen of the pharynx and esophagus, and the mucosa appears smooth and regular. When the peristaltic wave reaches the base of the esophagus, the cardiac sphincter opens, allowing the bolus to enter the stomach. After passage of the bolus, the cardiac sphincter closes.

As barium enters the stomach, it outlines the characteristic longitudinal folds called rugae, which are best observed using the double-contrast technique. When the stomach is completely filled with barium, its outer contour appears smooth and regular without evidence of flattened, rigid areas suggestive of intrinsic or extrinsic lesions.

After barium enters the stomach, it quickly empties into the duodenal bulb through relaxation of the pyloric sphincter. Although the mucosa of the duodenal bulb is relatively smooth, circular folds become apparent as barium enters the duodenal loop. These folds deepen and become more numerous in the jejunum. The barium temporarily lodges between these folds, producing a speckled pattern on the X-ray film. As barium enters the ileum, the circular folds become less prominent and, except for their broadness, resemble those in the duodenum. The film also shows that the diameter of the small intestine tapers gradually from the duodenum to the ileum.

Abnormal findings
X-ray studies of the esophagus may reveal strictures, tumors, hiatus hernia, diverticula, varices, and ulcers (particularly in the distal esophagus). Benign strictures usually dilate the esophagus, whereas malignant ones cause erosive changes in the mucosa. Tumors produce filling defects in the column of barium, but only malignant ones change the mucosal contour. Neverthe-

less, biopsy is necessary for definitive diagnosis of both esophageal strictures and tumors.

Motility disorders, such as esophageal spasm, are usually difficult to detect because spasms are erratic and transient; manometry, which measures the length and pressure of peristaltic contractions and evaluates the function of the cardiac sphincter, is generally performed to detect such disorders. However, achalasia (cardiospasm) is strongly suggested when the distal esophagus has a beaking appearance. Gastric reflux appears as a back flow of barium from the stomach into the esophagus.

X-ray studies of the stomach may reveal tumors and ulcers. Malignant tumors, usually adenocarcinomas, appear as filling defects on the X-ray film and usually disrupt peristalsis. Benign tumors, such as adenomatous polyps and leiomyomas, appear as outpouchings of the gastric mucosa and generally don't affect peristalsis. Ulcers occur most commonly in the stomach and duodenum (particularly in the duodenal bulb), and these two areas are thus examined together. Benign ulcers usually demonstrate evidence of partial or complete healing and are characterized by radiating folds extending to the edge of the ulcer crater. Malignant ulcers, usually associated with a suspicious mass, generally have radiating folds that extend beyond the ulcer crater to the edge of the mass. However, biopsy is necessary for definitive diagnosis of both tumors and ulcers.

Occasionally, this test detects signs that suggest pancreatitis or pancreatic carcinoma. Such signs include edematous changes in the mucosa of the antrum or duodenal loop or dilation of the duodenal loop. These findings mandate further studies for pancreatic disease, such as endoscopic retrograde cholangiopancreatography, abdominal ultrasonography, or computed tomography scanning.

X-ray studies of the small intestine may reveal regional enteritis, malabsorption syndrome, and tumors. Although regional enteritis may not be detected in its early stages, small ulcerations and edematous changes develop in the mucosa as the disease progresses. Edematous changes, segmentation of the barium column, and flocculation characterize malabsorption syndrome. Filling defects occur with Hodgkin's disease and lymphosarcoma.

BARIUM ENEMA

Also called lower GI examination, barium enema is the radiographic examination of the large intestine after rectal instillation of barium sulfate (single-contrast technique) or barium sulfate and air (double-contrast technique). It's indicated in patients with histories of altered bowel habits, lower abdominal pain, or the passage of blood, mucus, or pus in the stool. It may also be indicated after colostomy or ileostomy; in these patients, barium (or barium and air) is instilled through the stoma. Complications include perforation of the colon, water intoxication, barium granulomas and, rarely, intraperitoneal and extraperitoneal extravasation of barium and barium embolism.

The single-contrast technique provides a profile view of the large intestine; the double-contrast technique provides profile and frontal views. The latter technique best detects small intraluminal tumors (especially polyps), the early mucosal changes of inflammatory disease, and the subtle intestinal bleeding caused by ulcerated polyps or shallow ulcerations of inflammatory disease.

Although barium enema clearly outlines most of the large intestine, proctosigmoidoscopy provides the best view of the rectosigmoid region. Barium enema should precede the barium swallow and upper GI and small-bowel series because barium ingested in the latter procedure may take several days to pass through the GI tract and thus may interfere with subsequent X-ray studies.

Purpose
• To aid diagnosis of colorectal cancer and inflammatory disease
• To detect polyps, diverticula, and structural changes in the large intestine

Patient preparation
• Explain to the patient that this test permits examination of the large intestine through X-ray films taken after a barium enema.
• Describe the test, including who will perform it, where it will take place, and its expected duration (30 to 45 minutes).
• Because residual fecal material in the colon obscures normal anatomy on radiographs, carefully follow the prescribed bowel preparation.
• Diet, laxatives, or cleansing enemas may be used. However, in certain conditions, such as ulcerative colitis and active GI bleeding, their use may be prohibited.
• Stress that accurate test results depend on the patient's cooperation with prescribed dietary restrictions and bowel preparation. A common bowel preparation technique includes restricted intake of dairy products and maintenance of a liquid diet for 24 hours before the test. The patient is encouraged to drink five 8-oz glasses of water or clear liquids 12 to 24 hours before the test.
• Administer bowel preparation supplied by the X-ray department. An ene-

ma or repeat enemas may be prescribed until return is clear.
• Withhold breakfast before the procedure; if the test is scheduled for late afternoon (or delayed), clear liquids may be allowed.
• Tell the patient that he'll be placed on a tilting X-ray table and adequately draped. During the test, he'll be secured to the table and assisted to various positions.
• Tell the patient that he may experience cramping pains or the urge to defecate as the barium or air is introduced into the intestine. Instruct him to breathe deeply and slowly through his mouth to ease this discomfort.
• Tell him to keep his anal sphincter tightly contracted against the rectal tube; this holds the tube in position and helps prevent leakage of barium. Stress the importance of retaining the barium enema; if the intestinal walls aren't adequately coated with barium, test results may be inaccurate.
• Assure the patient that the barium enema is fairly easy to retain because of its cool temperature.

Procedure and posttest care
• After the patient is in a supine position on a tilting radiographic table, scout films of the abdomen are taken.
• The patient is assisted to Sims' position and a well-lubricated rectal tube is inserted through the anus. If the patient has anal sphincter atony or severe mental or physical debilitation, a rectal tube with a retaining balloon may be inserted.
• The barium is administered slowly, and the filling process is monitored fluoroscopically. To aid filling, the table may be tilted or the patient assisted to supine, prone, and lateral decubitus positions.
• As the flow of barium is observed, spot films are taken of significant findings. When the intestine is filled with

barium, overhead films of the abdomen are taken. The rectal tube is withdrawn, and the patient is escorted to the toilet or provided with a bedpan and is instructed to expel as much barium as possible.

• After evacuation, an additional overhead film is taken to record the mucosal pattern of the intestine and to evaluate the efficiency of colonic emptying.

• A double-contrast barium enema may directly follow this examination or may be performed separately. If it's performed immediately, a thin film of barium remains in the patient's intestine, coating the mucosa, and air is carefully injected to distend the bowel lumen.

• When the double-contrast technique is performed separately, a colloidal barium suspension is instilled, filling the patient's intestine to either the splenic flexure or the middle of the transverse colon. The suspension is then aspirated, and air is forcefully injected into the intestine. The intestine may also be filled to the lower descending colon and then air is forcefully injected, without prior aspiration of the suspension.

• The patient is then assisted to erect, prone, supine, and lateral decubitus positions in sequence. Barium filling is monitored fluoroscopically, and spot films are taken of significant findings. After the required films are taken, the patient is escorted to the toilet or provided with a bedpan.

• Make sure further studies haven't been ordered before allowing the patient food and fluids. Encourage extra fluid intake because bowel preparation and the test itself can cause dehydration.

• Encourage rest because this test and the bowel preparation that precedes it exhaust most patients.

• Because retention of barium after this test can cause intestinal obstruction or fecal impaction, administer a mild cathartic or a cleansing enema. Tell the patient his stool will be lightly colored for 24 to 72 hours. Record and describe any stool passed by the patient in the hospital.

Precautions

• Barium enema is contraindicated in patients with tachycardia, fulminant ulcerative colitis associated with systemic toxicity and megacolon, toxic megacolon, or suspected perforation.

• This test should be performed cautiously in patients with obstruction, acute inflammatory conditions (such as ulcerative colitis and diverticulitis), acute vascular insufficiency of the bowel, acute fulminant bloody diarrhea, and suspected pneumatosis cystoides intestinalis.

Normal findings

In the single-contrast enema, the intestine is uniformly filled with barium, and colonic haustral markings are clearly apparent. The intestinal walls collapse as the barium is expelled, and the mucosa has a regular, feathery appearance on the postevacuation film. In the double-contrast enema, the intestine is uniformly distended with air and has a thin layer of barium providing excellent detail of the mucosal pattern. As the patient is assisted to various positions, the barium collects on the dependent walls of the intestine by the force of gravity.

Abnormal findings

Although most colonic cancers occur in the rectosigmoid region and are best detected by proctosigmoidoscopy, X-ray films may reveal adenocarcinoma and, rarely, sarcomas occurring higher in the intestine. Carcinoma usually appears as a localized filling defect, with a sharp transition between the normal and the necrotic mucosa. These characteristics help distinguish carcinoma from the more diffuse lesions of inflammatory disease, but endoscopic biopsy may be necessary to confirm diagnosis.

X-ray studies demonstrate and define the extent of inflammatory disease, such as diverticulitis, ulcerative colitis, and granulomatous colitis. Ulcerative colitis usually originates in the anal region and ascends through the intestine; granulomatous colitis usually originates in the cecum and terminal ileum, and then descends through the intestine. However, biopsy may be necessary to confirm diagnosis. Barium X-ray films may also reveal saccular adenomatous polyps, broad-based villous polyps, structural changes in the intestine (such as intussusception, telescoping of the bowel, sigmoid volvulus [360-degree turn or greater], and sigmoid torsion [up to 180-degree turn]), gastroenteritis, irritable colon, vascular injury due to arterial occlusion, and selected cases of acute appendicitis.

HYPOTONIC DUODENOGRAPHY

Hypotonic duodenography is the fluoroscopic examination of the duodenum after instillation of barium sulfate and air through an intestinal catheter. This test is indicated in patients with symptoms of duodenal or pancreatic pathology, such as persistent upper abdominal pain.

After the catheter is passed through the patient's nose into the duodenum, I.V. infusion of glucagon or I.M. injection of propantheline bromide (or other anticholinergic) induces duodenal atony. Instillation of barium and air distends the relaxed duodenum, flattening its deep circular folds; spot films then record the precise delineation of the duodenal anatomy. Although these films

readily demonstrate small duodenal lesions and tumors of the head of the pancreas that impinge on the duodenal wall, differential diagnosis requires further studies.

Purpose
• To detect small postbulbar duodenal lesions, tumors of the head of the pancreas, and tumors of the ampulla of Vater
• To aid diagnosis of chronic pancreatitis

Patient preparation
• Explain to the patient that this test permits examination of the duodenum and pancreas after the instillation of barium and air.
• Instruct him to fast after midnight the night before the test.
• Describe the test, including who will perform it, where it will take place, and its expected duration (approximately 60 minutes).
• Inform the patient that a tube will be passed through his nose into the duodenum to serve as a channel for the barium and air.
• Tell him that he may experience a cramping pain as air is introduced into the duodenum. Instruct him to breathe deeply and slowly through his mouth if he experiences this pain to help relax the abdominal muscles.
• If glucagon or an anticholinergic is to be administered during the procedure, describe the possible adverse effects of glucagon (nausea, vomiting, hives, and flushing) or of anticholinergics (dry mouth, thirst, tachycardia, urinary retention, and blurred vision). If an anticholinergic is administered to an outpatient, advise him to have someone accompany him home.
• Just before the test, tell him to remove dentures, glasses, necklaces, hairpins, combs, and constricting undergarments.
• Instruct him to void.

Procedure and posttest care

• While the patient is in a sitting position, a catheter is passed through his nose into the stomach. He is then placed in a supine position on the radiographic table, and the catheter is advanced into the duodenum, under fluoroscopic guidance.

• Glucagon I.V. is administered, which quickly induces duodenal atony for approximately 20 minutes, or an anticholinergic is injected I.M.

• Barium is instilled through the catheter, and spot films are taken of the duodenum.

• Some of the barium is then withdrawn and air is instilled; then additional spot films are taken.

• When the required films have been obtained, the catheter is removed.

• Throughout the procedure, observe the patient for adverse reactions. Be aware that such reactions may follow administration of glucagon or an anticholinergic. If an anticholinergic was given, make sure the patient voids within a few hours after the test. Advise the outpatient to rest in a waiting area until his vision clears (about 2 hours) unless someone can take him home.

• Administer a cathartic, as prescribed.

• Tell the patient he may burp instilled air or pass flatus, and that the barium colors the stool chalky white for 24 to 72 hours.

• Record description of any stool passed by the patient in the hospital.

Precautions

• Anticholinergics are contraindicated in patients with severe cardiac disorders or glaucoma.

• Glucagon is contraindicated in brittle diabetics and relatively contraindicated in insulin-dependent diabetes mellitus.

• Patients with strictures in the upper GI tract, particularly those associated with ulcerations or large masses, shouldn't undergo this procedure.

• Monitor elderly or very ill patients for gastric reflux.

Normal findings

When barium and air distend the atonic duodenum, the mucosa normally appears smooth and even. The regular contour of the head of the pancreas also appears on the duodenal wall.

Abnormal findings

Irregular nodules or masses on the duodenal wall could mean duodenal lesions, tumors of the ampulla of Vater, tumors of the head of the pancreas, or chronic pancreatitis. Differential diagnosis requires further tests, such as endoscopic retrograde cholangiopancreatography, serum and urine amylase determinations, pancreas ultrasonography, and pancreatic computed tomography.

ORAL CHOLECYSTOGRAPHY

Oral cholecystography is the radiographic examination of the gallbladder after administration of a contrast medium. It's indicated in patients with symptoms of biliary tract disease, such as right upper quadrant epigastric pain, fat intolerance, and jaundice, and is most commonly performed to confirm gallbladder disease.

After the contrast medium is ingested, it is absorbed by the small intestine, filtered by the liver, excreted in the bile, and then concentrated and stored in the gallbladder. Full gallbladder opacification usually occurs 12 to 14 hours after ingestion, and a series of X-ray films then records gallbladder appearance. Additional information is obtained by giving the patient a fat stimulus, causing the gallbladder to contract and empty the contrast-laden bile into the common bile duct and small intestine. Films are then taken to record this emptying and to evaluate patency of the common bile duct.

Oral cholecystography should precede barium studies because retained barium may cloud subsequent X-ray films.

Purpose
• To detect gallstones
• To aid diagnosis of inflammatory disease and tumors of the gallbladder

Patient preparation
• Explain to the patient that this procedure permits examination of the gallbladder through X-ray films taken after ingestion of a contrast medium.
• Instruct the patient to eat a meal containing fat at noon the day before the test and a fat-free meal in the evening. The former stimulates release of bile from the gallbladder, preparing it to receive the contrast-laden bile; the latter inhibits gallbladder contraction, promoting accumulation of bile.
• After the evening meal, instruct the patient to restrict food and fluids, except water.
• Give the patient six tablets (3 g) of iopanoic acid 2 or 3 hours after the evening meal, as necessary. (Other commercial contrast agents are available, such as sodium ipodate, but iopanoic acid is most commonly used.) Have the patient swallow the tablets one at a time at 5-minute intervals, with one or two mouthfuls of water for a total of 8 oz (240 ml) of water. Thereafter, withhold water, cigarettes, and gum.
• Describe the test, including who will perform it, where it will take place, and its expected duration (usually 30 to 45 minutes, but a longer test may be necessary).

• Tell the patient he'll be placed on an X-ray table, and that films will be taken of his gallbladder.
• Check the patient's history for hypersensitivity to iodine, seafood, or contrast media used for other diagnostic tests.
• Inform him that the possible adverse effects of dye ingestion include diarrhea (common) and, rarely, nausea, vomiting, abdominal cramps, and dysuria. Tell him to report such symptoms immediately if they develop.
• Examine any emesis or diarrhea for undigested tablets. If any tablets were expelled, notify the X-ray department.
• Administer a cleansing enema the morning of the test, if prescribed. This clears the GI tract of interfering shadows that may obscure the gallbladder.

Procedure and posttest care
• After the patient is in a prone position on the radiographic table, the abdomen is examined fluoroscopically to evaluate gallbladder opacification, and films are taken of significant findings.
• The patient is then examined while in left lateral decubitus and erect positions to detect possible layering or mobility of any filling defects, and additional films are taken.
• The patient may then be given a fat stimulus, such as a high-fat meal or a synthetic fat-containing agent (for example, sincalide).
• Fluoroscopy is used to observe the emptying of the gallbladder in response to the fat stimulus, and spot films are taken at 15- and 30-minute intervals to visualize the common bile duct. If the gallbladder empties slowly or not at all, these films are also taken at 60 minutes.
• If the test results are normal, tell the patient he may resume his usual diet. Nonopacification and repeat cholecystography require continuation of a low-fat diet until definitive diagnosis can be made.

• If gallstones are discovered during opacification, the patient will need an appropriate diet — usually one that restricts fat intake — to help prevent acute attacks.

Precautions

• Oral cholecystography is contraindicated in patients with severe renal or hepatic damage, or with hypersensitivity to iodine, seafood, or contrast media used for other diagnostic tests.

Normal findings

The gallbladder is normally opacified and appears pear-shaped, with smooth, thin walls. Although its size is variable, its basic structure — neck, infundibulum, body, and fundus — is clearly outlined on film.

Abnormal findings

When the gallbladder is opacified, filling defects (typically appearing within the lumen as negative shadows that show mobility) indicate the presence of gallstones. Fixed defects, on the other hand, may indicate the presence of cholesterol polyps or a benign tumor such as an adenomyoma.

When the gallbladder fails to opacify or when only faint opacification occurs, inflammatory disease such as cholecystitis — with or without gallstone formation — may be present. Gallstones may obstruct the cystic duct and prevent the contrast medium from entering the gallbladder; inflammation may impair the concentrating ability of the gallbladder mucosa and prevent or diminish opacification.

When the gallbladder fails to contract following stimulation by a fatty meal, cholecystitis or common bile duct obstruction may be present. If the X-ray films are inconclusive, oral cholecystography will have to be repeated the following day.

PERCUTANEOUS TRANSHEPATIC CHOLANGIOGRAPHY

Percutaneous transhepatic cholangiography is the fluoroscopic examination of the biliary ducts after injection of an iodinated contrast medium directly into a biliary radicle. This test is especially useful for evaluating patients with persistent upper abdominal pain after cholecystectomy and for evaluating patients with severe jaundice.

Although computed tomography scan or ultrasonography is usually performed first when obstructive jaundice is suspected, percutaneous transhepatic cholangiography may provide the most detailed view of the obstruction; however, this invasive procedure carries a potential risk of complications that include bleeding, septicemia, bile peritonitis, extravasation of the contrast medium into the peritoneal cavity, and subcapsular injection.

Purpose

• To determine the cause of upper abdominal pain following cholecystectomy

• To distinguish between obstructive and nonobstructive jaundice

• To determine the location, the extent, and often the cause of mechanical obstruction

Patient preparation

• Explain to the patient that this procedure allows examination of the biliary ducts through X-ray films taken after a contrast medium is injected into the liver.

• Instruct him to fast for 8 hours before the test.

• Describe the test, including who will perform it, where it will take place, and its duration (about 30 minutes).

• Inform the patient that he'll be placed on a tilting X-ray table that rotates into vertical and horizontal positions during the procedure.

• Assure him that he will be adequately secured to the table and assisted to supine and side-lying positions throughout the procedure.

• Warn him that injection of the local anesthetic may sting the skin and produce transient pain when it punctures the liver capsule.

• Advise him that injection of the contrast medium may produce a sensation of pressure and epigastric fullness and may cause transient upper back pain on his right side.

• If appropriate, advise him that a sedative will be administered just before the procedure begins, and tell him that he must rest for at least 6 hours after the procedure.

• Make sure the patient or a responsible family member has signed a consent form.

• Check the patient's history for hypersensitivity to iodine, seafood, contrast media used in other diagnostic tests, and the local anesthetic. Describe the possible adverse effects of contrast medium administration, such as nausea, vomiting, excessive salivation, flushing, urticaria, sweating and, rarely, anaphylaxis; tachycardia and fever may accompany intraductal injection.

• Check the patient's history for normal bleeding, clotting, and prothrombin times, and a normal platelet count. If prescribed, administer 1 g of ampicillin I.V. every 4 to 6 hours for 24 hours before the procedure.

• Just before the procedure, administer a sedative, if prescribed.

Procedure and posttest care

• After the patient is placed in a supine position on the radiographic table and is adequately secured, the right upper quadrant of the abdomen is cleaned and draped, and the skin, subcutaneous tissue, and liver capsule are infiltrated with a local anesthetic.

• While the patient holds his breath at the end of expiration, the flexible needle is inserted under fluoroscopic guidance through the eighth or ninth intercostal space in the midaxillary line and into the liver.

• The needle is passed deeply into the liver substance and then slowly withdrawn, injecting the contrast medium to locate a biliary radicle. When fluoroscopy reveals placement in a radicle, the needle is held in position and the remaining contrast is injected. When the contrast medium enters a biliary radicle, it begins to outline the biliary tree.

• Using a fluoroscope and television monitor, the opacification of the biliary ducts is observed, and spot films of significant findings are taken with the patient in supine and lateral recumbent positions. When the required films have been taken, the needle is removed.

• Apply a sterile dressing to the puncture site.

• Check the patient's vital signs until they're stable.

• Enforce bed rest for at least 6 hours after the test, preferably with the patient lying on his right side, to help prevent hemorrhage.

• Check the injection site for bleeding, swelling, and tenderness. Watch for signs of peritonitis: chills, temperature of 102° to 103° F (38.8° to 39.4° C), and abdominal pain, tenderness, and distention.

• Tell the patient that he may resume his usual diet.

Precautions
• Percutaneous transhepatic cholangiography is contraindicated in patients with cholangitis, massive ascites, uncorrectable coagulopathy, or hypersensitivity to iodine.

Normal findings
The biliary ducts are of normal diameter and appear as regular channels homogeneously filled with contrast medium.

Abnormal findings
Distinguishing between obstructive and nonobstructive jaundice hinges on whether biliary ducts are dilated or of normal size. Obstructive jaundice is associated with dilated ducts; nonobstructive jaundice, with normal-sized ducts. When ducts are dilated, the obstruction site may be defined. Obstruction may result from cholelithiasis, biliary tract carcinoma, or carcinoma of the pancreas or papilla of Vater that impinges on the common bile duct, causing deviation or stricture. When ducts are of normal size and intrahepatic cholestasis is indicated, liver biopsy may be performed to distinguish among hepatitis, cirrhosis, and granulomatous disease.

POSTOPERATIVE CHOLANGIOGRAPHY

During cholecystectomy or common bile duct exploration, a T-shaped rubber tube may be inserted into the common bile duct to facilitate drainage. Seven to 10 days after surgery, postoperative cholangiography — the radiographic and fluoroscopic examination of the biliary ducts — may be performed.

This procedure requires injection of contrast medium through the T-tube.

The contrast medium flows through the biliary ducts and outlines the size and patency of the ducts, revealing any obstruction overlooked during surgery.

Purpose
• To detect calculi, strictures, neoplasms, and fistulae in the biliary ducts

Patient preparation
• Explain to the patient that this procedure permits examination of the biliary ducts through X-ray films taken after the injection of a contrast medium.
• Describe the test, including who will perform it, where it will take place, and its expected duration (approximately 15 minutes).
• Warn the patient that he may feel a bloating sensation (not pain) in the right upper quadrant as the contrast medium is injected.
• Clamp the T-tube the day before the procedure, if necessary. Because bile fills the tube after clamping, this helps prevent air bubbles from entering the ducts.
• Withhold the meal just before the test, and administer a cleansing enema about 1 hour before the procedure.
• Make sure the patient or a responsible family member has signed a consent form.
• Check the patient's history for hypersensitivity to iodine, seafood, or contrast media used in other diagnostic tests. Tell the patient that the adverse effects of intraductal administration may include nausea, vomiting, excessive salivation, flushing, urticaria, sweating and, rarely, anaphylaxis.

Procedure and posttest care
• After the patient is in supine position on the radiographic table, the injection area of the T-tube is cleaned with sponges soaked with povidone-iodine solution. The T-tube is held in a vertical position, which allows trapped air to

surface, and a needle attached to a long transparent catheter is carefully inserted into the end of the T-tube. Care must be taken to avoid injecting air into the biliary tree because air bubbles may affect the clarity of the X-ray films.

• Approximately 5 ml of contrast medium (usually sodium diatrizoate) is injected under fluoroscopic guidance, and a spot film is taken in the anteroposterior position. Additional injections are then administered, and spot films and plain films are taken with the patient in supine and right lateral decubitus positions.

• The T-tube is then clamped, and the patient is assisted to an erect position for additional films; in this position, air bubbles may be distinguished from calculi or other pathology.

• A final film is taken 15 minutes after contrast injection to record the emptying of contrast-laden bile into the duodenum. If emptying is delayed, additional films may be taken.

• If a sterile dressing is applied after removal of the T-tube, observe and record any drainage. Change the dressing, as necessary.

• If the T-tube is left in place, attach it to the drainage system.

Precautions
• Postoperative cholangiography is contraindicated in patients who are hypersensitive to iodine.

Normal findings
Biliary ducts demonstrate homogeneous filling with contrast medium and are normal in diameter. When Oddi's sphincter is functioning properly and the ducts are patent, the contrast flows unimpeded into the duodenum.

Abnormal findings
Negative shadows or filling defects within the biliary ducts associated with dilation may indicate calculi or neo-

plasms overlooked during surgery. Abnormal channels of contrast medium departing from the biliary ducts indicate fistulae.

ENDOSCOPIC RETROGRADE CHOLANGIO-PANCREATOGRAPHY

Endoscopic retrograde cholangiopancreatography (ERCP) is the radiographic examination of the pancreatic ducts and hepatobiliary tree after injection of a contrast medium into the duodenal papilla. It's indicated in patients with confirmed or suspected pancreatic disease or obstructive jaundice of unknown etiology. Complications may include cholangitis and pancreatitis.

Purpose
• To evaluate obstructive jaundice
• To diagnose cancer of the duodenal papilla, the pancreas, and the biliary ducts
• To locate calculi and stenosis in the pancreatic ducts and hepatobiliary tree

Patient preparation
• Explain to the patient that this procedure permits examination of the liver, the gallbladder, and the pancreas through X-ray films taken after injection of a contrast medium.
• Instruct him to fast after midnight before the test.
• Describe the test, including who will perform it, where it will take place, and its expected duration (30 to 60 minutes).
• Inform him that a local anesthetic will be sprayed into his mouth to calm the gag reflex. Warn him that the spray has

an unpleasant taste and makes the tongue and throat feel swollen, causing difficulty in swallowing.

• Instruct him to let saliva drain from the side of his mouth, and tell him that suction may be used to remove saliva. Tell him a mouth guard will be inserted to protect his teeth and the endoscope; assure him that it won't obstruct his breathing.

• Assure the patient that he'll receive a sedative before insertion of the endoscope to help him relax, but that he'll remain conscious.

• Tell him that he'll also receive an anticholinergic or glucagon I.V. after insertion of the scope. Describe the possible adverse effects of anticholinergics (dry mouth, thirst, tachycardia, urinary retention, and blurred vision) or of glucagon (nausea, vomiting, hives, and flushing).

• Warn him that he may experience transient flushing on injection of the contrast medium. Advise him that he may have a sore throat for 3 or 4 days after the examination.

• Make sure the patient or a responsible family member has signed a consent form.

• Check the patient's history for hypersensitivity to iodine, seafood, or contrast media used for other diagnostic procedures.

• Just before the procedure, obtain baseline vital signs. Instruct the patient to remove all metal or other radiopaque objects and constricting undergarments. Then, tell him to void, to minimize the discomfort of urinary retention that may follow the procedure.

Procedure and posttest care

• An I.V. is started with 150 ml of 0.9% sodium chloride solution. The local anesthetic is then administered and usually takes effect in about 10 minutes.

• If a spray is used, ask the patient to hold his breath while his mouth and throat are sprayed.

• Place the patient in a left lateral position, and give him an emesis basin; provide tissues. Because the anesthetic causes the patient to lose some control of his secretions and thus increases the risk of aspiration, encourage him to allow saliva to drain from the side of his mouth.

• Insert the mouth guard.

• While the patient remains in the left lateral position, 5 to 20 mg of diazepam is administered I.V.

• When ptosis or dysarthria develops, the patient's head is bent forward, and he is asked to open his mouth.

• The examiner inserts his left index finger in the patient's mouth and guides the tip of the endoscope along his finger to the back of the patient's throat. The scope is then deflected downward with the left index finger and advanced. As the endoscope passes through the posterior pharynx and cricopharyngeal sphincter, the patient's head is slowly extended to assist the advance of the endoscope. The patient's chin must be kept midline. When the endoscope has passed the cricopharyngeal sphincter, the scope is advanced under direct vision. When it's well into the esophagus, the patient's chin is moved toward the table so saliva can drain from the mouth. The endoscope is advanced through the remainder of the esophagus and into the stomach under direct vision.

• When the pylorus is located, a small amount of air is insufflated, and the tip of the endoscope is angled upward and passed into the duodenal bulb.

• After the endoscope is rotated clockwise to enter the descending duodenum, the patient is assisted to prone position.

• An anticholinergic or glucagon I.V. is administered to induce duodenal atony and to relax the ampullary sphincter.

• A small amount of air is insufflated, and the endoscope is manipulated until the optic lies opposite the duodenal papilla. Then, the cannula filled with contrast medium is passed through the biopsy channel of the endoscope, the duodenal papilla, and into the ampulla of Vater.

• The pancreas is visualized first under fluoroscopic guidance with injection of contrast medium.

• The cannula is repositioned at a more cephalad angle, and the hepatobiliary tree is visualized with injection of contrast medium.

• After each injection, rapid-sequence X-ray films are taken.

• Instruct the patient to remain prone while the films are developed and reviewed. If necessary, additional films may be taken.

• When the required radiographs have been obtained, the cannula is removed. Before the endoscope is withdrawn, a tissue specimen may be obtained or fluid aspirated for histologic and cytologic examination, respectively.

• Observe closely for signs of cholangitis and pancreatitis. Hyperbilirubinemia, fever, and chills are the immediate signs of cholangitis; hypotension associated with gram-negative septicemia may develop later. Left upper quadrant pain and tenderness, elevated serum amylase levels, and transient hyperbilirubinemia are the usual signs of pancreatitis. Draw blood samples for amylase and bilirubin determinations, if necessary, but remember that these levels usually rise after ERCP.

• Continue to watch for signs of respiratory depression, apnea, hypotension, excessive diaphoresis, bradycardia, and laryngospasm. Check vital signs every 15 minutes for 4 hours, then every hour for 4 hours, and then every 4 hours for 48 hours.

• Withhold food and fluids until the gag reflex returns. Test the gag reflex by touching the back of the throat with a tongue blade. When the gag reflex returns, allow fluids and a light meal.

• Discontinue or maintain I.V. as appropriate.

• Check for signs of urinary retention for the next 8 hours.

• If the patient has a sore throat, provide soothing lozenges and warm saline gargles to ease discomfort.

Precautions

• ERCP is contraindicated in patients with infectious disease, pancreatic pseudocysts, stricture or obstruction of the esophagus or duodenum, and acute pancreatitis, cholangitis, or cardiorespiratory disease.

• Monitor vital signs and airway patency throughout the procedure. Watch for signs of respiratory depression, apnea, hypotension, excessive diaphoresis, bradycardia, and laryngospasm. Be sure to have available emergency resuscitation equipment and a narcotic antagonist, such as naloxone.

Normal findings

The duodenal papilla appears as a small red (or sometimes pale) erosion protruding into the lumen. Its orifice is commonly bordered by a fringe of white mucosa, and a longitudinal fold running perpendicular to the deep circular folds of the duodenum helps mark its location. Although the pancreatic and the hepatobiliary ducts usually unite in the ampulla of Vater and empty through the duodenal papilla, separate orifices are sometimes present.

The contrast medium uniformly fills the pancreatic duct, the hepatobiliary tree, and the gallbladder.

Abnormal findings

Obstructive jaundice may result from various abnormalities of the hepatobiliary tree and pancreatic duct. Examination of the hepatobiliary tree may reveal stones, strictures, or irregular deviations that suggest biliary cirrhosis, primary sclerosing cholangitis, or carcinoma of the bile ducts.

Examination of the pancreatic ducts may also show stones, strictures, and irregular deviations that may indicate pancreatic cysts and pseudocysts, pancreatic tumor, carcinoma of the head of the pancreas, chronic pancreatitis, pancreatic fibrosis, carcinoma of the duodenal papilla, and papillary stenosis.

Depending on test findings, definitive diagnosis may require further studies.

SPLENOPORTOGRAPHY

Splenoportography (or transsplenic portography) is the cineradiographic examination of the splenic veins and portal system after injection of a contrast medium into the splenic pulp. The procedure begins with measurement of splenic pulp pressure. A contrast medium is then injected into the spleen, and cineradiography is used to record the subsequent filling of the splenic tributary veins, the splenic and portal veins, and the intrahepatic portal radicles. This test may cause excessive bleeding that requires transfusion or, occasionally, splenectomy.

Splenoportography generally provides clearer definition of the venous system than superior mesenteric arteriography; however, it fails to outline the portal vein and, often, the splenic vein in portal hypertension associated with reversed venous blood flow. Superior mesenteric arteriography offers the advantage of outlining the portal and splenic veins, even during reversed blood flow, and causes fewer complications.

Purpose

• To diagnose or assess portal hypertension

• To stage cirrhosis

Patient preparation

• Explain to the patient that this procedure permits examination of the veins supplying the spleen and liver through films taken after injection of a contrast medium.

• Instruct him to fast after the evening meal the day before the procedure. Tell him who will perform this procedure and where and that it takes 30 to 45 minutes.

• Explain that he may experience a brief stinging sensation on injection of the local anesthetic and a transient flushed feeling on injection of the contrast medium.

• Instruct him to report left upper quadrant pain (which indicates subcapsular injection) immediately.

• Make sure the patient or a responsible family member has signed a consent form.

• Check the patient's history for hypersensitivity to iodine, seafood, or contrast media used in other diagnostic tests.

• Describe the possible adverse effects of contrast administration, such as nausea, vomiting, excessive salivation, flushing, urticaria, sweating and, rarely, anaphylaxis. Because these reactions usually occur 5 to 10 minutes after injection of the contrast medium, tell the patient to report such signs if they develop.

• Make sure the patient's platelet count and bleeding, clotting, and prothrombin times are normal.

• About 30 minutes before the procedure, obtain baseline vital signs, and administer a mild sedative and an analgesic.

Procedure and posttest care
• The patient is placed in a supine position on the radiographic table, with his left hand under his head. The left side of his thorax and abdomen is cleaned with antiseptics.
• Using fluoroscopy, the spleen is located and palpated, and a scout film is taken.
• After a skin wheal is made with the local anesthetic to mark the puncture site — usually the intersection of the ninth or tenth intercostal space and the midline or posterior axillary line — the skin and subcutaneous tissue are infiltrated to the peritoneum.
• As the patient holds his breath midrespiration, a sheathed needle is rapidly inserted into the spleen and the inner needle withdrawn.
• The patient is instructed to maintain shallow respirations with the sheath in place. With flexible plastic tubing, a spinal manometer filled with 0.9% sodium chloride solution is connected to the sheath, and the splenic pulp pressure is measured.
• The manometer is replaced with a syringe containing 50 ml of sodium diatrizoate that's warmed to body temperature and the sheath is taped in place.
• Sheath placement is checked fluoroscopically by injection of a few milliliters of contrast medium.
• If the sheath is properly positioned, the patient is moved over the angiographic changer, the remaining contrast medium is injected, and films are ordered.
• When the required films have been obtained, the sheath is withdrawn, and pressure and a sterile dressing are applied to the puncture site.
• Check vital signs every 15 minutes for 1 hour, then every 30 minutes for 2

hours, and then every hour for 4 hours until stable. Observe for bleeding, swelling, and tenderness at the puncture site.
• Instruct the patient to lie on his left side for 24 hours to minimize the risk of bleeding. Advise an additional 24 hours of bed rest.
• Tell the patient he may resume his usual diet. Encourage fluids to promote excretion of the contrast medium.
• Draw a blood sample for hematocrit determination every 8 to 12 hours until hematocrit levels stabilize.

Precautions
• Splenoportography is contraindicated in patients with ascites, uncorrectable coagulopathy, splenomegaly due to infection, markedly impaired liver or kidney function, and hypersensitivity to iodine.

Normal findings
Splenic pulp pressure is normally 50 to 180 mm H_2O (3.5 to 13.5 mm Hg). After the contrast medium is injected into the splenic pulp, it outlines splenic tributary veins (splenography), then drains into the splenic and portal veins; venous flow is normally contained within these two vessels, without diversion into collateral veins. The contrast medium outlines the intrahepatic portal radicles (hepatography), with the radicles branching in an acute and homogeneous fashion throughout the liver. When the radicles empty, a dense hepatogram results.

Abnormal findings
In portal hypertension, splenic pulp pressure ranges from 200 to 450 mm H_2O (15 to 34 mm Hg). The presence of collateral veins, often associated with esophageal varices, splenomegaly, and in some cases, hepatomegaly — can also indicate portal hypertension resulting from intrahepatic or extrahepatic

CAUSES OF PORTAL HYPERTENSION

CAUSE	COMPLICATIONS	APPEARANCE
Suprahepatic • Tricuspid valve incompetence • Hepatic vein thrombosis • Constrictive pericarditis	• Enlarged liver • Moderately enlarged spleen • Few esophageal varices	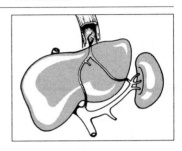
Intrahepatic • Liver cirrhosis	• Esophageal varices • Markedly enlarged spleen	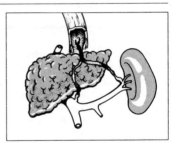
Intrahepatic • Portal vein thrombosis	• Esophageal varices • Decidedly enlarged spleen	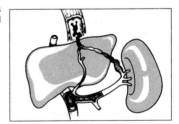

obstruction to portal venous flow. Results may also show thrombosis or occlusion in the splenic and portal veins provided venous flow isn't reversed. See *Causes of portal hypertension.*

In early-stage cirrhosis, a normal splenogram is characteristic, but emptying of the intrahepatic radicles is delayed. As cirrhosis progresses, collateral veins develop, the intrahepatic radicles become angular and shortened, and emptying is again delayed. In advanced cirrhosis, venous blood flow reverses, preventing visualization of the portal and, usually, the splenic veins. Numerous collateral veins in the hilum of the spleen and the immediate retroperitoneum are also characteristic. Actually, the presence of such collateral veins on a film that fails to show the portal vein generally indicates portal hypertension. However, superior mesenteric arteriography is then appropriate to confirm portal vein occlusion or thrombosis.

CELIAC AND MESENTERIC ARTERIOGRAPHY

This test involves the radiographic examination of the abdominal vasculature after intra-arterial injection of contrast medium through a catheter. Most commonly, the catheter is passed through the femoral artery into the aorta and then, using fluoroscopy, is positioned in the celiac, superior mesenteric, or inferior mesenteric artery. Injection of contrast medium into one or more of these arteries provides a map of abdominal vasculature; injection into specific arterial branches, called superselective angiography, permits detailed visualization of a particular area. As the contrast medium flows through the abdominal vasculature, serial radiographs outline abdominal vessels in the arterial, capillary, and venous phases of perfusion.

Celiac and mesenteric arteriography is indicated when endoscopy is unable to locate the source of GI bleeding or when barium studies, ultrasonography, and nuclear medicine or computed tomography scanning prove inconclusive in evaluating neoplasms. It's also used to evaluate cirrhosis and portal hypertension (especially when a portacaval shunt is being considered); to evaluate

vascular damage, particularly in the spleen and liver, after abdominal trauma; and to detect vascular abnormalities. Because arteriography can demonstrate the portal vein even when portal venous flow is reversed, it is used more often than splenoportography.

Complications associated with this test include hemorrhage, venous and intracardiac thrombosis, cardiac arrhythmia, and emboli caused by dislodging atherosclerotic plaques.

Purpose
• To locate the source of GI bleeding
• To help distinguish between benign and malignant neoplasms
• To evaluate cirrhosis and portal hypertension
• To evaluate vascular damage after abdominal trauma
• To detect vascular abnormalities

Patient preparation
• Explain to the patient that this test permits examination of the abdominal blood vessels after injection of a contrast medium.
• Instruct him to fast for 8 hours before the test.
• Tell him that he'll receive a local anesthetic and that he may feel a brief, stinging sensation as it's injected. He may also feel pressure when the femoral artery is palpated, but the local anesthetic will minimize the pain when the needle is introduced into the artery.
• Tell him he may feel a transient burning as the contrast medium is injected and that he may experience a transient headache, a salty taste in his mouth, and nausea and vomiting.
• Tell him that the X-ray equipment makes a loud, clacking sound as the films are taken.
• Instruct him to lie still during the test to avoid blurring the films, and inform him that restraints may be used to help him remain still.

• Warn him that he may feel some temporary stiffness after the test from lying still on the hard X-ray table.

• Tell him who will perform the test and where and that it takes 30 minutes to 3 hours depending on the number of vessels studied.

• Make sure the patient or a responsible family member has signed a consent form, if required.

• Check the patient's history for hypersensitivity to iodine, shellfish, or the contrast medium.

• Make sure blood studies (hemoglobin and hematocrit levels; clotting, prothrombin, and activated partial thromboplastin times; and platelet count) have been completed.

• Just before the procedure, instruct the patient to put on a hospital gown and to remove jewelry and other objects that might obscure anatomic detail on X-ray films.

• Tell the patient to void; then record baseline vital signs.

• Administer a sedative, if prescribed.

Procedure and posttest care

• After placing the patient in supine position on the radiographic table, an I.V. infusion is started to maintain hydration and to permit emergency administration of medication.

• Scout films of the patient's abdomen are taken, and the peripheral pulses are palpated and marked.

• The puncture site is cleaned with soap and water; the area is shaved, cleaned with povidone-iodine preparation, and surrounded by sterile drapes.

• The local anesthetic is injected and the femoral artery is located by palpation. The needle is gently inserted until a pulsing blood flow is obtained.

• A guide wire is passed through the needle into the aorta; then the needle is removed, leaving the guide wire in place.

• The angiographic catheter is inserted over the guide wire; the guide wire is withdrawn to inject the contrast medium to check for catheter placement. The guide wire is again inserted into the selected artery for fluoroscopic guidance.

• When the wire is in position, the catheter is advanced over it into the artery. The wire is then removed and placement verified by hand injection of contrast medium.

• The automatic injector is then attached to the catheter. As the contrast medium is injected, a series of films are taken in rapid sequence.

• After injecting into one or more major arteries, superselective catheterization may be performed. Using fluoroscopy, the catheter is repositioned in a specific branch of a major artery, contrast medium is injected, and rapid-sequence films are ordered. If necessary, several specific branches may be catheterized.

• After filming, the catheter is withdrawn, and firm pressure is applied to the puncture site for about 15 minutes.

• Observe the puncture site for hematoma formation and check peripheral pulses.

• Inform the patient that he'll be on bed rest for 4 to 6 hours and that he must keep the leg with the puncture site straight. Do not raise the bed further than 30 degrees. He will be able to log-roll and may use the unaffected leg to reposition himself to use the bedpan.

• Monitor vital signs until stable, and check peripheral pulses. Note the color and temperature of the leg that was used for the test.

• Check the puncture site for bleeding and hematoma. If bleeding develops, apply pressure to the site. If a hematoma develops, apply warm soaks.

• Confirm whether the patient can resume his usual diet. If the patient isn't receiving I.V. infusions, encourage intake of fluids to speed excretion of the contrast medium.

• Tell the patient that he must be careful when swallowing for 4 to 6 hours after surgery.

Precautions
• Celiac and mesenteric arteriography should be performed cautiously in patients with coagulopathy.
• Most reactions to the contrast medium occur within a half-hour. Watch carefully for cardiovascular shock or arrest, hives, flushing, laryngeal stridor, or urticaria.

Normal findings
X-ray films show the three phases of perfusion — arterial, capillary, and venous. The arteries normally taper regularly, becoming gradually smaller with subsequent divisions. The contrast medium then spreads evenly within the sinusoids. The portal vein appears 10 to 20 seconds after the injection, as the contrast medium empties from the spleen into the splenic vein or from the intestine into the superior mesenteric vein and further into the portal vein.

Abnormal findings
GI hemorrhage appears on the angiogram as the extravasation of contrast medium from the damaged vessels. Upper GI hemorrhage can result from conditions such as Mallory-Weiss syndrome, gastric or peptic ulcer, hemorrhagic gastritis, and eroded hiatal hernia. Esophageal hemorrhage rarely appears on the angiogram because the contrast medium usually fails to fill the esophageal vein. Lower GI hemorrhage can result from conditions such as bleeding diverticula and angiodysplasia.

Abdominal neoplasms — carcinoid tumors, adenomas, leiomyomas, angiomas, and adenocarcinomas — can disrupt the normal vasculature in several ways. Neoplasms can invade or encase nearby arteries and veins, distorting their regular channel-like appearance and, in late stages, displacing them. Vessels within the neoplasm, known as neovasculature, appear as abnormal vascular areas. Areas of necrosis appear as puddles of contrast medium. Contrast medium may also remain in the neoplasm longer during capillary perfusion, producing a tumor blush or stain on the angiogram. Arteriovenous shunting may also be present, depending on the size and location of the tumor. Because these characteristics aren't uniformly present in all neoplasms, combinations of these characteristics can often distinguish between benign and malignant neoplasms.

In early or mild cirrhosis, portal venous flow to the liver remains relatively unaffected, and the hepatic artery and its branches appear normal. As this disease progresses, portal venous flow diminishes, the hepatic artery and its branches become dilated and tortuous, and collateral veins develop. In advanced cirrhosis, portal venous flow reverses. However, the portal vein still appears on the X-ray film, which may also show thrombi.

Abdominal trauma often causes splenic and, less often, hepatic injury. Splenic rupture often displaces intrasplenic arterial branches, and contrast medium leaks from splenic arteries into the splenic pulp. When rupture occurs without subcapsular hematoma, the spleen usually maintains its normal size. However, in subcapsular hematoma, the spleen enlarges to displace the splenic artery and vein; the subcapsular hematoma itself appears as a large, avascular mass that stretches intrasplenic arteries and compresses the splenic pulp away from the capsule.

Hepatic injury causes similar vascular distortion, such as displacement of the common hepatic artery and extrahepatic branches. Intrahepatic and subcapsular hematomas displace and stretch intrahepatic arteries. As the hepatic vascular supply is disrupted, arteriovenous fistula may develop between the hepatic artery and the portal vein.

Various abnormalities affecting the diameter and course of an artery may appear on the angiogram. Atherosclerotic plaques or atheromas — lipid deposits on the intima — narrow the arterial lumen and may even occlude it, with formation of collaterals. Other identifiable vascular abnormalities include aneurysms, thrombi, and emboli.

GENITOURINARY SYSTEM

KIDNEY-URETER-BLADDER RADIOGRAPHY

Usually the first step in diagnostic testing of the urinary system, kidney-ureter-bladder (KUB) radiography surveys the abdomen to determine the position of the kidneys, ureters, and bladder, and to detect gross abnormalities.

This test does not require intact renal function and may aid differential diagnosis of urologic and GI diseases, which often produce similar signs and symptoms. However, a KUB has many limitations and nearly always must be followed by more elaborate tests, such as excretory urography or renal computed tomography. KUB should not follow recent instillation of barium.

Purpose
• To evaluate the size, structure, and position of the kidneys
• To screen for abnormalities, such as calcifications, in the region of the kidneys, ureters, and bladder

Patient preparation
• Explain to the patient that this test helps detect urinary system abnormalities.
• Inform him that he needn't restrict food or fluids. Tell him who will perform the test and where and that it takes only a few minutes.

Procedure and posttest care
• The patient is placed in a supine position in correct body alignment on an X-ray table. His arms are extended overhead, and the iliac crests are checked for symmetrical positioning.
• If the patient can't extend his arms or stand, he may lie on his left side with his right arm up.
• A single X-ray is taken.

Precautions
• Male patients should have gonadal shielding to prevent irradiation of the testes. Female patients' ovaries can't be shielded because they're too close to the kidneys, ureters, and bladder.

Normal findings
The shadows of the kidneys appear bilaterally, the right slightly lower than the left. Both kidneys should be approximately the same size, with the superior poles tilted slightly toward the vertebral column, paralleling the shadows (or stripes) produced by the psoas muscles. The ureters are only visible when an abnormality such as calcification is present. Visualization of the bladder depends on the density of its muscular wall and on the amount of urine in it.

Abnormal findings

Bilateral renal enlargement may result from polycystic disease, multiple myeloma, lymphoma, amyloidosis, hydronephrosis, or compensatory hypertrophy. Tumor, cyst, or hydronephrosis may cause unilateral enlargement. Abnormally small kidneys may suggest end-stage glomerulonephritis or bilateral atrophic pyelonephritis. An apparent decrease in the size of one kidney suggests possible congenital hypoplasia, atrophic pyelonephritis, or ischemia. Renal displacement may be due to a retroperitoneal tumor, such as an adrenal tumor. Obliteration or bulging of a portion of the psoas muscle stripe may result from tumor, abscess, or hematoma.

Congenital anomalies, such as abnormal location or absence of a kidney, may be detected. Horseshoe kidney may be suggested by renal axes that parallel the vertebral column, especially if the inferior poles of the kidneys cannot be clearly distinguished. A lobulated edge or border may suggest polycystic kidney disease or patchy atrophic pyelonephritis.

Opaque bodies may reflect calculi or vascular calcification due to aneurysm or atheroma; opacification may also suggest cystic tumors, fecaliths, foreign bodies, or abnormal fluid collection. Calcifications may appear anywhere in the urinary system, but positive identification requires further testing. The lone exception is staghorn calculus, which forms a perfect cast of the renal pelvis and calyces.

NEPHROTOMOGRAPHY

In nephrotomography, special films are exposed before and after opacification of the renal arterial network and parenchyma with contrast medium. The resulting tomographic slices clearly delineate various linear layers of the kidneys, while blurring structures in front of and behind these selected planes.

Nephrotomography can be performed as a separate procedure or as an adjunct to excretory urography. Nephrotomography is particularly helpful in visualizing space-occupying lesions suggested by excretory urography or retrograde ureteropyelography. Additional films are exposed to define the thickness of the wall of the mass and its interior. Other tests that may resolve nephrotomographic findings include renal angiography and radionuclide renal imaging.

Purpose

• To differentiate between a simple renal cyst and a solid neoplasm
• To assess renal lacerations as well as posttraumatic nonperfused areas of the kidneys
• To localize adrenal tumors when laboratory tests indicate their presence

Patient preparation

• Explain to the patient that this test provides images of sections or layers of the kidney tissues and blood vessels.
• Instruct him to fast for 8 hours before the test. Tell him who will perform the test and where and that the test takes less than 1 hour.
• Tell him that he'll be positioned on an X-ray table and that he may hear loud, clacking sounds as the films are exposed. Tell him that he may experience transient adverse effects from the injection of the contrast medium — usually a burning or stinging sensation at the injection site, flushing, and a metallic taste.
• Make sure that the patient or a responsible family member has signed a consent form if required.
• Check his history for hypersensitivity to iodine or iodine-containing foods or

to contrast media used in other diagnostic tests. If the patient has a history of sensitivity, provide anti-allergenic prophylaxis (such as diphenhydramine) or use non–iodine-containing contrast, as necessary.

Procedure and posttest care
• The test may be performed using either the infusion method or the bolus method. Complications resulting from either technique are minor and infrequent.
• A plain film of the kidneys is exposed to provide general information about their position, size, and shape, and preliminary anteroposterior tomograms are made to determine tomographic levels. Posterior oblique tomograms are made to rule out the presence of radiopaque renal calculi, which would be masked by the contrast.
Infusion method:
• After test tomograms are reviewed, five vertical slices of renal parenchyma $\frac{1}{3}''$ (1 cm) apart are selected for filming.
• Contrast medium is then administered through the antecubital vein — the first half in 4 to 5 minutes (rapid phase) and the second half in the following 8 to 10 minutes (slow phase). Serial tomograms are made as soon as the slow phase begins.
Bolus method:
• After test tomograms are reviewed, circulation time from arm to tongue is determined by injecting a bolus of a bitter-tasting agent (dehydrocholic acid or sodium dehydrocholate) into the antecubital vein. Arm-to-tongue circulation time is close to arm-to-kidney circulation time.
• With the needle still in place, a loading dose of a conventional urographic contrast medium is injected to perform excretory urography.
• Five minutes after this injection, a loading dose of a contrast medium (such as Renografin-76 or Hypaque-M

75%) is quickly injected to ensure a high concentration of the contrast medium in the kidneys. A multifilm tomographic cassette, exposed at the predetermined arm-to-kidney circulation time, visualizes the main renal vessels and possible vessels within tumors.
• A series of individual tomograms measuring $\frac{1}{3}''$ are then made in rapid succession through the opacified kidneys.
• If the exposures are poor, this method requires a second infusion of contrast medium because normal kidneys quickly clear the substance.
Both methods:
• If a hematoma develops at the injection site, apply warm soaks.
• Monitor vital signs and urine output for 24 hours after the test.
• Observe for signs of posttest allergic reaction (flushing, nausea, urticaria, and sneezing). Have epinephrine (1:1000) and an antihistamine readily available to counter allergic reactions.

Precautions
• Nephrotomography should be performed with extreme caution in patients with hypersensitivity to iodine-based compounds or in those with severe cardiovascular disease or multiple myeloma.

Normal findings
The size, shape, and position of the kidneys appear within normal range, with no space-occupying lesions or other abnormalities.

Abnormal findings
Among the abnormalities detectable through nephrotomography are simple cysts and solid tumors, renal sinus-related lesions, ectopic renal lobes, adrenal tumors, areas of nonperfusion, and renal lacerations following trauma. See *Simple cyst or solid tumor: Differential diagnosis in nephrotomography,* page 542.

SIMPLE CYST OR SOLID TUMOR: DIFFERENTIAL DIAGNOSIS IN NEPHROTOMOGRAPHY

FEATURE	CYST	TUMOR
Consistency	Homogeneous	Irregular
Contact with healthy renal tissue	Sharply distinct	Poorly resolved
Density	Radiolucent	Variable radiolucent patches (or same as normal renal parenchyma)
Shape	Spherical	Variable
Wall of lesion	Thin and well defined	Thick and irregular

RETROGRADE URETHROGRAPHY

Used almost exclusively in men, this radiographic study requires instillation or injection of a contrast medium into the urethra and permits visualization of its membranous, bulbar, and penile portions.

Although visualization of the anterior portion of the urethra is excellent with this test alone, the posterior portion is more effectively outlined by retrograde urethrography in tandem with voiding cystourethrography.

Purpose
• To diagnose urethral strictures, outlet obstruction, diverticula, and congenital anomalies
• To assess urethral lacerations or other trauma
• To assist with follow-up examination after surgical repair of the urethra

Patient preparation
• Explain to the patient that this test diagnoses urethral structural problems. Inform him that he needn't restrict food or fluids.
• Describe the test, including who will perform it, where it will take place, and its expected duration (about 30 minutes).
• Inform the patient that he may experience some discomfort when the catheter is inserted and when the contrast medium is instilled through the catheter.
• Tell him that he may hear loud, clacking sounds as the X-ray films are made.
• Make sure the patient or a responsible family member has signed a consent form if required.
• Check the patient's history for hypersensitivity to iodine-containing foods, like shellfish, or contrast media.
• Just before the procedure, administer any prescribed sedatives and instruct the patient to void before leaving the unit.

Equipment
Penile clamp, 50-ml syringe with tapered universal adapter, indwelling urinary catheter, 1″ (2.5-cm) roller gauze,

contrast medium (half-strength preparation).

Procedure and posttest care

For men:

• The patient is placed in a recumbent position on the examining table. Anteroposterior exposures of the bladder and urethra are made, and the resulting films studied for radiopaque densities, foreign bodies, or stones.

• The glans and meatus are cleaned with an antiseptic solution. The catheter is filled with the contrast medium before insertion to eliminate air bubbles.

• Although no lubricant should be used, the tip of the catheter may be dipped in sterile water to facilitate insertion.

• The catheter is inserted until the balloon portion is inside the meatus; the balloon is then inflated with 1 to 2 ml of water, which prevents the catheter from slipping during the procedure.

• The patient then assumes the right posterior oblique position, with his right thigh drawn up to a 90-degree angle and the penis placed along its axis. The left thigh is extended.

• The contrast medium is injected through the catheter. After three-fourths of the contrast medium has been injected, the first X-ray film is exposed while the remainder of the contrast medium is being injected. Left lateral oblique views may also be taken.

• Fluoroscopic control may be helpful, especially for evaluating urethral injury.

For women and children:

• In women, this test may be used when urethral diverticula are suspected. A double-balloon catheter is used, which occludes the bladder neck from above and the external meatus from below.

• In children, the procedure is the same as for adults except that a smaller catheter is used.

For all patients:

• Watch for chills and fever related to extravasation of contrast medium into the general circulation for 12 to 24 hours after retrograde urethrography. Also observe for signs of sepsis and allergic manifestations.

Precautions

• Retrograde urethrography should be performed cautiously in patients with urinary tract infection.

Normal findings

The membranous, bulbar, and penile portions of the urethra — and occasionally the prostatic portion — appear normal in size, shape, and course.

Abnormal findings

Radiographs obtained during retrograde urethrography may show the following abnormalities: urethral diverticula, fistulas, strictures, false passages, calculi, and lacerations; congenital anomalies, such as urethral valves and perineal hypospadias; and rarely, tumors (in less than 1% of patients).

RETROGRADE CYSTOGRAPHY

Retrograde cystography involves the instillation of contrast medium into the bladder, followed by radiographic examination. This procedure is used to diagnose bladder rupture without urethral involvement because it can determine the location and extent of the rupture. Other indications for retrograde cystography include neurogenic bladder, recurrent urinary tract infections (especially in children), suspected vesicoureteral reflux, and vesical fistulas, diverticula, and tumors. This test is also performed when cystoscopic examination is impractical, as in male infants, or when excretory urography has not adequately visualized the bladder. Voiding cystourethrography is often performed concomitantly.

Purpose
• To evaluate the structure and integrity of the bladder

Patient preparation
• Explain to the patient that the test permits radiographic examination (or X-ray films) of the bladder. Inform him that he needn't restrict food or fluids.
• Tell him who will perform the test and where and that the procedure takes about 30 to 60 minutes.
• Inform the patient that he may experience some discomfort when the catheter is inserted and when the contrast medium is instilled through the catheter.
• Tell him that he may hear loud, clacking sounds as the X-ray films are made.
• Make sure the patient or a responsible family member has signed a consent form.
• Check the patient's history for hypersensitivity to contrast media, iodine, or shellfish; mark it on the chart.

Equipment
Drip infusion set or syringes, standard contrast medium, urethral indwelling urinary catheters.

Procedure and posttest care
• The patient is placed in supine position on the examining table, and a preliminary kidney-ureter-bladder radiograph is taken.
• The radiograph is developed immediately and scrutinized for renal shadows, calcifications, contours of the bone and psoas muscles, and gas patterns in the lumen of the GI tract.
• The bladder is catheterized, and 200 to 300 ml of contrast medium (50 to 100 ml in an infant) is instilled by grav-

ity or gentle syringe injection. The catheter is then clamped.
• With the patient supine, an anteroposterior film is taken. The patient is then tilted to one side, then the other, and two posterior oblique (and sometimes lateral) views are taken.
• If the patient's condition permits, he is placed in the jackknife position and a posteroanterior film is taken. A space-occupying vesical lesion may require additional exposures. Rarely, to enhance visualization, 100 to 300 ml of air may be insufflated into the bladder by syringe after removal of the contrast medium (double-contrast technique).
• The catheter is then unclamped, the bladder fluid is allowed to drain, and a radiograph is obtained to detect urethral diverticula, fistulous tracts into the vagina, or intra- or extraperitoneal extravasation of the contrast medium.
• Monitor vital signs every 15 minutes for the first hour, every 30 minutes during the second hour, then every 2 hours for up to 24 hours.
• Record the time of the patient's voidings and the color and volume of the urine. Observe for hematuria that persists after the third voiding.
• Watch for signs of urinary sepsis from urinary tract infection (chills, fever, elevated pulse and respiration rates, and hypotension) or similar signs related to extravasation of contrast medium into the general circulation.

Precautions
• Retrograde cystography is contraindicated during exacerbation of an acute urinary tract infection or in patients with an obstruction that prevents passage of a urinary catheter.
• This test should not be performed in patients with urethral evulsion or transection, unless catheter passage and flow of contrast medium are monitored fluoroscopically.

Normal findings

Retrograde cystography shows a bladder with normal contours, capacity, integrity, and urethrovesical angle and with no evidence of tumor, diverticula, or rupture. Vesicoureteral reflux should be absent. The bladder should not be displaced or externally compressed; the bladder wall should be smooth, not thick.

Abnormal findings

Retrograde cystography can identify vesical trabeculae or diverticula, space-occupying lesions (tumors), calculi or gravel, blood clots, high- or low-pressure vesicoureteral reflux, and a hypo- or hypertonic bladder.

RETROGRADE URETEROPYELOGRAPHY

This test allows radiographic examination of the renal collecting system after injection of a contrast medium through a ureteral catheter during cystoscopy. The contrast medium is usually iodine-based and, although some of it may be absorbed through the mucous membranes, this test is preferred for patients with hypersensitivity to iodine (in whom I.V. administration of an iodine-based contrast medium, as in excretory urography, is contraindicated). This test is also indicated when visualization of the renal collecting system by excretory urography is inadequate due to inferior films or marked renal insufficiency because retrograde ureteropyelography is not influenced by impaired renal function.

Purpose

• To assess the structure and integrity of the renal collecting system (calyces, renal pelvis, and ureter)

Patient preparation

• Explain to the patient that this test permits visualization of the urinary collecting system.
• If a general anesthetic is to be used, instruct him to fast for 8 hours before the test. Generally, he should be well hydrated to ensure adequate urine flow.
• Tell him who will perform the test and where and that it takes about 1 hour.
• Inform the patient that he'll be positioned on an examining table, with his legs in stirrups, and that the position may be tiring.
• If he will be awake throughout the procedure, tell him he may feel pressure as the instrument is passed and a pressure sensation in the kidney area when the contrast medium is introduced. Also, he may feel an urgency to void.
• Make sure that the patient or a responsible family member has signed a consent form.
• Just before the procedure, administer any prescribed premedication.

Equipment

Cystoscopy setup, ureteral catheters, 10-ml syringes with ureteral adapters, contrast medium.

Procedure and posttest care

• Place the patient in lithotomy position. Care must be taken to avoid pressure points or impairment to circulation while his legs are in the stirrups.
• After the patient is anesthetized, the urologist first performs a cystoscopic examination.
• After visual inspection of the bladder, one or both ureters are catheterized with opaque catheters, depending on the condition or abnormality suspected. Radiographic monitoring allows cor-

SITES AND TYPES OF OBSTRUCTION INDICATED BY URETEROPYELOGRAPHY

Ureteropyelography may detect a stricture, neoplasm, blood clot, or calculus that obstructs urine flow in the calyces, pelvis, or ureter. Small calculi may remain in the calyces and pelvis or pass down the ureter. A staghorn calculus (a cast of the calyceal and pelvic collecting system) may form from calculus that stays in the kidney.

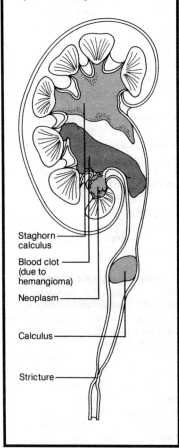

Staghorn calculus

Blood clot (due to hemangioma)

Neoplasm

Calculus

Stricture

rect positioning of the catheter tip in the renal pelvis.

• The renal pelvis is emptied by gravity drainage or aspiration. About 4 or 5 ml of contrast medium is then injected slowly through the catheter using the syringe fitted with a special adapter.

• When adequate filling and opacification have occurred, anteroposterior radiographic films are taken and immediately developed. Lateral and oblique films can be taken, as needed, after the injection of more contrast.

• After the radiographs of the renal pelvis are examined, a few more milliliters of contrast medium are injected to outline the ureters as the catheter is slowly withdrawn.

• Delayed films (10 to 15 minutes after complete catheter removal) are then taken to check for retention of the contrast medium, indicating urinary stasis.

• If ureteral obstruction is present, the ureteral catheter may be kept in place and, together with an indwelling urinary catheter, connected to a gravity drainage system until posttest urinary flow is corrected or returns to normal.

• Check vital signs every 15 minutes for the first 4 hours, then every hour for the next 4 hours, and then every 4 hours for 24 hours.

• Monitor fluid intake and urine output for 24 hours. Observe each specimen for hematuria. Gross hematuria or hematuria after the third voiding is abnormal and should be reported. If the patient doesn't void for 8 hours after the procedure, or immediately if the patient feels distress and his bladder is distended, urethral catheterization may be necessary.

• Be especially attentive to catheter output if ureteral catheters have been left in place because inadequate output may reflect catheter obstruction, requiring irrigation. Protect ureteral catheters from dislodgment.

• Administer prescribed analgesics, tub baths, and increased fluid intake for dysuria, which commonly occurs after retrograde ureteropyelography.
• Watch for and report severe pain in the area of the kidneys as well as any signs of sepsis (such as chills, fever, and hypotension).

Precautions
• Retrograde ureteropyelography must be done carefully in patients with urinary stasis caused by ureteral obstruction to prevent further injury to the ureter.

Normal findings
Following a normal cystoscopic examination, ureteral catheterization, and injection of contrast medium through the catheters, opacification of the renal pelves and calyces should occur immediately. Normal structures should be outlined clearly and should appear symmetrical in bilateral testing. Ureters should fill uniformly and appear normal in size and course. Inspiratory and expiratory exposures, when superimposed, normally create two outlines of the renal pelvis ¾″ (2 cm) apart.

Abnormal findings
Incomplete or delayed drainage reflects an obstruction, most commonly at the ureteropelvic junction. Enlargement of the components of the collecting system or delayed emptying of contrast medium may indicate obstruction due to tumor, blood clot, stricture, or calculi. See *Sites and types of obstruction indicated by ureteropyelography.*

Perinephric inflammation or suppuration often causes fixation of the kidney on the same side, resulting in a single sharp radiographic outline of the collecting system when inspiratory and expiratory exposures are superimposed. Upward, downward, or lateral renal displacement can result from re-nal abscess or tumor or from perinephric abscess. Neoplasms can cause displacement of either pole or of the entire kidney.

ANTEGRADE PYELOGRAPHY

This radiographic procedure allows examination of the upper collecting system when ureteral obstruction rules out retrograde ureteropyelography or when cystoscopy is contraindicated. It depends on percutaneous needle puncture for injection of contrast medium into the renal pelvis or calyces.

Renal pressure can be measured during this procedure. Also, urine can be collected for cultures and cytologic studies and for evaluation of renal functional reserve before surgery.

After completion of radiographic studies, a nephrostomy tube can be inserted to provide temporary drainage or access for other therapeutic or diagnostic procedures.

Purpose
• To evaluate obstruction of the upper collecting system by stricture, calculus, clot, or tumor
• To evaluate hydronephrosis revealed during excretory urography or ultrasonography and to enable placement of a percutaneous nephrostomy tube
• To evaluate the function of the upper collecting system after ureteral surgery or urinary diversion
• To assess renal functional reserve before surgery

Patient preparation
• Explain to the patient that this test allows radiographic examination of the kidney.

- Tell him that he may be required to fast for 6 to 8 hours before the test.
- Tell him he may receive antimicrobial drugs before and after the procedure.
- Inform the patient who will perform the test and where and that it will take approximately 1 to 2 hours.
- Explain that a needle will be inserted into the kidney after he is given a sedative and a local anesthetic. Explain that urine may be collected from the kidney for testing and that, if necessary, a tube will be left in the kidney for drainage.
- Tell him that he may feel mild discomfort during injection of the local anesthetic and contrast medium and that he may also feel transient burning and flushing from the contrast medium.
- Warn him that the X-ray machine makes loud, clacking sounds as films are taken.
- Check the patient's history for hypersensitivity reactions to contrast media, iodine, or shellfish. Mark any sensitivities clearly on the chart. Also check the history and recent coagulation studies for indications of bleeding disorders.
- Make sure that the patient or a responsible family member has signed an appropriate consent form.
- Just before the procedure, administer a sedative, if needed.

Equipment
Percutaneous nephrostomy tray, manometer, preparatory tray, gloves and sterile containers for specimens, syringes and needles, contrast medium, local anesthetic, emergency resuscitation equipment.

Procedure and posttest care
- The patient is placed prone on the X-ray table. The skin over the kidney is cleaned with antiseptic solution, and a local anesthetic is injected.
- Previous urographic films or ultrasound recordings are studied for anatomic landmarks. (It's important to de-termine if the kidney to be studied is in normal position. If not, the angle of the needle entry must be adjusted during percutaneous puncture.)
- Under guidance of fluoroscopy or ultrasonography, the percutaneous needle is inserted below the 12th rib at the level of the transverse process of the 2nd lumbar vertebra. Aspiration of urine confirms that the needle has reached the dilated collecting system.
- Flexible tubing is connected to the needle to prevent displacement during the procedure. If intrarenal pressure is to be measured, the manometer is connected to the tubing as soon as it's in place. Urine specimens are then taken if needed.
- An amount of urine equal to the amount of contrast medium to be injected is withdrawn to prevent overdistention of the collecting system.
- The contrast medium is injected under fluoroscopic guidance. Postero-anterior, oblique, and anteroposterior radiographs are taken. Ureteral peristalsis is observed on the fluoroscope screen to evaluate obstruction.
- A percutaneous nephrostomy tube is inserted if drainage is needed because of increased renal pressure, dilation, or intrarenal reflux. If drainage is not needed, the catheter is withdrawn and a sterile dressing is applied.
- Check vital signs every 15 minutes for the first hour, every 30 minutes for the second hour, and every 2 hours for the next 24 hours.
- Check dressings for bleeding, hematoma, or urine leakage at the puncture site at each check of vital signs. For bleeding, apply pressure. For a hematoma, apply warm soaks. Report urine leakage or the patient's failure to void within 8 hours.
- Monitor fluid intake and urine output for 24 hours. Observe each specimen for hematuria. Report hematuria if it persists after the third voiding.

• Watch for and report signs of sepsis or extravasation of contrast medium (chills, fever, rapid pulse or respirations, and hypotension).

• Also watch for and report signs that adjacent organs have been punctured: pain in the abdomen or flank, or pneumothorax (sudden onset of pleuritic chest pain, dyspnea, tachypnea, decreased breath sounds on the affected side, and tachycardia).

• If a nephrostomy tube is inserted, check to be sure that it is patent and draining well.

• Administer prescribed antibiotics for several days after the procedure as well as any prescribed analgesics.

Precautions

• Antegrade pyelography is contraindicated in patients with bleeding disorders.

• Watch for signs of hypersensitivity to the contrast medium.

Normal findings

After injection of contrast medium, the upper collecting system should fill uniformly and appear normal in size and course. Normal structures should be outlined clearly.

Abnormal findings

Enlargements of the upper collecting system and parts of the ureteropelvic junction indicate obstruction. Antegrade pyelography shows the degree of dilation, clearly defines obstructions, and demonstrates intrarenal reflux. In hydronephrosis, the ureteropelvic junction shows marked distention. Results of recent surgery or urinary diversion will be obvious; for example, a ureteral stent or a dilated stenotic area will be clearly visualized.

Intrarenal pressures greater than 20 cm H_2O indicate obstruction. Cultures or cytologic studies of urine specimens taken during antegrade pyelography can confirm antegrade pyelonephrosis or malignancy.

EXCRETORY UROGRAPHY

The cornerstone of a urologic workup, excretory urography (also called intravenous pyelography) requires I.V. administration of a contrast medium and allows visualization of the renal parenchyma, calyces, and pelvis, as well as the ureters, bladder and, in some cases, the urethra.

Purpose

• To evaluate the structure and excretory function of the kidneys, ureters, and bladder

• To evaluate suspected renal or urinary tract disease, renal calculi, space-occupying lesions, congenital anomalies, or trauma to the urinary system

• To support a differential diagnosis of renovascular hypertension

Patient preparation

• Explain to the patient that this test helps to evaluate the structure and function of the urinary tract.

• Make sure the patient is well hydrated; then instruct him to fast for 8 hours before the test. Tell him who will perform the test and where.

• Inform the patient that he may experience a transient burning sensation and metallic taste when the contrast medium is injected. Tell him to report any other sensations he may experience.

• Warn him that the X-ray machine may make loud, clacking sounds during the test.

• Make sure that the patient or a responsible family member has signed a consent form.

• Check the patient's history for hypersensitivity to iodine, iodine-containing foods, or contrast media containing iodine. Mark any sensitivities on the chart.

• Administer a laxative, if necessary, the night before the test, to minimize poor resolution of X-ray films due to feces and gas in the GI tract.

Equipment

Contrast medium (sodium diatrizoate or iothalamate, or meglumine diatrizoate or iothalamate); 50-ml syringe (or I.V. container and tubing); 19G to 21G needle, catheter, or butterfly needle; venipuncture equipment (tourniquet, antiseptic, adhesive bandage); emergency resuscitative equipment.

Procedure and posttest care

• The patient is placed in a supine position on the radiographic table.

• A kidney-ureter-bladder radiograph is exposed, developed, and studied for gross abnormalities of the urinary system. In the absence of any such abnormality, contrast medium is injected (dosage varies according to age), and the patient is observed for signs of hypersensitivity (flushing, nausea, vomiting, hives, or dyspnea).

• The first radiograph, visualizing the renal parenchyma, is obtained about 1 minute after the injection, possibly supplemented by tomography if small space-occupying masses like cysts or tumors are suspected.

• Films are then exposed at regular intervals — usually 5, 10, and 15 or 20 minutes after the injection.

• Ureteral compression is performed after the 5-minute film is exposed. This can be accomplished through inflation of two small rubber bladders placed on the abdomen on both sides of the midline, secured by a fastener wrapped around the patient's torso. The inflated bladders occlude the ureters, without causing the patient discomfort, and facilitate retention of the contrast medium by the upper urinary tract. (Ureteral compression is contraindicated by ureteral calculi, aortic aneurysm, pregnancy, or recent abdominal trauma or surgical procedure.)

• After the 10-minute film is exposed, ureteral compression is released. As the contrast flows into the lower urinary tract, another film is taken of the lower halves of both ureters and then, finally, one is taken of the bladder.

• At the end of the procedure, the patient voids, and another film is made immediately to visualize residual bladder content or mucosal abnormalities of the bladder or urethra.

• If a hematoma develops at the injection site, ease the patient's discomfort by applying warm soaks.

• Observe for delayed reactions to the contrast medium.

Precautions

• Premedication with corticosteroids may be indicated for patients with severe asthma or a history of sensitivity to the contrast medium.

Normal findings

The kidneys, ureters, and bladder show no gross evidence of soft- or hard-tissue lesions. Prompt visualization of the contrast medium in the kidneys demonstrates bilateral renal parenchyma and pelvicalyceal systems of normal conformity. The ureters and bladder should be outlined, and the postvoiding radiograph should show no mucosal abnormalities and minimal residual urine.

Abnormal findings

Excretory urography can demonstrate many abnormalities of the urinary system, including renal or ureteral calculi; abnormal size, shape, or structure of kidneys, ureters, or bladder; supernumerary or absent kidney; polycystic kidney disease associated with renal hypertrophy; redundant pelvis or ureter; space-occupying lesion; pyelonephritis; renal tuberculosis; hydronephrosis; and renovascular hypertension.

RENAL ANGIOGRAPHY

Renal angiography requires arterial injection of a contrast medium and permits radiographic examination of the renal vasculature and parenchyma. As the contrast pervades the renal vasculature, rapid-sequence radiographs show the vessels during three phases of filling: arterial, nephrographic, and venous.

This procedure virtually always follows standard bolus aortography, which shows individual variations in number, size, and condition of the main renal arteries, aberrant vessels, and the relationship of the renal arteries to the aorta.

Purpose
• To demonstrate the configuration of total renal vasculature before surgical procedures
• To determine the cause of renovascular hypertension, such as from stenosis, thrombotic occlusions, emboli, and aneurysms
• To investigate unilateral or bilateral kidney enlargement, nonfunctioning kidneys in patients with acute renal failure, and intrarenal calcifications of unexplained etiology
• To evaluate chronic renal disease or renal failure
• To investigate renal masses, vascular malformations, pseudotumors, and renal trauma
• To detect complications following renal transplantation, such as a non-

functioning shunt or rejection of the donor organ

Patient preparation
• Explain to the patient that this test permits visualization of the kidneys, blood vessels, and functional units and aids in diagnosing renal disease or masses.
• Instruct him to fast for 8 hours before the test.
• Tell him who will perform the test and where and that it takes approximately 1 hour.
• Describe the procedure to him, and inform him that he may experience transient discomfort (flushing, burning sensation, and nausea) during injection of the contrast medium.
• Make sure that the patient or a responsible family member has signed a consent form.
• Check the patient's history for hypersensitivity to iodine-based contrast media or iodine-containing foods, such as shellfish. Mark sensitivities on the chart. The patient may require prophylactic antiallergenics (diphenhydramine or steroids).
• Administer prescribed medications (usually a sedative and a narcotic analgesic) before the test.
• Instruct the patient to put on a hospital gown and to remove all metallic objects that may interfere with test results.
• Ask him to void before leaving the unit.

Equipment
Pressure-injection device; rapid cassette changer; polyethylene radiopaque vascular catheters; flexible guide wire; contrast material (such as Hypaque, Renografin, Conray, or Isopaque); preparation tray, with 70% alcohol or povidone-iodine solution; emergency resuscitative equipment.

Procedure and posttest care

• The patient is placed in supine position, and a peripheral I.V. infusion is started. The skin over the arterial puncture site is cleaned with antiseptic solution, and a local anesthetic is injected.

• The femoral artery is punctured and, under fluoroscopic visualization, cannulated. (If a femoral pulse is absent or the artery is convoluted or plaque-ridden, percutaneous transaxillary, transbrachial, or translumbar catheterization may be performed instead.)

• After passing the flexible guide wire through the artery, the cannula is withdrawn, leaving several inches of wire in the lumen.

• A polyethylene catheter is passed over the wire and advanced, under fluoroscopic guidance, up the femoroiliac vessels to the aorta. The guide wire is removed, and the catheter is flushed with heparin flush solution.

• The contrast medium is injected, and screening aortograms are taken before proceeding.

• On completion of the aortographic study, a renal catheter is exchanged for the vascular catheter.

• To determine the position of the renal arteries and ensure that the tip of the catheter is in the lumen, a test bolus of contrast medium is injected immediately.

• If the patient has no adverse reaction to the contrast agent, 20 to 25 ml of the substance is injected just below the origin of the renal arteries.

• A series of rapid-sequence X-ray films of the filling of the renal vascular tree is exposed.

• If additional selective studies are required, the catheter remains in place while the films are examined. If the films are satisfactory, the catheter is removed.

• Apply a sterile sponge firmly to the puncture site for 15 minutes.

• Before the patient is returned to his room, observe the puncture site for hematoma.

• Keep the patient flat in bed for at least 6 hours.

• Check vital signs every 15 minutes for 1 hour, then every 30 minutes for 2 hours, and then every hour until they stabilize.

• Monitor popliteal and dorsalis pedis pulses for adequate perfusion at least every hour for 4 hours.

• Watch for bleeding or hematomas at the injection site. Keep the pressure dressing in place, and check for bleeding when you check all vital signs. If bleeding occurs, act promptly and apply direct pressure to the site.

Precautions

• Renal angiography is contraindicated during pregnancy and in patients with bleeding tendencies, allergy to contrast media, and renal failure due to end-stage renal disease.

Normal findings

Renal arteriographs show normal arborization of the vascular tree and normal architecture of the renal parenchyma.

Abnormal findings

Renal tumors usually show hypervascularity; renal cysts typically appear as clearly delineated, radiolucent masses. Renal artery stenosis caused by arteriosclerosis produces a noticeable constriction in the blood vessels, usually within the proximal portion of its length; this is a crucial finding in confirming renovascular hypertension. Renal artery dysplasia, unlike renal artery stenosis, usually affects the middle and distal portions of the vessel. Alternating aneurysms and stenotic regions give this rare disorder a characteristic beads-on-a-string appearance.

In renal infarction, blood vessels may appear to be absent or cut off, with the normal tissue replaced by scar tissue. Another typical finding is the appearance of triangular areas of infarcted tissue near the periphery of the affected kidney. The kidney itself may appear shrunken due to tissue scarring.

Other disorders that may be discovered through renal angiography include renal artery aneurysms (saccular or fusiform) and renal arteriovenous fistula with abnormal widening of and direct passage between the renal artery and renal vein. Destruction, distortion, and fibrosis of renal tissue with areas of reduced and tortuous vascularity may be noted in severe or chronic pyelonephritis, and an increase in capsular vessels with abnormal intrarenal circulation may indicate renal abscesses or inflammatory masses.

When angiography is used to evaluate renal trauma, it may detect intrarenal hematoma, parenchymal laceration, shattered kidneys, and areas of infarction. Renal angiography may also be useful in distinguishing pseudotumors from tumors or cysts, in evaluating the volume of residual functioning renal tissue in hydronephrosis, and in evaluating donors and recipients before and after renal transplantation.

RENAL VENOGRAPHY

This relatively simple procedure allows radiographic examination of the main renal veins and their tributaries. In this test, contrast medium is injected by percutaneous catheter passed through the femoral vein and inferior vena cava into the renal vein. Indications for renal venography include renal vein thrombosis, tumor, and venous anomalies.

Purpose
• To detect renal vein thrombosis

• To evaluate renal vein compression due to extrinsic tumors or retroperitoneal fibrosis
• To distinguish renal parenchymal disease and aneurysms from pressure exerted by an adjacent mass
• To assess renal tumors and detect invasion of the renal vein or inferior vena cava
• To detect venous anomalies and defects
• To differentiate renal agenesis from a small kidney
• To collect renal venous blood samples for evaluation of renovascular hypertension

Patient preparation
• Explain to the patient that this test permits radiographic study of the renal veins.
• If prescribed, instruct him to fast for 4 hours before the test.
• Tell him who will perform the test and where and that it takes about 1 hour.
• Inform him that a catheter will be inserted into a vein in the groin area after he is given a sedative and a local anesthetic.
• Tell him that he may feel mild discomfort during injection of the local anesthetic and contrast medium and that he may feel transient burning and flushing from the contrast medium.
• Warn him that the X-ray equipment may make loud, clacking noises as the films are taken.
• Check his history for hypersensitivity to contrast media, iodine, or iodine-containing foods, such as shellfish. Mark sensitivities on the chart.
• Check his history and any coagulation studies for indications of bleeding disorders.
• If renin assays will be done, check the patient's diet and medications, and consult with the health care team. As necessary, restrict the patient's salt intake and discontinue antihypertensive drugs, di-

uretics, estrogen, and oral contraceptives.
• Make sure that the patient or a responsible family member has signed a consent form.
• Just before the procedure, administer a sedative if necessary.

Equipment
Renal venography tray with flexible guide wires, polyethylene radiopaque vascular catheters, needle and cannula or 18G needle, three-way stopcock, and flexible tubing; preparatory tray; syringes and needles; contrast medium; local anesthetic; emergency resuscitation equipment.

Procedure and posttest care
• The patient is placed in a supine position on the X-ray table, with his abdomen centered over the film. The skin over the right femoral vein near the groin is cleaned with antiseptic solution and draped. (The left femoral vein or jugular veins may be used.)
• A local anesthetic is injected, and the femoral vein is cannulated.
• Under fluoroscopic guidance, a guide wire is threaded a short distance through the cannula, which is then removed. A catheter is passed over the wire into the inferior vena cava.
• When catheterization of the femoral vein is contraindicated, the right antecubital vein is punctured, and the catheter is inserted and advanced through the right atrium of the heart into the inferior vena cava.
• A test bolus of contrast medium is injected to determine that the vena cava is patent. If so, the catheter is advanced into the right renal vein and contrast medium is injected.
• When studies of the right renal vasculature are completed, the catheter is withdrawn into the vena cava, rotated, and guided into the left renal vein.

• If visualization of the renal venous tributaries is indicated, epinephrine can be injected into the ipsilateral renal artery by catheter before contrast medium is injected into the renal vein. Epinephrine temporarily blocks arterial flow and allows filling of distal intrarenal veins. Obstructing the artery briefly with a balloon catheter produces the same effect.
• After anteroposterior films are made, the patient lies prone for posteroanterior films.
• For renin assays, blood samples are withdrawn under fluoroscopy within 15 minutes after venography. After catheter removal, apply pressure to the site for 15 minutes and put on a dressing.
• Check vital signs and distal pulses every 15 minutes for the first hour, then every 30 minutes for the second hour, and then every 2 hours for 24 hours.
• Observe the puncture site for bleeding or hematoma when checking vital signs; if bleeding occurs, apply pressure. Report bleeding as soon as possible.
• Report signs of vein perforation, embolism, and extravasation of contrast medium. These include chills, fever, rapid pulse and respiration, hypotension, dyspnea, and chest, abdominal, or flank pain. Also report complaints of paresthesia or pain in the catheterized limb — symptoms of nerve irritation or vascular compromise.
• Administer prescribed sedatives and antimicrobials.
• Instruct the patient to resume his normal diet and any discontinued medications.

Precautions
• Renal venography is contraindicated in severe thrombosis of the inferior vena cava.

- The guide wire and catheter should be advanced carefully if severe renal vein thrombosis is suspected.
- Watch for signs of hypersensitivity to the contrast medium.

Normal findings

After injection of the contrast medium, opacification of the renal vein and tributaries should occur immediately.

Normal renin content of venous blood in a supine adult is 1.5 to 1.6 ng/ml/hr.

Abnormal findings

Occlusion of the renal vein near the inferior vena cava or the kidney indicates renal vein thrombosis. If the clot is outlined by contrast medium, it may look like a filling defect. However, a clot can usually be identified because it is within the lumen and less sharply outlined than a filling defect. Collateral venous channels, which opacify with retrograde filling during contrast injection, often surround the occlusion. Complete occlusion prolongs transit of the contrast medium through the renal veins.

A filling defect of the renal vein may indicate obstruction or compression by extrinsic tumor or retroperitoneal fibrosis. A renal tumor that invades the renal vein or inferior vena cava usually produces a filling defect with a sharply defined border.

Venous anomalies are indicated by opacification of abnormally positioned or clustered vessels. Absence of a renal vein differentiates renal agenesis from a small kidney.

Elevated renin content in renal venous blood usually indicates essential renovascular hypertension when assay results correspond for both kidneys. Elevated renin levels in one kidney indicate a unilateral lesion and usually require further evaluation by arteriography.

VOIDING CYSTOURETHROGRAPHY

In voiding cystourethrography, a contrast medium is instilled by gentle syringe pressure or gravity into the bladder through a urethral catheter. Fluoroscopic films or overhead radiographs demonstrate bladder filling, and then show excretion of the contrast medium as the patient voids.

Purpose

- To detect abnormalities of the bladder and urethra, such as vesicoureteral reflux, neurogenic bladder, prostatic hyperplasia, or diverticula
- To investigate possible causes of chronic urinary tract infection
- To investigate a suspected congenital anomaly of the lower urinary tract, abnormal bladder emptying, and incontinence
- To assess hypertrophy of the lobes of the prostate, urethral stricture, and the degree of compromise of a stenotic prostatic urethra (in men)

Patient preparation

- Explain to the patient that this test permits assessment of the bladder and the urethra.
- Inform him that he needn't restrict food or fluids before the test.
- Tell him who will perform the test and where and that it takes approximately 30 to 45 minutes.
- Inform the patient that a catheter will be inserted into his bladder and that a contrast medium will be instilled through the catheter.
- Tell him he may experience a feeling of fullness and an urge to void when the contrast is instilled. Explain that X-ray films will be taken of his bladder and

urethra, and that he'll be asked to assume various positions.

• Make sure that the patient or a responsible family member has signed a consent form if required.

• Check the patient's history for hypersensitivity to contrast media or iodine-containing foods, such as shellfish; note sensitivities on the chart.

• Just before the procedure, administer a sedative, if prescribed.

Equipment
Accessories for spot-film radiography; indwelling urinary catheter; standard urographic contrast medium (up to 1,000 ml of 15% solution); 50-ml syringe (for infants) or gravity-feed apparatus.

Procedure and posttest care
• The patient is placed in a supine position, and an indwelling urinary catheter is inserted into the bladder.

• The contrast medium is instilled through the catheter until the bladder is full.

• The catheter is clamped, and X-ray films are exposed, with the patient in supine, oblique, and lateral positions.

• The catheter is removed, and the patient assumes right oblique position (right leg flexed to 90 degrees, left leg extended, penis parallel to right leg) and begins to void.

• Four high-speed exposures of the bladder and urethra, coned down to reduce radiation exposure, are usually made on one film during voiding.

• If the right oblique view does not delineate both ureters, the patient is asked to stop urinating and to begin again in the left oblique position.

• The most reliable voiding cystourethrograms are obtained with the patient recumbent. Patients who can't void recumbent may do so standing (not sitting).

• Expression cystourethrography may have to be performed, under a general anesthetic, for young children who cannot void on command.

• Observe and record the time, color, and volume of the patient's voidings. Report hematuria if present after the third voiding.

• Encourage the patient to drink large quantities of fluids to reduce burning on urination and to flush out any residual contrast medium.

• Monitor for chills and fever related to extravasation of contrast material or urinary sepsis.

Precautions
• Voiding cystourethrography is contraindicated in patients with an acute or exacerbated urethral or bladder infection, or an acute urethral injury.

• Hypersensitivity to the contrast medium may also contraindicate this test.

• Male patients should wear a lead shield over their testes to prevent irradiation of the gonads; female patients can't be shielded without blocking the urinary bladder.

Normal findings
Delineation of the bladder and urethra shows normal structure and function, with no regurgitation of contrast medium into the ureters.

Abnormal findings
Voiding cystourethrography may show urethral stricture, vesical or urethral diverticula, ureterocele, prostatic enlargement, vesicoureteral reflux, or neurogenic bladder. The severity and location of such abnormalities are then evaluated to determine whether surgical intervention is necessary.

WHITAKER TEST

Also called a pressure or flow study, this study of the upper urinary tract correlates radiographic findings with measurements of pressure and flow in the kidneys and ureters. It facilitates assessment of the upper tract's efficiency in emptying.

In this procedure, radiographs are taken after urethral catheterization, I.V. administration of a contrast medium, percutaneous cannulation of the kidney, and renal perfusion of the contrast medium. Intrarenal and bladder pressures are then measured.

Purpose

• To detect renal obstruction and to help determine if surgery is needed
• To further evaluate obstruction (following other procedures, such as percutaneous nephrostomy)

Patient preparation

• Explain to the patient that the test helps to evaluate kidney function.
• Instruct him to avoid food and fluids for at least 4 hours before the test.
• Tell him who will perform the test and where and that it will take about 1 hour.
• Describe the procedure to him. Inform him that he will be given a mild sedative before the test, that he may feel some discomfort during insertion of the urethral catheter and injection of the local anesthetic, and that he may sense transient burning and flushing after injection of the contrast medium.
• Warn him that the X-ray machine makes loud, clacking sounds as films are exposed.
• Make sure that the patient or a responsible family member has signed a consent form.

• Check his history and recent coagulation studies for bleeding disorders. Also check for hypersensitivity reactions to iodine, iodine-containing foods, such as shellfish, and contrast media. Mark any sensitivities on the chart.
• Just before the procedure, instruct the patient to void, and administer prescribed sedatives.
• Administer prophylactic antimicrobials as prescribed to prevent infection from instrumentation.

Equipment

Perfusion pump with 50-ml luer-lock syringe, transducer and recorder, manometer, three-way and four-way stopcocks, I.V. extension set, manometer lines, one double-male connector to connect urethral catheter and stopcock, sterile water and 0.9% sodium chloride solution, contrast medium, local anesthetic, percutaneous puncture tray with 4″ to 6″ 18G Longdwel cannula, gloves, preparatory tray, emergency resuscitation equipment.

Procedure and posttest care

• Place the patient in a supine position on the X-ray table. The table must be horizontal and must remain at the same height throughout the test.
• To prepare for measurement of bladder pressure, a urethral catheter is placed in the bladder. The patient's bladder may or may not be emptied, depending on his suspected condition.
• A plain film of the urinary tract is taken to obtain anatomic landmarks.
• The catheter is then connected to a three-way stopcock on a manometer line linked to the transducer and recorder. The line is then filled with sterile water.
• Contrast medium is injected I.V.
• The patient is placed prone and made comfortable with pillows. When urography demonstrates contrast medium in

the kidney, the skin is cleaned with antiseptic solution and draped.
• Pressure recording equipment is calibrated. The renal perfusion tubing is filled with sterile water or 0.9% sodium chloride solution and held at the level of the kidney.
• Local anesthetic is injected, and an incision is made through the flank for cannulation of the kidney.
• The patient is asked to hold his breath while the needle is inserted into the renal pelvis. Aspiration of urine confirms that the needle is in position.
• The cannula is then connected by a four-way stopcock to the perfusion tubing and the manometer line.
• Perfusion of the contrast medium is begun, serial X-rays are taken, and intrarenal pressure is measured. Bladder pressure is then measured.
• Perfusion continues until bladder pressure is constant. When pressure holds steady for a few minutes and adequate films have been taken, perfusion is discontinued. Residual fluid is aspirated from the kidney, the cannula is removed, and the wound is dressed.
• Keep the patient in a supine position for 12 hours after the test.
• Check vital signs every 15 minutes for the first hour, every 30 minutes for the next hour, and then every 2 hours for 24 hours.
• Check the puncture site for bleeding, hematoma, or urine leakage each time vital signs are checked. If bleeding occurs, apply pressure. If a hematoma develops, apply warm soaks. Report urine leakage.
• Monitor fluid intake and urine output for 24 hours. Report hematuria that persists after the third voiding.
• Watch for signs of sepsis (chills, fever, tachycardia, tachypnea, or hypotension) or similar signs of extravasation of the contrast medium.
• Inform the patient that colicky pains are transient.

• Administer prescribed analgesics.
• Administer antimicrobials for several days after the test as needed to prevent infection.

Precautions
• Contraindications include bleeding disorders and severe infection.

Normal findings
Visualization of the kidney after gradual perfusion of the contrast medium shows normal outlines of the renal pelvis and calyces. The ureter should fill uniformly and appear normal in size and course.

The normal value for intrarenal pressure is 15 cm H_2O. The normal value for bladder pressure may range from 5 to 10 cm H_2O.

Abnormal findings
Enlargement of the renal pelvis, calyces, or ureteropelvic junction may indicate obstruction. Subtraction of bladder pressure from intrarenal pressure results in a differential that aids diagnosis. A differential of 12 to 15 cm H_2O indicates obstruction. A differential of less than 10 cm H_2O indicates a bladder abnormality, such as hypertonia or neurogenic bladder.

REPRODUCTIVE SYSTEM

MAMMOGRAPHY

This radiographic technique helps to detect breast cysts or tumors, especially those not palpable on physical examination. Biopsy of suspicious areas may be required to confirm malignancy. Mammography can detect 90% to 95% of breast malignancies.

If a mass is present, a mammogram can be done during pregnancy. A shield is used to protect the fetus.

Purpose
• To screen for breast malignancy
• To investigate palpable and unpalpable breast masses, breast pain, or nipple discharge
• To help differentiate between benign breast disease and breast malignancy

Patient preparation
• Assess the patient's understanding of the test, answer her questions, and correct any misconceptions.
• Tell her who will perform the test and where.
• Inform her that although the test takes only about 15 minutes to perform, she may be asked to wait while the films are checked to make sure they're readable.
• Just before the test, give her a gown to wear that opens in the front, and ask her to remove all jewelry and clothing above the waist.

Procedure and posttest care
• The patient stands and is asked to rest one of her breasts on a table above an X-ray cassette.
• The compression plate is placed on the breast, and the patient is told to hold her breath. A radiograph is taken of the craniocaudal view. The machine is rotated, the breast is compressed again, and a radiograph of the lateral view is taken.
• The procedure is repeated on the other breast.
• After the films are developed, they are checked to make sure they're readable.

Normal findings
A normal mammogram reveals normal duct, glandular tissue, and fat architecture. No abnormal masses or calcifications should be seen.

Abnormal findings
Well-outlined, regular, and clear spots suggest benign cysts; irregular, poorly outlined, and opaque areas suggest malignancy. Findings that suggest cancer require further tests, such as additional mammographic views or, for confirmation, biopsy.

HYSTERO-SALPINGOGRAPHY

Hysterosalpingography is a radiologic examination for visualizing the uterine cavity, the fallopian tubes, and the peritubal area. The procedure consists of taking fluoroscopic X-ray films as a contrast medium flows through the uterus and the fallopian tubes.

This test is generally performed as part of an infertility study. Although ultrasonography has virtually replaced hysterosalpingography in the detection of foreign bodies, such as a dislodged intrauterine device, it can't evaluate tubal patency, which is the main purpose of hysterosalpingography. Risks of this test include uterine perforation, intravascular injection of the contrast medium, and exposure to potentially harmful radiation.

Purpose
• To confirm tubal abnormalities, such as adhesions and occlusion
• To confirm uterine abnormalities, such as the presence of foreign bodies, congenital malformations, and traumatic injuries

• To confirm the presence of fistulas or peritubal adhesions
• To help evaluate repeated fetal loss
• To assess the outcome of surgery, especially uterine unification procedures and tubal reanastomosis

Patient preparation
• Explain to the patient that this test confirms uterine and fallopian tube abnormalities.
• Tell her who will perform the test and where and that it takes about 15 minutes.
• Advise the patient that she may experience moderate cramping from the procedure; however, she may receive a mild sedative, such as diazepam.

Equipment
Povidone-iodine solution, sterile needle, contrast medium (oil- or water-based), vaginal speculum, tenaculum, cannula with acorn tip on one end and luer-lock on the other.

Procedure and posttest care
• With the patient in lithotomy position, a scout film is taken.
• A speculum is inserted in the vagina, the tenaculum is placed on the cervix, and the cervix is cleaned.
• The cannula is inserted into the cervix and anchored to the tenaculum. After the contrast medium is injected through the cannula, the uterus and the fallopian tubes are viewed fluoroscopically, and radiographs are taken. To take oblique views, the radiographic table may be tilted or the patient asked to change position.
• Watch for signs of infection, such as fever, pain, increased pulse rate, malaise, and muscle ache.
• Assure the patient that cramps and vagal reaction (slow pulse rate, nausea, and dizziness) are transient.

Precautions
• Hysterosalpingography is contraindicated in patients with menses, undiagnosed vaginal bleeding, or pelvic inflammatory disease.
• Watch for an allergic reaction to the contrast medium, such as hives, itching, or hypotension.

Normal findings
Normally, radiographs reveal a symmetrical uterine cavity; the contrast medium courses through fallopian tubes of normal caliber, spills freely into the peritoneal cavity, and doesn't leak from the uterus.

Abnormal findings
An asymmetrical uterus suggests intrauterine adhesions or masses, such as fibroids or foreign bodies; impaired contrast flow through the fallopian tubes suggests partial or complete blockage, resulting from intraluminal agglutination, extrinsic compression by adhesions, or perifimbrial adhesions; leakage of the contrast medium through the uterine wall suggests fistulas. Laparoscopy with contrast instillation confirms positive or equivocal findings.

SKELETAL SYSTEM

VERTEBRAL RADIOGRAPHY

Vertebral radiography visualizes all or part of the vertebral column. A commonly performed test, it is used to evaluate the vertebrae for deformities, fractures, dislocations, tumors, and other abnormalities. Bone films determine bone density, texture, erosion, and changes in bone relationships. X-rays of the cortex of the bone reveal the presence of any widening, narrowing, and signs of irregularity. Joint X-rays can reveal the presence of fluid, spur formation, narrowing, and changes in the joint structure.

Anatomically, the vertebral column is divided in descending order into five segments: cervical, thoracic, lumbar, sacral, and coccygeal. All vertebrae are similar in structure, but vary in size, shape, and articular surface, according to location. The type and extent of vertebral radiography depends on the patient's clinical condition. For example, a patient with lower back pain requires only study of the lumbar and sacral segments.

Purpose
• To detect vertebral fractures, dislocations, subluxations, and deformities
• To detect vertebral degeneration, infection, and congenital disorders
• To detect disorders of the intervertebral disks
• To determine the vertebral effects of arthritic and metabolic disorders

Patient preparation
• Explain to the patient that this test permits examination of the spine.
• Inform him that he needn't restrict food or fluids.
• Tell him the test requires X-ray films, who will perform the test and where, and that the procedure usually takes 15 to 30 minutes.
• Advise him that he'll be placed in various positions for the X-ray films.
• Tell him that although some positions may cause slight discomfort, his cooperation is needed to ensure accurate results.
• Stress that he must keep still and hold his breath during the procedure.

Procedure and posttest care
The procedure varies considerably depending upon the vertebral segment being radiographically examined.
• Initially, the patient is placed in a supine position on the radiograph table for an anteroposterior view.
• He may be repositioned for lateral or right and left oblique views; specific positioning depends on the vertebral segment or adjacent structure of interest.
• Analgesics or local heat applications may relieve pain.

Precautions
• Vertebral radiography is contraindicated during the first trimester of pregnancy, unless the benefits outweigh the risk of fetal radiation exposure.
• Exercise extreme caution when handling trauma patients with suspected spinal injuries, particularly of the cervical area. Such patients should be filmed while on the stretcher to avoid further injury during transfer to the radiographic table.

Normal findings
Normal vertebrae show no fractures, subluxations, dislocations, curvatures, or other abnormalities. Specific positions and spacing of the vertebrae vary with the patient's age.

In the lateral view, adult vertebrae are aligned to form four alternately concave and convex curves. The cervical and lumbar curves are convex anteriorly; the thoracic and sacral curves are concave anteriorly. Although the structure of the coccyx varies, it usually points forward and downward.

Neonatal vertebrae form only one curve, which is concave anteriorly.

Abnormal findings
The vertebral radiograph readily shows spondylolisthesis, fractures, subluxations, dislocations, wedging, and such

deformities as kyphosis, scoliosis, and lordosis.

To confirm other disorders, spinal structures and their spatial relationships on the radiograph must be examined, and the patient's history and clinical status must be considered. These disorders include congenital abnormalities, such as torticollis (wryneck), absence of sacral or lumbar vertebrae, hemivertebrae, and Klippel-Feil syndrome; degenerative processes, such as hypertrophic spurs, osteoarthritis, and narrowed disk spaces; tuberculosis (Pott's disease); benign or malignant intraspinal tumors; ruptured disk and cervical disk syndrome; and systemic disorders, such as rheumatoid arthritis, Charcot's disease, ankylosing spondylitis, osteoporosis, and Paget's disease. Depending on radiographic results, definitive diagnosis may also require additional tests, such as myelography or computed tomography scanning.

ARTHROGRAPHY

This test allows radiographic examination of a joint after the injection of a radiopaque dye, air, or both (double-contrast arthrogram) to outline soft-tissue structures and the contour of the joint. The joint is put through its range of motion while a series of radiographs are taken.

Indications for arthrography include persistent unexplained joint discomfort or pain. Complications may include persistent joint crepitus and allergic reactions to the contrast dye.

Purpose
• To identify acute or chronic tears or other abnormalities of the joint capsule or supporting ligaments of the knee, shoulder, ankle, hips, or wrist

• To detect internal joint derangements
• To locate synovial cysts

Patient preparation
• Describe the procedure to the patient, and answer any questions he may have. Explain that this test permits examination of a joint.
• Inform him he needn't restrict food or fluids.
• Tell him who will perform the procedure and where.
• Explain that the fluoroscope allows the doctor to track the contrast medium as it fills the joint space.
• Inform him that standard X-ray films will also be taken after diffusion of the contrast medium.
• Tell him that, while the joint area will be anesthetized, he may experience a tingling sensation or pressure in the joint on injection of the contrast medium.
• Instruct him to remain as still as possible during the procedure, except when following instructions to change position.
• Stress the importance of his cooperation in assuming various positions because films must be taken as quickly as possible to ensure optimum quality.
• Check the patient's history to determine if he is hypersensitive to local anesthetics, iodine, seafood, or the dyes used for other diagnostic tests.

Equipment
Fluoroscope, povidone-iodine solution, local anesthetic, two 2″ 20G needles, two 24G needles, three 3-ml syringes, short lumbar puncture needle (3″ 22G needle for arthrography of the shoulder), water-soluble radiopaque dye (5 to 15 ml), four sterile sponges, elastic knee bandage, sterile towels, sterile specimen container for fluid, culture tube, sterile adhesive bandage, collodion (optional), shave preparation kit.

Procedure and posttest care

Knee arthrography:

• The knee is cleaned with an antiseptic solution, and the area around the puncture site is anesthetized. (It's not usually necessary to anesthetize the joint space itself.)

• A 2″ needle is then inserted into the joint space between the patella and femoral condyle, and fluid is aspirated. The aspirated fluid is usually sent to the laboratory for analysis.

• While the needle is still in place, the aspirating syringe is removed and replaced with a syringe containing dye.

• If fluoroscopic examination demonstrates correct placement of the needle, the dye is injected into the joint space.

• After the needle is removed, the site is rubbed with a sterile sponge and the wound may be sealed with collodion.

• The patient is asked to walk a few steps or to move his knee through a range of motion to distribute the dye in the joint space. A film series is quickly taken with the knee held in various positions.

• If the films are clean and demonstrate proper dye placement, the knee is bandaged, possibly with an elastic bandage.

• Tell the patient to keep the bandage in place for several days, and teach him how to rewrap it.

Shoulder arthrography:

• The skin is prepared, and a local anesthetic is injected subcutaneously just in front of the acromioclavicular joint.

• Additional anesthetic is injected directly onto the head of the humerus.

• The short lumbar puncture needle is inserted until the point is embedded in the joint cartilage.

• The stylet is removed, a syringe of contrast medium attached, and using fluoroscopic guidance, about 1 ml of dye is injected into the joint space, as the needle is withdrawn slightly.

• If fluoroscopic examination demonstrates correct needle placement, the remainder of the dye is injected, while the needle is slowly withdrawn, and the site is wiped with a sterile sponge.

• A film series is taken quickly to achieve maximum contrast.

Both types:

• Tell the patient to rest the joint for at least 12 hours.

• Inform him that he may experience some swelling or discomfort, or may hear crepitant noises in the joint after the test, but that these symptoms usually disappear after 1 or 2 days; tell him to report persistent symptoms.

• Advise him to apply ice to the joint if swelling occurs and to take a mild analgesic for pain.

Precautions

• Arthrography is contraindicated during pregnancy.

• This procedure is also contraindicated in patients with active arthritis, joint infection, or previous sensitivity to radiopaque media.

Normal findings

A normal knee arthrogram shows a characteristic wedge-shaped shadow, pointed toward the interior of the joint, that indicates a normal medial meniscus. A normal shoulder arthrogram shows the bicipital tendon sheath, redundant inferior joint capsule, and subscapular bursa intact.

Abnormal findings

Arthrography accurately detects medial meniscal tears and lacerations in 90% to 95% of cases. Because the entire joint lining is opacified, arthrography can demonstrate extrameniscal lesions, such as osteochondritis dissecans, chondromalacia patellae, osteochondral fractures, cartilaginous abnormalities, synovial abnormalities, tears of the cruciate ligaments, and disruption of the joint capsule and collateral ligaments.

Arthrography can reveal shoulder abnormalities, such as adhesive capsulitis, bicipital tenosynovitis or rupture, and rotator cuff tears. It can also evaluate damage from recurrent dislocations.

MISCELLANEOUS TESTS

LYMPHANGIOGRAPHY

Lymphangiography (or lymphography) is the radiographic examination of the lymphatic system after the injection of an oil-based contrast medium into a lymphatic vessel in each foot or, less commonly, in each hand.

Injection into the foot allows visualization of the lymphatics of the leg, inguinal and iliac regions, and the retroperitoneum up to the thoracic duct.

Injection into the hand allows visualization of the axillary and supraclavicular nodes. This procedure may also be used to study the cervical region (retroauricular area), but this is less useful and less common.

X-ray films are taken immediately after injection to demonstrate the filling of the lymphatic system and then again 24 hours later to visualize the lymph nodes. Because the contrast medium remains in the nodes for up to 2 years, subsequent X-ray films can assess progression of disease and monitor effectiveness of treatment.

Purpose
• To detect and stage lymphomas, and to identify metastatic involvement of the lymph nodes
• To distinguish primary from secondary lymphedema
• To suggest surgical treatment or evaluate the effectiveness of chemotherapy and radiation therapy in controlling malignancy
• To investigate enlarged lymph nodes, detected by computed tomography or ultrasonography

Patient preparation
• Explain to the patient that this test permits examination of the lymphatic system through X-ray films taken after the injection of a contrast medium.
• Inform him he needn't restrict food or fluids before the test.
• Tell him who will perform this procedure and where and that it takes about 3 hours.
• Mention that additional X-ray films are also taken the following day, but these take less than 30 minutes.
• Inform the patient that blue contrast medium will be injected into each foot to outline the lymphatic vessels; that the injection causes transient discomfort; and that the contrast medium discolors urine and stool for 48 hours, and may give his skin and vision a bluish tinge for 48 hours.
• Tell him a local anesthetic will be injected before a small incision is made in each foot.
• Inform him that the contrast medium is then injected for the next $1\frac{1}{2}$ hours using a cannula inserted into a lymphatic vessel.
• Advise the patient that he must remain as still as possible during injection of the contrast medium, and that he may experience some discomfort in the popliteal or inguinal areas at the beginning of the injection of the contrast medium.

• If this test is performed on an outpatient basis, advise the patient to have a friend or relative accompany him.

• Warn him that the incision site may be sore for several days after lymphangiography.

• Make sure the patient or a responsible family member has signed a consent form.

• Check the patient's history to determine if he is hypersensitive to iodine, seafood, or the contrast media used in other diagnostic tests, such as intravenous pyelography.

• Just before the procedure, instruct the patient to void, and check his vital signs for a baseline. If prescribed, administer a sedative and an oral antihistamine (if hypersensitivity to the contrast medium is suspected).

Procedure and posttest care

• A preliminary X-ray of the chest is taken with the patient in an erect or a supine position.

• The skin over the dorsum of each foot is cleaned with antiseptics.

• Blue contrast dye is injected intradermally into the area between the toes, usually the first and fourth toe webs.

• The contrast medium infiltrates the lymphatic system and within 15 to 30 minutes the lymphatic vessels appear as small blue lines on the upper surface of the instep of each foot.

• A local anesthetic is then injected into the dorsum of each foot, and a transverse incision is made to expose the lymphatic vessel.

• Each vessel is cannulated with a 30G needle attached to polyethylene tubing and a syringe filled with ethiodized oil.

• Once the needles are positioned, the patient is instructed to remain still throughout the injection period to avoid dislodging the needles.

• The syringe is then placed within an infusion pump that injects the contrast medium.

• Fluoroscopy may be used to monitor filling of the lymphatic system.

• The needles are removed, the incisions sutured, and sterile dressings applied.

• X-ray films of the legs, pelvis, abdomen, and chest are taken.

• The patient is then taken to his room but must return 24 hours later for additional films.

• Check the patient's vital signs every 4 hours for 48 hours.

• Watch for pulmonary complications, such as shortness of breath, pleuritic pain, hypotension, low-grade fever, and cyanosis, due to embolization of the contrast medium.

• Enforce bed rest for 24 hours, with the patient's feet elevated to help reduce swelling.

• Apply ice packs to the incision sites to help reduce swelling, and administer prescribed analgesics.

• Check the incision sites for infection, and leave the dressings in place for 2 days, making sure the wounds remain dry. Tell the patient the sutures will be removed in 7 to 10 days.

• Prepare the patient for follow-up X-rays, as needed.

Precautions

• Lymphangiography is contraindicated in patients with hypersensitivities to iodine, pulmonary insufficiencies, cardiac diseases, and severe renal or hepatic diseases.

Normal findings

The lymphatic system normally demonstrates homogeneous and complete filling with contrast medium on the initial films. On the 24-hour films, the lymph nodes are fully opacified and well circumscribed; the lymphatic channels are emptied a few hours after injection of the contrast medium agent.

Abnormal findings

Enlarged, foamy-looking nodes indicate lymphoma, classified as Hodgkin's or non-Hodgkin's. Filling defects or lack of opacification indicates metastatic involvement of the lymph nodes. The number of nodes affected, unilateral or bilateral involvement, and the extent of extranodal involvement help determine staging of lymphoma. However, definitive staging may require additional diagnostic tests such as computed tomography, ultrasonography, selective biopsy, and laparotomy.

In differential diagnosis of primary and secondary lymphedema, shortened lymphatic vessels and a deficient number of vessels indicate primary lymphedema. Abruptly terminating lymphatic vessels, caused by retroperitoneal tumors impinging on the vessels, inflammation, filariasis, and trauma resulting from surgery or radiation, indicate secondary lymphedema.

CHAPTER 13

Computed Tomography and Magnetic Resonance Imaging

NEUROLOGIC SYSTEM

INTRACRANIAL COMPUTED TOMOGRAPHY

Intracranial computed tomography (CT) provides a series of tomograms, translated by a computer and displayed on a monitor, representing cross-sectional images of various layers of the brain. This technique can reconstruct cross-sectional, horizontal, sagittal, and coronal plane images. Hundreds of thousands of readings of radiation levels absorbed by brain tissues may be combined to depict anatomic slices of varying thickness. Intracranial tumors and other brain lesions may be identified as areas of altered density. Intracranial CT scanning may eliminate the need for painful and hazardous invasive procedures, such as pneumoencephalography and cerebral angiography.

Purpose
• To diagnose intracranial lesions and abnormalities
• To monitor the effects of surgery, radiotherapy, or chemotherapy on intracranial tumors
• To assess focal neurologic abnormalities and other clinical features that suggest an intracranial mass
• To provide early diagnosis of subdural hematoma in a patient with suspected head injury

Patient preparation
• Explain to the patient that this test permits assessment of the brain.

• Unless contrast enhancement is scheduled, inform him that there are no food or fluid restrictions. If contrast enhancement is scheduled, instruct him to fast for 4 hours before the test.
• Tell him that a series of X-ray films will be taken of his brain. Describe who will perform the test and where it will take place. Explain that the test will cause minimal discomfort and last 15 to 30 minutes.
• Tell him he'll be positioned on a moving CT bed, with his head immobilized and his face uncovered. The head of the table is moved into the scanner, which rotates around his head and makes clacking sounds.
• If a contrast agent is used, tell him that he may feel flushed and warm and may experience a transient headache, a salty taste, or nausea and vomiting after the dye's injected.
• Instruct him to wear a hospital gown (outpatients may wear any comfortable clothing) and to remove all metal objects from the CT scan field.
• If the patient is restless or apprehensive, a sedative may be prescribed.
• Check the patient's history for hypersensitivity to shellfish, iodine, or other contrast media, and mark your findings on his chart. Report this information as necessary.

Equipment
Contrast medium (meglumine iothalamate or sodium diatrizoate), 60-ml syringe, 19G to 21G needle, tourniquet.

Procedure and posttest care
• Place patient in a supine position on a radiographic table, with his head immobilized by straps, and ask him to lie still.
• The head of the table is moved into the scanner, which rotates around the patient's head, taking radiographs at 1-degree intervals in a 180-degree arc.
• When this series of radiographs is completed, contrast enhancement is

performed. Monitor for hypersensitivity reactions, such as urticaria, respiratory difficulty, or rash. Reactions usually develop within 30 minutes.
• After injection of the contrast medium, another series of scans is taken. Information from the scans is stored on magnetic tapes, fed into a computer, and converted into images on an oscilloscope screen. Photographs of selected views are taken for further study.
• If a contrast agent was used, watch for residual adverse reactions (headache, nausea, and vomiting), and inform the patient that he may resume his usual diet.

Precautions
• Intracranial CT scanning with contrast enhancement is contraindicated in persons who are hypersensitive to iodine or contrast medium.
• Iodine or contrast medium may be harmful or fatal to a fetus, especially during the first trimester.

Normal findings
The density of tissue determines the amount of radiation that passes through it. Tissue densities appear as white, black, or shades of gray on the computed image obtained by intracranial CT scanning. Bone, the densest tissue, appears white; ventricular and subarachnoid cerebrospinal fluid, the least dense, appears black. Brain matter appears in shades of gray. Structures are evaluated according to their density, size, shape, and position.

Abnormal findings
Areas of altered density (they may be lighter or darker) or displaced vasculature or other structures may indicate intracranial tumor, hematoma, cerebral atrophy, infarction, edema, or congenital anomalies, such as hydrocephalus.
  Intracranial tumors vary significantly in appearance and characteristics.

Metastatic tumors generally cause extensive edema in early stages and can usually be defined by contrast enhancement. Primary tumors vary in density and in their capacity to cause edema, displace ventricles, and absorb dye in contrast enhancement. Astrocytomas, for example, usually have low densities; meningiomas have higher densities and can generally be defined with contrast enhancement; glioblastomas, usually ill-defined, are also enhanced after injection of a contrast medium.
  Because the high density of blood contrasts markedly with low-density brain tissue, it's normally easy to detect both subdural and epidural hematomas and other acute hemorrhages. Contrast enhancement helps locate subdural hematomas.
  Cerebral atrophy customarily appears as enlarged ventricles with large sulci. Cerebral infarction may appear as low-density areas at the obstruction site or may not be apparent if the infarction is small or doesn't cause edema. With contrast enhancement, the infarcted area may not show in the acute phase, but will show clearly after resolution of the lesion. Cerebral edema usually appears as an area of marked generalized lucency. In children, enlargement of the fourth ventricle generally indicates hydrocephalus.
  Normally, the cerebral vessels don't appear on computed tomogram images. However, in patients with arteriovenous malformation, cerebral vessels may appear with slightly increased density. Contrast enhancement allows a better view of the abnormal area, but magnetic resonance imaging is now the preferred procedure for imaging cerebral vessels.
  Another emerging technology for obtaining images of the brain in positron emission tomography. See *Positron emission tomography,* page 570.

POSITRON EMISSION TOMOGRAPHY

Like computed tomography (CT) scanning and magnetic resonance imaging (MRI), positron emission tomography (PET) provides images of the brain through sophisticated computer reconstruction algorithms. However, PET images detail brain function as well as structure and thus differ significantly from the images provided by these other advanced techniques.

How it works

During positron emission, pairs of gamma rays are emitted; the PET scanner detects these and relays the information to a computer for reconstruction as an image. Positron-emitters can be chemically "tagged" to biologically active molecules such as carbon monoxide, neurotransmitters, hormones, and metabolites (particularly glucose), enabling study of their uptake and distribution in brain tissue. For example, blood tagged with ^{11}C-carbon monoxide allows study of hemodynamic patterns in brain tissue, whereas tagged neurotransmitters, hormones, and drugs allow map-ping of receptor distribution. Isotope-tagged glucose (which penetrates the blood-brain barrier rapidly) allows dynamic study of brain function because PET can pinpoint the sites of glucose metabolism in the brain under various conditions. This may prove to be useful in the diagnosis of psychiatric disorders, transient ischemic attacks, amyotrophic lateral sclerosis, Parkinson's disease, Wilson's disease, multiple sclerosis, seizure disorders, cerebrovascular disease, and Alzheimer's disease. The reason: All of these disorders may alter the location and patterns of cerebral glucose metabolism.

Cost factors

PET is a costly test because the radioisotopes used have very short half-lives and must be produced at an onsite cyclotron and attached quickly to the desired tracer molecules. So far, this prohibitive cost has limited PET's use. However, PET has already provided significant information about the brain and may someday have widespread clinical applications.

INTRACRANIAL MAGNETIC RESONANCE IMAGING

Magnetic resonance imaging (MRI) produces cross-sectional images of the brain and spine in multiple planes. MRI images are highly detailed. MRI's advantages include its ability to "see through" bone and to delineate fluid-filled soft tissue. Thus far, it's proved useful in the diagnosis of cerebral infarction, tumors, abscesses, edema, hemorrhage, nerve fiber demyelination (as in multiple sclerosis), and other disorders that increase the fluid content of affected tissues. It can also show irregularities of the spinal cord with a resolution and detail previously unobtainable. It can also produce images of organs and vessels in motion.

MRI technology makes use of magnetic fields and radiofrequency (RF) waves, which are imperceptible by the patient; no harmful effects have been documented. Research is continuing on the optimal magnetic fields and RF waves for each type of tissue. See *Current techniques for monitoring cerebral function,* page 572.

Purpose
• To aid diagnosis of intracranial and spinal lesions and soft-tissue abnormalities

Patient preparation
• Explain to the patient that this test assesses bone and soft tissue. Tell him who will perform the test, where it will be done, and that it takes up to 90 minutes.
• Explain that although MRI is painless and involves no exposure to radiation from the scanner, a radioactive contrast dye may be used, depending on the type of tissue being studied.
• Emphasize that the opening for the patient's head and body in the MRI scanner is quite small and deep. Ask if claustrophobia has ever been a problem; if so, he might not be able to tolerate the scan, or he may need sedation.
• Tell him that he'll hear the scanner clicking, whirring, and thumping as it moves inside its housing.
• Reassure him that he'll be able to communicate with the technician at all times.
• Instruct him to remove all metallic objects, including jewelry, hair pins, or watch, and ask if he has any surgically implanted joints, pins, clips, valves, pumps, or pacemakers containing metal that could be attracted to the strong MRI magnet. If he does, he won't be able to undergo the test.
• Obtain a signed consent form from the patient or his family.

Procedure and posttest care
• The patient is placed in a supine position on a narrow bed, which then slides him to the desired position inside the scanner where RF energy is directed at his head or spine.
• The resulting images are displayed on a monitor and recorded on film or magnetic tape for permanent storage.
• The radiologist may vary RF waves and use the computer to manipulate and enhance the images.
• During the procedure the patient must remain still.
• Tell the patient that he may resume normal activity after the test.
• If the test took a long time, observe the patient for postural hypotension.
• Provide emotional support to the patient with claustrophobic anxiety or anxiety over his diagnosis.

Precautions
• Because MRI works through a powerful magnetic field, it can't be performed on patients with pacemakers, intracranial aneurysm clips, or other ferrous metal implants or on a patient with gunshot wounds to the head.
• Because of the strong magnetic field, metallic or computer-based equipment (for example, ventilators and intravenous pumps) can't enter the MRI area.

Normal findings
MRI can show normal anatomic details of the central nervous system in any plane, without bone interference. Brain and spinal cord structures should appear distinct and sharply defined. Tissue color and shading will vary, depending on the RF energy, magnetic strength, and degree of computer enhancement. MRI can detect white matter abnormalities, especially multiple sclerosis.

Abnormal findings
Because MRI depicts the density (water content) of tissue, it clearly shows structural changes resulting from disorders that increase tissue water content, such as cerebral edema, demyelinating

CURRENT TECHNIQUES FOR MONITORING CEREBRAL FUNCTION

Magnetic resonance imaging (MRI) is used to provide clear images of parts of the brain, such as the brain stem and cerebellum, that are difficult to image by other methods. Ongoing research into MRI applications has produced valuable methods of investigating the brain more completely. The following technologies represent the most recent developments in magnetic field technology.

Fast MRI

This highly sensitive process quickly produces a series of images depicting blood flow in the brain and vascular changes that occur as the patient performs tasks. It is currently used to detect vascular lesions and extramedullary spinal disease and to depict areas abnormally susceptible to magnetic resonance, possibly indicating hemorrhage, occult cerebrovascular malformations, hemorrhagic metastasis, or calcification.

Fast MRI distinguishes between oxygen-laden blood and oxygen-depleted blood. And, because active areas of the brain consume more oxygen than inactive areas, this technology may prove useful in identifying areas of the brain that are active during specific activities or emotional states.

MR-angiogram

MR-angiogram provides images of cerebral blood vessels. MRA is more expensive than conventional angiography and does not represent a replacement technology. However, this noninvasive technique may help determine whether conventional angiography is needed.

MR-spectroscopy

MR-spectroscopy creates images over time that show the metabolism of certain chemical markers in a specific area of the brain. Some researchers have dubbed this test a "metabolic biopsy" because it reveals pathologic neurochemistry over time.

Diffusion-perfusion imaging

This MRI techniques uses a stronger-than-normal magnetic gradient to reveal areas of focal cerebral ischemia within minutes. Currently used in stroke research, diffusion-perfusion imaging may some day be used by diagnosticians to distinguish permanent from reversible ischemia.

Neurograms

The most recent breakthrough in magnetic field technology, neurograms produce a three-dimensional image of nerves. Although the technology enabling neurograms is still in development, they may be used in the future to find the exact location of nerves that are damaged, crimped, or in disarray.

disease, and pontine and cerebellar tumors. Edematous fluid, for example, generally appears cloudy or gray, whereas blood generally appears dark. Lesions of multiple sclerosis appear as areas of demyelination (curdlike, gray or gray-white areas) around the edges of ventricles. Tumors show as changes in normal anatomy, which computer enhancement may further delineate.

GASTROINTESTINAL SYSTEM

LIVER AND BILIARY TRACT COMPUTED TOMOGRAPHY

In computed tomography (CT) of the biliary tract and liver, multiple X-rays pass through the upper abdomen and are measured while detectors record differences in tissue attenuation. A computer reconstructs this data as a two-dimensional image on a television screen. CT scanning accurately distinguishes the biliary tract and the liver if the ducts are large. Use of I.V. contrast media during CT scanning can accentuate different densities.

Although CT scanning and ultrasonography both detect biliary tract and liver disease equally well, the latter technique is performed more often. CT scanning is more expensive than ultrasonography and requires exposure to moderate amounts of radiation. However, it's the test of choice in patients who are obese and in those with livers positioned high under the rib cage because bone and excessive fat hinder ultrasound transmission.

Barium studies should precede this test by at least 4 days because barium may hinder visualization.

Purpose
• To distinguish between obstructive and nonobstructive jaundice
• To specify focal defects detected by liver-spleen scanning as solid, cystic, inflammatory, and vascular lesions (biopsy may be necessary to rule out malignancy or to distinguish between metastatic and primary tumors)
• To detect suspected hematoma after abdominal trauma

Patient preparation
• Explain to the patient that this test helps detect biliary tract and liver disease.
• Instruct the patient to fast after midnight before the test if receiving an oral contrast medium. If contrast isn't ordered, fasting isn't necessary.
• Tell him who will perform the test and where and that it takes approximately 90 minutes.
• Inform him that he'll be placed on an adjustable table, which is positioned inside a scanning gantry. Assure him that the test will be painless.
• Tell him he'll be asked to remain still during the test and to hold his breath when instructed. Stress the importance of remaining still during the test, because movement can cause artifacts, thereby prolonging the test and limiting its accuracy.
• If I.V. contrast medium is being used, inform the patient that he may experience transient discomfort from the needle puncture and a localized feeling of warmth on injection. Tell him to immediately report nausea, vomiting, dizziness, headache, and urticaria.
• Check his history for hypersensitivity to iodine, seafood, or the contrast media used in other diagnostic tests.
• If a contrast agent is used, give him the oral contrast agent supplied by the radiology department.

Procedure and posttest care
• The patient is placed in supine position on a radiographic table, and the table is positioned within the opening in the scanning gantry.
• A series of transverse X-ray films are taken and recorded on magnetic tape. This information is reconstructed by a

computer and appears as images on a television screen.

• These images are studied, and selected ones are photographed. When the first series of films is completed, the images are reviewed.

• Contrast enhancement may be performed. After the contrast medium is injected, a second series of films is taken, and the patient is carefully observed for allergic reaction.

• Following the procedure, tell the patient that he may resume his usual diet.

Precautions
• CT scanning of the biliary tract and liver is usually contraindicated during pregnancy.

• If an I.V. contrast medium is used, the test is contraindicated for patients with hypersensitivity to iodine or with severe renal or hepatic disease.

Normal findings
Normally, the liver has a uniform density that's slightly greater than that of the pancreas, kidneys, and spleen. Linear and circular areas of slightly lower density, representing hepatic vascular structures, may interrupt this uniform appearance. The portal vein is usually visible; the hepatic artery usually isn't. I.V. contrast medium enhances the isodensity of both vascular structures and the liver parenchyma.

Typically, intrahepatic biliary radicles are not visible, but the common hepatic and bile ducts may be visible as low-density structures. Because bile has the same density as water, use of an I.V. contrast medium improves demarcation of the biliary tract by enhancing surrounding parenchyma and vascular structures.

Like the biliary ducts, the gallbladder is visible as a round or elliptic low-density structure. A contracted gallbladder may be impossible to visualize.

Abnormal findings
Most focal hepatic defects appear less dense than the normal parenchyma, and CT scans can detect small lesions. Use of rapid-sequence scanning with an I.V. contrast medium helps distinguish between the two because the normal parenchyma shows greater enhancement than focal defects.

Primary and metastatic neoplasms may appear as well-circumscribed or poorly defined areas of slightly lower density than the normal parenchyma. However, some lesions have the same density as the liver parenchyma and may be undetectable. Neoplasms that are especially large may distort the liver's contour. Hepatic abscesses appear as relatively low-density, homogeneous areas, usually with well-defined borders. Hepatic cysts appear as sharply defined round or oval structures and have a density lower than abscesses and neoplasms.

The density of a hepatic hematoma varies with its age. A recent clot is as dense as or slightly more dense than the normal parenchyma; a resolving clot is somewhat less dense than the normal parenchyma. Intrahepatic hematomas vary in shape; subcapsular hematomas are usually crescent-shaped and compress the liver away from the capsule.

When distinguishing between obstructive and nonobstructive jaundice, biliary duct dilation indicates the former and an absence of dilation indicates the latter. Dilated intrahepatic bile ducts appear as low-density linear and circular branching structures. Dilation of the common hepatic duct, common bile duct, and gallbladder may also be apparent, depending on the site and severity of obstruction. Use of an I.V. contrast medium helps detect biliary dilation, especially when the ducts are only slightly dilated.

Usually, CT scanning can identify the cause of obstruction — for example, calculi or pancreatic carcinoma. However, if the site of obstruction must be located before surgery, percutaneous transhepatic cholangiography or endoscopic retrograde cholangiopancreatography (less common) may be performed as well.

PANCREATIC COMPUTED TOMOGRAPHY

In computed tomography (CT) of the pancreas, multiple X-rays penetrate the upper abdomen while a detector records the differences in tissue attenuation, which is then displayed as an image on a television screen. A series of cross-sectional views can provide a detailed look at the pancreas. CT scanning accurately distinguishes the pancreas and surrounding organs and vessels if enough fat is present between the structures. Use of an I.V. or oral contrast medium can further accentuate differences in tissue density.

Purpose
• To detect pancreatic carcinoma or pseudocysts
• To detect or evaluate pancreatitis (CT scans may fail to distinguish between carcinoma and pancreatitis)
• To distinguish between pancreatic disorders and disorders of the retroperitoneum

Patient preparation
• Explain to the patient that this test helps detect disorders of the pancreas.
• Instruct him to fast after midnight before the day of the test.
• Describe the test, including who will perform it, where it will take place, and its duration (about 30 minutes).

• Tell him that he'll be placed on an adjustable table that is positioned inside a scanning gantry. Assure him that the procedure is painless.
• Explain that he'll have to remain still during the test and periodically hold his breath.
• Inform him that he may be given an I.V. contrast medium, oral contrast medium, or both to enhance visualization of the pancreas. Describe possible adverse reactions of the agent, such as nausea, flushing, dizziness, and sweating, and tell him to report any of these symptoms.
• Check his history for recent barium studies and for hypersensitivity to iodine, seafood, or contrast media used in prior tests.
• Administer the oral contrast agent.

Procedure and posttest care
• Help the patient into the supine position on the radiographic table and position the table within the opening in the scanning gantry.
• A series of transverse X-rays is taken and recorded on magnetic tape. The varying tissue absorption is calculated by a computer, and the information is reconstructed as images on a television screen. These images are studied, and selected ones are photographed.
• After the first series of films is completed, the images are reviewed. Then contrast enhancement may be ordered. After the contrast medium is administered, another series of films is taken, and the patient is observed for an allergic reaction — itching, hypotension, hypertension, diaphoresis, or dyspnea.
• After the procedure, tell the patient he may resume his usual diet.

Precautions
• CT scanning of the pancreas should not be performed during pregnancy or, if a contrast medium is indicated, on patients with a history of hypersensitivity

NORMAL CT SCAN OF THE PANCREAS

This normal pancreatic computed tomography (CT) scan shows the pancreas opacified by contrast medium.

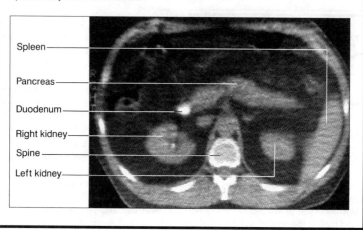

to iodine or severe renal or hepatic disease.

Normal findings

Usually, the pancreatic parenchyma displays a uniform density, especially when an I.V. contrast medium is used. The gland normally thickens from tail to head and has a smooth surface. A contrast medium administered orally opacifies the adjacent stomach and duodenum and helps outline the pancreas, particularly in patients with little peripancreatic fat, such as children and thin adults. See *Normal CT scan of the pancreas.*

Abnormal findings

Because the tissue density of pancreatic carcinoma resembles that of the normal parenchyma, changes in pancreatic size and shape help demonstrate carcinoma and pseudocysts. Usually, carcinoma first appears as a localized swelling of the head, body, or tail of the pancreas

and may spread to obliterate the fat plane, dilate the main pancreatic duct and common bile duct by obstructing them, and produce low-density focal lesions in the liver from metastasis. Use of an I.V. contrast medium helps detect metastases by opacifying the pancreatic and hepatic parenchyma.

Adenocarcinoma and islet cell tumor are the most common carcinomas of the pancreas. Cystadenomas and cystadenocarcinomas, usually multilocular, occur most frequently in the body and tail of the pancreas and appear as low-density focal lesions marked by internal septa. Contrast medium administered by mouth helps distinguish between bowel loops and tumors in the tail of the pancreas.

Acute pancreatitis, either edematous (interstitial) or necrotizing (hemorrhagic), produces diffuse enlargement of the pancreas. In acute edematous pancreatitis, the density of the parenchyma is uniformly decreased. In acute necrotizing pancreatitis, the density is nonuniform because of the presence of both necrosis and hemorrhage. The areas of tissue necrosis have diminished density. In acute pancreatitis, inflammation often spreads into the peripancreatic fat and blurs the margin of the gland. Abscesses, phlegmons, and pseudocysts may occur as complications of acute pancreatitis. Abscesses, either within or outside of the pancreas, appear as low-density areas and are most readily detected when they contain gas. Pseudocysts, which may be unilocular or multilocular, appear as sharply circumscribed, low-density areas that may contain debris. Ascites and pleural effusion may also be apparent in acute pancreatitis.

In chronic pancreatitis, the pancreas may appear normal, enlarged (localized or generalized), or atrophic, depending on the severity of the disease. Calcification of the ducts and dilation of the main pancreatic duct are characteristic. Pseudocysts, obliteration of the fat plane, and secondary complications (such as biliary obstruction) may occur.

MUSCULOSKELETAL SYSTEM

SPINAL COMPUTED TOMOGRAPHY

Much more versatile than conventional radiography, computed tomography (CT) of the spine provides detailed high-resolution images in the cross-sectional, longitudinal, sagittal, and lateral planes. Multiple X-ray beams from a computerized body scanner are directed at the spine from different angles; these pass through the body and strike radiation detectors, producing electrical impulses. A computer then converts these impulses into digital information, which is displayed as a three-dimensional image on a video monitor. Storage of the digital information allows electronic recreation and manipulation of the image, creating a permanent record of the images to enable reexamination without repeating the procedure.

Two variations of spinal CT scanning further expand the procedure's diagnostic capabilities. Contrast-enhanced CT scans accentuate spinal vasculature and highlight even subtle differences in tissue density. Air CT scanning, which involves removing a small amount of cerebrospinal fluid (CSF) and injecting air via lumbar puncture, intensifies the contrast between the subarachnoid space and surrounding tissue.

Purpose
• To diagnose spinal lesions and abnormalities
• To monitor the effects of spinal surgery or therapy

Patient preparation
• Explain to the patient that this procedure allows visualization of his spine.
• If contrast enhancement isn't ordered, tell him that he needn't restrict food or fluids. If contrast is ordered, instruct him to fast for 4 hours before the test.
• Tell the patient that a series of scans will be taken of his spine. Explain who will perform the procedure and where and that the test takes 30 to 60 minutes.
• Reassure him that the procedure is painless, but that he may find having to remain still for a prolonged period uncomfortable.
• Explain that he will be positioned on an X-ray table inside a CT body scanning unit and told to lie still because movement during the procedure may cause distorted images. The computer-

controlled scanner will revolve around him taking multiple scans.

• If contrast dye is used, tell him that he may feel flushed and warm and may experience a transient headache, a salty taste, and nausea or vomiting after injection of the contrast dye. Reassure him that these reactions are normal.

• Instruct the patient to wear a radiologic examining gown and to remove all metal objects and jewelry.

• Check the patient's history for hypersensitivity reactions to iodine, shellfish, or contrast media. If such reactions have occurred, mark them on the patient's chart. The doctor may order prophylactic medications or choose not to use contrast enhancement.

• If the patient appears restless or apprehensive about the procedure, a mild sedative may be prescribed.

Equipment
Recording equipment, contrast medium (meglumine iothalamate or sodium diatrizoate), 60-ml syringe, 19G to 20G needle, tourniquet.

Procedure and posttest care
• Place the patient in a supine position on a radiographic table and tell him to lie as still as possible.

• The table slides into the circular opening of the CT scanner and the scanner revolves around the patient, taking radiographs at preselected intervals.

• After the first set of scans is taken, the patient is removed from the scanner. Contrast medium may be administered.

• Observe the patient for signs and symptoms of a hypersensitivity reaction, including pruritus, rash, and respiratory difficulty, for 30 minutes after the contrast dye has been injected.

• After dye injection, the patient is moved back into the scanner, and another series of scans is taken. The images obtained from the scan are displayed on a video monitor during the procedure and stored on magnetic tape.

• After testing with contrast enhancement, observe the patient for residual effects, such as headache, nausea, and vomiting, and inform him that he may resume his usual diet.

Precautions
• Body CT scanning with contrast enhancement is contraindicated in patients who are hypersensitive to iodine, shellfish, or contrast media used in radiographic studies.

• Some patients may experience strong feelings of claustrophobia or anxiety when inside the body CT scanner. For such patients, a mild sedative to help reduce anxiety may be ordered.

• For patients with significant back pain, administer prescribed analgesics before the scan.

Normal findings
In the CT image, spinal tissue appears white, black, or gray, depending on its density. Vertebrae, the densest tissues, are white; CSF is black; soft tissues appear in shades of gray.

Abnormal findings
By highlighting areas of altered density and depicting structural malformation, CT scanning can reveal all types of spinal lesions and abnormalities. It's particularly useful in detecting and localizing tumors, which appear as masses varying in density. Measuring this density and noting the configuration and location relative to the spinal cord can often identify the type of tumor. For example, a neurinoma (schwannoma) appears as a spherical mass dorsal to the cord. A darker, wider mass lying more laterally or ventrally to the cord may be a meningioma.

CT scans also reveal degenerative processes and structural changes in detail. Herniated nucleus pulposus shows as an obvious herniation of disk material with unilateral or bilateral nerve root compression; if the herniation is midline, spinal cord compression will be evident. Cervical spondylosis shows as cervical cord compression due to bony hypertrophy of the cervical spine; lumbar stenosis as hypertrophy of the lumbar vertebrae, causing cord compression by decreasing space within the spinal column. Facet disorders show as soft-tissue changes, bony overgrowth, and spurring of the vertebrae, which result in nerve root compression. Fluid-filled arachnoidal and other paraspinal cysts show as dark masses displacing the spinal cord. Vascular malformations, evident after contrast enhancement, show as masses or clusters, usually on the dorsal aspect of the spinal cord.

Congenital spinal malformations, such as meningocele, myelocele, and spina bifida, show as abnormally large, dark gaps between the white vertebrae.

SKELETAL COMPUTED TOMOGRAPHY

Skeletal computed tomography (CT) provides a series of tomograms, translated by a computer and displayed on an oscilloscope screen, representing cross-sectional images of various layers (or slices) of bone. This technique can reconstruct cross-sectional, horizontal, sagittal, and coronal plane images.

Taking collimated (parallel) radiographs increases the number of radiation density calculations the computer makes, thereby improving the degree of resolution and thus specificity and accuracy. Hundreds of thousands of readings of radiation levels absorbed by tissues may be combined to depict anatomic slices of varying thickness.

Purpose
• To determine the existence and extent of primary bone tumors, skeletal metastases, and soft-tissue tumors
• To diagnose joint abnormalities difficult to detect by other methods

Patient preparation
• Explain to the patient that this procedure allows visualization of bones and joints. If contrast medium isn't ordered, tell him that he needn't restrict food or fluids. If contrast enhancement is ordered, instruct him to fast for 4 hours before the test.
• Explain who will perform the procedure and where and that the test takes 30 to 60 minutes. Reassure him that the procedure is painless.
• Explain that he'll be positioned on an X-ray table inside a CT scanner and asked to lie still; the computer-controlled scanner will revolve around him taking multiple scans. Stress that he should lie as still as possible because movement may cause distorted images.
• If contrast dye is used, tell him that he may feel flushed and warm and may experience a transient headache, a salty taste, and nausea or vomiting after its injection. Reassure him that these reactions are normal.
• Instruct him to wear a radiologic examining gown and to remove all metal objects and jewelry that may appear in the X-ray field.
• Make sure the patient or a responsible family member has signed an appropriate consent form.
• Check his history for hypersensitivity reactions to iodine, shellfish, or contrast media. Mark any such reactions on the chart. The doctor may order prophylactic medications or choose not to use a contrast dye.

• If the patient appears restless or apprehensive about the procedure, a mild sedative may be prescribed.

Equipment
Recording equipment, contrast medium (either meglumine iothalamate or sodium diatrizoate), 60-ml syringe, 19G to 20G needle, tourniquet.

Procedure and posttest care
• Place the patient in a supine position on a radiographic table and tell him to lie as still as possible.
• The table is slid into the circular opening of the CT scanner. The scanner revolves around the patient, taking radiographs at preselected intervals.
• After the first set of scans is taken, the patient is removed from the scanner and contrast dye is administered if necessary.
• Observe the patient for signs and symptoms of a hypersensitivity reaction, including pruritus, rash, and respiratory difficulty, for 30 minutes after the contrast dye has been injected.
• After dye injection, the patient is moved back into the scanner, and another series of scans is taken. The images obtained from the scan are displayed on a video monitor during the procedure and stored on magnetic tape to create a permanent record for subsequent study.
• If contrast media is used, observe for a delayed allergic reaction and treat as necessary. (Diphenhydramine is the drug of choice.)
• Encourage fluids to assist in dye elimination.
• Tell the patient that he may resume his usual activity level and diet, if appropriate.

Precautions
• A CT scan with contrast enhancement is contraindicated in patients who are hypersensitive to iodine, shellfish, or radiographic contrast dye.

• Some patients may experience strong feelings of claustrophobia or anxiety when inside the body CT scanner. For such patients, a mild sedative may be ordered to help reduce anxiety.
• For patients with significant bone or joint pain, administer analgesics so that the patient can lie still comfortably during the scan.

Normal findings
The scan should reveal no pathology in the bones or joints. It produces crisp images of the structure while blurring or eliminating details of surrounding structures.

Abnormal findings
Because of its ability to display cross-sectional anatomy, CT scanning is useful for detecting the shoulder, spine, hip, and pelvis. This cross-sectional view eliminates the confusing shadows of superimposed structures that occur with conventional radiographs. The scan can reveal primary bone tumors and soft-tissue tumors as well as skeletal metastasis. It can also reveal joint abnormalities difficult to detect by other methods.

SKELETAL MAGNETIC RESONANCE IMAGING

A noninvasive technique, magnetic resonance imaging (MRI) produces clear and sensitive tomographic images of bone and soft tissue. The scan provides superior contrast of body tissues and allows imaging of multiple planes, including direct sagittal and coronal views in regions that can't be easily visualized with X-rays or computed tomography (CT) scans. MRI eliminates any risks associated with exposure to

X-ray beams and causes no known harm to cells.

During an MRI scan, the patient is placed on a table that slides into a cylindrical magnet. A radiofrequency beam is then introduced into the magnetic field. Resulting energy changes are measured and used to generate images on a television screen.

Purpose

• To evaluate bony and soft-tissue tumors
• To identify changes in bone marrow composition
• To identify spinal disorders

Patient preparation

• Explain to the patient that this test assesses bone and soft tissue. Tell him who will perform the test, where it will be done, and that it takes up to 90 minutes.
• Explain that although MRI is painless and involves no exposure to radiation from the scanner, a radioactive contrast dye may be used, depending on the type of tissue being studied.
• Emphasize that the opening for the patient's head and body in the MRI scanner is quite small and deep. Ask if claustrophobia has ever been a problem; if so, sedation may help him to tolerate the scan.
• Explain that he'll hear the scanner clicking, whirring, and thumping as it moves inside its housing.
• Reassure him that he'll be able to communicate with the technician at all times.
• Instruct him to remove all metallic objects, including jewelry, hair pins, or watch.
• Ask if he has any surgically implanted joints, pins, clips, valves, pumps, or pacemakers containing metal. If he does, he won't be able to have the test.
• Make sure that an appropriate consent form has been signed by the patient or a responsible family member.

Procedure and posttest care

• At the scanner room door, check the patient one last time for metal objects.
• The patient is placed on a narrow, padded, nonmetallic table that moves into the scanner tunnel. Fans continuously circulate air in the tunnel, and a call bell or intercom is used to maintain verbal contact.
• Remind the patient to remain still throughout the procedure.
• While the patient lies within the strong magnetic field, the area to be studied is stimulated with radiofrequency waves.
• If the test is prolonged, monitor the patient for postural hypotension.
• After the test, tell the patient that he may resume normal activity.
• Provide emotional support to the patient with claustrophobic anxiety or anxiety over his diagnosis.

Precautions

• MRI can't be performed on patients with pacemakers, intracranial aneurysm clips, or other ferrous metal implants. Ventilators, I.V. infusion pumps, and other metallic or computer-based equipment must be kept out of the MRI area.
• If the patient is unstable, make sure an I.V. line without metal components is in place and that all equipment is compatible with MRI imaging. If necessary, monitor oxygen saturation, cardiac rhythm, and respiratory status during the test. An anesthesiologist may be needed to monitor a heavily sedated patient.
• A technician should maintain verbal contact with the conscious patient.

Normal findings

MRI should reveal no pathology in bone, muscles, and joints.

Abnormal findings

MRI is excellent for visualizing diseases of the spinal canal and cord and for identifying primary and metastatic bone tumors. It's beneficial in anatomic delineation of muscles, ligaments, and bones. The images show superior contrast of body tissues and sharply define healthy, benign, and malignant tissues.

MISCELLANEOUS TESTS

ORBITAL COMPUTED TOMOGRAPHY

Orbital computed tomography (CT) allows visualization of abnormalities not readily seen on standard radiographs, delineating their size, position, and relationship to adjoining structures. A series of tomograms reconstructed by a computer and displayed as anatomic slices on an oscilloscope screen, the orbital CT scan identifies space-occupying lesions earlier and more accurately than other radiographic techniques and provides three-dimensional images of orbital structures, especially the ocular muscles and the optic nerve.

Purpose
• To evaluate pathologies of the orbit and eye — especially expanding lesions and bone destruction
• To evaluate fractures of the orbit and adjoining structures
• To determine the cause of unilateral exophthalmos
• To aid diagnosis of intracranial lesions that affect vision
• To evaluate a patient with conditions such as suspected circulatory disorders, hemangioma, or subdural hematoma (with contrast enhancement)

Patient preparation
• Describe the procedure to the patient, and explain that this test visualizes the anatomy of the eye and its surrounding structures.
• If contrast enhancement isn't scheduled, inform him that he needn't restrict food or fluids. If contrast enhancement is scheduled, withhold food and fluids from the patient for 4 hours before the test.
• Tell the patient that a series of X-ray films will be taken of his eye and who will perform the test and where.
• Reassure him that the test will cause him no discomfort and will take 15 to 30 minutes to perform.
• Tell the patient that he'll be positioned on an X-ray table and that the head of the table will be moved into the scanner, which will rotate around his head and make loud, clacking sounds.
• If a contrast agent will be used for the procedure, tell the patient that he may feel flushed and warm and experience a transient headache, a salty taste, and nausea or vomiting after the dye is injected. Reassure him that these reactions to contrast medium are typical.
• Make sure the patient or a responsible family member has signed a consent form.
• Check his history for hypersensitivity reactions to iodine, shellfish, or radiographic dyes.
• Instruct him to remove jewelry, hairpins, or other metal objects in the X-ray field to allow for precise imaging of the orbital structures.

Procedure and posttest care
• The patient is placed in a supine position on the radiographic table, with his head immobilized by straps. Ask him to lie still.
• The head of the table is moved into the scanner, which rotates around the patient's head taking radiographs.

• Information obtained is stored on magnetic tapes, and the images are displayed on an oscilloscope screen. Photographs may be made if a permanent record is desired.

• When this series of radiographs has been taken, contrast enhancement is performed. The contrast agent is injected and a second series of scans is recorded.

• If a contrast agent was used, watch for its residual adverse effects, including headache, nausea, or vomiting. Following the procedure, advise the patient that he may resume his usual diet.

Precautions

• Use of contrast enhancement is contraindicated in those patients with known hypersensitivity reactions to iodine, shellfish, or radiographic dyes used in other tests.

Normal findings

Orbital structures are evaluated for size, shape, and position. Dense orbital bone provides a marked contrast to less dense periocular fat. The optic nerve and the medial and lateral rectus muscles are clearly defined. The rectus muscles appear as thin dense bands on each side, behind the eye. The optic canals should be equal in size.

Abnormal findings

Orbital CT scans can identify intra- and extraorbital space-occupying lesions that obscure the normal structures or cause orbital enlargement, indentation of the orbital walls, or bone destruction. This test can also help determine the type of lesion. For example, infiltrative lesions, such as lymphomas and metastatic carcinomas, appear as irregular areas of density. However, encapsulated tumors, such as benign hemangiomas and meningiomas, appear as clearly defined masses of consistent density. CT scans can also visu-alize intracranial tumors that invade the orbit, thickening of the optic nerve that may occur with gliomas, meningiomas, and secondary tumors that may cause enlargement of the optic canal.

In evaluating fractures, CT scans allow a complete three-dimensional view of the affected structures. In determining the cause of unilateral exophthalmos, CT scans can show early erosion or expansion of the medial orbital wall that may arise from lesions in the ethmoidal cells. It can also detect space-occupying lesions in the orbit or paranasal sinuses that cause exophthalmos. CT scans can also show thickening of the medial and lateral rectus muscles in proptosis, resulting from Graves' disease.

Enhancement with a contrast agent may provide information about the circulation through abnormal ocular tissues.

THORACIC COMPUTED TOMOGRAPHY

Thoracic computed tomography (CT) provides cross-sectional views of the chest by passing an X-ray beam from a computerized scanner through the body at different angles. CT scanning may be done with or without an injected radio-iodine contrast agent, which is primarily used to highlight blood vessels and to allow greater visual discrimination.

This test provides a three-dimensional image and is especially useful in detecting small differences in tissue density. The thoracic CT scan may replace mediastinoscopy in diagnosis of mediastinal masses and Hodgkin's disease; its value in the evaluation of pulmonary pathology is proven.

Purpose

- To locate suspected neoplasms (such as in Hodgkin's disease), especially with mediastinal involvement
- To differentiate coin-sized calcified lesions (indicating tuberculosis) from tumors
- To distinguish tumors adjacent to the aorta from aortic aneurysms
- To detect the invasion of a neck mass in the thorax
- To evaluate primary malignancy that may metastasize to the lungs, especially in patients with primary bone tumors, soft-tissue sarcomas, and melanomas
- To evaluate the mediastinal lymph nodes

Patient preparation

- Explain to the patient that this test provides cross-sectional views of the chest and distinguishes small differences in tissue density.
- If a contrast agent will not be used, inform him that he needn't restrict food or fluids. If the test is to be performed with contrast enhancement, instruct the patient to fast for 4 hours before the test.
- Tell him who will perform the test and where and that the procedure usually takes 90 minutes and will not cause him any discomfort.
- Tell him he'll be positioned on an X-ray table that moves into the center of a large ring-shaped piece of X-ray equipment and that the equipment may be noisy.
- Inform him that a radiographic contrast agent may be injected into a vein in his arm. If so, he may experience nausea, warmth, flushing of the face, or a salty taste. Reassure him that radiation exposure is minimal.
- Tell him not to move during the test, but to breathe normally. Instruct him to remove all jewelry and metal in the X-ray field.

- Make sure the patient or a responsible family member has signed a consent form.
- Check the patient's history for hypersensitivity to iodine, shellfish, or radiographic contrast agents.

Procedure and posttest care

- After the patient is placed in a supine position on the radiographic table and the contrast agent has been injected, the machine scans the patient at different angles, while the computer calculates small differences in the densities of various tissues, water, fat, bone, and air.
- This information is displayed as a printout of numerical values and as a projection on an oscilloscope screen. Images may be recorded for further study.
- Watch for signs of delayed hypersensitivity to the contrast agent (itching, hypotension or hypertension, or respiratory distress).
- Following the test, encourage fluid intake.

Precautions

- Thoracic CT scanning is contraindicated during pregnancy and, if a contrast agent is used, in persons who have a history of hypersensitivity reactions to iodine, shellfish, or radiographic contrast agents.

Normal findings

Black and white areas on a thoracic CT scan refer, respectively, to air and bone densities. Shades of gray correspond to water, fat, and soft-tissue densities.

Abnormal findings

Abnormal thoracic CT findings include tumors, nodules, cysts, aortic aneurysms, enlarged lymph nodes, pleural effusion, and accumulations of blood, fluid, or fat.

CARDIAC MAGNETIC RESONANCE IMAGING

A great asset in the diagnosis of cardiac disorders, magnetic resonance imaging (MRI) has the ability to "see through" bone and to delineate fluid-filled soft tissue in great detail, as well as produce images of organs and vessels in motion.

In this noninvasive procedure, the patient is placed in a magnetic field, into which a radiofrequency beam is introduced. Resulting energy changes are measured and used by the MRI computer to generate images on a television screen. Cross-sectional images of the anatomy are viewed in multiple planes and recorded for permanent record.

Purpose
• To identify anatomic sequelae related to myocardial infarction (MI), such as formation of ventricular aneurysm, ventricular wall thinning, and mural thrombus
• To detect and evaluate cardiomyopathy
• To detect and evaluate pericardial disease
• To identify paracardiac or intracardiac masses
• To detect congenital heart disease, such as atrial or ventricular septal defects, and the degree of malposition of the great vessel
• To identify vascular disease, such as thoracic aneurysm and thoracic dissection
• To assess the structure of the pulmonary vasculature

Patient preparation
• Explain to the patient that this test assesses the heart's function and structure.

• Tell him who will perform the test, where it will be done, and that it takes up to 90 minutes.
• Inform the patient that he'll be positioned on a narrow bed, which slides into a large cylinder that houses the MRI magnets. Tell him that the scanner will make clicking, whirring, and thumping noises as it moves inside its housing.
• Explain that although MRI is painless, he may feel uncomfortable because he must remain still inside a small space throughout the test. Ask if he suffers from claustrophobia; if so, he might not be able to tolerate the procedure or may need sedation.
• Reassure him that he'll be able to communicate with the technician at all times and that the procedure will be stopped if he feels claustrophobic.
• Immediately before the test, have the patient remove all metal objects. Double check to be sure he doesn't have a pacemaker or any surgically implanted joints, pins, clips, valves, or pumps containing metal that could be attracted to the strong MRI magnet. If he does, he won't be able to undergo the test.
• Make sure the patient or a responsible family member signs a consent form.
• Administer prescribed sedation.

Procedure and posttest care
• At the scanner room door, check the patient one last time for metal objects.
• The patient is placed supine on a narrow, padded, nonmetallic bed that slides to the desired position inside the scanner. Radiofrequency (RF) waves are directed at his chest. The resulting images are displayed on a monitor and recorded on film or magnetic tape for permanent storage.
• The radiologist may vary RF waves and use the computer to manipulate and enhance the images.
• Remind the patient to remain still throughout the procedure.

CARDIAC POSITRON EMISSION TOMOGRAPHY

Positron emission tomography (PET) combines elements of computed tomography (CT) scanning and conventional radionuclide imaging. PET is used to detect coronary artery disease, to evaluate myocardial metabolism and contractility, and to distinguish viable from infarcted cardiac tissue, especially during early stages of myocardial infarction.

PET technology

Like radionuclide imaging, PET scans measure emissions of injected radioisotopes and convert these values to tomographic images. However, PET uses radioisotopes of biologically important elements — oxygen, nitrogen, carbon, and fluorine, which emit particles called *positrons*. During positron emissions, gamma rays are detected by the PET scanner and reconstructed to form an image. One distinct advantage to PET is that positron emitters can be chemically "tagged" to biologically active molecules such as carbon monoxide, neurotransmitters, hormones, and metabolites (particularly glucose), enabling study of their uptake and distribution in tissue.

Preparing the cardiac patient

When preparing a patient for PET scan, explain the following key points:
• If the test is ordered to assess myocardial contractility, explain to the patient that the test distinguishes viable tissue from tissue injured by infarction and may also help the doctor assess mitochondrial impairment associated with ischemia or evaluate coronary artery obstruction.
• Explain that he'll be given a radioactive substance, either by injection, inhalation, or I.V., and that a highly specialized camera will detect the radioactive decay of this substance and send this data to a computer, which converts it to a visual image.
• Describe the test, including who will administer it, where it will take place, and its duration (typically 60 to 90 minutes). Take time to describe the equipment.
• Tell him that the test is painless, unless an I.V. infusion is planned, in which case he may experience some discomfort from the needle puncture and the tourniquet. If the radioisotope will be inhaled, explain this painless procedure.
• If a fast is ordered, describe food and fluid restrictions (the necessity of fasting is still under investigation).
• Tell him that he will undergo an attenuation scan for about 30 minutes. Then he'll receive the appropriate positron emitter and undergo PET scanning.

The radioisotope may be harmful to a fetus, so female patients of childbearing age should be screened carefully before undergoing this procedure.

• Assess how he responds to the enclosed environment. Provide reassurance if necessary.
• Monitor the sedated patient's hemodynamic, cardiac, respiratory, and mental status until the effects of the sedative have worn off.

Precautions
• Claustrophobic patients may experience anxiety. Monitor cardiac patients for signs of ischemia (chest pressure, shortness of breath, or changes in hemodynamic status).

• MRI can't be performed on patients with pacemakers, intracranial aneurysm clips, or other ferrous metal implants.

• If the patient is unstable, make sure an I.V. line with *no metal components* is in place and that all equipment is compatible with MRI imaging. If necessary, monitor the patient's oxygen saturation, cardiac rhythm, and respiratory status during the test.

• An anesthesiologist may be needed to monitor a heavily sedated patient.

• A nurse or radiology technician should maintain verbal contact with the conscious patient.

Normal findings

MRI should reveal no anatomic or structural dysfunctions in cardiovascular tissue.

Abnormal findings

MRI can detect cardiomyopathy and pericardial disease. It can also detect atrial or ventricular septal defects or other congenital defects. MRI is useful for identifying paracardiac or intracardiac masses. In addition, it can evaluate the extent of pericardial or vascular disease.

Another emerging technology for evaluating cardiac pathology is positron emission tomography. See *Cardiac positron emission tomography.*

RENAL COMPUTED TOMOGRAPHY

Renal computed tomography (CT) provides a useful image of the kidneys made from a series of tomograms or cross-sectional slices, which are then translated by a computer and displayed on an oscilloscope screen. The image density reflects the amount of radiation absorbed by renal tissue and permits identification of masses and other lesions. An I.V. contrast medium may be injected to accentuate the renal parenchyma's density and help differentiate renal masses. This highly accurate test is usually performed to investigate diseases found by other diagnostic procedures, such as excretory urography.

Purpose

• To detect and evaluate renal pathology, such as tumor, obstruction, calculi, polycystic kidney disease, congenital anomalies, and abnormal fluid accumulation around the kidneys

• To evaluate the retroperitoneum

• To guide needle placement before percutaneous biopsy

• To determine the kidney's size and location in relation to the bladder following a kidney transplant

• To localize renal or perinephric abscesses for drainage

Patient preparation

• Explain to the patient that this test permits examination of the kidneys.

• If contrast enhancement isn't scheduled, inform the patient that he needn't restrict food or fluids. If contrast enhancement is scheduled, instruct him to fast for 4 hours before the test.

• Tell him who will perform the test and where and that the procedure takes about an hour, depending on the purpose of the scan.

• Inform the patient that he'll be positioned on an X-ray table, and that a scanner will take films of his kidneys.

• Warn him that the scanner may make loud, clacking sounds as it rotates around his body.

• Tell him that he may experience transient adverse effects, such as flushing, metallic taste, and headache, following injection of the contrast medium.

• Make sure that the patient or a responsible family member has signed a consent form.

• Check the patient's history for hypersensitivity to shellfish, iodine, or contrast media. Mark any sensitivities clearly on the patient's chart.

• Just before the procedure, instruct the patient to put on a hospital gown and to remove any metallic objects that could interfere with the scan.

• Administer prescribed sedatives.

Procedure and posttest care

• The patient is placed in supine position on the scanning table and secured with straps.

• The table is moved into the scanner.

• Instruct the patient to lie still.

• The scanner then rotates around the patient, taking multiple images at different angles within each cross-sectional slice.

• When one series of tomograms is complete, contrast enhancement may be performed. Another series of tomograms is then taken.

• After the I.V. contrast medium is administered, monitor for allergic reactions, such as respiratory difficulty, urticaria, or other skin eruption.

• Information from the scan is stored on a disk or on magnetic tape, fed into a computer, and converted into an image for display on an oscilloscope screen. Radiographs and photographs are taken of selected views.

• After the test, tell the patient he may resume his usual diet if a contrast dye was used.

Precautions

• Watch for signs of hypersensitivity to the contrast medium if contrast enhancement is required.

Normal findings

Normally, the density of the renal parenchyma is slightly higher than that of the liver, but less dense than bone, which appears white on a CT scan. The density of the collecting system is generally low (black), unless a contrast medium is used to enhance it to a higher (whiter) density. The position of the kidneys is evaluated according to the surrounding structures; the size and shape of the kidneys are determined by counting cuts between the superior and inferior poles and following the contour of the renal outline.

Abnormal findings

Renal masses appear as areas of different density than normal parenchyma, possibly altering the kidneys' shape or projecting beyond their margins. Renal cysts, for example, appear as smooth, sharply defined masses, with thin walls and a lower density than normal parenchyma. Tumors such as renal cell carcinoma, however, are usually not as well delineated; they tend to have thick walls and nonuniform density. With contrast enhancement, solid tumors show a higher density than renal cysts but lower density than normal parenchyma. Tumors with hemorrhage, calcification, or necrosis show higher densities. Vascular tumors are more clearly defined with contrast enhancement. Adrenal tumors are confined masses, usually detached from the kidneys and from other retroperitoneal organs.

Renal CT may also identify other abnormalities, including obstructions, calculi, polycystic kidney disease, congenital anomalies, and abnormal accumulations of fluid around the kidneys, such as hematomas, lymphoceles, and abscesses. After nephrectomy, CT can detect abnormal masses, such as recurrent tumors, in a renal fossa that should be empty.

Nuclear Medicine Scans

THYROID

RADIOACTIVE IODINE UPTAKE TEST

The radioactive iodine uptake (RAIU) test evaluates thyroid function by measuring the amount of orally ingested ^{123}I or ^{131}I that accumulates in the thyroid gland after 6 and 24 hours. An external single counting probe measures the radioactivity in the thyroid as a percentage of the original dose, thus indicating its ability to trap and retain iodine. The test accurately diagnoses hyperthyroidism but is less accurate for hypothyroidism. Indications for this test include abnormal results of chemical tests used to evaluate thyroid function.

Purpose
• To evaluate thyroid function
• To help diagnose hyperthyroidism or hypothyroidism
• To help distinguish between primary and secondary thyroid disorders
• To help differentiate Graves' disease from hyperfunctioning toxic adenoma (performed concurrently with radionuclide thyroid imaging and the T_3 resin uptake test)

Patient preparation
• Tell the patient that RAIU testing assesses thyroid function.
• Instruct him to fast beginning at midnight the night before the test.
• Explain that he'll receive radioactive iodine (capsule or liquid) and then be scanned after 6 hours and again after 24 hours.
• Assure him that the test is painless and that the small amount of radioactivity used is harmless.

• Tell him that test results will be available within 24 hours.
• Check patient history for iodine exposure, which may interfere with test results. Note any prior radiologic tests using contrast media, nuclear medicine procedures or current use of iodine preparations or thyroid medications on the film request slip. Iodine hypersensitivity is not considered a contraindication because the amount of iodine used is similar to the amount consumed in a normal diet.

Equipment
Oral dose of ^{123}I or ^{131}I, external single counting probe.

Procedure and posttest care
• After ingesting an oral dose of radioactive iodine, the patient's thyroid is scanned at 6 hours and 24 hours by placing the anterior portion of his neck in front of an external single counting probe.
• The amount of radioactivity detected by the probe is compared to the amount of radioactivity contained in the original dose to determine the percent of radioactive iodine retained by the thyroid.
• Instruct the patient to resume a light diet 2 hours after taking the oral dose of radioactive iodine. When the study is complete, the patient may resume a normal diet.

Precautions
• Radioactive iodine uptake testing is contraindicated during pregnancy and lactation because of possible teratogenic effects.

Reference values
At 6 hours, 3% to 16% of the radioactive iodine should accumulate in the thyroid; at 24 hours, accumulation should be 8% to 29%. The balance of the radioactive iodine is excreted in the urine. Local variations in the normal range of iodine uptake may occur due

to regional differences in dietary iodine intake and procedural differences among laboratories.

Abnormal findings

Below-normal iodine uptake may indicate hypothyroidism, subacute thyroiditis, or iodine overload. Above-normal uptake may indicate hyperthyroidism, early Hashimoto's thyroiditis, hypoalbuminemia, lithium ingestion, or iodine-deficient goiter. However, in hyperthyroidism, the rate of turnover may be so rapid that a false normal measurement occurs at 24 hours.

RADIONUCLIDE THYROID IMAGING

In radionuclide thyroid imaging, the thyroid is studied by gamma camera after the patient receives a radioisotope (^{123}I, ^{99m}Tc pertechnetate, or ^{131}I). Thyroid imaging typically follows discovery of a palpable mass, enlarged gland, or asymmetric goiter and is performed concurrently with thyroid uptake tests and measurement of serum triiodothyronine (T_3) and serum thyroxine (T_4) levels. Later, thyroid ultrasonography may be performed.

Purpose

• To assess the size, structure, and position of the thyroid gland
• To evaluate thyroid function (in conjunction with specific thyroid uptake studies)

Patient preparation

• Tell the patient that this test helps determine the cause of thyroid dysfunction.
• If ^{123}I or ^{131}I will be used, tell him to fast after midnight the night before the test. Fasting isn't required if an I.V. injection of ^{99m}Tc pertechnetate is used.
• Explain that after he receives the radiopharmaceutical, a gamma camera will be used to produce an image of his thyroid. Tell him that the imaging procedure will take about 30 minutes and assure him that his exposure to radiation is minimal.
• Ask the patient if he has undergone tests that used radiographic contrast media within the past 60 days. Note previous radiographic contrast media exposure on the X-ray request slip.
• Check the patient's diet and medication history. Medications such as thyroid hormones, thyroid hormone antagonists, and iodine preparations (Lugol's solution, some multivitamins, and cough syrups) should be discontinued 2 to 3 weeks before the test. Phenothiazines, corticosteroids, salicylates, anticoagulants, and antihistamines should be discontinued one week before the test. Instruct the patient to stop consuming iodized salt, iodinated salt substitutes, and seafood during this period.
• The patient receives ^{123}I or ^{131}I (oral) or ^{99m}Tc pertechnetate (I.V.). Record the date and the time of administration.
• Imaging follows oral administration (^{123}I or ^{131}I) by 24 hours, and I.V. injection (^{99m}Tc pertechnetate) by 20 to 30 minutes.
• Just before the test, tell the patient to remove dentures, jewelry, or other materials that may interfere with the imaging process.

Procedure and posttest care

• The patient is placed in a supine position with his neck extended; the thyroid gland is palpated. The gamma camera is positioned above the anterior portion of his neck.
• Images of the patient's thyroid gland are projected on an oscilloscope screen and are recorded on X-ray film. Three views of the thyroid are obtained: a

RESULTS OF THYROID IMAGING IN THYROID DISORDERS

CONDITION	FINDINGS	CAUSES
Hypothyroidism	• Glandular damage or absent gland	• Surgical removal of gland • Inflammation • Radiation • Neoplasm (rare)
Hypothyroid goiter	• Enlarged gland • Decreased uptake if glandular destruction is present • Increased uptake possible from congenital error in thyroxine synthesis	• Insufficient iodine intake • Hypersecretion of thyroid-stimulating hormone (TSH) caused by thyroid hormone deficiency
Myxedema (cretinism in children)	• Normal or slightly reduced gland size • Uniform pattern • Decreased uptake	• Defective embryonic development, resulting in congenital absence or underdevelopment of thyroid gland • Maternal iodine deficiency
Hyperthyroidism (Graves' disease)	• Enlarged gland • Uniform pattern • Increased uptake	• Unknown, but may be hereditary • Production of thyroid-stimulating immunoglobulins
Toxic nodular goiter	• Multiple hot spots	• Long-standing simple goiter
Hyperfunctioning adenomas	• Solitary hot spot	• Adenomatous production of T_3 and T_4, suppressing TSH secretion and producing atrophy of other thyroid tissue
Hypofunctioning adenomas	• Solitary cold spot	• Cyst or nonfunctioning nodule
Benign multinodular goiter	• Multiple nodules with variable or no function	• Local inflammation • Degeneration
Thyroid carcinoma	• Usually a solitary cold spot with occasional or no function	• Neoplasm

straight-on anterior view and two bilateral oblique views.

• Following the procedure, tell the patient he may resume medications suspended for the test. Instruct him to resume his normal diet.

Precautions

• Radionuclide thyroid imaging is contraindicated during pregnancy and lactation.

Normal findings

Normally, radionuclide thyroid imaging reveals a thyroid gland that is about 2″ (5 cm) long and 1″ (2.5 cm) wide, with a uniform uptake of the radioisotope and without tumors. The gland is butterfly-shaped, with the isthmus located at the midline. Occasionally, a third lobe called the pyramidal lobe may be present; this is a normal variant.

Abnormal findings

During radionuclide thyroid imaging, hyperfunctioning nodules (areas of excessive iodine uptake) appear as black regions called "hot spots." The presence of hot spots requires a follow-up T_3 (Cytomel) thyroid suppression test to determine if the hyperfunctioning areas are autonomous. Hypofunctioning nodules (areas of little or no iodine uptake) appear as white or light gray regions called "cold spots." If a cold spot appears, subsequent thyroid ultrasonography may be performed to rule out cysts; in addition, fine needle aspiration and biopsy of such nodules may be performed to rule out malignancy. See *Results of thyroid imaging in thyroid disorders.*

RESPIRATORY SYSTEM

LUNG PERFUSION SCAN

A lung perfusion scan produces an image of pulmonary blood flow after I.V. injection of a radiopharmaceutical, either human serum albumin microspheres or macroaggregated albumin bonded to technetium.

Purpose

- To assess arterial perfusion of the lungs
- To detect pulmonary emboli
- To aid preoperative evaluation of the pulmonary function of a patient with marginal lung reserves
- To help confirm pulmonary vascular obstruction, such as pulmonary emboli
- To help determine ventilation-perfusion ratios (when performed in conjunction with a lung ventilation scan)

Patient preparation

- Tell the patient that this test helps evaluate respiratory function.
- Explain that there are no food or fluid restrictions before the test.
- Describe the test, including who will perform it, where it will take place, and its expected duration (15 to 30 minutes).
- Tell the patient that a radiopharmaceutical will be injected into a vein in his arm and then he'll sit in front of a camera or lie under it. Explain that neither the camera nor the uptake probe emits radiation and that the amount of radioactivity in the radiopharmaceutical is minimal.
- Assure the patient that he'll be comfortable during the test and that he doesn't have to remain perfectly still.
- On the test request slip, note if he has conditions such as chronic obstructive pulmonary disease, vasculitis, pulmonary edema, tumor, sickle cell disease, or parasitic disease.

Procedure and posttest care

- Half of the radiopharmaceutical is injected I.V. while the patient is in a supine position; the remaining half is injected while the patient is in a prone position.
- After the injection, the gamma camera takes a series of single stationary images in the anterior, posterior, oblique, and both lateral chest views.

- Images, which are projected on an oscilloscope screen, show the distribution of radioactive particles.
- If a hematoma develops at the injection site after the test, apply warm soaks.

Precautions
- A lung scan is contraindicated in patients hypersensitive to the radiopharmaceutical.

Normal findings
Hot spots — areas with normal blood perfusion — show a high uptake of the radioactive substance; a normal lung shows a uniform uptake pattern.

Abnormal findings
Cold spots — areas of low radioactive uptake — indicate poor perfusion, suggesting an embolism; however, a ventilation scan is necessary to confirm diagnosis. Decreased regional blood flow that occurs without vessel obstruction may indicate pneumonitis.

LUNG VENTILATION SCAN

This nuclear scan is performed after the patient inhales a mixture of air and radioactive gas that delineates areas of the lung ventilated during respiration. The scan records the distribution of the gas during three phases: the buildup of radioactive gas (wash-in phase), the time after rebreathing when radioactivity reaches a steady level (equilibrium phase), and after removal of the radioactive gas from the lungs (wash-out phase).

Purpose
- To help diagnose pulmonary emboli, identify areas of the lung capable of ventilation, help evaluate regional respiratory function, and locate regional hypoventilation (usually caused by smoking or chronic obstructive pulmonary disease)
- To distinguish between parenchymal disease, such as emphysema, sarcoidosis, bronchogenic carcinoma, and tuberculosis and conditions due to vascular abnormalities such as pulmonary emboli (performed with a lung perfusion scan)

Patient preparation
- Describe the procedure to the patient and explain that this test helps evaluate respiratory function.
- Tell him there are no food or fluid restrictions.
- Tell him who will perform the test, where it will take place, and that it takes 15 to 30 minutes.
- Ask the patient to remove all jewelry or metal from the scanning field.
- Explain that he'll be asked to hold his breath for a short time after inhaling a gas and to remain still while a machine scans his chest.
- Reassure him that a minimal amount of radioactive gas is used.

Procedure and posttest care
- After the patient inhales air mixed with a small amount of radioactive gas through a mask, its distribution in the lungs is monitored on a nuclear scanner.
- The patient's chest is scanned as he exhales.

Precautions
- Watch for leaks in the closed system of radioactive gas, such as through the mask, which can contaminate the surrounding atmosphere.
- In a patient on mechanical ventilation, krypton gas must be used instead of xenon gas.

Normal findings

Normal findings include an equal distribution of gas in both lungs and normal wash-in and wash-out phases.

Abnormal findings

Unequal gas distribution in both lungs indicates poor ventilation or airway obstruction in areas with low radioactivity. When compared with a lung scan (perfusion scan), in vascular obstructions such as pulmonary embolism, the perfusion to the embolized area is decreased, but the ventilation to this area is maintained; in parenchymal disease such as pneumonia, ventilation is abnormal within the areas of consolidation.

CARDIOVASCULAR SYSTEM

TECHNETIUM PYRO-PHOSPHATE SCANNING

Technetium pyrophosphate scanning (also called hot spot myocardial imaging or infarct avid imaging) is used to detect a recent myocardial infarction (MI) and to determine its extent. This test uses an I.V. tracer isotope (technetium-99m pyrophosphate). This isotope accumulates in damaged myocardial tissue (possibly by combining with calcium in the damaged myocardial cells), where it forms a hot spot on a scan made with a scintillation camera. Such hot spots first appear within 12 hours of infarction, are most apparent after 48 to 72 hours, and usually disappear after 1 week. Hot spots that persist longer than

1 week usually suggest ongoing myocardial damage.

Purpose

• To confirm recent MI in patients suffering from obscure cardiac pain or when electrocardiography or serum enzyme studies do not provide sufficient information
• To help define the size and location of an MI
• To aid in determining prognosis after acute MI

Patient preparation

• Explain to the patient that this test helps assess if the heart muscle is injured.
• Inform the patient that he needn't restrict food or fluids. Tell him who will perform the 30- to 60-minute test and where.
• Inform him that he'll receive a tracer isotope I.V., 2 or 3 hours before the procedure, and that multiple images of his heart will be made.
• Reassure him that the injection causes only transient discomfort, that the scan itself is painless, and that the test involves less exposure to radiation than chest radiography.
• Instruct him to remain quiet and motionless while he's being scanned.
• Make sure the patient or a responsible family member has signed a consent form.

Procedure and posttest care

• Usually, 20 millicuries (mC) of technetium-99m pyrophosphate are injected into the antecubital vein.
• After 2 or 3 hours, the patient is placed in supine position and electrocardiography electrodes are attached for continuous monitoring during the test.
• Generally, scans are taken with the patient in several positions, including anterior, left anterior oblique, right an-

terior oblique, and left lateral. Each
scan takes 10 minutes.

Normal findings
A normal technetium scan shows no
isotope in the myocardium.

Abnormal findings
The isotope is taken up by the sternum
and ribs, and their activity is compared
with the heart's; 2+, 3+, and 4+ activity
(equal to or greater than bone) indicates
a positive myocardial scan. The technetium scan can reveal areas of isotope
accumulation, or hot spots, in damaged
myocardium, particularly 48 to 72
hours after onset of acute MI; however,
hot spots are apparent as early as 12
hours after acute MI. In most patients
with MI, hot spots disappear after 1
week; in some, they persist for several
months if necrosis continues in the area
of infarction.

Knowing where the infarct is makes
it possible to anticipate complications
and to plan patient care. About one-
fourth of patients with unstable angina
pectoris show hot spots due to subclinical myocardial necrosis, and may require coronary arteriography and bypass grafting.

THALLIUM IMAGING

Also called cold spot myocardial imaging or thallium scintigraphy, this test
evaluates myocardial blood flow after
I.V. injection of the radioisotope thalli-
um-201 (thallous chloride Tl 201, or
^{201}TlCl). Because thallium, the physiologic analogue of potassium, concentrates in healthy myocardial tissue but
not in necrotic or ischemic tissue, areas
of the heart with normal blood supply
and intact cells rapidly take it up. Areas
with poor blood flow and ischemic cells

fail to take up the isotope and appear as
cold spots on a scan.

This test is performed in a resting
state or after stress. Possible complications of stress testing include arrhythmias, angina pectoris, and MI.

Purpose
Resting imaging:
• To assess myocardial scarring and
perfusion
• To demonstrate the location and ex-
tent of acute or chronic MI, including
transmural and postoperative infarction
Stress imaging:
• To diagnose coronary artery disease
(CAD)
• To evaluate the patency of grafts after
coronary artery bypass surgery
• To evaluate the effectiveness of anti-
anginal therapy or balloon angioplasty

Patient preparation
• Explain to the patient that these tests
help determine if any areas of the heart
muscle aren't receiving an adequate
supply of blood.
• For stress imaging, instruct him to restrict alcohol, tobacco, and unpre-
scribed medications for 24 hours before
the test and to have nothing by mouth
for 3 hours before the test (advise him
to eat a light meal beforehand).
• Describe the test, including who will
perform it, where it will take place, and
its expected duration (45 to 90 minutes). Explain that additional scans may
be required.
• Tell him that he will receive a radioactive tracer I.V. and that multiple images of his heart will be scanned.
• Warn him that he may experience discomfort from skin abrasion during
preparation for electrode placement.
Assure him the test involves minimal
radiation exposure.
• Make sure the patient or a responsible
family member has signed a consent
form.

• For stress imaging, instruct the patient to wear walking shoes during the treadmill exercise and to report fatigue, pain, or shortness of breath immediately.

Procedure and posttest care
For resting imaging:
• Within the first few hours of symptoms of MI, the patient receives an injection of thallium I.V. and scanning begins after 3 to 5 minutes.
• If further scanning is required, have the patient rest and restrict food and fluids.
For stress imaging:
• The patient, wired with electrodes, walks on a treadmill at a regulated pace that's gradually increased, while the electrocardiogram (ECG), blood pressure, and heart rate are monitored.
• When the patient reaches peak stress, the examiner injects 1.5 to 3 mC of thallium into the antecubital vein and then flushes it with 10 to 15 ml of 0.9% sodium chloride solution.
• The patient exercises an additional 45 to 60 seconds to permit circulation and uptake of the isotope, and then lies on his back under the scintillation camera.
• If the patient is asymptomatic, the precordial leads are removed. Scanning begins after 3 to 5 minutes with the patient in anterior, 45-degree and 60-degree left anterior oblique, and left lateral positions.
• Additional scans may be taken after the patient rests 3 to 6 hours.

Precautions
• Contraindications include impaired neuromuscular function, pregnancy, locomotor disturbances, acute MI and myocarditis, aortic stenosis, acute infection, unstable metabolic conditions (like diabetes), digitalis toxicity, and recent pulmonary infarction.
• Stop stress imaging at once if the patient develops chest pain, dyspnea, fatigue, syncope, hypotension, ischemic ECG changes, significant arrhythmias, or critical signs (pale, clammy skin, confusion, or staggering).

Normal findings
Imaging should show normal distribution of the isotope throughout the left ventricle and no defects (cold spots).

Abnormal findings
Persistent defects indicate MI; transient defects (which disappear after 3- to 6-hour rest) indicate ischemia from CAD. After coronary artery bypass surgery, improved regional perfusion suggests patency of the graft. Increased perfusion after ingestion of antianginal drugs can show that they relieve ischemia. Improved perfusion after balloon angioplasty suggests increased coronary flow.

PERSANTINE-THALLIUM IMAGING

This imaging test is an alternative method of assessing coronary vessel function for patients who can't tolerate exercise or stress electrocardiography. Persantine (dipyridamole) infusion simulates the effects of exercise by increasing blood flow to the collateral circulation and away from the coronary arteries, thereby inducing ischemia. Then thallium infusion evaluates the cardiac vessels' response. The heart is scanned immediately after the thallium infusion and again 2 to 4 hours later. Diseased vessels can't deliver thallium to the heart, and thallium lingers in diseased areas of the myocardium.

Purpose
• To identify exercise- or stress-induced arrhythmias
• To assess the presence and degree of cardiac ischemia

Patient preparation
• Tell the patient that a painless, 5- to 10-minute baseline electrocardiogram (ECG) will precede the test.
• Explain that he'll need to restrict food and fluids before the test. Tell him to avoid caffeine and other stimulants (which may cause arrhythmias).
• Instruct him to continue to take all his regular medications, with the possible exception of beta blockers, as prescribed.
• Explain that an I.V. line infuses the medications for study. Tell him who will start the I.V. and when and that the needle insertion and pressure of the tourniquet may cause some discomfort.
• Inform him that he may experience mild nausea, headache, dizziness, or flushing after Persantine administration. Reassure him that these usually temporary adverse reactions rarely need treatment.
• Make sure that the patient or a responsible family member has signed a consent form.

Procedure and posttest care
• The patient reclines or sits while a resting ECG is performed. Then Persantine is given either orally or I.V. over 4 minutes. Blood pressure, pulse, and cardiac rhythm are monitored continuously.
• After administration of the Persantine, the patient is asked to get up and walk. After Persantine takes effect, thallium is injected.
• The patient is placed in a supine position for about 40 minutes while the scan is performed. Then the scan is reviewed. If necessary, a second scan is performed.

• If the patient must return for further scanning, tell him to rest and to restrict food and fluids in the interim.

Precautions
• The patient may experience arrhythmias, angina, ST-segment depression, or bronchospasm. Make sure resuscitative equipment is readily available.
• More common adverse reactions are nausea, headache, flushing, dizziness, and epigastric pain.

Normal findings
Imaging should reveal characteristic distribution of the isotope throughout the left ventricle and no visible defects.

Abnormal findings
The presence of ST-segment depression, angina, and arrhythmias strongly suggests coronary artery disease. Persistent ST-segment depression generally indicates myocardial infarction. In contrast, transient ST-segment depression indicates ischemia from coronary artery disease.

Cold spots are usually due to coronary artery disease, but may result from sarcoidosis, myocardial fibrosis, cardiac contusion, attenuation due to soft tissue (for example, breast and diaphragm) apical cleft, and coronary spasm. The absence of cold spots in the presence of coronary artery disease may result from insignificant obstruction, single-vessel disease, and collateral circulation.

CARDIAC BLOOD POOL IMAGING

Cardiac blood pool imaging evaluates regional and global ventricular performance after I.V. injection of human serum albumin or red blood cells (RBCs) tagged with the isotope technetium-99m (^{99m}Tc) pertechnetate. In first-pass imaging, a scintillation camera records the radioactivity emitted by the isotope in its initial pass through the left ventricle. Higher counts of radioactivity occur during diastole because there is more blood in the ventricle; lower counts occur during systole as the blood is ejected. The portion of isotope ejected during each heartbeat can then be calculated to determine the ejection fraction; the presence and size of intracardiac shunts can also be determined.

Gated cardiac blood pool imaging, performed after first-pass imaging or as a separate test, has several forms; however, most forms use signals from an electrocardiogram (ECG) to trigger the scintillation camera. In two-frame gated imaging, the camera records left ventricular end-systole and end-diastole for 500 to 1,000 cardiac cycles; superimposition of these gated images allows assessment of left ventricular contraction to find areas of dyskinesia or akinesia.

In multiple-gated acquisition (MUGA) scanning, the camera records 14 to 64 points of a single cardiac cycle, yielding sequential images that can be studied like motion picture films to evaluate regional wall motion and determine the ejection fraction and other indices of cardiac function. In the stress MUGA test, the same test is performed at rest and after exercise to detect changes in ejection fraction and cardiac output. In the nitro MUGA test, the scintillation camera records points in the cardiac cycle after the sublingual administration of nitroglycerin to assess its effect on ventricular function.

Blood pool imaging is more accurate and involves less risk to the patient than left ventriculography in assessing cardiac function.

Purpose
• To evaluate left ventricular function
• To detect aneurysms of the left ventricle and other motion abnormalities of the myocardial wall (areas of akinesia or dyskinesia)
• To detect intracardiac shunting

Patient preparation
• Explain to the patient that this test permits assessment of the heart's left ventricle.
• Describe the test, including who will perform it, where it will take place, and its expected duration, and tell him there are no food or fluid restrictions.
• Explain that he will receive an I.V. injection of a radioactive tracer and that a detector positioned above his chest will record the circulation of this tracer through the heart.
• Reassure him that the tracer poses no radiation hazard and rarely produces adverse effects.
• Inform him that he may experience transient discomfort from the needle puncture, but that the imaging itself is painless.
• Instruct him to remain silent and motionless during imaging, unless otherwise instructed.
• Make sure the patient or a responsible family member has signed a consent form.

Procedure and posttest care
• The patient is placed in supine position beneath the detector of a scintillation camera, and 15 to 20 mC of albumin or RBCs tagged with technetium-99m pertechnetate are injected.
• For the next minute, the scintillation camera records the first pass of the isotope through the heart so that the aortic and mitral valves can be located.
• Then, using an ECG, the camera is gated for selected 60-millisecond intervals, representing end-systole and end-diastole, and 500 to 1,000 cardiac cy-

cles are recorded on X-ray or Polaroid film.

• To observe septal and posterior wall motion, the patient may be assisted to modified left anterior oblique position; or he may be assisted to right anterior oblique position and given 0.4 mg of nitroglycerin sublingually. The scintillation camera then records additional gated images to evaluate abnormal contraction in the left ventricle.

• The patient may be asked to exercise as the scintillation camera records gated images.

Precautions
• Cardiac blood pool imaging is contraindicated during pregnancy.

Normal findings
Normally, the left ventricle contracts symmetrically, and the isotope appears evenly distributed in the scans. The normal ejection fraction is 55% to 65%.

Abnormal findings
Patients with coronary artery disease usually have asymmetric blood distribution to the myocardium, which produces segmental abnormalities of ventricular wall motion; such abnormalities may also result from preexisting conditions, such as myocarditis. In contrast, patients with cardiomyopathies show globally reduced ejection fractions. In patients with left-to-right shunts, the recirculating radioisotope prolongs the downslope of the curve of scintigraphic data; early arrival of activity in the left ventricle or aorta signifies a right-to-left shunt.

MISCELLANEOUS TESTS

BONE SCAN

Bone scan is a test that permits imaging of the skeleton by a scanning camera after I.V. injection of a radioactive tracer compound. The tracer of choice, radioactive technetium diphosphonate, collects in bone tissue in increased concentrations at sites of abnormal metabolism. When scanned, these sites appear as "hot spots" that are often detectable months before a radiograph can reveal any lesion. To promote early detection of lesions, this test may be performed with a gallium scan.

Purpose
• To detect or rule out malignant bone lesions when radiographic findings are normal but cancer is confirmed or suspected
• To detect occult bone trauma due to pathologic fractures
• To monitor degenerative bone disorders
• To detect infection
• To evaluate unexplained bone pain

Patient preparation
• Describe the procedure to the patient. Explain that this test may detect abnormal skeletal pathology sooner than is possible with ordinary X-ray films.
• Because the patient is required to drink 4 to 6 glasses of water or tea in the interval between injection of the tracer and the actual scanning, advise him not to drink large amounts of fluids before the test.
• Tell him who will perform the test and where and that he may have to assume

various positions on a scanner table. Emphasize that he must keep still for the scan.

• Assure the patient that the scan itself, which takes about 1 hour, is painless and that the isotope, although radioactive, emits less radiation than a standard X-ray machine.

• Make sure the patient or a family member has signed a consent form.

• If a bone scan is ordered to diagnose cancer, evaluate the patient's emotional state and offer support.

• Administer prescribed analgesics.

• After the patient receives an I.V. injection of the tracer and imaging agent, encourage him to increase his intake of fluids for the next 1 to 3 hours to facilitate renal clearance of the circulating free tracer.

Equipment

Bone mineral tracer, 3-ml syringe, 21G needle, 70% alcohol or povidone-iodine solution, sterile sponge, tourniquet, scanning camera.

Procedure and posttest care

• Instruct the patient to void immediately before the procedure; then position him on the scanner table.

• As the scanner head moves back and forth over the patient's body, it detects low-level radiation emitted by the skeleton and translates this into a film or paper chart, or both, to produce two-dimensional pictures of the area scanned.

• The scanner takes as many views as needed to cover the specified area. The patient may have to be repositioned several times during the test to obtain adequate views.

• Check the injection site for redness or swelling. If a hematoma develops, apply warm soaks.

• Don't schedule any other radionuclide tests for 24 to 48 hours.

Precautions

• To avoid exposing the fetus or infant to radiation, a bone scan is contraindicated during pregnancy or lactation.

• Allergic reactions to radionuclides may occur.

Normal findings

The tracer concentrates in bone tissue at sites of new bone formation or increased metabolism. The epiphyses of growing bone are normal sites of high concentration, or hot spots.

Abnormal findings

Although a bone scan demonstrates hot spots that identify sites of bone formation, it doesn't distinguish between normal and abnormal bone formation. But scan results can identify all types of bone malignancy, infection, fracture, and other disorders, if viewed in light of the patient's medical and surgical history, radiographs, and other laboratory tests.

LIVER-SPLEEN SCANNING

In this test, a gamma camera records the distribution of radioactivity within the liver and spleen after I.V. injection of a radioactive colloid. The colloid most commonly used, technetium sulfide-99m (^{99m}Tc), concentrates in the reticuloendothelial cells through phagocytosis. About 80% to 90% of the injected colloid is taken up by Kupffer's cells in the liver, 5% to 10% by the spleen, and 3% to 5% by bone marrow. The gamma camera images either organ instantaneously without moving.

While the indications for this test include the detection of focal disease, such as tumors, cysts, and abscesses, liver-spleen scanning demonstrates focal disease nonspecifically as a cold spot (a defect that fails to take up the colloid) and may fail to detect focal lesions smaller than ¾″ (2 cm) in diameter. Although clinical signs and symptoms may aid diagnosis, liver-spleen scanning frequently requires confirmation by ultrasonography, computed tomography, gallium scanning, or biopsy.

Purpose

• To screen for hepatic metastases and hepatocellular disease, such as cirrhosis and hepatitis
• To detect focal disease, such as tumors, cysts, and abscesses in the liver and spleen
• To demonstrate hepatomegaly or splenomegaly (in patients with palpable abdominal masses)
• To assess splenic infarcts
• To assess the condition of the liver and spleen after abdominal trauma

Patient preparation

• Explain to the patient that this procedure permits examination of the liver and spleen through scintigraphs or scans taken after I.V. injection of a radioactive substance.
• Inform him that he needn't restrict food or fluids before the test.
• Tell him who will perform the test and where it will take place and that it takes about 1 hour.
• Explain that he may experience transient discomfort from the needle puncture.
• Make sure the patient isn't scheduled for more than one radionuclide scan on the same day.
• Assure him that the injection isn't dangerous because the test substance contains only trace amounts of radioactivity and allergic reactions to it are rare.
• Explain that the detector head of the gamma camera may touch his abdomen

(if appropriate), and reassure him that this isn't dangerous.
• Advise him that he'll be asked to lie still and to breathe quietly during the procedure to ensure images of good quality; he may also be asked to hold his breath briefly. Explain that this technique helps to evaluate liver mobility and pliability.

Procedure and posttest care

• The ^{99m}Tc is injected I.V.; after 10 to 15 minutes, the patient's abdomen is scanned with the patient placed in supine, left and right lateral, left and right anterior oblique, and prone positions to ensure optimal visualization of the liver and spleen.
• The left anterior oblique position provides the best view of the spleen separate from the left lobe of the liver. With the patient supine, liver mobility and pliability may be evaluated by marking the costal margin and scanning as the patient breathes deeply (fixation suggests pathology).
• The scintigraphs are reviewed for clarity before the patient is allowed to leave. If necessary, additional views are obtained.
• Watch for anaphylactoid or pyrogenic reactions that may result from a stabilizer, such as dextran or gelatin, added to ^{99m}Tc.

Precautions

• Liver-spleen scanning is usually contraindicated in children and during pregnancy and lactation.

Normal findings

Because the liver and spleen contain equal numbers of reticuloendothelial cells, both organs normally appear equally bright on the image. However, distribution of radioactive colloid is generally more uniform and homogeneous in the spleen than in the liver. The liver has various normal indentations and impressions, such as the gallbladder fossa and falciform ligament, that may mimic focal disease. For more information, see *Identifying liver indentations in nuclear imaging,* page 604.

Abnormal findings

Although liver-spleen scanning may fail to detect early hepatocellular disease, it shows characteristic, distinct patterns as such disease progresses. The most prominent sign of hepatocellular disease is a shift of the radioactive colloid that's caused by reduced hepatic blood flow and impaired function of Kupffer's cells. This inhibits distribution of the colloid in the liver, causing it to appear uniformly decreased or patchy. The spleen and bone marrow then take up the abnormally large amounts of the colloid unabsorbed by the liver, thus concentrating more radioactivity than the liver, and appear brighter on the scan. This same distribution pattern (colloid shift) also accompanies portal hypertension due to extrahepatic causes.

Hepatitis and cirrhosis are both associated with hepatomegaly and a colloid shift, but certain characteristics help distinguish them. In hepatitis, distribution of the colloid is usually uniformly decreased; in cirrhosis, it's patchy. Splenomegaly is typical in cirrhosis but not in hepatitis.

Metastasis to the liver or spleen may appear on the scan as a focal defect and requires biopsy to confirm diagnosis. Liver metastasis usually originates in the gastrointestinal or genitourinary tract, the breasts, or the lungs and is more common than metastasis to the spleen. After metastasis is confirmed, serial liver-spleen studies are useful in evaluating effectiveness of therapy.

Because cysts, abscesses, and tumors fail to take up the radioactive colloid, they appear on the scan as solitary or multiple focal defects. Hepatic cysts may appear as solitary defects; poly-cystic hepatic disease, as multiple defects. Splenic cysts are rarer than hepatic cysts and may have a parasitic or nonparasitic origin. Ultrasonography can confirm hepatic or splenic cysts.

Intrahepatic abscesses are usually pyogenic or amoebic. Subphrenic abscesses, located beneath the diaphragm, may distort the dome of the right lobe. Splenic abscesses are characteristic in bacterial endocarditis. All abscesses require gallium scanning or ultrasonography to confirm diagnosis.

Benign hepatic tumors — such as hemangiomas, adenomas, and hamartomas — require confirming biopsy or flow studies. Primary malignant tumors, such as hepatomas, also require biopsy. Benign splenic tumors are rare and include hemangiomas, fibromas, myomas, and hamartomas. Primary malignant splenic tumors are also rare, except in lymphoreticular malignancies such as Hodgkin's disease. Splenic tumors also require biopsy to confirm diagnosis. Although focal disease usually inhibits uptake of radioactive colloid, both obstruction of the superior vena cava and Budd-Chiari syndrome cause markedly increased uptake.

A left upper quadrant mass may result from splenomegaly, or from hepatomegaly if the liver is grossly extended across the abdomen. A right upper quadrant mass may result from hepatomegaly; a right lower quadrant mass may be a Riedel's lobe or a large dependent gallbladder. Splenic infarcts, often associated with bacterial endocarditis and massive splenomegaly, appear as peripheral defects, with decreased and irregular colloid distribution.

Scanning can assess hepatic injury after abdominal trauma. Intrahepatic hematoma appears as a focal defect; subcapsular hematoma, as a lentiform defect on the periphery of the liver; hepatic laceration, as a linear defect.

IDENTIFYING LIVER INDENTATIONS IN NUCLEAR IMAGING

In nuclear imaging, normal indentations and impressions may be mistaken for focal lesions. These drawings of the liver —anterior view and posterior view — identify the contours and impressions that may be misread.

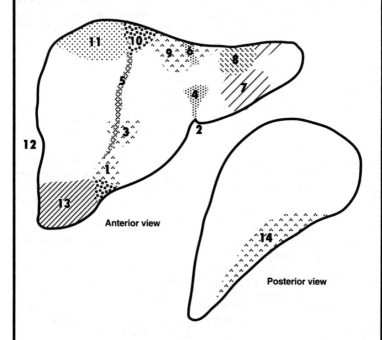

Anterior view

Posterior view

KEY.

1. Gallbladder fossa
2. Ligamentum teres and falciform ligament
3. Hilum, main branching of the portal vein
4. Pars umbilicalis portion, left portal vein
5. Variable stripe of lobar fissure between right and left lobes
6. Variable stripe of segmental fissure, left lobe
7. Thinning of left lobe
8. Impression of pectus excavatum
9. Cardiac impression
10. Hepatic veins and inferior vena cava
11. Shielding from right female breast
12. Harrison's groove or costal impression
13. Impression of hepatic flexure of colon
14. Right renal impression

Scanning can also detect splenic injury after abdominal trauma. Splenic hematoma appears as a focal defect in or next to the spleen and may transect it. Subcapsular hematoma appears as a lentiform defect on the periphery of the spleen; splenic laceration appears as a linear defect.

GALLIUM SCANNING

This test, a total body scan, is used to assess certain neoplasms and inflammatory lesions that attract gallium. It is usually performed 24 to 48 hours after the I.V. injection of radioactive gallium (^{67}Ga) citrate; occasionally, it's performed 72 hours after the injection or, in acute inflammatory disease, after 4 to 6 hours.

Because gallium has an affinity for both benign and malignant neoplasms and inflammatory lesions, exact diagnosis requires additional confirming tests, such as ultrasonography and computerized tomography scanning. Also be aware that many neoplasms and a few inflammatory lesions may fail to demonstrate abnormal gallium activity.

Purpose
• To detect primary or metastatic neoplasms and inflammatory lesions when the site of the disease hasn't been clearly defined and when the patient's condition won't be jeopardized by the time required for the procedure
• To evaluate malignant lymphoma and identify recurrent tumors following chemotherapy or radiation therapy
• To clarify focal defects in the liver when liver-spleen scanning and ultrasonography prove inconclusive
• To evaluate bronchogenic carcinoma when sputum culture proves positive for malignancy but other tests are nor-

mal or when hydrothorax is present and bronchoscopy is contraindicated

Patient preparation
• Explain to the patient that this test helps detect abnormal or inflammatory tissue.
• Tell him he need not restrict food or fluids before the test.
• Explain that the test requires a total body scan (usually performed 24 to 48 hours after the I.V. injection of radioactive gallium).
• Tell him who will perform the test, where it will take place, and that the scan takes 30 to 60 minutes.
• Warn him that he may experience transient discomfort from the needle puncture during injection of the radioactive gallium. Reassure him, however, that the dosage is only slightly radioactive and isn't harmful.
• If a gamma scintillation camera is to be used, assure the patient that while the uptake probe and detector head may touch his skin, he will experience no discomfort.
• If a rectilinear scanner is to be used, mention that it makes a soft, irregular clicking noise as it registers the radiation emissions.
• Make sure the patient or a responsible family member has signed a consent form.
• Administer a laxative, cleansing enema, or both.

Procedure and posttest care
• The patient may be positioned erect or recumbent or in an appropriate combination of these positions, depending on his physical condition.
• Scans or scintigraphs of the patient are taken 24 to 48 hours after ^{67}Ga citrate injection, from anterior and posterior views and, occasionally, lateral views.
• If the initial gallium scan suggests bowel disease and additional scans are

necessary, give the patient a cleansing enema before continuing the test.

Precautions
• This test should precede barium studies because barium retention may hinder visualization of gallium activity in the bowel.
• Gallium scanning is usually contraindicated in children and during pregnancy or lactation; however, it may be performed if the potential diagnostic benefit outweighs the risks of exposure to radiation.

Normal findings
Gallium activity is normally demonstrated in the liver, spleen, bones, and large bowel. Activity in the bowel results from mucosal uptake of gallium and the fecal excretion of gallium.

Abnormal findings
Gallium scanning may reveal inflammatory lesions — discrete abscesses or diffuse infiltration. In pancreatic or perinephric abscess, gallium activity is relatively localized; in bacterial peritonitis, gallium activity is spread diffusely within the abdomen.

Abnormally high gallium accumulation is characteristic in inflammatory bowel diseases, such as ulcerative colitis and regional ileitis (Crohn's disease), and in carcinoma of the colon. However, because gallium normally accumulates in the colon, the detection of inflammatory and neoplastic diseases is sometimes difficult.

Abnormal gallium activity may be present in various sarcomas, Wilms' tumor, and neuroblastomas; carcinoma of the kidney, uterus, vagina, and stomach; and testicular tumors, such as seminoma, embryonal carcinoma, choriocarcinoma, and teratocarcinoma, which often metastasize via the lymphatic system. In Hodgkin's disease and malignant lymphoma, gallium scanning can demonstrate abnormal activity in one or more lymph nodes or in extranodal locations. However, gallium scanning supported by results of lymphangiography can gauge the extent of metastases more accurately than either test alone because neither test consistently identifies all neoplastic nodes.

After chemotherapy or radiation therapy, gallium scanning may be used to detect new or recurrent tumors. However, these forms of therapy tend to diminish tumor affinity for gallium without necessarily eliminating the tumor.

In the differential diagnosis of focal hepatic defects, abnormal gallium activity may help narrow the diagnostic possibilities. Gallium localizes in hepatomas, but not in pseudotumors; in abscesses, but not in pleural effusions; and in tumors, but not in cysts or hematomas.

In examining patients with suspected bronchogenic carcinoma, abnormal activity confirms the presence of tumor. However, because gallium also localizes in inflammatory pulmonary diseases, such as pneumonia and sarcoidosis, chest radiography should be performed to distinguish a tumor from an inflammatory lesion.

RED BLOOD CELL SURVIVAL TIME

Normally, red blood cells (RBCs) are only destroyed when they reach senility. However, in hemolytic diseases, RBCs of all ages are randomly destroyed, resulting in anemia. This test measures the survival time of circulating RBCs and detects sites of abnormal RBC sequestration and destruction.

Survival time is measured by labeling a random sample of RBCs with radioactive chromium-51 sodium chromate (^{51}Cr). This labeled group of RBCs is then injected back into the patient. Serial blood samples measure the percent of labeled cells per unit volume over 3 to 4 weeks until 50% of the cells disappear (disappearance rate corresponds to destruction of a random cell population).

During the test period, a gamma camera scans the body for sites of abnormally high radioactivity, which indicate sites of excessive RBC sequestration and destruction. Other tests performed with the RBC survival time test may include spot-checks of the stool to detect GI blood loss; hematocrit; blood volume studies; and radionuclide iron uptake and clearance tests to aid differential diagnosis of anemia.

Purpose
• To help evaluate unexplained anemia, particularly hemolytic anemia
• To identify sites of abnormal RBC sequestration and destruction

Patient preparation
• Explain to the patient that this test helps identify the cause of his anemia.
• Advise him that he needn't restrict food or fluids.
• Explain that the test involves labeling a blood sample with a radioactive substance and requires regular blood samples at 3-day intervals for 3 to 4 weeks. Tell him who will perform the testing and where it will take place.
• Tell him that he may experience slight discomfort from the needle punctures. Reassure him that collecting each sample takes less than 3 minutes and that the small amount of radioactive substance used is harmless.
• If a stool collection is required to test for GI bleeding, teach the patient the proper collection technique.

Procedure and posttest care
• A 30-ml blood sample is drawn and mixed with 100 microcuries (µC) of ^{51}Cr for an adult, less for a child.
• After an incubation period, the mixture is injected I.V. into the patient. A blood sample is drawn 30 minutes after injection to determine blood and RBC volumes.
• A 6-ml sample is collected in a *green-top* tube after 24 hours; follow-up samples are collected at 3-day intervals for 3 to 4 weeks. (Intervals between samples may vary, depending on the laboratory.)
• To avoid error from physical decay of the ^{51}Cr, each sample is measured with a scintillation well counter on the day it's drawn.
• Radioactivity per milliliter of RBCs is calculated and the values are plotted to determine mean RBC survival time. Simultaneous gamma camera scans of the precordium, sacrum, liver, and spleen detect radioactivity at sites of excess RBC sequestration. A hematocrit test is done on a small portion of each blood sample to check for blood loss.
• At the end of the study, a sample is drawn to compare ending blood and RBC volumes with beginning volumes.
• If a hematoma develops at the venipuncture site, apply warm soaks.

Precautions
• This test is contraindicated during pregnancy because it exposes the fetus to radiation.
• Because excess blood loss can invalidate test results, this test is usually contraindicated for a patient with active bleeding or poor clotting function. However, if the test is necessary for a patient with poor clotting function, observe the venipuncture sites carefully for signs of hemorrhage.
• The patient should not receive blood transfusions during the test period and

should not have blood samples drawn for other tests.

Normal findings
Normal half-life for RBCs labeled with ^{51}Cr is 25 to 35 days. Normal gamma camera scans reveal slight radioactivity in the spleen, liver, and sometimes the bone marrow.

Abnormal findings
Decreased RBC survival time indicates a hemolytic disease, such as chronic lymphocytic leukemia, congenital non-spherocytic hemolytic anemia, hemoglobin C disease, hereditary spherocytosis, idiopathic acquired hemolytic anemia, paroxysmal nocturnal hemoglobinuria, elliptocytosis, pernicious anemia, sickle cell anemia, sickle cell hemoglobin C disease, or hemolytic-uremic syndrome. If hemolytic anemia is diagnosed, additional tests using cross transfusion of labeled RBCs can determine if anemia results from an intrinsic RBC defect or an extrinsic factor.

A gamma camera scan that detects a site of excess RBC sequestration provides direction for treatment. For example, abnormally high RBC sequestration in the spleen may require a splenectomy.

RADIONUCLIDE RENAL IMAGING

This test, involving I.V. injection of a radionuclide followed by scintiphotography, can provide a wealth of information for evaluating the kidneys. Observing the uptake concentration and transit of the radionuclide during this test allows assessment of renal blood flow, nephron and collecting system function, and renal structure. Depend-ing on the patient's clinical presentation, this procedure may include dynamic scans to assess renal perfusion and function or static scans to assess structure.

The radioisotope injected depends on the specific information required and the examiner's preference. However, this procedure often includes double isotope technique to obtain a sequence of perfusion and function studies, followed by static images. This test may also be substituted for excretory urography in patients with hypersensitivity to contrast agents.

Purpose
• To detect and assess functional and structural renal abnormalities (such as lesions)
• To detect renovascular hypertension and acute and chronic renal disease (such as pyelonephritis and glomerulonephritis)
• To assess renal transplantation or renal injury due to trauma and obstruction of the urinary tract

Patient preparation
• Explain to the patient that this test permits evaluation of the structure, blood flow, and function of the kidneys.
• Tell him who will perform the test and where and that it takes about 90 minutes. (If static scans are ordered, there will be a delay of several hours before the images are taken.)
• Inform him that he'll receive an injection of a radionuclide and that he may experience transient flushing and nausea.
• Emphasize that only a small amount of radionuclide is administered and that it's usually excreted within 24 hours.
• Tell him several series of films will be taken of his bladder.
• Make sure the patient or a responsible family member has signed a consent form.

• Make sure the patient isn't scheduled for other radionuclide scans on the same day as this test.
• If the patient receives antihypertensive medication, it may be withheld before the test.
• Women who are pregnant and young children may receive supersaturated solution of potassium iodide (SSKI) 1 to 3 hours before the test to block thyroid uptake of iodine.

Equipment
Computerized gamma scintillation camera, ^{99m}Tc-DTPA (technetium and diethylenetriaminepentaacetic acid) for perfusion study, ^{131}I-orthoiodohippurate (Hippuran) for function study, oscilloscope, magnetic tape, I.V. equipment.

Procedure and posttest care
• The patient is commonly placed in prone position so posterior views may be obtained. If the test is being performed to evaluate transplantation, the patient is positioned supine for anterior views.
• Instruct the patient not change his position.
• A perfusion study (radionuclide angiography) is performed first to evaluate renal blood flow. ^{99m}Tc-DTPA is administered I.V., and rapid-sequence photographs (one per second) are taken for 1 minute.
• Next, a function study is performed to measure the transit time of the radionuclide through the kidneys' functional units. After ^{131}I-orthoiodohippurate is administered I.V., images are obtained at a rate of one per minute for 20 minutes. Alternatively, this entire procedure can be recorded on computer-compatible magnetic tape and concurrent renogram curves plotted.
• Finally, static images are obtained 4 or more hours later, after the radionuclide has drained through the pelvicalyceal system.

• Instruct the patient to flush the toilet immediately after each voiding for 24 hours as a radiation precaution.

Normal findings
Because 25% of cardiac output goes directly to the kidneys, renal perfusion should be evident immediately following uptake of the radionuclide (^{99m}Tc-DTPA) in the abdominal aorta. Within 1 to 2 minutes, a normal pattern of renal circulation should appear. The radionuclide should delineate the kidneys simultaneously, symmetrically, and with equal intensity.

^{131}I-orthoiodohippurate administered for the function study rapidly outlines the kidneys—which should be normal in size, shape, and position—and also defines the collecting system and bladder. Maximum counts of the radionuclide in the kidneys occur within 5 minutes after injection (and within 1 minute of each other) and should fall to approximately one-third or less of the maximum counts of the same kidney within 25 minutes. Within this time, the function of both kidneys can be compared as the concentration of radionuclide shifts from the cortex to the pelvis and, finally, to the bladder.

Renal function is best evaluated by comparing these images to the renogram curves. Total function is considered normal when the effective renal plasma flow is 420 ml/minute or greater and the percentage of the dose excreted in the urine at 30 to 35 minutes is greater than 66%.

Abnormal findings
Images from the perfusion study can identify impeded renal circulation, such as that caused by trauma and renal artery stenosis or renal infarction. These conditions may occur in patients with renovascular hypertension and abdominal aortic disease. Because malignant renal tumors are usually vascular, these

images can help differentiate tumors from cysts. In evaluating a transplant, abnormal perfusion may indicate obstruction of the vascular grafts. The function study can detect abnormalities of the collecting system and extravasation of the urine. Markedly decreased tubular function causes reduced radionuclide activity in the collecting system; outflow obstruction causes decreased radionuclide activity in the tubules, with increased activity in the collecting system. This test can also define the level of ureteral obstruction.

Static images can demonstrate lesions, congenital abnormalities, and traumatic injury. These images also detect space-occupying lesions within or surrounding the kidney, such as tumors, infarcts, and inflammatory masses (abscesses, for example); they can also identify congenital disorders, such as horseshoe kidney and polycystic kidney disease. They can define regions of infarction, rupture, or hemorrhage after trauma.

A lower than normal total concentration of the radionuclide, as opposed to focal defects, suggests a diffuse renal disorder, such as acute tubular necrosis, severe infection, or ischemia. In a patient who has had a kidney transplant, decreased radionuclide uptake generally indicates organ rejection. Failure of visualization may indicate congenital ectopia or aplasia.

Definitive diagnosis usually requires the combined analysis of static images, perfusion studies, and function studies.

CHAPTER 15

Monitoring and Catheterization

FETAL MONITORING

EXTERNAL FETAL MONITORING

In this noninvasive test, an electronic transducer and a cardiotachometer amplify and record fetal heart rate (FHR) while a pressure-sensitive transducer (tokodynamometer) records uterine contractions. Fetal monitoring records the baseline FHR (average FHR over two contraction cycles or 10 minutes), periodic fluctuations in the baseline FHR, and beat-to-beat heart rate variability. (See *Understanding fetal monitoring terminology.*) External fetal monitoring is also used during other tests of fetal health, notably the nonstress test and the contraction stress test (CST).

Purpose
• To measure FHR and the frequency of uterine contractions
• To evaluate antepartum and intrapartum fetal health during stress and nonstress situations
• To detect fetal distress
• To determine the necessity for internal fetal monitoring

Patient preparation
• Explain to the patient that this test assesses fetal health. Describe the procedure and answer all questions. Assure her that external fetal monitoring is painless and won't hurt the fetus or interfere with normal labor.
• For antepartum monitoring, instruct the patient to eat a meal just before the test. This increases fetal activity and thus reduces the test time.

• Explain that she may have to restrict movement during baseline readings, but that she may change position between the readings.
• Make sure she or a responsible family member has signed a consent form.

Equipment
Mineral oil or ultrasound transmission jelly, elastic band, stockinette, or abdominal strap.

Procedure and posttest care
• Place the patient in the semi-Fowler or left lateral position, with her abdomen exposed. Cover the ultrasound transducer receiver crystal with ultrasound transmission jelly.
• Palpate the patient's abdomen to identify the fetal chest area, locate the most distinct fetal heart sounds, and then secure the ultrasound transducer over this area with the elastic band, stockinette, or abdominal strap.
• Check the recording equipment for calibration, adequate paper, and alarm boundaries.
• During monitoring, check the elastic band, stockinette, or abdominal strap to ensure that the fit is comfortable yet tight enough to produce a good tracing.
• As labor progresses, reposition the pressure transducer as necessary so that it remains on the fundal portion of the uterus. You may have to reposition the ultrasound transducer as fetal position changes.
• Repeat antepartum monitoring weekly as long as indications, such as pregnancy over 42 weeks' gestation or fetal growth retardation, persist.
• If FHR patterns indicate distress, fetal oxygenation can often be improved by turning the mother on her side (preferably left) to alleviate supine hypoxia, administering oxygen to the mother, or loading maternal fluids to increase placental perfusion. If the FHR returns to normal, labor may continue. If abnor-

mal FHR patterns persist, cesarean birth may be required.

Antepartum monitoring with non-stress tests:

• Tell the patient to hold the pressure transducer in her hand and to push it each time she feels the fetus move.

• Monitor baseline FHR until you record two fetal movements that last longer than 15 seconds each and cause heart rate accelerations of more than 15 beats/minute from the baseline. If you can't obtain two FHR accelerations within 20 to 30 minutes, shake the patient's abdomen to stimulate the fetus, and repeat the test.

Antepartum monitoring with CST:

• Induce contractions by oxytocin infusion or nipple stimulation (endogenous oxytocin).

• When administering oxytocin, infuse a dilute solution at a rate of 1 mU/minute, increasing the oxytocin rate until the patient experiences three contractions within 10 minutes, each lasting longer than 45 seconds.

• When using nipple stimulation, tell the patient to stimulate one nipple by hand until contractions begin. If a second contraction doesn't occur in 2 minutes, have her stimulate the nipple again. Stimulate both nipples if contractions don't occur in 15 minutes. Continue until three contractions occur in 10 minutes.

• If no decelerations occur during three contractions, the patient may be discharged. Late decelerations during any of the contractions require notification of the doctor and additional testing.

Intrapartum monitoring:

• Secure the pressure transducer with an elastic band, stockinette, or abdominal strap over the area of greatest uterine electrical activity during contractions (usually the fundus).

• Adjust the machine to record 0 to 10 mm Hg pressure between palpable contractions.

UNDERSTANDING FETAL MONITORING TERMINOLOGY

• *Baseline fetal heart rate:* Average fetal heart rate (FHR) over two contraction cycles or 10 minutes
• *Baseline changes:* Fluctuations in FHR unrelated to uterine contractions
• *Periodic changes:* Fluctuations in FHR related to uterine contractions
• *Amplitude:* Difference in beats per minute between baseline readings and fluctuation in FHR
• *Recovery time:* Difference between the end of the contraction and the return to the baseline FHR
• *Acceleration:* Transient rise in FHR lasting longer than 15 seconds and associated with a uterine contraction
• *Deceleration:* Transient fall in FHR related to a uterine contraction
• *Lag time:* Difference between the peak of the contraction and the lowest point of deceleration

• Reposition the ultrasound and pressure transducers as necessary to ensure continuous accurate readings. Review the tracings frequently for baseline abnormalities, periodic changes, variability of changes, and uterine contraction abnormalities.

• Record maternal movement, administration of drugs, and procedures performed directly on the tracing, to assist evaluation of changes in the tracing.

• Report any abnormalities immediately.

Precautions

• During CST, watch for fetal distress with oxytocin infusion or nipple stimulation.

Normal findings

Normal FHR baseline ranges from 120 to 160 beats/minute, with a variability of 5 to 25 beats/minute. For the antepartum nonstress test, the fetus is considered healthy and should remain so for another week if two fetal movements causing a heart rate acceleration of more than 15 beats/minute from baseline FHR occur in a 20-minute period.

For the CST, the fetus is assumed to be healthy and should remain so for another week if three contractions occur during a 10-minute period, with no late decelerations.

Abnormal findings

Bradycardia (FHR of less than 120 beats/minute) may indicate fetal heart block, malposition, or hypoxia. Fetal bradycardia may also be drug-induced. Tachycardia (FHR of more than 160 beats/minute) may result from vagolytic drugs; maternal fever, tachycardia, or hyperthyroidism; early fetal hypoxia; or fetal infection or arrhythmia.

Decreased variability (a fluctuation of less than 5 beats/minute in the FHR) may be caused by fetal arrhythmia or heart block; by fetal hypoxia, central nervous system malformation, or infections; or by vagolytic drugs. FHR accelerations may result from early hypoxia. They may precede or follow variable decelerations and may indicate a breech position.

For the antepartum nonstress test, a positive result (less than two accelerations of FHR that last longer than 15 seconds each, with a heart rate acceleration over 15 beats/minute) indicates an exaggerated risk of perinatal morbidity and mortality and usually necessitates CST.

For the CST, persistent late decelerations during two or more contractions may indicate increased risk of fetal

morbidity or mortality. Hyperstimulation (long or frequent uterine contractions) or suspicious results require repetition of the test on the following day. If results are still positive, internal fetal monitoring or cesarean birth may be necessary.

INTERNAL FETAL MONITORING

Internal fetal monitoring is an invasive procedure that involves attaching an electrode to the fetal scalp to directly monitor fetal heart rate (FHR). A fluid-filled catheter introduced into the uterine cavity measures the frequency and pressure of uterine contractions. Internal monitoring is only performed during labor, after the membranes have ruptured and the cervix has dilated $1\frac{1}{4}''$ (3 cm), with the fetal head lower than the -2 station and only if external monitoring fails to provide adequate data.

Internal monitoring provides more accurate information about fetal health than external monitoring and is especially useful in determining if cesarean birth is necessary. The procedure carries minimal risks to the mother (perforated uterus or intrauterine infection) and fetus (scalp abscess or hematoma).

Purpose

• To monitor FHR, especially beat-to-beat variability

• To measure the frequency and pressure of uterine contractions to assess the progress of labor

• To evaluate intrapartum fetal health

• To supplement or replace external fetal monitoring

Patient preparation

- Explain to the patient that this test accurately assesses fetal health and that it does not necessarily mean that there is a problem. Describe the procedure and answer all questions.
- Warn her that she may feel mild discomfort when the uterine catheter and scalp electrode are inserted.
- Make sure she has signed a consent form.

Equipment

Sterile fetal scalp electrode and guide tube, intrauterine pressure catheter, catheter guide, pressure transducer, fetal heart monitor.

Procedure and posttest care

Measuring FHR:

- Place the patient in the dorsal lithotomy position, and prepare her perineal area for a vaginal examination, explaining each step of the procedure as it's performed. As the procedure begins, ask the patient to breathe through her mouth and relax her abdominal muscles.
- After the vaginal examination, the fetal scalp is palpated and an appropriate site is identified. A plastic tube carrying the small electrode is introduced into the cervix, pressed firmly against the fetal scalp, and rotated clockwise to attach the electrode to the scalp. The electrode wire is tugged gently to ensure proper attachment and the tube is withdrawn.
- The electrode wire is attached to a leg plate, which is strapped securely to the mother's thigh, and another cable attaches the leg plate to the fetal monitor.

Measuring uterine contractions:

- Fill the uterine catheter with sterile 0.9% sodium chloride solution. As you prepare, explain each step of the procedure to the patient.

- Ask her to breathe deeply through her mouth and to relax her abdominal muscles.
- After the vagina has been examined and the presenting part of the fetus palpated, the fluid-filled catheter and catheter guide are inserted $\frac{3}{8}''$ to $\frac{3}{4}''$ (1 to 2 cm) into the cervix, usually between the fetal head and the posterior cervix.
- The catheter is then gently advanced into the uterus until the black mark on the catheter is flush with the vulva (the catheter guide should *never* be passed deeply into the uterus).
- The guide is removed and the catheter is connected to a transducer that interprets intrauterine pressure.
- After the fetal scalp electrode is removed, apply antiseptic or antibiotic solution to the site.
- Watch for signs of fetal scalp abscess or maternal intrauterine infection.

Precautions

- Internal fetal monitoring is contraindicated if there is uncertainty about the fetus's presenting part or a technical impediment to attaching the lead.
- This procedure is also contraindicated if the mother has cervical or vaginal herpes lesions.
- Prevent artifacts in pressure readings by flushing the pressure transducer with 0.9% sodium chloride solution. Relieve catheter obstruction (by vernix caseosa, for example) by injecting a small amount of sterile 0.9% sodium chloride solution into the catheter (while the transducer is isolated from the system).
- Make sure a low heart rate is actually the FHR; it's possible that the fetal cardiotachometer may be recording a maternal heart rate.
- If FHR patterns indicate fetal distress, fetal oxygenation often can be improved by loading maternal fluids to increase placental perfusion, turning the mother on her side (preferably left) to

NORMAL INTRAUTERINE PRESSURE READINGS DURING LABOR

STAGE OF LABOR	FREQUENCY (Number of contractions per 10 minutes)	BASELINE PRESSURE (mm Hg)	PRESSURE DURING CONTRACTION (mm Hg)
Prelabor	1 to 2	—	25 to 40
First stage	3 to 5	8 to 12	30 to 40 (or more)
Second stage	5	10 to 20	50 to 80

alleviate supine hypotension, and administering oxygen to the mother. If these measures return heart rate patterns to normal, labor may continue. If abnormal patterns persist, cesarean birth may be necessary.
• Make sure that the fetal scalp electrode and the uterine catheter are removed before cesarean birth.

Reference values
Normal FHR ranges from 120 to 160 beats/minute, with a variability of 5 to 25 beats/minute. (See *Normal intrauterine pressure readings during labor.*)

Abnormal findings
Bradycardia (FHR of less than 120 beats/minute) may indicate fetal heart block, malposition, or hypoxia. Fetal bradycardia may also result from maternal ingestion of certain drugs, such as propranolol or narcotic analgesics.

Tachycardia (FHR greater than 160 beats/minute) may result from vagolytic drugs; maternal fever, tachycardia, or hyperthyroidism; early fetal hypoxia; fetal infection or arrhythmia; or prematurity.

Decreased variability (fluctuation of less than 5 beats/minute from baseline) may result from vagolytic drugs; fetal arrhythmia or heart block; or fetal hypoxia, central nervous system malformation, or infections.

Early decelerations (slowing of FHR at the onset of a contraction with recovery to baseline within no more than 15 seconds after the contraction ends) are related to fetal head compression and usually ensure fetal health.

Late decelerations (slowing of FHR after a contraction begins, a lag time greater than 20 seconds, and a recovery time of more than 15 seconds) may be related to uteroplacental insufficiency, fetal hypoxia, or acidosis. Recurrent and persistently late decelerations with decreased variability usually indicate serious fetal distress, possibly resulting from conduction (spinal, caudal, or epidural) anesthesia or fetal hypoxia.

Variable decelerations (sudden precipitous drops in FHR unrelated to uterine contractions) are commonly related to cord compression. A severe drop in FHR (to less than 70 beats/minute for more than 60 seconds) with a decrease in variability indicates fetal distress and may result in a compromised neonate. Poor beat-to-beat variability without periodic patterns may indicate fetal distress, requiring further evaluation, such as analysis of fetal blood gas levels.

Decreased intrauterine pressure during labor that's not progressing normally may require oxytocin stimulation. Elevated intrauterine pressure readings may indicate abruptio placentae or overstimulation from oxytocin, possibly resulting in fetal distress due to decreased placental perfusion.

NEUROLOGIC MONITORING

ELECTROENCEPHALOG-RAPHY

In this test, electrodes attached to areas of the patient's scalp record a portion of the brain's electrical activity and transmit this information to an electroencephalograph, which records the resulting brain waves on recording paper. The procedure may be performed in a special lab or by a portable unit at the bedside.

Purpose
• To determine the presence and type of seizure disorder
• To aid diagnosis of intracranial lesions, such as abscesses and tumors
• To evaluate the brain's electrical activity in metabolic disease, head injury, meningitis, encephalitis, mental retardation, and psychological disorders
• To confirm brain death

Patient preparation
• Explain to the patient that this test records the brain's electrical activity. Describe the procedure to the patient and

family members and answer all questions.
• Tell him that he must forgo caffeine prior to the test; other than this, there are no food or fluid restrictions.
• Thoroughly wash and dry his hair to remove hair sprays, creams, or oils.
• Explain that during the test, he'll relax in a reclining chair or lie on a bed, and that electrodes will be attached to his scalp with a special paste. Assure him that the electrodes won't shock him.
• If needle electrodes are used, explain that he'll feel a pricking sensation as they're inserted; however, flat electrodes are used more commonly.
• Do your best to allay the patient's fears because nervousness can affect brain wave patterns.
• Check his medication history for drugs that may interfere with test results — for example, anticonvulsants, antianxiety agents, sedative-hypnotics, and antidepressants — and withhold these medications for 24 to 48 hours before the test.
• A patient with a seizure disorder may require a "sleep EEG." In this case, keep the patient awake the night before the test, and administer a sedative (such as chloral hydrate) to help him sleep during the test.
• If the test is performed to confirm brain death, provide family members with emotional support.

Procedure and posttest care
• Position the patient on the bed or reclining chair. Reassure him as the electrodes are attached to his scalp.
• Before the recording procedure begins, instruct the patient to close his eyes, relax, and remain still.
• During the recording, observe the patient carefully; note blinking, swallowing, talking, or other movements that may cause artifacts on the tracing.

• The recording may be stopped at intervals to let the patient rest or reposition himself. This is important because restlessness and fatigue can alter brain wave patterns.

• After an initial baseline recording, the patient may be tested under various stress-producing conditions to elicit patterns not observable while he is at rest. For example, he may be asked to breathe deeply and rapidly for 3 minutes (hyperventilation), which may elicit brain wave patterns typical of seizure disorders or other abnormalities. This technique is commonly used to detect absence seizures. Also, photic stimulation tests central cerebral activity in response to bright light, accentuating abnormal activity in absence or myoclonic seizures.

• Review carefully the reinstatement of anticonvulsant medication or other drugs withheld before the test.

• Carefully observe the patient for seizure activity and provide a safe environment.

• Help the patient remove electrode paste from his hair.

• If the patient received a sedative before the test, take safety precautions, such as raising the bed's side rails.

Precautions
• Observe the patient carefully for seizure activity.

• If seizure activity occurs, record seizure patterns and be prepared to provide assistance. Have suction equipment and diazepam for I.V. injection readily available.

Normal findings
Electroencephalography (EEG) records a portion of the brain's electrical activity as waves; some are irregular, while others demonstrate frequent patterns. Among the basic waveforms are the alpha, beta, theta, and delta rhythms.

Alpha waves occur at a frequency of 8 to 12 cycles/second in a regular rhythm. They're present only in the waking state when the patient's eyes are closed but he's mentally alert; usually, they disappear with visual activity or mental concentration. *Beta waves* (13 to 30 cycles/second) — generally associated with anxiety, depression, or use of sedatives — are seen most readily in the frontal and central regions of the brain. *Theta waves* (4 to 7 cycles/second) are most common in children and young adults, and appear in the frontal and temporal regions. *Delta waves* (0.5 to 3.5 cycles/second) normally occur only in young children and during sleep.

Abnormal findings
Usually, about 100 pages of recording paper are evaluated, with particular attention paid to basic waveforms, symmetry of cerebral activity, transient discharges, and responses to stimulation. A specific diagnosis depends on the patient's clinical status.

In seizures disorders, EEG patterns may identify the specific disorder. In *absence seizures,* the EEG shows spikes and waves at a frequency of 3 cycles/second. In *generalized tonic-clonic seizures*, it generally shows multiple, high-voltage, spiked waves in both hemispheres. In *complex partial seizures*, the EEG usually shows spiked waves in the affected temporal region. And in patients with *focal seizures*, it usually shows localized, spiked discharges.

In patients with intracranial lesions, such as tumors or abscesses, the EEG may show slow waves (usually delta waves, but possibly unilateral beta waves). Vascular lesions, such as cerebral infarcts and intracranial hemorrhages, generally produce focal abnormalities in the injured area.

Generally, any condition that causes a diminishing level of consciousness alters the EEG pattern in proportion to the degree of consciousness lost. For example, in a patient with a metabolic disorder, an inflammatory process (such as meningitis or encephalitis), or increased intracranial pressure, the EEG shows generalized, diffuse, and slow brain waves.

EVOKED POTENTIAL STUDIES

These tests evaluate the integrity of visual, somatosensory, and auditory nerve pathways by measuring evoked potentials — the brain's electrical response to stimulation of the sensory organs or peripheral nerves. Evoked potentials are recorded as electronic impulses by surface electrodes attached to the scalp and skin over various peripheral sensory nerves. A computer extracts these low-amplitude impulses from background brain wave activity and averages the signals from repeated stimuli.

Three types of responses are measured:
• Visual evoked potentials, produced by exposing the eye to a rapidly reversing checkerboard pattern, help evaluate demyelinating diseases, traumatic injury, and puzzling visual complaints.
• Somatosensory evoked potentials, produced by electrically stimulating a peripheral sensory nerve, help diagnose peripheral nerve disease and locate brain and spinal cord lesions.
• Auditory brain stem evoked potentials, produced by delivering clicks to the ear, help locate auditory lesions and evaluate brain stem integrity.

Purpose
• To aid diagnosis of nervous system lesions and abnormalities
• To assess neurologic function
• To monitor comatose patients and patients under anesthesia
• To monitor spinal cord function during spinal cord surgery
• To evaluate neurologic function in infants whose sensory systems can't be adequately assessed

Patient preparation
• Tell the patient that this group of tests measures the electrical activity of his nervous system. Explain who will perform the test, where it will take place, and that it usually lasts 45 to 60 minutes.
• Tell him that he'll sit in a reclining chair or lie on a bed. If visual evoked potentials will be measured, electrodes will be attached to his scalp; if somatosensory evoked potentials will be measured, electrodes will be placed on his scalp, neck, lower back, wrist, knee, and ankle.
• Assure him that the electrodes won't hurt him. Encourage him to relax; tension can affect neurologic function and interfere with test results.
• Have him remove all jewelry.

Procedure and posttest care
• Position the patient in the reclining chair or on the bed and tell him to relax and remain still.
To measure visual evoked potentials:
• Electrodes are attached to the patient's scalp at occipital, parietal, and vertex locations; a reference electrode is placed on the midfrontal area or on the ear.
• The patient is positioned 3′ (1 m) from the pattern-shift stimulator.
• One eye is occluded, and the patient is instructed to fix his gaze on a dot in the center of the screen.

• A checkerboard pattern is projected and then rapidly reversed or shifted 100 times, once or twice per second.
• A computer amplifies and averages the brain's response to each stimulus, and the results are plotted as a waveform.
• The procedure is repeated for the other eye.

To measure somatosensory evoked potentials:
• Electrodes are attached to the patient's skin over somatosensory pathways — typically the wrist, knee, and ankle — to stimulate peripheral nerves. Recording electrodes are placed on the scalp over the sensory cortex of the hemisphere opposite the limb to be stimulated. Additional electrodes may be placed at Erb's point (above the clavicle overlying the brachial plexus), at the second cervical vertebra, and over the lower lumbar vertebrae. Midfrontal or noncephalic electrodes are placed for reference.
• Painless electrical stimulation is delivered to the peripheral nerve through the electrode. The intensity is adjusted to produce a minor muscle response, such as a thumb twitch upon median nerve stimulation at the wrist.
• Electrical stimuli are delivered 500 or more times, at a rate of five per second.
• A computer measures and averages the time it takes for the electrical current to reach the cortex; the results, expressed in milliseconds (msec), are recorded as waveforms.
• The test is repeated once to verify results; then the electrodes are repositioned and the entire procedure is repeated for the other side.

Normal findings
Visual evoked potentials:
On the waveform, the most significant wave is P100, a positive wave appearing about 100 msec after the pattern-shift stimulus is applied. The most clinically

significant measurements are absolute P100 latency (the time between stimulus application and peaking of the P100 wave) and the difference between the P100 latencies of each eye. Because many physical and technical factors affect P100 latency, normal results vary greatly among laboratories and patients.

Somatosensory evoked potentials:
Waveforms obtained vary, depending on locations of the stimulating and recording electrodes. The positive and negative peaks are labeled in sequence, based on normal time of appearance. For example, N19 is a negative peak normally recorded 19 msec after application of the stimulus. Each wave peak arises from a discrete location: N19 is generated mainly from the thalamus, P22 from the parietal sensory cortex, and so on. Interwave latencies (time between waves), rather than absolute latencies, are used as a basis for clinical interpretation. Latency differences between sides are significant. (See *Visual and somatosensory evoked potentials.*)

Abnormal findings
Information from evoked potential studies is useful but insufficient to confirm a specific diagnosis. Test data must be interpreted in light of clinical information.

Visual evoked potentials:
Generally, abnormal (extended) P100 latencies confined to one eye indicate a visual pathway lesion anterior to the optic chiasm. A lesion posterior to the optic chiasm usually doesn't produce abnormal P100 latencies. Because each eye projects to both occipital lobes, the unaffected pathway transmits sufficient impulses to produce a normal latency response. Bilateral abnormal P100 latencies have been found in patients with multiple sclerosis, optic neuritis, retinopathies, amblyopia (although abnormal latencies don't correlate well with impaired visual acuity), spinocerebellar

VISUAL AND SOMATOSENSORY EVOKED POTENTIALS

Visual (pattern-shift) evoked potentials: In this test, visual neural impulses are recorded as they travel along the pathway from the eye to the occipital cortex. Wave P100 is the most significant component of the resultant waveform. Normal P100 latency is approximately 100 msec after the application of a visual stimulus, as shown in the top diagram. Increased P100 latency, shown in the bottom diagram, is an abnormal finding indicating a lesion along the visual pathway.

Normal tracing

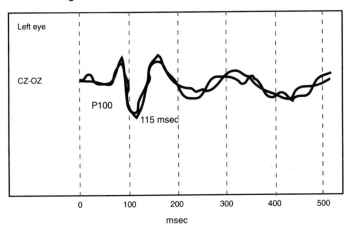

Tracing in multiple sclerosis

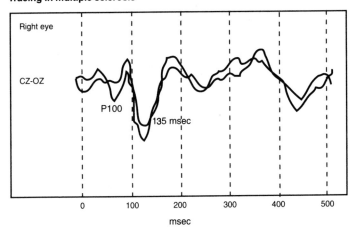

CZ = vertex; OZ = midocciput

(continued)

VISUAL AND SOMATOSENSORY EVOKED POTENTIALS *(continued)*

Somatosensory evoked potentials: These tests measure the conduction time of an electrical impulse traveling along a somatosensory pathway to the cortex. Interwave latency is the most significant component of the resultant waveform. On the set of upper- and lower-limb tracings shown below, the top tracings represent normal interwave latencies; the bottom tracings, typical abnormal latencies found in a patient with multiple sclerosis. Because of the close correlation between waveforms and the anatomy of somatosensory pathways, such tracings allow precise location of lesions that produce conduction defects.

Upper limb

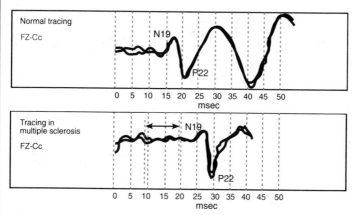

Lower limb

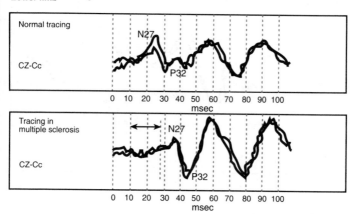

CZ = vertex; Cc = sensoparietal cortex contralateral to stimulated limb; FZ = mid-frontal

degeneration, adrenoleukodystrophy, sarcoidosis, Parkinson's disease, and Huntington's disease.

Somatosensory evoked potentials:
Because somatosensory evoked potential components are assumed to be linked in series, an abnormal interwave latency indicates a conduction defect between the generators of the two peaks involved. This often allows precise location of a neurologic lesion. Abnormal upper-limb interwave latencies may indicate cervical spondylosis, intracerebral lesions, or sensorimotor neuropathies. Abnormalities in the lower limb demonstrate peripheral nerve and root lesions, such as those in Guillain-Barré syndrome, compressive myelopathies, multiple sclerosis, transverse myelitis, and traumatic spinal cord injury.

ELECTROMYOGRAPHY

This test records the electrical activity of selected skeletal muscle groups at rest and during voluntary contraction. It involves percutaneous insertion of a needle electrode into a muscle. The electrical discharge of the muscle is then measured by an oscilloscope. Nerve conduction time is often measured simultaneously.

Purpose
• To aid differentiation between primary muscle disorders, such as the muscular dystrophies, and secondary disorders
• To help assess diseases characterized by central neuronal degeneration, such as amyotrophic lateral sclerosis
• To aid diagnosis of neuromuscular disorders, such as myasthenia gravis

Patient preparation
• Explain to the patient that this test measures the electrical activity of his muscles.

• Tell him there are usually no restrictions on food or fluids (in some cases, cigarettes, coffee, tea, and cola may be restricted for 2 or 3 hours before the test).
• Describe the test, including who will perform it, where it will take place, and its duration (1 hour).
• Tell him he may wear a hospital gown or any comfortable clothing that permits access to the muscles to be tested.
• Advise him that a needle will be inserted into selected muscles and that he may experience some discomfort. Reassure him that adverse effects or complications are rare.
• Make sure the patient or a responsible family member has signed a consent form.
• Check the patient's history for medications that may interfere with the results of the test, for example, cholinergics, anticholinergics, and skeletal muscle relaxants. If the patient is receiving such medications, note this on the chart.

Procedure and posttest care
• Position the patient on a stretcher or bed, or in a chair, depending on the muscles to be tested. Position his arm or leg so that the muscle to be tested is at rest.
• Needle electrodes are quickly inserted and a metal plate is placed under the patient to serve as a reference electrode. Then the muscle's electrical signal (motor unit potential) is recorded during rest and contraction.
• The oscilloscope display is photographed for a permanent record. Frequently, the leadwires of the recorder are attached to an audio-amplifier so that the fluctuation of voltage within the muscle can be heard.
• If the patient experiences residual pain, apply warm compresses and administer prescribed analgesics.
• Resume administration of any medications withheld for the test.

Precautions
• Electromyography is contraindicated in patients with bleeding disorders.

Normal findings
At rest, a normal muscle exhibits minimal electrical activity. During voluntary contraction, however, electrical activity increases markedly. A sustained contraction or one of increasing strength causes a rapid "train" of motor unit potentials that can be heard as a crescendo of sounds over the audio-amplifier.

At the same time, the oscilloscope screen displays a sequence of waveforms that vary in amplitude (height) and frequency. Waveforms that are close together indicate a high frequency, while waveforms that are far apart signify a low frequency.

Normal findings must be correlated with the patient's history and clinical features and with the results of other neurologic tests.

Abnormal findings
In primary muscle diseases, such as the muscular dystrophies, motor unit potentials are short (low amplitude), with frequent, irregular discharges. In disorders such as amyotrophic lateral sclerosis (as well as in peripheral nerve disorders), motor unit potentials are isolated and irregular but show increased amplitude and duration. In myasthenia gravis, motor unit potentials initially may be normal but progressively diminish in amplitude with continuing contractions. The interpreter makes a distinction between waveforms that indicate a muscle disorder and those that indicate denervation.

CARDIAC MONITORING AND CATHETERIZATION

ELECTROCARDIOGRAPHY

A common test for evaluating cardiac status, electrocardiography (ECG) graphically records the electrical current (electrical potential) generated by the heart. This current radiates from the heart in all directions and, on reaching the skin, is measured by electrodes connected to an amplifier and strip chart recorder. The standard resting (scalar) ECG uses 5 electrodes to measure the electrical potential from 12 different leads: the standard limb leads (I, II, III), the augmented limb leads (aVR, aV_L, and aV_F), and the precordial, or chest, leads (V_1 through V_6).

Purpose
• To help identify primary conduction abnormalities, cardiac arrhythmias, cardiac hypertrophy, pericarditis, electrolyte imbalances, myocardial ischemia, and the site and extent of myocardial infarction (MI)
• To monitor recovery from MI
• To evaluate the effectiveness of cardiac medication (cardiac glycosides, antiarrhythmics, antihypertensives, and vasodilators)
• To assess pacemaker performance

Patient preparation
• Explain to the patient that this test evaluates the heart's electrical activity.

Inform him that there are no food or fluid restrictions.

• Describe the test, including who will perform it, where it will take place, and its expected duration (5 to 10 minutes).

• Tell him that electrodes will be attached to his arms, legs, and chest and that the procedure is painless. Explain that during the test, he'll be asked to relax, lie still, and breathe normally.

• Advise him not to talk during the test because the sound of his voice may distort the ECG tracing.

• Check the patient's medication history for use of cardiac drugs, and note your findings on the chart.

Equipment

Recording paper, pregelled disposable electrodes or reusable electrodes with suction bulbs, electrode gel, rubber straps, 4″ × 4″ gauze pads, moist cloth towel, sterile drape.

Procedure and posttest care

• Place the patient in the supine position. If he can't tolerate lying flat, help him to assume semi-Fowler's position.

• Have him expose his chest, both ankles, and both wrists for electrode placement. If the patient is a woman, provide a chest drape until the chest leads are applied.

• Turn on the machine to warm up the stylus mechanism and check the paper supply.

Multichannel ECG:

• Place electrodes on the inner aspect of the wrists, the medial aspect of the lower legs, and the chest. If using disposable electrodes, remove the paper backing before positioning. For reusable electrodes, apply electrode gel and affix the electrodes with suction bulbs.

• Connect the leadwires after all electrodes are in place. Secure the limb electrodes with rubber straps, but avoid tightening them to prevent circulatory impairment and distortion on the recording.

• If frequent ECGs will be necessary, use a marking pen to indicate lead positions on the patient's chest to ensure consistent placement.

• Set the paper speed (usually 25mm/second). Calibrate the machine by adjusting the sensitivity to normal and checking the quality and baseline position of the tracing. Press the START button and record any required information (for example, patient's name and room number).

• The machine produces a printout showing all 12 leads simultaneously. Check to be sure that all leads are represented in the tracing. If not, determine which one has come loose, reattach it, and restart the tracing.

• Check for artifacts in the tracing and be sure that the wave doesn't peak beyond the top edge of the recording grid. If it does, adjust the machine to bring the wave inside the boundaries.

• When the machine finishes the tracing, remove the electrodes and reposition the patient's gown and bed covers.

Single-channel ECG:

• Apply either disposable or standard electrodes to the inner aspects of the wrists and medial aspects of the lower legs. Connect each leadwire to the corresponding electrode by inserting the wire prong into the terminal post and tightening the screw.

• Set the paper speed (usually 25 mm/second) and calibrate the machine by adjusting the sensitivity to normal. Recalibrate the machine after running each lead to provide a consistent test standard.

• Turn the lead selector to I. Then mark the lead by writing "I" on the paper strip or by depressing the marking button on the machine (some machines do this automatically). Record for 3 to 6 seconds and then return the machine to the standby mode. Repeat this procedure for leads II, III, aV$_R$, aV$_L$, and aV$_F$.

• Determine proper placement for the chest electrodes. (If frequent ECGs are necessary, mark these spots on the patient's chest to ensure consistent placement.)

• Connect the chest leadwire to the suction bulb, apply gel to each of the six chest positions, and then firmly press the suction bulb to attach the chest lead to the V$_1$ position. Mark the strips as before.

• Turn the lead selector to V and record V$_1$ for 3 to 6 seconds. Return the lead selector to standby. Reposition the electrode and repeat the procedure for V$_2$ to V$_6$.

• After completing V$_6$, run a rhythm strip on lead II for at least 6 seconds. Assess the quality of the tracings and repeat any that are unclear.

• Disconnect the equipment, remove the electrodes, and wipe the gel from the patient with a moist cloth towel. Wash the gel from the electrodes and dry them thoroughly.

Both types:

• Label each ECG strip with the patient's name and room number (if applicable), the date and time of the procedure, and the doctor's name. Note whether the ECG was performed during or upon resolution of a chest pain episode.

• Disconnect the equipment. The electrode patches are usually left in place if the patient is having recurrent chest pain or if serial ECGs are ordered, as with the use of thrombolytics. If using suction cups, be sure to wash the conductive gel from the patient's skin.

Precautions

• The recording equipment and other nearby electrical equipment should be properly grounded to prevent electrical interference.

• Double-check color codes and lead markings to be sure connectors match.

• Check to make sure that suction cups are firmly attached, and reattach electrodes if loose skin contact is suspected.

• Be sure the patient is quiet and motionless during the test because talking or limb movement distorts the recordings.

• If the patient has a pacemaker in place, an ECG may be performed with or without a magnet. Indicate the presence of a pacemaker and whether or not a magnet is used. (Many pacemakers function only when the heartbeat falls below a preset rate; a magnet makes the pacemaker fire regularly, which permits evaluation of pacemaker performance.)

Normal findings

ECG tracings normally consist of three identifiable waveforms: the P wave, the QRS complex, and the T wave. The P wave depicts atrial depolarization; the QRS complex, ventricular depolarization; and the T wave, ventricular repolarization.

The lead II waveform, known as the rhythm strip, depicts the heart's rhythm more clearly than any other waveform. In lead II, the normal P wave does not exceed 2.5 mm (0.25 millivolt) in height or last longer than 0.11 second. The PR interval, which includes the P wave plus the PR segment, persists for 0.12 to 0.2 second for heart rates over 60 beats/minute. The QT interval varies with the heart rate and lasts 0.4 to 0.52 second for rates above 60; the voltage of the R wave in the V$_1$ through V$_6$ leads doesn't exceed 27 mm. The total QRS complex lasts 0.06 to 0.1 second. (See *Normal ECG waveforms.*)

(Text continues on page 630.)

NORMAL ECG WAVEFORMS

Because each lead takes a different view of heart activity, it generates its own characteristic tracing. The traces shown here are representative of each of the 12 leads. Leads aV_R, V_1, V_2, and V_3 normally show strong negative deflections below the baseline. Negative deflections indicate that the current is flowing away from the positive electrode; positive deflections, that the current is flowing toward the positive electrode.

Lead I

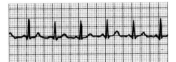

Lead V₁

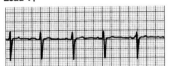

Lead II

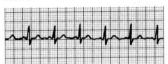

Lead V₂

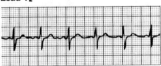

Lead III

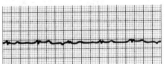

Lead V₃

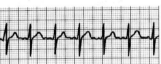

Lead aV_R

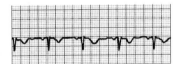

Lead V₄

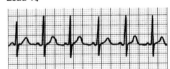

Lead aV_L

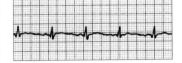

Lead V₅

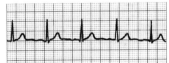

Lead aV_F

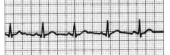

Lead V₆

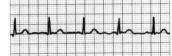

EXAMPLES OF ABNORMAL ECG WAVEFORMS

Premature ventricular contractions (PVCs) originate in an ectopic focus of the ventricular wall. They can be unifocal (having the same single focus), as shown in this tracing from lead V_1, or they can be multifocal (arising from more than one ectopic focus). In PVCs, the P wave is absent, and the QRS complex shows considerable distortion, usually deflecting in the opposite direction from the patient's normal QRS. The T wave also deflects in the opposite direction from the QRS complex, and the PVC usually precedes a compensatory pause. Some examples of abnormalities causing PVCs include electrolyte imbalances (especially hypokalemia), an old myocardial infarction, hypoxia, and drug toxicity (digitalis glycosides, beta-adrenergics).

PREMATURE VENTRICULAR CONTRACTION — LEAD V_1

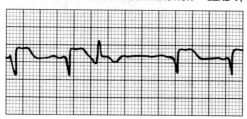

First-degree heart block — the most common conduction disturbance — occurs in healthy hearts as well as diseased hearts and usually is clinically insignificant. It's often characteristic in elderly patients with chronic degeneration of the cardiac conduction system, and it occasionally occurs in patients receiving digitalis glycosides or antiarrhythmic drugs, such as procainamide or quinidine. In children, first-degree heart block may be the earliest sign of acute rheumatic fever. In this lead V_1 tracing, the interval between the P wave and QRS complex (the PR interval) exceeds 0.20 second.

FIRST-DEGREE HEART BLOCK — LEAD V_1

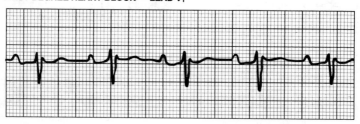

Hypokalemia is a common electrolyte imbalance that's caused by low blood potassium levels and that affects the electrical activity of the myocardium. Mild hypokalemia may cause only muscle weakness, fatigue, and possibly atrial or ventricular irritability; a severe imbalance causes pronounced muscle weakness, paralysis, atrial tachycardia with varying degrees of block, and PVCs that may progress to ventricular tachycardia and fibrillation.

Early signs of hypokalemia, as shown on this V_1 tracing, include prominent
U waves, a prolonged QU interval, and flat or inverted T waves. Usually,
T waves do not flatten or invert until potassium depletion becomes severe.

HYPOKALEMIA — LEAD V_1

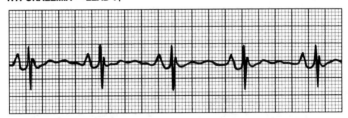

Myocardial infarction (MI) produces typical ECG changes in several leads at
once, enabling the doctor to determine accurately the location and extent of tissue damage. MI causes three changes: an inner zone of tissue necrosis, a surrounding zone of inflamed tissue, and an outer zone of ischemia (see diagram).
As the infarction progresses, the first ECG change is an elevated ST segment,
which indicates formation of an ischemic zone. Then the T wave begins to flat-

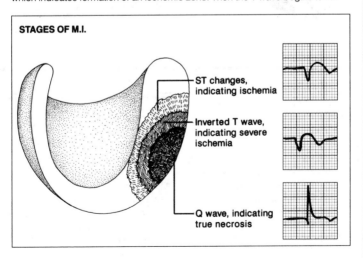

STAGES OF M.I.

ST changes,
indicating ischemia

Inverted T wave,
indicating severe
ischemia

Q wave, indicating
true necrosis

(continued)

ten and finally inverts, and enlarged Q waves appear, indicating developing necrosis — a true infarction. (Abnormal Q waves should be larger than one small square on the chart — 0.04 second by 0.1 millivolt.) The T wave may stay inverted for the rest of the patient's life or it can revert to normal, whereas the deep Q wave remains as a permanent indicator of necrosis. The infarction can be located by studying the characteristic ST, T, and Q wave changes in various lead combinations. In the three tracings shown below, the ST segments elevated in leads II, III, and aV_F indicate an infarction in the inferior (diaphragmatic) area of the heart.

E.C.G. CHANGES WITH AN INFERIOR M.I.

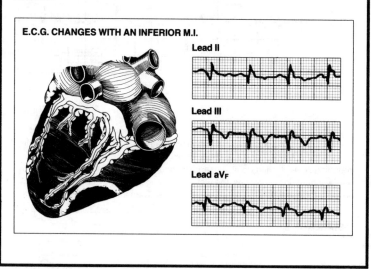

Lead II

Lead III

Lead aV_F

Abnormal findings

An abnormal ECG may show MI, right or left ventricular hypertrophy, arrhythmias, right or left bundle-branch block, ischemia, conduction defects or pericarditis, electrolyte abnormalities (such as hypokalemia), or the effects of cardioactive drugs. Sometimes an ECG may reveal abnormal waveforms only during angina episodes or during exercise. (See *Examples of abnormal ECG waveforms*, pages 628 to 630.)

EXERCISE ELECTRO-CARDIOGRAPHY

Also referred to as a stress test, an exercise electrocardiogram (ECG) evaluates the heart's response to physical stress, providing important diagnostic information that can't be obtained from a resting ECG alone.

An ECG and blood pressure readings are taken while the patient walks on a treadmill or pedals a stationary bicycle, and his response to a constant or an increasing workload is observed. Unless complications develop, the test continues until the patient reaches the target heart rate (determined by an established protocol) or experiences chest pain or fatigue. The patient with recent myocardial infarction (MI) or coronary artery surgery may walk the treadmill at a slow pace to determine his activity tolerance before discharge from the hospital.

Purpose

• To help diagnose the cause of chest pain or other possible cardiac pain
• To determine the functional capacity of the heart after surgery or MI
• To screen for asymptomatic coronary artery disease (particularly in men over age 35)
• To help set limitations for an exercise program
• To identify arrhythmias that develop during physical exercise
• To evaluate the effectiveness of antiarrhythmic or antianginal therapy

Patient preparation

• Explain to the patient that this test records the heart's electrical activity and performance under stress.
• Instruct him not to eat, smoke, or drink alcoholic or caffeinated beverages for 3 hours before the test, but to continue his prescribed drug regimen unless directed otherwise.
• Describe who will perform the test, where it will take place, and its expected duration.
• Tell him that the test will cause fatigue and he'll be slightly breathless and sweaty, but assure him that it poses few risks. He may, in fact, stop the test if he experiences fatigue or chest pain.
• Advise him to wear comfortable socks and shoes and loose, lightweight shorts or slacks. Men usually don't wear a shirt during the test, and women generally wear a bra and a lightweight short-sleeved blouse or a patient gown with a front closure.
• Explain that electrodes will be attached to several areas on his chest and, possibly, his back. Reassure him that he will not feel any current from the electrodes; however, they may itch slightly.
• Tell him that his blood pressure will be checked periodically throughout the procedure, and assure him that his heart rate will be monitored continuously.
• If the patient is scheduled for a multistage *treadmill test,* explain that the speed and incline of the treadmill will increase at predetermined intervals and that he'll be informed of each adjustment.
• If he's scheduled for a *bicycle ergometer test,* explain that the resistance he experiences in pedaling increases gradually as he tries to maintain a specific speed.
• Encourage him to report his feelings during the test. Tell him his blood pressure and ECG will be monitored for 10 to 15 minutes after the test.
• Check the patient's history for a recent physical examination (within 1 week) and for baseline 12-lead ECG results.
• Be sure that the patient or a responsible family member has signed a consent form.

Procedure and posttest care

• The electrode sites are cleaned with an alcohol swab, and superficial epidermal cell layers and excess skin oils are removed with a gauze pad, fine sandpaper, or a dental burr.
• Chest electrodes are placed according to the lead system selected and are secured with adhesive tape or a rubber belt. The leadwire cable is placed over the patient's shoulder and the leadwire box is placed on his chest. The cable is secured by pinning it to the patient's

clothing or taping it to his shoulder or back. Then the leadwires are connected to the chest electrodes.

• The monitor is started, and a stable baseline tracing is obtained. A baseline rhythm strip is checked for arrhythmias. A blood pressure reading is taken, and the patient is auscultated for the presence of S_3 or S_4 gallops or crackles.

• In a treadmill test, the treadmill is turned on to a slow speed, and the patient is shown how to step onto it and how to use the support railings to maintain balance, but not to support weight. Then the treadmill is turned off. The patient is instructed to step onto the treadmill, and it is turned on to slow speed until he gets used to walking on it.

• For a bicycle ergometer test, the patient is instructed to sit on the bicycle while the seat and handlebars are adjusted to comfortable positions. The patient is instructed not to grip the handlebars tightly, but to use them only for maintaining balance, and to pedal until he reaches the desired speed, as shown on the speedometer.

• In both tests, a monitor is observed continuously for changes in the heart's electrical activity. The rhythm strip is checked at preset intervals for arrhythmias, premature ventricular contractions (PVCs), ST-segment changes, or T-wave changes. The test level and the time elapsed in the test level are marked on each strip. Blood pressure is monitored at predetermined intervals, usually at the end of each test level, and changes in systolic readings are noted. Some common responses to maximal exercise are dizziness, light-headedness, leg fatigue, dyspnea, diaphoresis, and a slightly ataxic gait. If symptoms become severe, the test is stopped.

• Usually, testing stops when the patient reaches the target heart rate. As the treadmill speed slows, he may be instructed to continue walking for several minutes to prevent nausea or dizziness.

Then the treadmill is turned off, the patient is helped to a chair, and his blood pressure and ECG are monitored for 10 to 15 minutes or until the ECG returns to baseline.

• Auscultate for the presence of S_3 or S_4 gallops. An S_4 gallop commonly develops after exercise because of increased blood flow volume and turbulence. However, an S_3 gallop is more significant than an S_4 gallop, indicating transient left ventricular dysfunction.

• Tell the patient that he may resume his usual diet.

• If any drugs were discontinued before the test, tell the patient that he may resume taking them.

• Remove electrodes and clean the electrode sites before the patient leaves.

Precautions

• Because an exercise ECG places considerable stress on the heart, it may be contraindicated in patients with ventricular or dissecting aortic aneurysm, uncontrolled arrhythmias, pericarditis, myocarditis, severe anemia, uncontrolled hypertension, unstable angina, or congestive heart failure.

• Stop the test immediately if the ECG shows three consecutive PVCs or any significant increase in ectopy, if systolic blood pressure falls below resting level, if heart rate falls to 10 beats/minute below resting level, or if the patient becomes exhausted. Depending on the patient's condition, the test may be stopped if the ECG shows bundle-branch block, ST-segment depression that exceeds 1.5 mm, persistent ST-segment elevation, or frequent or complicated PVCs; if blood pressure fails to rise above resting level; if systolic pressure exceeds 220 mm Hg; or if the patient experiences angina.

Normal findings

In a normal exercise ECG, the P and T waves, the QRS complex, and the ST

EXERCISE ECG TRACINGS

These tracings are from an abnormal exercise electrocardiogram (ECG) obtained during a treadmill test performed on a patient who had just undergone a triple coronary artery bypass graft. The first tracing shows the heart at rest, with a blood pressure of 124/80 mm Hg. In the second tracing, the patient worked up to a 10% grade at 1.7 mph before experiencing angina at 2 minutes, 25 seconds. The tracing shows a depressed ST segment; heart rate was 85 beats/minute and blood pressure was 140/70 mm Hg. The third tracing shows the heart at rest 6 minutes after the test; blood pressure was 140/90 mm Hg.

Resting

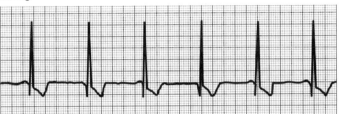

Angina

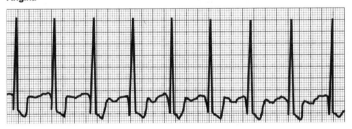

Recovery

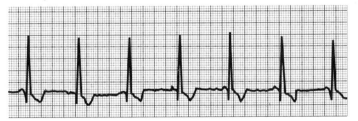

segment change slightly; slight ST-segment depression occurs in some patients, especially women. Heart rate rises in direct proportion to the workload and metabolic oxygen demand; systolic blood pressure also rises as workload increases. The normal patient attains the endurance levels predicted by his age and the appropriate exercise protocol. (See *Exercise ECG tracings,* page 633.)

Abnormal findings

Although criteria for judging test results vary, two findings strongly suggest an abnormality: a flat or downsloping ST-segment depression of 1 mm or more for at least 0.08 second after the junction of the QRS and ST segments (J point); and a markedly depressed J point, with an upsloping but depressed ST segment of 1.5 mm below the baseline 0.08 second after the J point. T-wave inversion also signifies ischemia. Initial ST-segment depression on the resting ECG must be further depressed by 1 mm during exercise to be considered abnormal.

Hypotension resulting from exercise, ST-segment depression of 3 mm or more, downsloping ST segments, and ischemic ST segments appearing within the first 3 minutes of exercise and lasting 8 minutes into the posttest recovery period may indicate multivessel or left coronary artery disease. ST-segment elevation may indicate dyskinetic left ventricular wall motion or severe transmural ischemia.

The predictive value of this test for coronary artery disease varies with the patient's history and sex; however, false-negative and false-positive test results are common. To detect coronary artery disease accurately, thallium imaging and stress testing, exercise multiple-gated acquisition scanning, or coronary angiography may be necessary.

Ambulatory Electrocardiography

Also called Holter monitoring, this test involves the continuous recording of heart activity as the patient follows his normal routine. It is usually performed for 24 hours, during which the patient wears a small reel-to-reel or cassette tape recorder connected to electrodes placed on his chest and keeps a diary of his activities and any associated symptoms. At the end of the recording period, the tape is analyzed by a computer that correlates cardiac irregularities, such as arrhythmias and ST-segment changes, with the activities in the patient's diary.

Purpose

• To detect cardiac arrhythmias missed by an exercise or resting electrocardiogram (ECG)

• To evaluate chest pain

• To evaluate cardiac status after acute myocardial infarction (MI) or pacemaker implantation

• To evaluate effectiveness of antiarrhythmic drug therapy

• To assess and correlate dyspnea, central nervous system symptoms (such as syncope and light-headedness) and palpitations with actual cardiac events and the patient's activities

Patient preparation

• Explain to the patient that this test helps determine how the heart responds to normal activity or, if appropriate, to cardioactive medication. Tell him that electrodes will be attached to his chest and that his chest may be shaved.

• Explain that he will wear a small tape recorder for 24 hours (for 5 to 7 days if a patient-activated monitor is being used), and show him how to position the recorder when he lies down.

• Encourage him to continue his routine activities during the monitoring period. Stress the importance of logging his usual activities (such as walking, climbing stairs, urinating, sleeping, and sexual activity), emotional upsets, physical symptoms (dizziness, palpitations, fatigue, chest pain, and syncope), and ingestion of medication; show the patient a sample diary.

• Tell him to wear loose-fitting clothing with front-buttoning tops during monitoring.

• Demonstrate the proper use of specific equipment, including how to mark the tape (if applicable) at the onset of symptoms.

• If a patient-activated monitor is being used, show the patient how to press the event button to activate the monitor if he experiences any unusual sensations. Instruct him not to tamper with the monitor or to disconnect the leadwires or electrodes.

• Advise him to avoid magnets, metal detectors, high-voltage areas, and electric blankets. Show him how to check the recorder to make sure it's working properly. Explain that if the monitor light flashes, one of the electrodes may be loose and he should depress the center of each one. Tell him to notify you if one comes off.

• If the patient won't be returning to the office or hospital immediately after the monitoring period, show him how to remove and store the equipment. Remind him to bring the diary when he returns.

Procedure and posttest care

• Clean and gently abrade the electrode sites. Peel the backings from the electrodes and apply them to the correct sites, making sure to press the sides and bottom of each electrode firmly to ensure proper adhesion.

• Attach the electrode cable securely to the monitor.

• Position the monitor and case as the patient will wear it and then attach the leadwires to the electrodes.

• Make sure the recorder has a new or fully charged battery, insert the tape, and turn the recorder on.

• The electrode attachment circuit is tested by connecting the recorder to a standard ECG machine. Watch for artifacts while the patient moves normally (stands, sits).

• After the testing period, remove all chest electrodes, and clean the electrode sites.

Precautions

• To eliminate muscle artifact, make sure the lead cable is firmly plugged in. Check to ensure that electrodes aren't placed over large muscle masses such as the pectorals.

Normal findings

When compared with the patient's diary, the normal ECG pattern shows no significant arrhythmias or ST-segment changes. Changes in heart rate normally occur during various activities.

Abnormal findings

Abnormalities of the heart detected by ambulatory ECG include premature ventricular contractions (PVCs), conduction defects, tachyarrhythmias, bradyarrhythmias, and brady-tachyarrhythmia syndrome. Arrhythmias may be associated with dyspnea and central nervous system symptoms, such as dizziness and syncope.

During recovery from an MI, this test can monitor for PVCs to help determine the prognosis and the effectiveness of drug therapy.

ST-T wave changes associated with ischemia may coincide with chest pain or increased patient activity. ST-segment changes associated with an acute

MI require careful study, because smoking, eating, postural changes, certain drugs, Wolff-Parkinson-White syndrome, bundle-branch block, myocarditis, myocardial hypertrophy, anemia, hypoxemia, and abnormal hemoglobin binding can produce a similar tracing on the ECG. Monitoring the MI patient 1 to 3 days before discharge and again 4 to 6 weeks after discharge may detect ST-T wave changes associated with ischemia or arrhythmias; such information aids patient therapy and rehabilitation and refines the prognosis. Monitoring a patient with an artificial pacemaker may detect an arrhythmia, such as bradycardia, that the pacemaker fails to override.

Although ambulatory ECG correlates patient symptoms and ECG changes, it doesn't always identify the symptoms' causes. If initial monitoring proves inconclusive, the test may be repeated.

IMPEDANCE PLETHYSMOGRAPHY

Also called impedance phlebography, this reliable, widely used, noninvasive test measures venous flow in the limbs. Electrodes from a plethysmograph are applied to the patient's leg to record changes in electrical resistance (impedance) caused by blood volume variations that may result from respiration or venous occlusion.

Purpose
• To detect deep vein thrombosis (DVT) in the proximal deep veins of the leg
• To screen patients at high risk for thrombophlebitis
• To evaluate patients with suspected pulmonary embolism (because most pulmonary emboli are complications of DVT in the leg)

Patient preparation
• Explain to the patient that this test helps detect DVT. Inform him that there are no food, fluid, or medication restrictions.
• Explain that the test requires that both legs be tested and that three to five tracings may be made for each leg.
• Tell him who will perform the test and where and that it takes 30 to 45 minutes.
• Assure him that the test is painless and safe.
• Emphasize that accurate testing requires that leg muscles be relaxed and breathing be normal. Reassure him that if he experiences pain that interferes with leg relaxation, a mild analgesic will be administered.
• Just before the test, instruct him to void and to put on a hospital gown.

Procedure and posttest care
• Place the patient in a supine position, elevating the leg to be tested 30 to 35 degrees. To promote venous drainage, the calf should be above heart level.
• Ask him to flex his knee slightly and to rotate his hips by shifting weight to the same side as the leg being tested.
• After the electrodes have been loosely attached to the calf, the pressure cuff is wrapped snugly around the thigh.
• The pressure cuff is inflated to 45 to 60 cm H_2O, allowing full venous distention without interfering with arterial blood flow. Pressure is maintained for 45 seconds or until the tracing stabilizes. (In a patient with reduced arterial blood flow, pressure is maintained for 2 minutes or longer, after which the pressure cuff is rapidly deflated.)
• The strip chart tracing, which records the increase in venous volume following cuff inflation and the decrease in venous volume 3 seconds after defla-

tion, is checked. Then the test is repeated for the other leg. If necessary, three to five tracings for each leg are obtained to confirm full venous filling and outflow; the tracing showing the greatest rise and fall in venous volume is used as the test result.

• If the result is ambiguous, the position of the patient's leg, and cuff and electrode placement are checked.

• After the test, make sure the conductive gel is removed from the patient's skin.

Normal findings

Temporary venous occlusion normally produces a sharp rise in venous volume; release of the occlusion produces rapid venous outflow.

Abnormal findings

When clots in a major deep vein obstruct venous outflow, the pressure in the distal leg (calf) veins rises, and these veins become distended. Such veins are unable to expand further when additional pressure is applied with an occlusive thigh cuff. Blockage of major deep veins also decreases the rate at which blood flows from the leg. If significant thrombi are present in a major deep vein of the lower leg (popliteal, femoral, or iliac), both calf vein filling and venous outflow rate are reduced. Note that this test is less sensitive for calf vein clots or partially occlusive thrombi because these are less likely to cause detectable obstruction in veins below the knee.

CARDIAC CATHETERIZATION

This test involves passing a catheter into the right or left side of the heart.

Catheterization can determine blood pressure and blood flow in the chambers of the heart, permit collection of blood samples, or record films of the heart's ventricles (contrast ventriculography) or arteries (coronary arteriography or angiography).

In catheterization of the left side of the heart, a catheter is inserted into an artery in the antecubital fossa or into the femoral artery through a puncture or cutdown procedure and, guided by fluoroscopy, the catheter is advanced retrograde through the aorta into the coronary artery orifices and left ventricle. Then, a contrast medium is injected into the ventricle, permitting radiographic visualization of the ventricle and coronary arteries and filming (cineangiography) of heart activity.

Catheterization of the left side of the heart assesses the patency of the coronary arteries, mitral and aortic valve function, and left ventricular function. It aids diagnosis of left ventricular enlargement, aortic stenosis and insufficiency, aortic root enlargement, mitral insufficiency, aneurysm, and intracardiac shunt.

In catheterization of the right side of the heart, the catheter is inserted into an antecubital vein or into the femoral vein and advanced through the inferior vena cava or right atrium into the right side of the heart and into the pulmonary artery. Catheterization of the right side of the heart assesses tricuspid and pulmonic valve function and pulmonary artery pressures.

Purpose

• To evaluate valvular insufficiency or stenosis, septal defects, congenital anomalies, myocardial function and blood supply, and cardiac wall motion.

Patient preparation

• Explain to the patient that this test evaluates the function of the heart and its vessels.

• Instruct him to restrict food and fluids for at least 6 hours before the test but to continue his prescribed drug regimen unless directed otherwise.

• Describe the test, including who will perform it, where it will take place, and its duration (2 to 3 hours).

• Inform the patient that he may receive a mild sedative but will remain conscious during the procedure. He'll be strapped to a padded table, and the table may be tilted so his heart can be examined from different angles.

• Warn him that the catheterization team will wear gloves, masks, and gowns to protect him from infection and that the changing X-ray plates and advancing film will make clacking noises.

• Inform him that he will have an I.V. needle inserted in his arm to allow administration of medication. Assure him that the electrocardiography (ECG) electrodes attached to his chest during the procedure will cause no discomfort.

• Tell him that the catheter will be inserted into an artery or vein in his arm or leg; if the skin above the vessel is hairy, it will be shaved and cleaned with an antiseptic.

• Explain that he'll experience a transient stinging sensation when a local anesthetic is injected to numb the incision site for catheter insertion, and he may feel pressure as the catheter moves along the blood vessel; assure him these sensations are normal.

• Inform him that injection of a contrast medium through the catheter may produce a hot, flushing sensation or nausea that quickly passes; instruct him to follow directions to cough or breathe deeply.

• Explain that he'll be given medication if he experiences chest pain during the procedure and may also receive nitroglycerin periodically to dilate coronary vessels and aid visualization. Assure him that complications, such as myocardial infarction or thromboemboli, are rare.

• Make sure the patient or a responsible family member has signed a consent form.

• Check the patient's history for hypersensitivity to shellfish, iodine, or the contrast media used in other diagnostic tests; notify the doctor of any hypersensitivities.

• If the patient is scheduled for catheterization of the right side of the heart, discontinue any anticoagulant therapy to reduce the risk of complications from venous bleeding. If he's scheduled for catheterization of the left side of the heart, begin or continue anticoagulant therapy to reduce the risk of arterial catheter-tip clotting.

• Just before the procedure, tell the patient to void and put on a hospital gown.

Procedure and posttest care

• The patient is placed in the supine position on a tilt-top table and secured by restraints. ECG leads are applied for continuous monitoring and an I.V. line, if not already in place, is started, with dextrose 5% in water or 0.9% sodium chloride solution at a keep-vein-open rate.

• After a local anesthetic is injected at the catheterization site, a small incision or percutaneous puncture is made into the artery or vein, and the catheter is passed through the needle into the vessel; the catheter is guided to the cardiac chambers or coronary arteries using fluoroscopy.

• When the catheter is in place, the contrast medium is injected through it.

• The patient may be asked to cough or breathe deeply. Coughing helps counteract nausea or light-headedness caused by the contrast medium and can correct arrhythmias produced by its depressant effect on the myocardium; deep breathing can ease catheter placement into the pulmonary artery or the wedge position and moves the diaphragm downward, making the heart easier to visualize.

• During the procedure, the patient may be given nitroglycerin to eliminate catheter-induced spasm or measure its effect on the coronary arteries. Ergonovine maleate, a vasoconstrictor, may be administered to provoke coronary artery spasm (a risky but valuable test in Prinzmetal's angina).

• Monitor heart rate and rhythm, respiration, pulse rate, and blood pressure frequently during the procedure.

• After completing the procedure, the catheter is removed, and a pressure dressing is applied to the incision site.

• Monitor vital signs every 15 minutes for the first hour after the procedure, then every hour until stable. If unstable, check every 5 minutes and notify the doctor.

• Observe the insertion site for a hematoma or blood loss, and reinforce the pressure dressing as needed.

• Check the patient's color, skin temperature, and peripheral pulse below the puncture site every 15 minutes for the first hour. Once the patient is stable, check every hour.

• Enforce bed rest for 8 hours. If the femoral route was used for catheter insertion, keep the patient's leg extended for 6 to 8 hours; if the antecubital fossa was used, keep the patient's arm extended for at least 3 hours.

• If medications were withheld before the test, check with the doctor about resuming administration.

• Administer prescribed analgesics.

• Unless the patient is scheduled for surgery, encourage intake of fluids high in potassium, such as orange juice, to counteract the diuretic effect of the contrast medium.

• Make sure a posttest ECG is scheduled to check for possible myocardial damage.

Precautions

• Coagulopathy, impaired renal function, or debilitation usually contraindicates catheterization of both sides of the heart. Unless a temporary pacemaker is inserted to counteract induced ventricular asystole, left bundle-branch block contraindicates catheterization of the right side of the heart.

• If the patient has valvular heart disease, prophylactic antimicrobial therapy may be indicated to guard against subacute bacterial endocarditis.

Normal findings

Cardiac catheterization should reveal no abnormalities of heart chamber size or configuration, wall motion or thickness, direction of blood flow, or valve motion; the coronary arteries should have a smooth and regular outline.

Cardiac catheterization provides information on pressures in the heart's chambers and vessels. Higher pressures than normal are clinically significant; lower pressures, except in shock, usually aren't significant. (See *Normal pressure curves,* page 640, and *Upper limits of normal pressures in cardiac chambers and great vessels in recumbent adults,* page 641.)

Cardiac catheterization also provides information for determining the injection fraction, a comparison of the amount of blood ejected from the left ventricle during systole with the amount of blood remaining in the left ventricle at the end of diastole. A normal ejection fraction (60% to 70%) is a good indicator for successful cardiac surgery.

Abnormal findings

Common abnormalities and defects confirmable by cardiac catheterization

NORMAL PRESSURE CURVES

Chambers of the right side of the heart

Two pressure complexes are represented for each chamber. Complexes at far right in this diagram represent simultaneous recordings of pressures from the right atrium, right ventricle, and pulmonary artery.

Chambers of the left side of the heart

Overall pressure configurations are similar to those of the right side of the heart, but pressures in the left side of the heart are significantly higher because systemic flow resistance is much greater than pulmonary resistance.

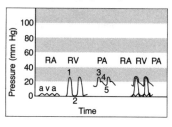

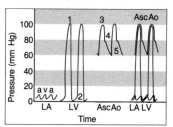

KEY

PA	=	Pulmonary artery
RV	=	Right ventricle
RA	=	Right atrium
a wave	=	Contraction
v wave	=	Passive filling
LV	=	Left ventricle

LA	=	Left atrium
AscAo	=	Ascending aorta
1	=	RV peak systolic pressure
2	=	RV end-diastolic pressure
3	=	PA peak systolic pressure
4	=	PA dicrotic notch
5	=	PA diastolic pressure

include coronary artery disease, myocardial incompetence, valvular heart disease, and septal defects.

In *coronary artery disease,* catheterization shows constriction of the lumen of the coronary arteries. Constriction greater than 70% is especially significant, particularly in proximal lesions. Narrowing of the left main coronary artery and occlusion or narrowing high in the left anterior descending artery is often an indication for revascularization surgery. (This lesion responds best to coronary artery bypass grafting.)

Impaired wall motion can indicate *myocardial incompetence* from coronary artery disease, aneurysm, cardiomyopathy, or congenital anomalies.

Comparing the size of the left ventricle in systole and diastole helps assess the efficiency of cardiac muscle contraction, segmental wall motion, chamber size, and ejection fraction. An ejection fraction under 35% generally increases the risk of complications and decreases the probability of successful surgery.

Valvular heart disease is indicated by a gradient, or difference in pressures, above and below a heart valve. For example, systolic pressure measurements on both sides of a stenotic aortic valve show a gradient across the valve. The higher the gradient, the greater the degree of stenosis. If left ventricular systolic pressure measures 200 mm Hg and aortic systolic pressure

UPPER LIMITS OF NORMAL PRESSURES IN CARDIAC CHAMBERS AND GREAT VESSELS IN RECUMBENT ADULTS

CHAMBER OR VESSEL	PRESSURE (mm Hg)
Right atrium	6 (mean)
Right ventricle	30/6*
Pulmonary artery	30/12* (mean, 18)
Left atrium	12 (mean)
Left ventricle	140/12*
Ascending aorta	140/90* (mean, 105)
Pulmonary artery wedge	Almost identical (±1 to 2 mm Hg) to left atrial mean pressure

* Peak systolic and end-diastolic

measures 120 mm Hg, the gradient across the valve is 80 mm Hg. Because these pressures should normally be equal during systole, when the aortic valve is open, a gradient of this magnitude indicates the need for corrective surgery. Incompetent valves can be visualized during ventriculography by watching retrograde flow of the contrast medium across the valve during systole.

Septal defects (both atrial and ventricular) can be confirmed by measuring blood oxygen content in both sides of the heart. Elevated blood oxygen on the right side indicates a left-to-right atrial or ventricular shunt; decreased oxygen on the left side indicates a right-to-left shunt.

Cardiac output can be measured by analyzing blood oxygen levels in the cardiac chambers. This may be accomplished by drawing blood from cardiac chambers or by injecting contrast medium into the venous circulation and measuring its concentration as it moves past a thermodilution catheter.

HIS BUNDLE ELECTROGRAPHY

His bundle electrography permits measurement of discrete conduction intervals by recording electrical conduction during the slow withdrawal of a bipolar or tripolar electrode catheter from the right ventricle through the bundle of His to the sinoatrial node. The catheter is introduced into the femoral vein, passing through the right atrium and across the septal leaflet of the tricuspid valve.

Possible complications of His bundle electrography include arrhythmias, phlebitis, pulmonary emboli, thromboemboli, and catheter-site hemorrhage.

Purpose
• To diagnose arrhythmias and conduction disturbances
• To determine the need for implanted pacemakers and cardioactive drugs and to evaluate their effects on the conduction system and ectopic rhythms
• To localize disturbances within the atrioventricular conduction system
• To locate the site of a bundle-branch block, especially in asymptomatic patients with conduction disturbances
• To identify an ectopic site that has taken over as pacemaker of the heart
• To evaluate syncope
• To determine the presence and location of accessory conducting structures

Patient preparation
• Explain to the patient that this test evaluates the heart's conduction system.
• Instruct him to restrict food and fluids for at least 6 hours before the test.
• Describe the test, including who will perform it, where it will take place, and its duration (1 to 3 hours).
• Inform him that after the groin area is shaved, a catheter will be inserted into the femoral vein and an I.V. line may be started. Explain that although he'll receive a local anesthetic, he may still feel some pressure upon catheter insertion.
• Assure him that he'll be conscious during the test, and urge him to report any discomfort or pain.
• Make sure the patient or a responsible family member has signed a consent form.
• Check the patient's history, and inform the doctor of any ongoing drug therapy.
• Just before the test, advise the patient to void.

Procedure and posttest care
• The patient is placed in the supine position on a special X-ray table. Limb electrodes and precordial leads are applied for electrocardiogram (ECG) recording during catheterization, and the insertion site is shaved, scrubbed, and sterilized.
• The local anesthetic is injected, and a J-tip electrode is introduced I.V. into the femoral vein (occasionally, into a vein in the antecubital fossa).
• Guided by a fluoroscope, the catheter is advanced until it crosses the tricuspid valve and enters the right ventricle. Then the catheter is slowly withdrawn from the tricuspid area, and recordings of conduction intervals are made from each pole of the catheter, either simultaneously or sequentially.
• After recordings and measurements are completed, the catheter is removed and a pressure dressing is applied to the site.
• Monitor the patient's vital signs every 15 minutes for 1 hour and then hourly for 4 hours. If they're unstable, check every 15 minutes and alert the doctor.
• Observe for shortness of breath, chest pain, pallor, or changes in pulse rate or blood pressure. Enforce bed rest for 4 to 6 hours.
• Check the catheter insertion site for bleeding every 30 minutes for 8 hours; apply a pressure bandage until the bleeding stops.
• Advise the patient that he may resume his usual diet.
• Make sure the patient is scheduled for a 12-lead resting ECG.

Precautions
• Bundle of His electrography is contraindicated in patients with severe coagulopathy, recent thrombophlebitis, or acute pulmonary embolism.
• Be sure emergency medication is available in case the patient develops arrhythmias during the test.
• Have resuscitation equipment at hand.

Reference values

Normal conduction intervals in adults: conduction time from the bundle of His to the Purkinje fibers (H-V interval), 35 to 55 milliseconds; atrioventricular conduction time (A-H interval), 45 to 150 milliseconds; and intra-atrial conduction time (P-A interval), 20 to 40 milliseconds.

Abnormal findings

A prolonged H-V interval can result from acute or chronic disease. A-H interval delays can stem from atrial pacing, chronic conduction system disease, carotid sinus pressure, recent myocardial infarction, and use of certain drugs. P-A interval delays can result from acquired, surgically induced, or congenital atrial disease and atrial pacing.

PULMONARY ARTERY CATHETERIZATION

In this procedure, also known as Swan-Ganz or right-heart catheterization, a balloon-tipped, flow-directed catheter is threaded through the right atrium to provide intermittent occlusion of the pulmonary artery. Pulmonary artery catheterization permits measurement of both pulmonary artery pressure (PAP) and pulmonary artery wedge pressure (PAWP, also known as pulmonary capillary wedge pressure).

The PAWP reading accurately reflects left atrial pressure and left ventricular end-diastolic pressure, although the catheter itself never enters the left side of the heart. Obtaining this information is possible because the heart momentarily relaxes during diastole as it fills with blood from the pulmonary veins; at this instant, the pulmonary vasculature, left atrium, and left ventricle act as a single chamber, and all have identical pressures. Thus, changes in PAP and PAWP reflect changes in left ventricular filling pressure, permitting detection of left ventricular impairment.

The procedure is usually performed at bedside in an intensive care unit. The catheter is inserted through the cephalic vein in the antecubital fossa or the subclavian (sometimes, femoral) vein. In addition to measuring atrial and pulmonary arterial pressures, this procedure evaluates pulmonary vascular resistance and tissue oxygenation, as indicated by mixed venous oxygen content. It should be performed cautiously in patients with left bundle-branch block or implanted pacemakers.

Purpose

• To help assess right and left ventricular failure
• To monitor therapy during treatment of complications of acute myocardial infarction. Such complications may include cardiogenic shock, pulmonary edema, fluid-related hypovolemia and hypotension, systolic murmur, unexplained sinus tachycardia, and various cardiac arrhythmias.
• To monitor fluid status in patients with serious burns, renal disease, or noncardiogenic pulmonary edema after open heart surgery
• To monitor the effects of cardiovascular drugs, such as nitroglycerin and nitroprusside

Patient preparation

• Explain to the patient that this test evaluates heart function and provides information necessary to determine appropriate therapy or to manage fluid status.
• Tell him there are no food or fluid restrictions.
• Describe the test, including who will perform it and where.

• Tell him he'll be conscious during catheterization and may feel transient local discomfort from the administration of the local anesthetic.

• Explain that catheter insertion takes about 30 minutes but that the catheter will remain in place, causing little or no discomfort, for 48 to 72 hours. Tell him that he will need to stay in bed to avoid dislodging the catheter.

• Instruct him to report any discomfort immediately.

• Be sure the patient or a responsible family member has signed a consent form.

Equipment

Pressure cuff; balloon-tipped, flow-directed pulmonary artery catheter; bag of heparinized 0.9% sodium chloride solution (usually 500 ml of 0.9% sodium chloride solution with 500 to 1,000 units of heparin); alcohol sponges; medication-added label; pressure tubing with flush device and disposable transducer; I.V. pole with transducer mount; emergency resuscitation equipment; armboard (for antecubital insertion); lead aprons (if fluoroscope is used during insertion); sutures; 4″ × 4″ gauze pads or other dry occlusive dressing material; prepackaged introducer kit; dextrose 5% in water; shaving materials (optional).

If a prepackaged introducer kit is unavailable, obtain the following: an introducer (one size larger than the catheter), sterile tray containing instruments for procedure, masks, sterile gowns and gloves, povidone-iodine ointment, sutures, two 10-ml syringes, local anesthetic (1% to 2% lidocaine), one 5-ml syringe, 25G ½″ needle, 1″ and 3″ tape.

Procedure and posttest care

• Choose an appropriate flexible pulmonary artery catheter. Catheters used in this test comes in two-lumen to five-lumen modes and in various lengths.

One lumen contains the balloon and the balloon inflation valve.

• Before catheterization, set up the equipment according to the manufacturer's directions and the hospital's procedure.

• If the insertion site is being prepared for a cutdown procedure, prepare the patient's skin and cover it with a sterile drape.

• Assist the patient to a supine position. For antecubital insertion, his arm is abducted with palm upward on an overbed table for support; for subclavian insertion, the patient is placed in the supine position with his head and shoulders slightly lower than his trunk to make the vein more accessible. If the patient can't tolerate the supine position, assist him to semi-Fowler's position. During the test, monitor all pressures with the patient in the same position.

• Check the catheter balloon for defects using sterile technique, and flush all ports to ensure patency.

• The catheter is introduced into the vein percutaneously or by cutdown.

• The catheter is directed to the right atrium, and the catheter balloon is partially inflated so that venous flow carries the catheter tip through the right atrium and tricuspid valve into the right ventricle and into the pulmonary artery.

• Observe the monitor for characteristic waveform changes. Obtain a printout of each stage of catheter insertion.

• Instruct the patient to extend the appropriate arm (or leg, if the catheter is inserted into femoral vein).

• As the catheter is passed into the chambers of the right side of the heart, observe the monitor screen for frequent premature ventricular contractions or tachycardia (including ventricular tachycardia), which may result from right ventricular catheter irritation. If irritation occurs, the catheter may be partial-

ly withdrawn or medication administered to suppress the arrhythmia or right
bundle-branch block.

• To record the PAWP, carefully inflate
the catheter balloon with the specified
amount of air or carbon dioxide, using
no more than 5 cc; the catheter tip will
float into the wedge position, as indicated by an altered waveform on the monitor screen. If a PAWP waveform occurs
with less than the recommended inflation volume, do not inflate the balloon
further.

• After the balloon is inflated, record
the wedge pressure. Then allow the balloon to deflate passively. This allows
the catheter to float back into the pulmonary artery. Observe the monitor
screen for a pulmonary artery waveform.

• Do not overinflate the balloon catheter. Overinflation could distend the pulmonary artery, causing vessel rupture.

• If the balloon can't be fully deflated
after recording the PAWP, do not rein-
flate it unless the doctor is present; balloon rupture may cause a life-threatening air embolism. Check all connections for air leaks that may have pre-
vented balloon inflation, particularly if
the patient is confused or uncooperative.

• When the catheter's correct positioning and function is established, it is sutured to the skin. Antimicrobial ointment and an airtight dressing are applied to the insertion site. A chest X-ray
is obtained to verify catheter placement.

• Set alarms on the electrocardiogram
(ECG) and pressure monitors.

• Monitor vital signs.

• Document PAP waveforms at the beginning of each shift, and monitor them
frequently throughout each shift and
with changes in treatment. Check
PAWP and cardiac output regularly
(usually every 6 hours).

• Take routine aseptic precautions to
prevent infection.

• When the catheter is no longer needed, the balloon is deflated, the dressing
is removed, and the catheter is slowly
withdrawn. The ECG is monitored for
arrhythmias. If any difficulty is encoun-
tered in removing the catheter, stop the
procedure and notify the doctor. In
some institutions, the doctor is required
to remove the catheter.

• After the catheter is withdrawn, apply
pressure and a sterile dressing to the insertion site.

• Observe the catheterization insertion
site for signs of infection, such as redness, swelling, and discharge.

• Watch for complications, such as pulmonary emboli, pulmonary artery perforation, heart murmurs, thrombi, and
arrhythmias.

Precautions

• After each PAWP reading, flush and
recalibrate the monitoring system and
make sure the balloon is completely deflated; if you encounter difficulty in
flushing the system, notify the doctor.

• Maintain 300 mm Hg of pressure in
the pressure bag to permit fluid flow of
3 to 6 ml/hour. Instruct the patient to
extend the appropriate arm (or leg, if
the catheter is inserted in the femoral
vein).

• If a damped waveform occurs, the
catheter may need to be withdrawn a
small amount. Pulmonary infarct may
occur if the catheter is allowed to remain in a wedged position.

• Make sure stopcocks are properly positioned and connections are secure.
Loose connections may introduce air
into the system or cause blood backup,
leakage of deoxygenated blood, or inaccurate pressure readings.

• Be sure the lumen hubs are properly
identified to serve the appropriate catheter ports. Don't add or remove fluids
from the distal pulmonary artery port;

this may cause pulmonary extravasation or damage the artery.

• If the catheter has not been sutured to the skin, tape it securely to prevent dislodgment.

• If the patient shows signs of sepsis, treat the catheter as the source of infection, and send it for culture when removed.

Reference values
Normal pressures:
• Right atrial: 1 to 6 mm Hg
• Systolic right ventricular (RV): 20 to 30 mm Hg
• End-diastolic RV: < 5 mm Hg
• Systolic PAP: 20 to 30 mm Hg
• Diastolic PAP: about 10 mm Hg
• Mean PAP: < 20 mm Hg
• PAWP: 6 to 12 mm Hg
• Left atrial: about 10 mm Hg

Abnormal findings
An abnormally high right atrial pressure can indicate pulmonary disease, failure of the right side of the heart, fluid overload, cardiac tamponade, tricuspid stenosis and insufficiency, or pulmonary hypertension.

Elevated right ventricular pressure can result from pulmonary hypertension, pulmonary valvular stenosis, right ventricular failure, pericardial effusion, constrictive pericarditis, chronic congestive heart failure, or ventricular septal defects.

An abnormally high PAP is characteristic in increased pulmonary blood flow, as occurs in a left-to-right shunt secondary to atrial or ventricular septal defect; increased pulmonary artery resistance, as occurs in pulmonary hypertension or mitral stenosis; chronic obstructive pulmonary disease; pulmonary edema or embolus; and left ventricular failure from any cause. Pulmonary artery systolic pressure is the same as right ventricular systolic pressure. Pulmonary artery diastolic pressure is the same as left atrial pressure, except in patients with severe pulmonary disease causing pulmonary hypertension; in such patients, catheterization is still important diagnostically.

Elevated PAWP can result from left ventricular failure, mitral stenosis and insufficiency, cardiac tamponade, or cardiac insufficiency; depressed PAWP can result from hypovolemia.

Special Function Tests

EYES AND VISION

Visual Acuity Tests

A visual acuity test evaluates the patient's ability to distinguish the form and detail of an object. In this test, the patient is asked to read letters on a standardized visual chart, commonly called the Snellen chart, from a distance of 20′ (6 m). Charts showing the letter E in various positions and sizes are used for young children and other people who can't read. The smaller the symbol the patient can identify, the sharper his visual acuity. A patient's near (reading) vision may be tested as well, using a standardized chart such as the Jaeger card (a card with print in graded sizes). The Snellen test should be performed on all patients with eye complaints. Near-vision testing is routine for those complaining of eyestrain or reading difficulty and for everyone over age 40. Results serve as a baseline for treatments, follow-up examinations, and referrals.

Purpose
• To test distance and near visual acuity
• To identify refractive errors in vision

Patient preparation
• Tell the patient that these tests evaluate distant and near vision.
• Explain that the tests take only a few minutes. If he wears glasses, tell him to bring them to the examination.

Equipment
Standardized eye charts, including the Snellen or E chart and Jaeger card; occlusion supplies, including a hand-held occluder, and disposable tissues for insertion between the patient's eyes and glasses; disposable eyepatches; standard 20′ (6-m) room or equipment to simulate correct distance (mirrors or chart with proportionately reduced letters).

Procedure and posttest care
Distance visual acuity:
• Have the patient sit 20′ away from the eye chart. If he's wearing glasses, tell him to remove them so his uncorrected vision can be tested first.
• Begin with the right eye unless vision in the left eye is known to be more acute. Have the patient occlude the left eye; then ask him to read the smallest line of letters he can see on the chart. Encourage him to try to read lines he can't see clearly because intelligent guesses usually indicate the patient can recognize some of the symbols' details.
• Record the number of the smallest line the patient can read. This number is expressed as a fraction. The numerator is the distance between the patient and the chart; the denominator is the distance from which a patient with normal vision can read the line. The greater the denominator, the poorer the vision.
• If the patient makes an error on a line, record the results with a minus number. For example, if the patient reads the 20/40 line but makes one error, record his vision as 20/40-1. If the patient reads the 20/40 line and one symbol on the following line, record his vision as 20/40+1.
• Have the patient occlude the right eye, and repeat the test for the left eye. To minimize recall, use a different set of symbols or have the patient read the lines backward.
• If the patient wears glasses, test his corrected vision using the same procedure. If he normally wears glasses but doesn't have them with him, note this on the test results.
• In recording the patient's responses, indicate which eye was tested and

whether it was tested with or without corrective lenses.

• If the patient can't read the largest letter on the chart, further testing is necessary.

Near visual acuity:

• Have the patient remove his glasses and occlude the left eye. Ask him to read the Jaeger card at his customary reading distance. Both eyes are tested with and without corrective lenses.

• In reporting near visual acuity, specify both the size of the smallest print legible to the patient and the nearest distance at which reading is possible.

Normal findings

Most charts for distance visual acuity are read at 20′ (6 m). If the patient's vision is normal, results are expressed as 20/20, which means that the smallest symbol he can identify at 20′ is the same symbol a patient with normal vision can identify from the same distance.

If the patient reads the 20/20 line on the Snellen chart, he has normal distance visual acuity. If the denominator is more than 20 — for example, 40 — the patient's visual acuity is less than normal. In this case, it means he reads at 20′ what a person with normal vision can read at 40′ (12 m). A person with visual acuity of 20/200 in the better corrected eye is considered legally blind. Similarly, if the denominator is less than 20, the patient's distance visual acuity is better than normal. For example, 20/15 vision means the patient can read at 20′ what a person with normal visual acuity can see at 15′ (4.5 m).

Normal near visual acuity is usually recorded as 14/14 because standard testing charts, such as the Jaeger card, are generally held 14″ (35 cm) from the patient's eyes. Decreased near visual acuity is indicated by a larger denominator. For example, 14/20 near vision means the patient can read at 14″ what a

person with normal vision can read at 20″ (50 cm).

Normal or better-than-normal visual acuity doesn't necessarily indicate normal vision, however. For example, a visual field defect may be present if the patient consistently misses the letters on one side of all the lines. A field defect is present if the patient states that one or more of the letters disappear or become illegible when he is looking at a nearby letter. Such findings indicate the need for further visual field testing, such as the Amsler grid test and the tangent screen examination.

Abnormal findings

Patients with less-than-normal visual acuity require further testing, including refraction and a complete ophthalmologic examination, to determine whether visual loss is due to injury, disease, or a need for corrective lenses.

SLIT-LAMP EXAMINATION

The slit lamp is an instrument equipped with a special lighting system and a binocular microscope that allows an ophthalmologist to visualize in detail the anterior segment of the eye, including the eyelids, eyelashes, conjunctiva, sclera, cornea, tear film, anterior chamber, iris, crystalline lens, and vitreous face. To evaluate normally transparent or near-transparent ocular fluids and tissues, the size, shape, intensity, and depth of the light source as well as the magnification of the microscope may be altered. If abnormalities are noted, special devices are attached to the slit lamp to allow more detailed investigation.

Purpose

• To detect and evaluate abnormalities of anterior segment tissues and structures.

Patient preparation

• Explain to the patient that this examination evaluates the front portion of the eyes. Tell him that the test takes 5 to 10 minutes and requires that he remain still. Reassure him that the examination is painless.

• If he wears contact lenses, tell him to remove them for the test, unless the test is being performed to evaluate the fit of the lens.

• If the test calls for dilating eyedrops, check the patient's history for adverse reactions to mydriatics or for the presence of narrow-angle glaucoma before administering the drops. Dilating eyedrops are not used in routine eye examinations; however, some diseases require pupillary dilation before slit-lamp examination.

Procedure and posttest care

• Seat the patient in the examining chair. Have him place both feet on the floor and position his chin on the rest and his forehead against the bar. Dim the lights in the room.

• The ophthalmologist examines the patient's eyes starting with the lids and lashes and progressing to the vitreous face, altering light and magnification as necessary. In some cases, a special camera can be attached to the slit lamp to photograph portions of the eye.

• If dilating drops were instilled, tell the patient that his near vision will be blurred for 40 minutes to 2 hours.

Precautions

• Don't instill mydriatic drops into the eyes of a patient who has had a hypersensitivity reaction to them or who has narrow-angle glaucoma.

Normal findings

Slit-lamp examination should reveal no abnormalities of anterior segment tissues and structures.

Abnormal findings

Slit-lamp examination may detect pathologic conditions, such as corneal abrasions and ulcers, lens opacities, iritis, and conjunctivitis, as well as irregularly shaped corneas. A parchment-like consistency of the lid skin, with redness, minor swelling, and moderate itching, may indicate a hypersensitivity reaction. If a corneal abrasion or ulcer is detected, a fluorescein stain may be applied to allow better viewing of the area. If a tearing deficiency is suspected, the ophthalmologist may examine the eye after applying a fluorescein or rose bengal stain; he may also perform the Schirmer tearing test. Some abnormal findings may indicate impending disorders. For example, early-stage lens opacities may signal the development of cataracts.

OPHTHALMOSCOPY

Ophthalmoscopy allows magnified examination of the vascular and nerve tissue of the fundus, including the optic disk, retinal vessels, macula, and retina. This test is conducted with either a direct or indirect ophthalmoscope — one of the most important diagnostic tools in ophthalmology. Generally, examiners use the direct ophthalmoscope — a small, hand-held instrument consisting of a light source, viewing device, reflecting device to channel light into the patient's eyes, and spherical lenses to correct refractive error of the patient or examiner. If a slit lamp is not available, the examiner may also use the ophthalmoscope to examine the patient's cornea, iris, and lens.

Purpose
• To detect and evaluate eye disorders as well as ocular manifestations of systemic disease

Patient preparation
• Explain to the patient that this test permits examination of the back of the eye.
• Describe the test, including who will perform it, where it will take place, and its duration (usually less than 5 minutes).
• Advise him that eyedrops may be instilled to dilate the pupils for a clearer examination, but reassure him that he'll feel no discomfort during the test.
• When using eyedrops, check the patient's history for previous use of dilating eyedrops, indications of possible hypersensitivity, and narrow-angle glaucoma.

Procedure and posttest care
• Routine examination of the ocular media and fundus is usually conducted without dilating the pupil if there is sufficient light in the ophthalmoscope and room lighting is subdued. However, if indicated, two instillations of mydriatic eyedrops are usually necessary to achieve maximum dilation.
• Have the patient sit upright in the examination chair. Dim the room lights to keep irregular reflections from interfering with the examination.
• The examiner sits about 2′ (60 cm) away from the patient and slightly to his right. The examination begins with the patient's right eye. The ophthalmoscope is held in the right hand in front of the examiner's right eye. A small adjustment near the forefinger allows him to select different lenses quickly.
• The patient is told to look straight ahead at a specific object 20′ (6 m)

away, for example, a large symbol on a standardized vision chart, for the duration of the examination.
• Remaining on the patient's right side, the examiner moves forward until he is within 6″ (15 cm) of the patient. At this point, he directs the light beam into the pupil and looks for the red reflex (red reflection from the fundus), which is visible without magnification. Then he focuses on the optic disk, noting its size, shape, and color.
• Next, the examiner looks for a white central depression in the optic disk — the physiologic cup — and observes the retinal vessels that emerge from the disk.
• Finally, the examiner focuses on the macula — a yellowish depression slightly below the center of the optic disk — and its center, the fovea.
• The procedure is then repeated for the left eye.

Precautions
• Don't administer dilating eyedrops to a patient who has a history of hypersensitivity reactions to them or who has narrow-angle glaucoma.
• Make sure the patient maintains fixation throughout the procedure.

Normal findings
With the beam of light from the ophthalmoscope directed into the patient's pupil, the red reflex should be visible through the aperture. The slightly oval optic disk, measuring approximately 1.5 mm vertically, lies to the nasal side of the fundus center. Although its color varies widely, it's usually pink, with darker edges at its nasal border. The physiologic cup, a pale depression in the center of the optic disk, varies widely in size; it tends to be larger in patients with myopia and smaller in those with hyperopia.

The semitransparent retina surrounds the optic disk. Branching out from the disk are the retinal vessels, including venules and the slightly smaller arterioles. Vessel diameter progressively decreases with distance from the optic disk. Retinal arterioles generally have a medium red color; venules appear dark red or blue.

The macula is the most darkly pigmented area of the retina. In its center lies a small, even darker spot — the fovea. A tiny light reflex can be seen at the center of the fovea, caused by reflection of the ophthalmoscopic light from the concave inner surface of the area.

Abnormal findings

An absent or diminished red reflex may be due to gross corneal lesions, dense opacities of the aqueous or vitreous (such as from blood following hemorrhage), cataracts, or detached retina. A cloudy vitreous that obscures the fundus may be caused by inflammatory disease of the optic disk, retina, or uvea. Fundal lesions should be sketched or photographed for further study.

Optic neuritis causes the optic disk to become elevated and more vascular; small hemorrhages may also occur. Optic nerve atrophy causes the disk to appear white. Papilledema, which may result from increased intracranial pressure, causes abnormal elevation of the disk, blurring of disk margins, engorged vessels, and hemorrhages.

In glaucoma, the physiologic cup may appear enlarged and gray, with white edges. A milky-white retina characterizes the acute phase of a central retinal artery occlusion; the fovea, in contrast to the ischemic macula, appears as a bright red spot. Central retinal vein occlusion is marked by widespread retinal hemorrhaging, patches of white exudate, and disk elevation.

Retinal detachments appear as gray elevated areas, possibly with areas of red vascular choroid exposed by retinal tears. A choroidal tumor appears as a dark lesion.

The integrity of retinal vessels is commonly evaluated to aid diagnosis of systemic disease. Hypertension, for example, causes vasospasm, sclerosis, and eventual occlusion of retinal arterioles, leading to retinal edema and hemorrhage and papilledema. Diabetes mellitus may be complicated by retinal fibroses, patches of white exudate, and microaneurysms. Other systemic disorders present similar findings.

Interpretation of ophthalmoscopic findings depends largely on the examiner's knowledge and experience, because an abnormality can arise from several sources. After an ophthalmoscopic evaluation, referral for complete medical evaluation may be necessary.

EARS AND HEARING

OTOSCOPY

Otoscopy is the direct visualization of the external auditory canal and the tympanic membrane through an otoscope. It's a basic part of any physical examination of the ear and should be performed before other auditory or vestibular tests. Otoscopy indirectly provides information about the eustachian tube and the middle ear cavity.

Purpose

• To detect foreign bodies, cerumen, or stenosis in the external canal
• To detect external or middle ear pathology, such as infection or tympanic membrane perforation

COMMON ABNORMALITIES OF THE TYMPANIC MEMBRANE

ABNORMAL FINDINGS	USUAL CAUSE
Bright red color	Inflammation (otitis media)
Yellowish color	Pus or serum behind the tympanic membrane (acute or chronic otitis media)
Bubble behind tympanic membrane	Serous fluid in middle ear (serous otitis media)
Absent light reflection	Bulging tympanic membrane (acute otitis media)
Absent or diminishing landmarks	Thickened tympanic membrane (chronic otitis media, otitis externa, or tympanosclerosis)
Oval dark areas	Perforated or scarred tympanic membrane (otitis media or trauma)
Very prominent malleus	Retracted tympanic membrane (nonfunctional eustachian tube)
Reduced mobility	Stiffened middle ear system (serous otitis media or, less frequently, middle ear adhesions)

Patient preparation
• Describe the procedure to the patient, and explain that this test permits visualization of the ear canal and eardrum.
• Reassure him that the examination is usually painless and takes less than 5 minutes to perform.
• Tell him that his ear will be pulled upward and backward to straighten the canal, to facilitate insertion of the otoscope.

Procedure and posttest care
• When assembling the otoscope, test the lamp and be sure to attach the largest speculum that fits comfortably into the patient's ear.
• With the patient seated, tilt his head slightly away from you so that the ear to be examined is pointed upward.
• Pull the auricle up and back (pull downward if the patient is under age 3); insert the otoscope gently into the ear canal, with a downward and forward motion. If insertion is difficult, replace the speculum with a smaller one.
• Look through the lens, and gently advance the speculum until you see the eardrum. Obtain as full a view as possible, and note redness, swelling, lesions, discharge, foreign bodies, or scaling in the canal. Check the eardrum for color, contours, and perforation.
• Locate the malleus, partially visible through the translucent tympanic membrane. Examine the membrane itself and the surrounding fibrous rim (annulus).

Precautions
• The otoscope should be advanced slowly and gently through the medial portion of the ear canal to avoid irritation of the canal lining, especially if an infection is suspected.
• Continuing to insert an otoscope against resistance may cause perforation or damage.

Normal findings

The normal tympanic membrane is thin, translucent, shiny, and slightly concave. It appears as a pearl-gray or pale pink disk that reflects light in its inferior portion. The short process, manubrium mallei, and umbo should be visible but not prominent.

Abnormal findings

Scarring, discoloration, or retraction or bulging of the tympanic membrane indicates pathology. (See *Common abnormalities of the tympanic membrane,* page 653.) Movement of the tympanic membrane in tandem with respiration suggests abnormal patency of the eustachian tube.

TUNING FORK TESTS

The Weber, Rinne, and Schwabach tuning fork tests are quick, valuable screening tools for detecting hearing loss and obtaining preliminary information as to its type. The Weber test determines whether a patient lateralizes the tone of the tuning fork to one ear. The Rinne test compares air and bone conduction in both ears. The Schwabach test compares the patient's bone conduction response with that of the examiner, who is assumed to have normal hearing.

Test results are most reliable when a low-frequency tuning fork is used; however, results are not definitive because they depend on subjective factors, such as the examiner's ability to strike the fork with equal force each time and the patient's ability to report audible tones correctly.

Results of the Weber test may be misleading, and the Rinne test frequently doesn't detect a mild conductive hearing loss (10 to 35 dB). Thus, abnormal test results require confirmation by pure tone audiometry.

Purpose

• To screen for or confirm hearing loss
• To help distinguish conductive from sensorineural hearing loss

Patient preparation

• Describe the procedure to the patient and explain that these tests help detect and assess hearing loss. Tell him who will conduct the tests and reassure him that they are painless and take only a few minutes.
• Explain that concentration and prompt responses are essential for accurate testing. Have the patient use hand signals to indicate whether a tone is louder in his right ear or left ear and also when he stops hearing the tone.
• Inform him that tuning fork tests are not definitive and that further testing may be necessary to confirm abnormal results.

Procedure and posttest care

• Using a low-frequency tuning fork (256 or 512 Hz), practice achieving a consistent tone by gently striking a prong against your elbow or the heel of your hand, by stroking the prongs upward, or by pinching them together.
• When performing each test, be careful to strike the tuning fork with equal force. Hold the fork at its base to allow the prongs to vibrate freely. Record the name of the test, the result, and the vibrating frequency of the tuning fork.
   Weber test:
• Vibrate the fork and place its base on the midline of the patient's skull at the forehead.
• Ask the patient if the tone is louder in his left ear or his right ear or is equally loud in both. Describe the results as Weber left, Weber right, or Weber midline according to his response.

Rinne test:

• Test bone conduction by holding the tuning fork between your thumb and index finger and placing the base of the vibrating fork against the patient's mastoid process.

• Test air conduction by moving the vibrating prongs next to (not touching) the external ear. Ask the patient which location has the louder or longer sound. Repeat the procedure for the other ear.

• Record results as Rinne-positive if the air-conducted sound is heard louder or longer or Rinne-negative if the bone-conducted sound is heard louder or longer.

Schwabach test:

• Holding the tuning fork between thumb and index finger, place the base of the vibrating tuning fork against the patient's left mastoid process and ask if he hears the tone. If affirmative, immediately place the tuning fork on your left mastoid process and listen for the tone.

• Alternate the tuning fork between the patient's left mastoid process and your own until one of you stops hearing the sound. Record the length of time the patient continues to hear it.

• Repeat the procedure on the right mastoid process.

• Refer the patient for further audiologic testing if tuning fork tests suggest a hearing loss.

Normal findings

A patient with normal hearing will respond to the Weber test by hearing the same tone equally loud in both ears (Weber-midline result); to the Rinne test by hearing the air-conducted tone louder or longer than the bone-conducted tone (Rinne-positive result); and to the Schwabach test by hearing the tone for the same duration as the examiner.

Abnormal findings

In the Weber test, lateralization of the tone to one ear suggests a conductive loss on that side or a sensorineural loss on the other side. Lateralization results if the tone is louder in one ear (Stenger effect) or reaches one ear sooner (phase effect). If one ear has a sensorineural loss, the Stenger effect causes lateralization to the unaffected ear; if one ear has a conductive loss, either the Stenger or phase effect produces lateralization to that ear. If a patient's hearing loss is unilateral, the Weber test may suggest the type of loss. If a patient's hearing loss is bilateral, this test may help to identify the ear with the better bone conduction.

In the Rinne test, hearing the bone-conducted tone louder or longer than the air-conducted tone indicates a conductive loss. In unilateral hearing loss, the tone may be heard louder when conducted by bone, but in the opposite ear; this is a false-negative Rinne test result. A sensorineural loss is indicated when the sound is heard louder by air conduction.

In the Schwabach test, hearing the tone longer than the examiner hears it suggests a conductive loss; conversely, a shorter duration indicates a sensorineural loss. A conductive loss attenuates (decreases the energy of) air-conducted sound in a room with ambient noise, enabling patients with this type of loss to hear bone-conducted sound longer than the examiner can hear such sound.

If the patient has abnormal results upon retesting, pure tone audiometry is indicated to confirm hearing loss and determine its type and severity.

PURE TONE AUDIOMETRY

This test, performed with an audiometer, provides a record of the thresholds (the lowest intensity levels) at which a patient can hear a set of test tones introduced through earphones or a bone conduction (sound) vibrator. The energy of these pure tones is concentrated at discrete frequencies. The octave frequencies between 125 and 8,000 Hz are used to obtain air conduction thresholds; frequencies between 250 and 4,000 Hz, to obtain bone conduction thresholds.

Comparison of air and bone conduction thresholds can suggest a conductive, sensorineural, or mixed hearing loss but does not indicate the cause of the loss; further audiologic and vestibular tests and X-rays may be needed. Pure tone audiometry results may also suggest a need to consult an audiologist for evaluation of communication difficulties. (See *Pure tone audiograms*.)

Pure tone audiometry is indicated for any patient requiring quantitative hearing assessment. There are no contraindications; however, results depend on the cooperation of the patient. Acoustic emission test results may provide additional information.

Purpose
• To determine the presence, type, and degree of hearing loss
• To assess communication abilities and rehabilitation needs

Patient preparation
• Describe the procedure to the patient, and explain that this test helps to determine the presence and degree of hearing loss. Explain who will perform the test, where it will take place, and that it takes about 20 minutes.
• Tell him that each ear will be tested, beginning with the ear with the better hearing acuity. Explain that he will hear tones at various intensities and that he should signal (or press the response button) each time he hears the tone. Emphasize that he should respond even if the tone is very faint.
• Just before the test, ask the patient to remove any jewelry or apparel that obstructs proper earphone placement.

• If he has been exposed to loud noises (loud enough to cause tinnitus or make face-to-face communication difficult) within the past 16 hours, postpone the test.

Equipment
Otoscope, calibrated audiometer with earphones and bone conduction vibrator. Note that the test environment must be quiet; a sound-treated room is recommended.

Procedure and posttest care
• The patient's ear canal is checked with the otoscope for impacted cerumen.
• The examiner presses a finger on the auricle and then the tragus to rule out possible closure of the ear canal under pressure from the earphones. If the canal tends to close, a stiff-walled plastic tube is carefully inserted into the canal. This modification is recorded on the audiogram.
• The earphones are positioned properly and the headband is tightened.
• A test tone is presented to the patient's better ear.

In air conduction testing:
• A 1,000 Hz tone is presented to the patient's better ear. Intensity of the tone is decreased in 10-dB steps until the patient fails to respond. Then intensity is increased in 5-dB steps until he hears the tone again. Sequences of 10-dB decrements and 5-dB increments are repeated until the patient responds to at least two of three presentations at a single level. The threshold level is the lowest decibel level at which the response rate is at least 50%.
• Using this procedure, tones are presented to the better ear in this order: 1,000 Hz, 2,000 Hz, 4,000 Hz, 8,000 Hz, 1,000 Hz, 500 Hz, and 250 Hz.
• After testing the better ear, the other ear is tested.

In bone conduction testing:
• The earphones are removed and the vibrator is placed on the mastoid pro-

PURE TONE AUDIOGRAMS

Sensorineural hearing loss depresses both air (circles) and bone (arrows) conduction thresholds to about the same degree. No matter how sound vibrations reach the inner ear, they must be transmitted to higher neural centers through the sensorineural system.

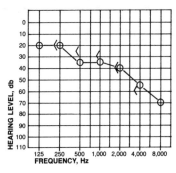

Conductive hearing loss, produced by interference with the conductive mechanism, depresses air conduction thresholds but generally doesn't affect bone thresholds.

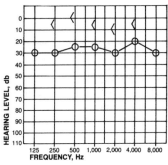

Mixed hearing loss involves abnormal air and bone conduction thresholds. Air conduction thresholds demonstrate a greater loss due to a conductive lesion.

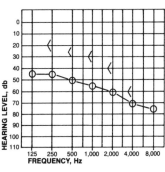

cess of the better ear (the auricle shouldn't touch the vibrator).

• Ascending and descending tones are presented, as in air conduction testing, using 250, 500, 1,000, 2,000, and 4,000 Hz.

In both tests:

• If test results are inconsistent or if they are confounded by possible crossover, refer the patient to an audiologist.

RELATING PURE TONE AVERAGE TO HEARING LOSS AND SPEECH AUDIBILITY

PURE TONE AVERAGE	DEGREE OF HEARING LOSS	SPEECH AUDIBILITY
0 to 25 dB	Normal limits	No significant difficulty
26 to 40 dB	Mild	Difficulty with faint or distant speech
41 to 55 dB	Moderate	Difficulty with conversational speech
56 to 70 dB	Moderately severe	Speech must be loud; difficulty with group conversation
71 to 90 dB	Severe	Difficulty with loud speech; understands only shouted or amplified speech
91 dB +	Profound	May not understand amplified speech

Precautions

• Any modifications of standard testing procedure — for example, inserting a plastic tube to prevent ear canal collapse — must be recorded on the audiogram.

Normal findings

The normal range of hearing sensitivity is 0 to 25 dB for adults and 0 to 15 dB for children. However, normal test results do not rule out pathology; a mild middle ear infection or other pathology may exist without interfering with auditory function.

Abnormal findings

The pure tone average — the average of pure tone air conduction thresholds obtained at 500 Hz, 1,000 Hz, and 2,000 Hz — quantifies the degree of hearing loss. When these three thresholds vary widely, the mean of the best two — the Fletcher average — indicates the degree of hearing loss.

The relationship between threshold responses for air and bone conduction tones determines the type of hearing loss. In *sensorineural* loss, both thresholds are depressed; in *conductive* loss, air thresholds are depressed, but bone thresholds are unchanged; and in *mixed* hearing loss, both thresholds are abnormal, with air conduction more depressed than bone conduction. (See *Relating pure tone average to hearing loss and speech audibility*.)

SCREENING TESTS FOR VESTIBULAR AND CEREBELLAR DYSFUNCTION

A patient who reports dizziness, disequilibrium, or nystagmus may undergo screening tests for vestibular or cerebellar dysfunction. These tests evaluate balance and coordination as the patient performs various maneuvers with eyes open and closed. Abnormal results suggest the need for further evaluation.

Purpose
• To help identify vestibular or cerebellar disorders affecting the entire body (balance tests)
• To help identify vestibular or cerebellar disorders affecting the arms (coordination tests)

Patient preparation
• Explain to the patient that these tests help identify neurologic dysfunction and that some evaluate his sense of balance.
• Describe the tests, including who will perform them, where they will take place, and their duration.
• Reassure him that there is no danger of falling during the test.
• Assess the patient's general physical condition, which will influence his ability to perform the maneuvers.
• Check the patient's history for use of drugs that affect the central nervous system and for recent alcohol consumption.

Procedure and posttest care
To assess balance:
Ask the patient to perform as many of the following test maneuvers as possible, and observe for a tendency to sway or fall:
• Have him stand with his feet together, arms at his sides, and eyes open for 20 seconds. Tell him to maintain this position for another 20 seconds with eyes closed.
• Have the patient stand on one foot for 5 seconds, then on the other foot for 5 seconds; instruct him to repeat the procedure with eyes closed.
• Tell him to stand heel to toe for 20 seconds with eyes opened, then to maintain the same position with eyes closed for another 20 seconds.
• Instruct him to walk forward and backward in a straight line, heel to toe, first with eyes open, then with eyes closed.

To assess coordination:
• With the patient seated and facing you, hold out your index finger at his shoulder level.
• Tell him to touch your finger with his right index finger.
• Then tell him to lower his arm and close his eyes. Have him touch your finger again.
• The patient then repeats the entire maneuver using his left index finger.
• Failure to perform this maneuver rapidly and accurately is called past-pointing. Observe the degree and direction of past-pointing.

Precautions
• Any of these tests may be contraindicated if the patient is physically incapable of performing some or all of the required maneuvers.
• When assessing balance, the examiner should stand close to the patient to catch him if he falls. If the patient is tall or heavy, someone should assist the examiner.

Normal findings
During tests for balance, a healthy person maintains his balance with eyes open and closed. When testing coordination, a healthy person touches the examiner's finger with eyes open and closed; past-pointing does not occur.

Abnormal findings
A peripheral vestibular lesion can cause swaying or falling in the direction opposite to the nystagmus when the patient's eyes are closed; a cerebellar lesion causes swaying or falling when eyes are open or closed.

A labyrinthine disorder can lead to past-pointing in the opposite direction to the nystagmus when the patient's eyes are closed; a cerebellar lesion can lead to past-pointing when eyes are open or closed; and a lateralized lesion can lead to past-pointing only with the arm on the affected side.

GASTROINTESTINAL FUNCTION

ESOPHAGEAL ACIDITY TEST

This test evaluates the competence of the lower esophageal sphincter — the major barrier to reflux — by measuring intraesophageal pH with an electrode attached to a manometric catheter.

Purpose
• To evaluate competence of the lower esophageal sphincter
• To evaluate gastric reflux in patients who complain of persistent heartburn with or without regurgitation

Patient preparation
• Explain to the patient that this test evaluates the function of the sphincter between the esophagus and stomach. Tell him to fast and avoid smoking after midnight before the test.
• Describe the test, including who will perform it, where it will take place, and its duration (about 45 minutes).
• Tell him that a tube will be passed through his mouth into his stomach and that he may experience slight discomfort, a desire to cough, or a gagging sensation.
• Just before the test, check the patient's pulse rate and blood pressure, and instruct him to void.
• Withhold antacids, anticholinergics, cholinergics, adrenergic blockers, alco-

hol, corticosteroids, cimetidine, and reserpine for 24 hours before the test. If these medications must be continued, note this on the laboratory slip.

Procedure and posttest care
• After the patient is placed in high Fowler's position, the catheter with electrode is introduced into his mouth.
• The patient is instructed to swallow when the electrode reaches the back of his throat.
• Using a manometer, the examiner locates the lower esophageal sphincter. The catheter is raised ¼" (2 cm). The patient is told to perform Valsalva's maneuver or lift his legs to stimulate reflux. After he does so, intraesophageal pH is measured.
• If the pH is normal, the catheter is passed into the patient's stomach. A prescribed acid solution is instilled over 3 minutes. Then the catheter is raised ¼" above the sphincter. Again, the patient is asked to perform Valsalva's maneuver or lift his legs and intraesophageal pH is measured.
• After the test, tell the patient he may resume his usual diet and restart any medications withheld for the test.
• Provide lozenges if the patient complains of a sore throat.

Precautions
• During insertion, the electrode may enter the trachea instead of the esophagus. If the patient develops cyanosis or paroxysms of coughing, move the electrode immediately.
• Observe the patient closely during intubation because arrhythmias may develop.
• Clamp the catheter before removing it, to prevent aspiration of fluid into the lungs.

Reference values
The pH of the esophagus normally exceeds 5.0.

Abnormal findings

An intraesophageal pH of 1.5 to 2.0 indicates gastric acid reflux resulting from incompetence of the lower esophageal sphincter. Persistent reflux leads to chronic reflux esophagitis. Additional studies, such as barium swallow and esophagogastroduodenoscopy, are necessary to diagnose and determine the extent of esophagitis.

ACID PERFUSION TEST

Also called the Bernstein test, this procedure helps to distinguish pain caused by esophagitis (burning epigastric or retrosternal pain that radiates to the back or arms) from pain caused by angina pectoris or other disorders. It requires perfusion of saline and acidic solutions into the esophagus through a nasogastric (NG) tube.

Purpose

• To distinguish chest pains caused by esophagitis from those caused by cardiac disorders

Patient preparation

• Tell the patient that this test helps determine the cause of chest pain. Explain the following food, fluid, and medication restrictions: no antacids for 24 hours, no food for 12 hours, and no fluids or smoking for 8 hours before the test.

• Describe the test, including who will perform it, where it will take place, and its duration (about 1 hour).

• Explain that the test involves passing a tube through his nose into the esophagus and that he may experience some discomfort, a desire to cough, or a gagging sensation during intubation.

• Tell him that liquid is slowly perfused through the tube into the esophagus and

that he should immediately report any pain or burning during perfusion.

• Just before the test, check the patient's pulse rate and blood pressure. Ask him if he's experiencing any chest pain and, if so, to describe it.

Procedure and posttest care

• After the patient is seated, insert an NG tube that has been marked 12″ (30 cm) from the tip into his stomach. Attach a 20-ml syringe to the tube and aspirate stomach contents. Withdraw the tube into the esophagus (to the 12″ mark).

• Hang labeled containers of 0.9% sodium chloride solution and a prescribed acidic solution on an I.V. pole behind the patient; then connect the NG tube to I.V. tubing.

• Open the line from the 0.9% sodium chloride solution, and infuse it at a rate of 60 to 120 drops/minute. Continue perfusion for 5 to 10 minutes.

• Ask the patient if he's experiencing any discomfort and record his response.

• Without the patient's knowledge, close the line from the 0.9% sodiium chloride solution and open the line from the acidic solution. Infuse the acidic solution into the esophagus at the same rate used for the saline solution. Continue perfusion for 30 minutes.

• Ask the patient again if he's experiencing any discomfort, and record his response.

• If the patient experiences discomfort, close the line from the acidic solution immediately and open the line from the 0.9% sodium chloride solution. Continue to perfuse this solution until the discomfort subsides.

• Unless perfusion of the acidic solution is to be repeated, the NG tube is withdrawn.

• If the patient complains of pain or burning, administer an antacid. If he complains of a sore throat, provide soothing lozenges or an ice collar.

• Tell him he may resume his usual diet and any medications withheld for the test.

Precautions

• The acid perfusion test is contraindicated in patients with esophageal varices, congestive heart failure, acute myocardial infarction, or other cardiac disorders.

• During intubation, make sure the tube enters the esophagus and not the trachea. Withdraw the tube immediately if the patient develops cyanosis or paroxysmal coughing.

• Assess the patient's pulse rate and rhythm to detect any arrhythmias that may develop.

• Clamp the tube before removing it to prevent aspiration of fluid into the lungs.

Normal findings

Absence of pain or burning during perfusion of either solution indicates a healthy esophageal mucosa.

Abnormal findings

In patients with esophagitis, the acidic solution causes pain or burning, whereas the 0.9% sodium chloride solution should produce no adverse effects. Occasionally, both solutions cause pain in patients with esophagitis, but they may cause no pain in patients with asymptomatic esophagitis.

RENAL FUNCTION

UROFLOWMETRY

This simple noninvasive test uses a uroflowmeter to detect and evaluate dysfunctional voiding patterns. The uroflowmeter, contained in a funnel into which the patient voids, measures flow rate (volume of urine voided per second), continuous flow (time of measurable flow), and intermittent flow (total voiding time, including any interruptions).

Types of uroflowmeters include rotary disc, electromagnetic, spectrophotometric, and gravimetric systems. The gravimetric system, which weighs urine as it's voided and plots the weight against time, is the simplest to use.

Purpose

• To evaluate lower urinary tract function
• To demonstrate bladder outlet obstruction

Patient preparation

• Explain to the patient that this test evaluates his pattern of urination. Advise him not to urinate for several hours before the test and to increase fluid intake so he'll have a full bladder and a strong urge to void.

• Describe the test, including who will perform it, where it will take place, and its duration (10 to 15 minutes).

• Instruct him to remain still while voiding during the test to help ensure accurate results. Assure him that he will have complete privacy during the test.

• Discontinue drugs that may affect bladder and sphincter tone, such as urinary spasmolytics and anticholinergics.

Equipment

Commode chair with funnel containing a uroflowmeter or beaker to hold urine, transducer, start and flow cables, data recording module.

Procedure and posttest care

• Check cable connections prior to the test.

- Remind the patient not to strain while voiding.
- Ask a male patient to void while standing and a female patient to void while sitting.
- The patient pushes the start button on the commode chair, counts for 5 seconds (1 one-thousand, 2 one-thousand, and so on), and voids. When finished, he counts for 5 seconds and pushes the button again. The volume of urine voided is then recorded and plotted as a curve over the time of voiding. The patient's position and the route of fluid intake (oral or I.V.) are noted.
- Instruct the patient to resume any medications that were discontinued for the test.

Precautions
- The transducer must be level, and the beaker must be centered beneath the funnel.
- The beaker must be large enough to hold all urine; overflow can invalidate results and damage the transducer.

Reference values
Flow rate varies according to the patient's age and sex and the volume of urine voided. The chart below lists minimum volumes needed to obtain adequate recordings.

AGE	MINIMUM VOLUME (ml)	MALE (ml/sec)	FEMALE (ml/sec)
4 to 7	100	10	10
8 to 13	100	12	15
14 to 45	200	21	18
46 to 65	200	12	15
66 to 80	200	9	10

CHARACTERISTIC UROFLOW CURVES

A. Normal curve

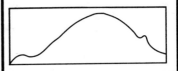

B. Normal peak with hesitancy may result from the patient's embarrassment or advanced age.

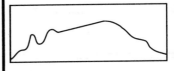

C. High peak flow over short voiding time may indicate incontinence.

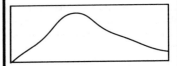

D. Many peaks over normal voiding time indicate abdominal straining and detrusor muscle weakness.

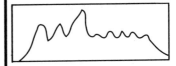

E. Low peak with long voiding time and urethral dribbling indicates obstruction.

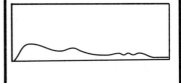

Abnormal findings

Increased flow rate indicates reduced urethral resistance, possibly associated with external sphincter dysfunction. A high peak on the curve plotted over the voiding time indicates decreased outflow resistance, possibly due to stress incontinence. Decreased flow rate indicates outflow obstruction or hypotonia of the detrusor muscle. More than one distinct peak in a normal curve indicates abdominal straining, possibly due to pushing against an obstruction to empty the bladder. (See *Characteristic uroflow curves,* page 663.)

CYSTOMETRY

Cystometry assesses the bladder's neuromuscular function by measuring efficiency of the detrusor muscle reflex, intravesical pressure and capacity, and the bladder's reaction to thermal stimulation. Because results from cystometry can be ambiguous, they are typically supported by results of other tests, such as cystourethrography, excretory urography, and voiding cystourethrography.

Purpose

• To evaluate detrusor muscle function and tonicity
• To help determine the cause of bladder dysfunction
• To detect the cause of involuntary bladder contractions in an unstable bladder

Patient preparation

• Explain to the patient that this test evaluates bladder function. Tell him that there are no food or fluid restrictions for the test.
• Describe the procedure, including who will perform it, where it will take place, and its duration (about 40 minutes unless additional tests are ordered).
• Tell him that he'll feel a strong urge to void during the test and may feel embarrassed or uncomfortable. Provide reassurance.
• Make sure that the patient or a responsible family member has signed a consent form.
• Check the patient's medication history for drugs, such as antihistamines, that may affect test results.
• Just before the procedure, tell the patient to urinate.

Equipment

Four-channel gas cystometer, set of catheters.

Procedure and posttest care

• Place the patient in the supine position on the examination table.
• A catheter is passed into the bladder to measure residual urine level. Any difficulty with insertion of the catheter may reflect meatal or urethral obstruction.
• To test the patient's response to thermal sensation, 30 ml of room temperature physiologic saline solution or sterile water is instilled into the bladder. Then an equal volume of warm fluid (110° to 115° F [43.3° to 46.1° C]) is instilled into the bladder. The patient is asked to report his sensations, such as the need to void, nausea, flushing, discomfort, and a feeling of warmth.
• After the fluid is drained from the patient's bladder, the catheter is connected to the cystometer, and 0.9% sodium chloride solution, sterile water, or gas (usually carbon dioxide) is slowly introduced into the bladder. The flow of gas is adjusted automatically to the desired reading (100 ml/minute) by a four-channel cystometer.
• The patient is asked to indicate when he *first* feels an urge to void, then when he feels he *must* urinate. The related

CYSTOMETRY: NORMAL AND ABNORMAL FINDINGS

Because cystometry assesses micturition and vesical function, it can aid diagnosis of neurogenic bladder dysfunction. The five main types of neurogenic bladder, as presented in the following chart, result from lesions of the central or peripheral nervous system. Uninhibited neurogenic bladder results from a lesion to the upper motor neuron and causes frequent, often uncontrollable micturition in the presence of even a small amount of urine. A complete upper motor neuron lesion characterizes reflex neurogenic bladder and causes total loss of conscious sensation and vesical control.

FEATURE OR RESPONSE	NORMAL BLADDER FUNCTION	UNINHIBITED NEUROGENIC BLADDER (mild spastic, incomplete upper motor neuron)	REFLEX NEUROGENIC BLADDER (complete spastic, complete upper motor neuron)
Micturition			
Start	+	+/0	0
Stop	+	0	0
Residual urine	0	0	+
Vesical sensation	+	+	0
First urge to void	150 to 200 ml	E (< 150 ml)	0
Bladder capacity	400 to 500 ml	↓	↓
Bladder contractions	0	+	+
Intravesical pressure	L	↑	↑
Bulbocavernosus reflex	+	+	↑
Saddle sensation	+	+	0
Bethanechol test (exaggerated response)	0	+	0
Ice water test	+	+	+
Anal reflex	+	+	+
Heat sensation and pain	+	+	0

KEY: + Present/Positive   ↑ Increased   V Variable   D Delayed
　　　 0 Absent/Negative   ↓ Decreased   E Early   L Low

(continued)

CYSTOMETRY: NORMAL AND ABNORMAL FINDINGS *(continued)*

In autonomous neurogenic bladder, a lower motor neuron lesion produces a flaccid bladder that fills without contracting. The patient can't perceive bladder fullness or initiate and maintain urination without applying external pressure. Lower motor neuron lesions can cause sensory or motor paralysis of the bladder. In sensory paralysis, the patient experiences chronic urine retention because he can't perceive bladder fullness. In motor paralysis, the patient has full sensation but can't initiate or control urination.

FEATURE OR RESPONSE	AUTONOMOUS NEUROGENIC BLADDER (flaccid, incomplete lower motor neuron)	SENSORY PARALYTIC BLADDER (lower motor neuron—sensory)	MOTOR PARALYTIC BLADDER (lower motor neuron—motor)
Micturition			
Start	0	+	0
Stop	0	+	0
Residual urine	+	+	+ +
Vesical sensation	0	0	+
First urge to void	0	D	+
Bladder capacity	↑	↑ (< 1,000 ml)	V
Bladder contractions	0	0	0
Intravesical pressure	↓	↓	L
Bulbocavernosus reflex	0	+/↓/0	+
Saddle sensation	0	V	+
Bethanechol test (exaggerated response)	+	+	0
Ice water test	0	0	0
Anal reflex	0	V	V
Heat sensation and pain	0	0	+

KEY: + Present/Positive ↑ Increased V Variable D Delayed
     0 Absent/Negative ↓ Decreased E Early L Low

pressure and volume are automatically plotted on the graph.

• When the bladder reaches its full capacity, the patient is asked to urinate so that the maximal intravesical voiding pressure can be recorded. The patient's bladder is then drained and, if no additional tests are required, the catheter is removed.

• Administer a sitz bath or warm tub bath if the patient experiences discomfort after the test.

• Measure fluid intake and urine output for 24 hours. Watch for hematuria that persists after the third voiding and for signs of sepsis (such as fever or chills).

Precautions

• Cystometry is contraindicated in patients with acute urinary tract infections because uninhibited contractions may cause erroneous readings and the test may lead to pyelonephritis and septic shock.

• Tell the patient not to strain at voiding; it can cause ambiguous cystometric readings.

• If the patient has a spinal cord injury that has caused motor impairment, transport him on a stretcher so that the test can be performed without transferring him to the examination table.

Normal findings

For characteristic findings, see *Cystometry: Normal and abnormal findings,* pages 665 and 666.

EXTERNAL SPHINCTER ELECTROMYOGRAPHY

This procedure measures electrical activity of the external urinary sphincter using needle electrodes inserted in perineal or periurethral tissues, electrodes in an anal plug, or skin electrodes. Skin electrodes are the most common method used.

Incontinence is the primary indication for external sphincter electromyography. Often, the test is done with cystometry and voiding urethrography as part of a full urodynamic study.

Purpose

• To assess neuromuscular function of the external urinary sphincter

• To assess the functional balance between bladder and sphincter muscle activity

Patient preparation

• Explain to the patient that this test will determine how well his bladder and sphincter muscles work together.

• Describe the test, including who will perform it, where it will take place, and its duration (30 to 60 minutes).

• If skin electrodes are used, describe their placement and explain the preparatory procedure, which may include shaving a small area.

• If needle electrodes are used, describe their placement and explain that the discomfort is equivalent to an intramuscular injection. Assure him that he'll feel discomfort only during insertion. Explain that wires connect the needles to the recorder but that there is no danger of electric shock. If the patient is a woman, tell her that she may notice slight bleeding at the first voiding.

• If an anal plug is used, tell the patient that only the tip of the plug will be inserted into the rectum and that he may feel fullness but no discomfort.

• Check the patient's medications. Note if he is taking cholinergic or anticholinergic drugs.

Equipment

Electromyograph and recorder; skin, needle, or anal plug electrodes; ground plate; electrode paste; tape; antiseptic solution such as povidone-iodine; preparatory tray if shaving is necessary.

Procedure and posttest care
• Place the patient in the lithotomy position for electrode placement. After placement, he may lie supine. Record the patient's position, type of electrode and measuring equipment used, and any other tests done at the same time.
• Electrode paste is applied to the ground plate, which is taped to the thigh and grounded. The electrodes are positioned and connected to electrode adaptors.
• When using skin electrodes, clean the skin with antiseptic solution and then dry the area. If necessary, shave a small area to optimize electrode contact. Apply electrode paste and tape the electrodes in place. For women, electrodes are placed in the periurethral area; for men, in the perineal area beneath the scrotum.
• To position needle electrodes on a male patient, a gloved finger is inserted in the rectum. The needles and wires are inserted 1½″ (3.75 cm) through the perineal skin toward the apex of the prostate. Needle positions are 3:00 and 9:00. While the needles are withdrawn, the wires are held in place and then taped to the thigh.
• To position needle electrodes on a female patient, the labia are spread, and the needles and wires inserted periurethrally at 2:00 and 10:00. The needles are withdrawn and the wires taped to the thigh.
• When using anal plug electrodes, the plug is lubricated and the patient is asked to breathe slowly and deeply and to relax the anal sphincter to accommodate the plug by bearing down.
• After electrode placement, the adapters are inserted in the preamplifier and recording starts. The patient is asked to alternately relax and tighten the sphincter.

• When sufficient data have been recorded, the patient is asked to bear down and exhale while anal plug and needle electrodes are removed. Remove skin electrodes gently to avoid pulling hair and tender skin.
• Clean and dry the area before the patient dresses.
• In some urodynamic laboratories, cystometrography is done with electromyography for thorough evaluation of detrusor and sphincter coordination.
• For women, watch for and report hematuria after the first voiding if needle electrodes were used.
• Watch for and report symptoms of mild urethral irritation, such as dysuria, hematuria, and urinary frequency.
• Advise the patient to take a warm sitz bath, and encourage fluid intake of 2 to 3 liters/day unless contraindicated.

Precautions
• Insert needles quickly to minimize discomfort.
• The ground plate should be properly applied and anchored; wires should be taped securely to prevent artifacts.

Normal findings
The electromyogram shows increased muscle activity when the patient tightens the external urinary sphincter and decreased muscle activity when he relaxes it. If electromyography and cystometrography are performed simultaneously, a comparison of results shows that muscle activity of the normal sphincter increases as the bladder fills. During voiding and bladder contraction, muscle activity decreases as the sphincter relaxes. This comparison is important in assessing external sphincter efficiency and functional balance between bladder and sphincter muscle activity.

Abnormal findings
Failure of the sphincter to relax or increased muscle activity during voiding

demonstrates detrusor-external sphincter dyssynergia. Confirmation of such muscle activity by electromyography may indicate neurogenic bladder, spinal cord injury, multiple sclerosis, Parkinson's disease, or stress incontinence.

MISCELLANEOUS TESTS

TENSILON TEST

This test involves careful observation of the patient following I.V. administration of Tensilon (edrophonium chloride), a rapid, short-acting anticholinesterase that improves muscle strength by increasing muscle response to nerve impulses.

Purpose
• To aid diagnosis of myasthenia gravis (results of other procedures, including electromyography, may supplement Tensilon test findings)
• To aid in differentiation between myasthenic and cholinergic crises
• To monitor oral anticholinesterase therapy

Patient preparation
• Explain to the patient that this test helps determine the cause of muscle weakness.
• Describe the test, including who will perform it, where it will take place, and its duration (15 to 30 minutes).
• Don't describe the exact response that will be evaluated; foreknowledge can affect the test's objectivity.
• Explain to the patient that a small tube will be inserted into a vein in his arm

and that a drug will be administered periodically. He will be asked to make repetitive muscle movements and his reactions will be observed. To ensure accuracy, the test may be repeated several times.
• Advise him that Tensilon may produce some unpleasant adverse effects, but reassure him that someone will be with him at all times and that any reactions will quickly disappear.
• Check the patient's history for medications that affect muscle function, anticholinesterase therapy, drug hypersensitivities, and respiratory disease. Withhold medications. If the patient is receiving anticholinesterase therapy, note this on the requisition slip; include the time of the most recent dose.

Equipment
Standard: 10 mg Tensilon, 0.4 mg atropine (may be prescribed for patients with respiratory distress), one tuberculin and one 3-ml syringe, I.V. infusion set, 50-ml bag of I.V. solution (dextrose 5% in water [D_5W] or 0.9% sodium chloride solution), tape, tourniquet, alcohol swabs.
Emergency: 0.5 to 1 mg atropine I.V. for cholinergic crisis, 0.5 to 2 mg neostigmine methylsulfate I.V. for myasthenic crisis (may be repeated up to a total of 5 mg), extra tuberculin and 3-ml syringes (for atropine or neostigmine injections), resuscitation equipment, including a tracheotomy tray.

Procedure and posttest care
• Begin I.V. infusion of D_5W or 0.9% sodium chloride solution.
• When performing the test on an adult patient suspected of having myasthenia gravis, 2 mg of Tensilon are administered initially. Before the rest of the dose is administered, the doctor may want to fatigue the muscles by asking the patient to perform various exercises, such as looking up until ptosis de-

velops, counting to 100 until his voice diminishes, or holding his arms above his shoulders until they drop. When the muscles are fatigued, the remaining 8 mg of Tensilon are administered over 30 seconds.

• The test may begin with a placebo injection to evaluate the patient's muscle response more accurately. The placebo isn't necessary if cranial muscles are being tested because cranial strength can't be simulated voluntarily.

• After Tensilon is administered, the patient is asked to perform repetitive muscle movements, such as opening and closing his eyes and crossing and uncrossing his legs. Closely observe the patient for improved muscle strength. If muscle strength doesn't improve within 3 to 5 minutes, the test may be repeated.

• To differentiate between myasthenic crisis and cholinergic crisis, 1 to 2 mg of Tensilon is infused. After infusion, continually monitor the patient's vital signs. Watch closely for respiratory distress, and be prepared to provide respiratory assistance.

• If muscle strength doesn't improve, more Tensilon is infused cautiously, 1 mg at a time up to a maximum of 5 mg, and the patient is observed for distress.

• Neostigmine is administered immediately if the test demonstrates myasthenic crisis; atropine is administered for cholinergic crisis.

• To evaluate oral anticholinesterase therapy, 2 mg of Tensilon is infused 1 hour after the patient's last dose of the anticholinesterase. The patient is observed carefully for adverse effects and muscle response.

• After Tensilon administration, the I.V. line is kept open at a rate of 20 ml/hour until all the patient's responses have been evaluated.

• When the test is complete, discontinue the I.V., and check the patient's vital signs.

• Check the puncture site for hematoma, excessive bleeding, and swelling.

• Tell the patient to resume any medications withheld for the test.

Precautions

• Because of the systemic adverse reactions Tensilon may produce, this test may be contraindicated in patients with hypotension, bradycardia, apnea, and mechanical obstruction of the intestine or urinary tract.

• Patients with respiratory ailments such as asthma should receive atropine during the test to minimize adverse reactions to Tensilon.

• Stay with the patient during the test, and observe him closely for adverse reactions.

• Keep resuscitation equipment handy in case of respiratory failure.

Normal findings

People who don't have myasthenia gravis usually develop fasciculation in response to Tensilon. The doctor must interpret the responses carefully to distinguish a normal person from one with myasthenia gravis.

Abnormal findings

If the patient has myasthenia gravis, muscle strength should improve promptly after administration of Tensilon. The degree of improvement depends on the muscle group being tested; however, improvement is usually obvious within 30 seconds. Although the maximum benefit lasts only several minutes, lingering effects may persist — up to 2 hours in a patient receiving prednisone, for example. All patients with myasthenia gravis show improved muscle strength in this test; some patients, however, respond slightly and the test may need to be repeated to confirm the diagnosis.

The test may yield inconsistent results if myasthenia gravis affects only ocular muscles, as in mild or early forms of the disorder. It may produce a positive response in motor neuron disease and in some neuropathies and my-opathies. However, the response is usu-ally less dramatic and less consistent than in myasthenia gravis.

Patients in myasthenic crisis show brief improvement in muscle strength after Tensilon administration. Patients in cholinergic crisis (anticholinesterase overdose) may experience exaggerated muscle weakness. If Tensilon increases the patient's muscle strength without increasing adverse effects, oral anticho-linesterase therapy can be increased. If Tensilon decreases muscle strength in a person with severe adverse reactions, therapy should be reduced. If the test shows no change in muscle strength and only mild adverse effects occur, therapy should remain the same.

COLD STIMULATION TEST FOR RAYNAUD'S SYNDROME

This test demonstrates Raynaud's syndrome by recording temperature changes in the patient's fingers before and after submersion in ice water. Note that digital blood pressure recording or examination of the arteries in the arm and palmar arch should precede this test to rule out arterial occlusive disease.

Purpose
• To detect Raynaud's syndrome, an arteriospastic disorder characterized by intense vasospasm of the small cutane-ous arteries and arterioles of the hands after exposure to cold or stress

Patient preparation
• Explain to the patient that this test de-tects a vascular disorder.

• Tell him that he need not restrict food or fluids for the test.
• Describe the test, including who will perform it, where it will take place, and its duration (20 to 40 minutes).
• Explain that he may experience dis-comfort when his hands are briefly im-mersed in ice water.
• Have him remove his watch and other jewelry and encourage him to relax.

Procedure and posttest care
• To minimize extraneous environmen-tal stimuli, make sure the test room is neither too warm nor too cold.
• Tape a thermistor to each of the patient's fingers and record the temperature.
• Have the patient submerge his hands in an ice-water bath for 20 seconds.
• When he removes his hands from the water, record the temperature of his fin-gers immediately and every 5 minutes thereafter until it returns to the baseline temperature.

Precautions
• The cold stimulation test is contrain-dicated in patients with gangrenous fin-gers or open, infected wounds.

Normal findings
Normally, digital temperature returns to baseline levels within 15 minutes.

Abnormal findings
If digital temperature takes longer than 20 minutes to return to the baseline level, Raynaud's syndrome is indicated. Its be-nign form, Raynaud's disease, requires no specific treatment and has no serious se-quelae. Its more serious form, Raynaud's phenomenon, is associated with connec-tive tissue disorders — scleroderma, sys-temic lupus erythematosus, and rheuma-toid arthritis — which may not be clini-cally apparent for several years. However, distinguishing between Raynaud's phe-nomenon and Raynaud's disease is diffi-cult.

PULMONARY FUNCTION TESTS

Pulmonary function tests (volume and capacity tests) are a series of measurements that evaluate ventilatory function through spirometric measurements; they are performed on patients with suspected pulmonary dysfunction.

Of the seven tests to determine volume, tidal volume (V_T) and expiratory reserve volume (ERV) are direct spirographic measurements; minute volume (MV), CO_2 response, inspiratory reserve volume (IRV), and residual volume (RV) are calculated from the results of other pulmonary function tests; and thoracic gas volume (TGV) is calculated from body plethysmography.

Of the pulmonary capacity tests, vital capacity (VC), inspiratory capacity (IC), functional residual capacity (FRC), total lung capacity (TLC), and forced expiratory flow (FEF) may be measured directly or calculated from the results of other tests. Forced vital capacity (FVC), flow-volume curve, forced expiratory volume (FEV), peak expiratory flow rate (PEFR), and maximal voluntary ventilation (MVV) are direct spirographic measurements. The diffusing capacity for carbon monoxide (DL_{CO}) is calculated from the amount of carbon monoxide exhaled.

Purpose

- To determine the cause of dyspnea
- To assess the effectiveness of specific therapeutic regimens
- To determine whether a functional abnormality is obstructive or restrictive
- To measure pulmonary dysfunction
- To evaluate a patient before surgery

Patient preparation

- Explain to the patient that these tests evaluate pulmonary function. Instruct him to eat only a light meal before the tests and not to smoke for 4 to 6 hours before the tests.
- Describe the tests and equipment. Explain who will perform the tests, where they will take place, and their duration.
- Describe the operation of a spirometer.
- Advise him that the accuracy of the tests depends on his cooperation.
- Assure him that the procedures are painless and that he will be able to rest between tests.
- Inform the laboratory if the patient is taking an analgesic that depresses respiration.
- Withhold bronchodilators and intermittent positive-pressure breathing therapy.
- Just before the test, tell the patient to void and to loosen tight clothing. If he wears dentures, tell him to wear them during the test to help form a seal around the mouthpiece.

Equipment

For direct spirography: spirometer, recording paper, nose clip, mouthpiece.

For body plethysmography: body plethysmograph, mouthpiece, transducer.

Procedure and posttest care

- When measuring *tidal volume,* tell the patient to breathe normally into the mouthpiece 10 times.
- When measuring *expiratory reserve volume,* tell the patient to breathe normally for several breaths and then to exhale as completely as possible.
- When measuring *vital capacity,* tell the patient to inhale as deeply as possible and to exhale into the mouthpiece as completely as possible. This procedure is repeated three times, and the test result showing the largest volume is used.

INTERPRETING PULMONARY FUNCTION TESTS

MEASUREMENT OF PULMONARY FUNCTION	METHOD OF CALCULATION	IMPLICATIONS
Tidal volume (VT): amount of air inhaled or exhaled during normal breathing	Determine the spirographic measurement for 10 breaths, and then divide by 10.	Decreased V_T may indicate restrictive disease and requires further testing, such as full pulmonary function studies or chest X-rays.
Minute volume (MV): total amount of air expired per minute	Multiply V_T by the respiratory rate.	Normal MV can occur in emphysema; decreased MV may indicate other diseases, such as pulmonary edema. Increased MV can occur with acidosis, increased CO_2, decreased PaO_2, exercise, and low compliance states.
CO_2 response: increase or decrease in MV after breathing various CO_2 concentrations	Calculate by plotting changes in MV against increasing inspired CO_2 concentrations.	Reduced CO_2 response may occur in emphysema, myxedema, obesity, hypoventilation syndrome, and sleep apnea.
Inspiratory reserve volume (IRV): amount of air inspired over above-normal inspiration	Subtract V_T from inspiratory capacity.	Abnormal IRV alone doesn't indicate respiratory dysfunction; IRV decreases during normal exercise.
Expiratory reserve volume (ERV): amount of air exhaled after normal expiration	Direct spirographic measurement	ERV varies, even in healthy people, but usually decreases in the obese.
Residual volume (RV): amount of air remaining in the lungs after forced expiration	Subtract ERV from functional residual capacity (FRC).	RV greater than 35% of total lung capacity after maximal expiratory effort may indicate obstructive disease.
Vital capacity (VC): total volume of air that can be exhaled after maximum inspiration	Direct spirographic measurement, or add V_T, IRV, and ERV.	Normal or increased VC with decreased flow rates may indicate any condition that causes a reduction in functional pulmonary tissue, such as pulmonary edema. Decreased VC with normal or increased flow rates may indicate decreased respiratory effort resulting from neuromuscular disease, drug overdose, or head injury; decreased thoracic expansion; or limited movement of the diaphragm.

(continued)

INTERPRETING PULMONARY FUNCTION TESTS *(continued)*

MEASUREMENT OF PULMONARY FUNCTION	METHOD OF CALCULATION	IMPLICATIONS
Inspiratory capacity (IC): amount of air that can be inhaled after normal expiration	Direct spirographic measurement, or add IRV and V_T.	Decreased IC indicates restrictive disease.
Thoracic gas volume (TGV): total volume of gas in lungs from both ventilated and nonventilated airways	Body plethysmography	Increased TGV indicates air trapping, which may result from obstructive disease.
Functional residual capacity (FRC): amount of air remaining in lungs after normal expiration	Nitrogen washout, helium dilution technique, or add ERV and RV.	Increased FRC indicates overdistention of lungs, which may result from obstructive pulmonary disease.
Total lung capacity (TLC): total volume of the lungs when maximally inflated	Add V_T, IRV, ERV, and RV; or FRC and IC; or VC and RV.	Low TLC indicates restrictive disease; high TLC indicates overdistended lungs caused by obstructive disease.
Forced vital capacity (FVC): the amount of air exhaled forcefully and quickly after maximum inspiration	Direct spirographic measurement; expressed as a percentage of the total volume of gas exhaled	Decreased FVC indicates flow resistance in respiratory system from obstructive disease, such as chronic bronchitis, or from restrictive disease, such as pulmonary fibrosis.
Flow-volume curve (also called flow-volume loop): greatest rate of flow (V_{max}) during FVC maneuvers versus lung volume change	Direct spirographic measurement at 1-second intervals; calculated from flow rates (expressed in liters/second) and lung volume changes (expressed in liters) during maximal inspiratory and expiratory maneuvers	Decreased flow rates at all volumes during expiration indicate obstructive disease of the small airways, such as emphysema. A plateau of expiratory flow near TLC, a plateau of inspiratory flow at mid-VC, and a square wave pattern through most of VC indicate obstructive disease of large airways. Normal or increased peak expiratory flow rate, decreased flow with decreasing lung volumes, and markedly decreased VC indicate restrictive disease.
Forced expiratory volume (FEV): volume of air expired in the 1st, 2nd, or 3rd second of FVC maneuver	Direct spirographic measurement; expressed as percentage of FVC	Decreased FEV_1, and increased FEV_2 and FEV_3 may indicate obstructive disease; decreased or normal FEV_1 may indicate restrictive disease.

INTERPRETING PULMONARY FUNCTION TESTS *(continued)*

MEASUREMENT OF PULMONARY FUNCTION	METHOD OF CALCULATION	IMPLICATIONS
Forced expiratory flow (FEF): average rate of flow during middle half of FVC	Calculated from the flow rate and the time needed for expiration of middle 50% of FVC	Low FEF (25% to 75%) indicates obstructive disease of the small and medium-sized airways.
Peak expiratory flow rate (PEFR): V_{max} during forced expiration	Calculated from flow-volume curve, or by direct spirographic measurement, using a pneumotachometer or electronic tachometer with a transducer to convert flow to electrical output display	Decreased PEFR may indicate a mechanical problem, such as upper airway obstruction, or obstructive disease. PEFR is usually normal in restrictive disease but decreases in severe cases. Because PEFR is effort-dependent, it's also low in a person who has poor expiratory effort or doesn't understand the procedure.
Maximal voluntary ventilation (MVV), also called maximum breathing capacity: greatest volume of air breathed per unit of time	Direct spirographic measurement	Decreased MVV may indicate obstructive disease; normal or decreased MVV may indicate restrictive disease such as myasthenia gravis
Diffusing capacity for carbon monoxide (DL_{CO}): milliliters of carbon monoxide diffused per minute across the alveocapillary membrane	Calculated from analysis of amount of carbon monoxide exhaled compared with amount inhaled	Decreased DL_{CO} due to a thickened alveocapillary membrane occurs in interstitial pulmonary diseases, such as pulmonary fibrosis, asbestosis, and sarcoidosis; DL_{CO} is reduced in emphysema because of the loss of alveocapillary membrane.

• When measuring *inspiratory capacity,* tell the patient to breathe normally for several breaths and then to inhale as deeply as possible.

• When measuring *functional residual capacity,* tell the patient to breathe normally into a spirometer that contains a known concentration of an insoluble gas (usually helium or nitrogen) in a known volume of air. After a few breaths, the concentrations of gas in the spirometer and in the lungs reach equilibrium. Then the point of equilibrium and the concentration of gas in the spirometer are recorded.

• When measuring *thoracic gas volume,* the patient is put in an airtight box (or *body plethysmograph*) and told to breathe through a tube connected to a transducer. At end-expiration the tube is occluded, the patient is told to pant, and changes in intrathoracic and plethysmographic pressures are measured. The results are used to calculate total TGV and FRC.

• When measuring *forced vital capacity* and *forced expiratory volume,* tell the patient to inhale as slowly and deeply as possible and then exhale into the mouthpiece as quickly and completely as possible. This procedure is repeated three times, and the largest volume is recorded. The volume of air expired at 1 second (FEV_1), at 2 seconds (FEV_2), and at 3 seconds (FEV_3) during all three repetitions is also recorded.

• When measuring *maximal voluntary ventilation,* tell the patient to breathe into the mouthpiece as quickly and deeply as possible for 15 seconds.

• When measuring *diffusing capacity for carbon monoxide,* the patient inhales a gas mixture with a low concentration of carbon monoxide, and then holds his breath for 10 seconds before exhaling.

• After the tests, tell the patient to resume his usual diet and daily activities as well as any medications withheld for the test.

Precautions

• Pulmonary function tests are contraindicated in patients with acute coronary insufficiency, angina, or recent myocardial infarction. During such tests, watch for respiratory distress, changes in pulse rate and blood pressure, and coughing or bronchospasm.

Reference values

Normal values are predicted for each patient based on age, height, weight, and sex and are expressed as a percentage. Usually, results are considered abnormal if they're less than 80% of these values.

The following reference values can be calculated at bedside with a portable spirometer: V_T, 5 to 7 ml/kg of body weight; ERV, 25% of VC; IC, 75% of VC; FEV_1, 83% of VC (after 1 second); FEV_2, 94% of VC (after 2 seconds); and FEV_3, 97% of VC (after 3 seconds).

Abnormal findings

See *Interpreting pulmonary function tests,* pages 673 to 675.

D-XYLOSE ABSORPTION

This test evaluates patients with symptoms of malabsorption, such as weight loss and generalized malnutrition, weakness, and diarrhea. D-xylose is a pentose sugar that's absorbed in the small intestine without the aid of pancreatic enzymes, passes through the liver without being metabolized, and is excreted in the urine. Because of its absorption in the small intestine without digestion, measurement of D-xylose in the urine and blood indicates the absorptive capacity of the small intestine.

Purpose

• To aid differential diagnosis of malabsorption

• To determine the cause of malabsorption syndrome

Patient preparation

• Tell the patient that this test helps evaluate digestive function by analyzing blood and urine specimens after ingestion of a sugar solution.

• Explain that he must fast overnight before the test and that he will have to fast and remain in bed during the test.

• Explain that several blood samples will be taken; tell him who will perform the venipunctures and when.

• Advise him that he may experience some discomfort from the needle punctures and the pressure of the tourniquet but that collecting each blood sample takes less than 3 minutes.

• Inform him that all his urine will be collected for 5 or 24 hours.

• Withhold medications that alter test results, such as aspirin and indomethacin. Record any medications the patient is taking on the laboratory slip.

Procedure and posttest care

• Perform a venipuncture to obtain a fasting blood sample. Collect a first-voided morning urine specimen. Label these specimens, and send them to the laboratory immediately to serve as a baseline.

• Give the patient 25 g of D-xylose dissolved in 8 oz (240 ml) of water, followed by an additional 8 oz of water. If the patient is a child, administer 0.5 g of D-xylose per pound of body weight, up to 25 g. Record the time of D-xylose ingestion.

• For an adult, draw a blood sample 2 hours after D-xylose ingestion; for a child, 1 hour after ingestion. Collect the sample in a 10-ml *red-top* tube. Occasionally, a 5-hour sample may be drawn to support the findings of the 1- or 2-hour sample.

• Collect and pool all urine during the 5 or 24 hours following D-xylose ingestion.

• If a hematoma develops at the venipuncture site, apply warm soaks.

• Observe the patient for abdominal discomfort or mild diarrhea caused by D-xylose ingestion.

• After the test, tell him he may resume his usual diet and any medications withheld for the test.

Precautions

• The patient must have adequate renal function for the absorption and excretion of D-xylose.

• Handle the blood collection tubes gently to prevent hemolysis.

• Tell the patient not to contaminate the urine specimens with toilet tissue or stool.

• Be sure to collect all urine and refrigerate the specimen during the collection period.

• Because patients age 65 and older and those with borderline or elevated creatinine levels tend to have low 5-hour urine levels but normal 24-hour levels, the doctor will have to establish the length of the collection period. At the end of the collection period, send the urine specimen to the laboratory immediately.

• Maintain bed rest and withhold food and fluids (other than D-xylose) throughout the test period.

Reference values

Normal values are as follows:

• Children: blood concentration greater than 30 mg/dl in 1 hour; urine, 16% to 33% of ingested D-xylose excreted in 5 hours

• Adults under age 65: blood concentration 25 to 40 mg/dl in 2 hours; urine, more than 4 g excreted in 5 hours

• Adults over age 65: blood concentration 25 to 40 mg/dl in 2 hours; urine, more than 3.5 g excreted in 5 hours and more than 5 g excreted in 24 hours.

Abnormal findings

Depressed blood and urine D-xylose levels most commonly result from malabsorption disorders affecting the proximal small intestine, such as sprue and celiac disease. However, depressed levels may also result from regional enteritis involving the jejunum, Whipple's disease, multiple jejunal diverticula, myxedema, diabetic neuropathic diarrhea, rheumatoid arthritis, alcoholism, severe congestive heart failure, and ascites.

DEXAMETHASONE SUPPRESSION TEST

This test requires administration of dexamethasone, an oral steroid. Dexamethasone suppresses levels of circulating adrenal steroid hormones in normal people, but fails to suppress them in patients with Cushing's syndrome and some forms of depression.

Purpose
• To diagnose Cushing's syndrome
• To aid diagnosis of clinical depression

Patient preparation
• Explain the purpose of the test.
• Inform the patient that the test requires two blood samples drawn after administration of dexamethasone. Tell him who will perform the venipuncture and when and that he may experience transient discomfort from the needle puncture and the pressure of the tourniquet.
• Restrict food and fluids for 10 to 12 hours before the test.
• Many medications, including corticosteroids, oral contraceptives, lithium, methadone, aspirin, diuretics, morphine, and monoamine oxidase inhibitors, can affect the accuracy of test results. If possible, don't administer any of these medications after midnight the night before the test.

Procedure and posttest care
• On the first day, give the patient 1 mg of dexamethasone at 11 p.m. On the next day, collect blood samples at 4 p.m. and 11 p.m. More frequent sampling may increase the likelihood of measuring a nonsuppressed cortisol peak.

• If a hematoma develops at the venipuncture site, apply warm soaks.

Reference values
A cortisol level of 5 μg/dl (140 nmol/L) or greater indicates failure of dexamethasone suppression.

Abnormal findings
A normal test result doesn't rule out major depression, but an abnormal result strengthens a clinically based diagnosis. Failure of suppression occurs in patients with Cushing's syndrome, severe stress, and depression that's likely to respond to treatment with antidepressants.

INDEX

Antithyroid antibodies, **256-257**
incidence of, 257t
Aortic insufficiency, 6-7
Aortic stenosis, 7
Aplastic anemias, 7
Aplitest, 289-290
Appendicitis, 7
APTT. *See* Activated partial thromboplastin time.
Arginine test, **184-185**
Argininosuccinicaciduria, chromatographic identification of, 331t
Arm fractures, 7
Arterial blood gas analysis, **121-123**
Arterial blood gases, 121-124
Arterial ischemia index, 479
Arterial occlusive disease, 7
Arthrocentesis, 394, 396-398
Arthrography, **562-564**
Arthroscopy, **467, 469-470**
of the knee, 468i
Arylsulfatase A, **306**
Asbestosis, 8
Ascariasis, 8
Ascending contrast phlebography, **515-517**
Ascorbic acid. *See* Vitamin C.
ASO. *See* Antistreptolysin-O test.
Aspartate aminotransferase, **135-136**
Aspergillosis, 8
implications of serology tests in, 280t
Asphyxia, 8
AST. *See* Aspartate aminotransferase.
Asthma, 8
Asystole, 8
Ataxia-telangiectasia, 8
Atelectasis, 8-9
Atopic dermatitis, 9
Atrial fibrillation, 9
Atrial flutter, 9
Atrial septal defect, 9
Atrial tachycardia, 9-10

Atrionatriuretic peptides. *See* Plasma atrial natriuretic factor.
Atriopeptins. *See* Plasma atrial natriuretic factor.
Atrioventricular block, third-degree, 10
Australia antigen. *See* Hepatitis B surface antigen.
Autoantibodies, 251-264

B

Bacterial meningitis antigen, **281-282**
Barium enema, **521-524**
Barium swallow, **517-518**
Basal cell carcinoma, 10
Basal gastric secretion test, **361-363**
Basophils
influence of disease on, 102t
reference values for, 101i
B cell deficiency, 10
Bee sting, 39
Bell's palsy, 10
Bence Jones protein, **327-328**
Benign prostatic hyperplasia, 10-11
Bernstein test, 661-662
Berylliosis, 11
Beta-subunit assay for hCG, 218-219
β-Hydroxybutyrate, **173-174**
Bile duct carcinoma, 26
Biliary ducts
fluoroscopic examination of, 527-529
radiographic study of, 529-530
Biliary system, ultrasonography of, **481-483**
Biliary tract computed tomography, **573-575**
Bilirubin, serum, **166-167**
Bilirubin, urine, **341, 343**
as aid in identifying cause of jaundice, 342t
Biopsy, 426-450
Black widow spider bite, 39-40

Bladder, radiographic examination of, 543-545, 555-556
Bladder cancer, 11
Blastomycosis, 11
implications of serology tests in, 279t
Bleeding time, **104-105**
methods of measuring, 104-105
Blepharitis, 11
Blood chemistry tests, 121-176
Blood culture, **413-414**
Blood transfusion reaction, 11
Blood urea nitrogen, **164-165**
Blunt abdominal injuries, 11
Blunt chest injuries, 12
B-lymphocyte assay, **239-240**
Body section roentgenography, 509-510
Bone biopsy, **437-438**
Bone marrow aspiration and biopsy, **438-440**
implications of findings of, 441-442t
Bone scan, **600-601**
Bone tumor, primary malignant, 12
Botulism, 12
Brain abscess, 12
Breast, radiographic examination of, 558-559
Breast biopsy, **432-434**
Breast cancer, 12
Breast engorgement, 45
Bronchiectasis, 12
Bronchitis, chronic, 12-13
Bronchography, **510-512**
Bronchoscopy, **453-455**
Brown recluse (violin) spider bite, 39
Brucellosis, 13
Brush biopsy, 449
Buerger's disease, 13
BUN. *See* Blood urea nitrogen.
Burns, 13
Bursitis, 73